AF183328

Addiction: A Clinical Approach

Addiction: A Clinical Approach

Edited by James Burke

hayle medical

New York

Hayle Medical,
750 Third Avenue, 9th Floor,
New York, NY 10017, USA

Visit us on the World Wide Web at:
www.haylemedical.com

© Hayle Medical, 2019

This book contains information obtained from authentic and highly regarded sources. Copyright for all individual chapters remain with the respective authors as indicated. All chapters are published with permission under the Creative Commons Attribution License or equivalent. A wide variety of references are listed. Permission and sources are indicated; for detailed attributions, please refer to the permissions page and list of contributors. Reasonable efforts have been made to publish reliable data and information, but the authors, editors and publisher cannot assume any responsibility for the validity of all materials or the consequences of their use.

ISBN: 978-1-63241-744-2

The publisher's policy is to use permanent paper from mills that operate a sustainable forestry policy. Furthermore, the publisher ensures that the text paper and cover boards used have met acceptable environmental accreditation standards.

Trademark Notice: Registered trademark of products or corporate names are used only for explanation and identification without intent to infringe.

Printed in China.

Cataloging-in-Publication Data

Addiction : a clinical approach / edited by James Burke.
p. cm.
Includes bibliographical references and index.
ISBN 978-1-63241-744-2
1. Drug abuse--Treatment. 2. Substance abuse--Treatment.
3. Drug addiction. I. Burke, James.
RC564 .A23 2019
616.86--dc23

Table of Contents

Preface IX

Chapter 1 **Multifaceted academic detailing program to increase pharmacotherapy for alcohol use disorder: interrupted time series evaluation of effectiveness** 1
Alex H. S. Harris, Thomas Bowe, Hildi Hagedorn, Andrea Nevedal, Andrea K. Finlay, Risha Gidwani, Craig Rosen, Chad Kay and Melissa Christopher

Chapter 2 **Prenatal treatment for opioid dependency: observations from a large inner-city clinic** 8
Kelley Saia, Sarah M. Bagley, Elisha M. Wachman, Payal P. Patel, Marisa D. Nadas and Susan B. Brogly

Chapter 3 **A qualitative study of treatment-seeking heroin users** 16
Anna Lembke and Niushen Zhang

Chapter 4 **Implementation of integrated stepped care for unhealthy alcohol use in HIV clinics** 24
E. Jennifer Edelman, Nathan B. Hansen, Christopher J. Cutter, Cheryl Danton, Lynn E. Fiellin, Patrick G. O'Connor, Emily C. Williams, Stephen A. Maisto, Kendall J. Bryant and David A. Fiellin

Chapter 5 **Emerging adults in substance misuse intervention: preintervention characteristics and responses to a motivation-enhancing program** 38
Blair Beadnell, Michele A. Crisafulli, Pamela A. Stafford and Erin A. Casey

Chapter 6 **The association between age of onset of opioid use and comorbidity among opioid dependent patients receiving methadone maintenance therapy** 50
Leen Naji, Brittany Burns Dennis, Monica Bawor, Michael Varenbut, Jeff Daiter, Carolyn Plater, Guillaume Pare, David C. Marsh, Andrew Worster, Dipika Desai, James MacKillop, Lehana Thabane and Zainab Samaan

Chapter 7 **Feasibility of a computer-assisted social network motivational interviewing intervention for substance use and HIV risk behaviors for housing first residents** 57
Karen Chan Osilla, David P. Kennedy, Sarah B. Hunter and Ervant Maksabedian

Chapter 8 **Seek, test, treat: substance-using women in the HIV treatment cascade** 68
Wendee M. Wechsberg, Charles van der Horst, Jacqueline Ndirangu, Irene A. Doherty, Tracy Kline, Felicia A. Browne, Jennifer M. Belus, Robin Nance and William A. Zule

Chapter 9 **Health evaluation and referral assistant: a randomized controlled trial to improve smoking cessation among emergency department patients**.....78
Edwin D. Boudreaux, Beau Abar, Brianna Haskins, Brigitte Bauman and Grant Grissom

Chapter 10 **How do people with mood and anxiety disorders perceive and interpret the Drinking Motives Questionnaire? A think-aloud study in a clinical setting**.....88
Christina Nehlin, Margareta Wennberg and Caisa Öster

Chapter 11 **Comparison of DSM-IV and DSM-5 criteria for alcohol use disorders in VA primary care patients with frequent heavy drinking**.....94
Traci Takahashi, Gwen Lapham, Laura J. Chavez, Amy K. Lee, Emily C. Williams, Julie E. Richards, Diane Greenberg, Anna Rubinsky, Douglas Berger, Eric J. Hawkins, Joseph O. Merrill and Katharine A. Bradley

Chapter 12 **Physician versus non-physician delivery of alcohol screening, brief intervention and referral to treatment in adult primary care**.....104
Jennifer R. Mertens, Felicia W. Chi, Constance M. Weisner, Derek D. Satre, Thekla B. Ross, Steve Allen, David Pating, Cynthia I. Campbell, Yun Wendy Lu and Stacy A. Sterling

Chapter 13 **Prevalence and factors associated with use of khat: a survey of patients entering HIV treatment programs**.....121
Alan R. Lifson, Sale Workneh, Tibebe Shenie, Desalegn Admassu Ayana, Zenebe Melaku, Lemlem Bezabih, Hiwot Tekle Waktola, Behailu Dagne, Rose Hilk, Ken C. Winters and Lucy Slater

Chapter 14 **Predictive validity of two process-of-care quality measures for residential substance use disorder treatment**.....128
Alex H. S. Harris, Shalini Gupta, Thomas Bowe, Laura S. Ellerbe, Tyler E. Phelps, Anna D. Rubinsky, John W. Finney, Steven M. Asch, Keith Humphreys and Jodie Trafton

Chapter 15 **HIV treatment cascade among female entertainment and sex workers in Cambodia: impact of amphetamine use and an HIV prevention program**.....136
Sokunny Muth, Aynar Len, Jennifer L. Evans, Maly Phou, Sophal Chhit, Yuthea Neak, Song Ngak, Ellen S. Stein, Adam W. Carrico, Lisa Maher and Kimberly Page

Chapter 16 **Insights from individuals successfully recovered from cannabis use disorder: natural versus treatment-assisted recoveries and abstinent versus moderation outcomes**.....146
David C. Hodgins and Jonathan N. Stea

Chapter 17 **Patterns of HIV testing, drug use and sexual behaviors in people who use drugs: findings from a community-based outreach program**.....155
Gitau Mburu, Chanrith Ngin, Sovannary Tuot, Pheak Chhoun, Khuondyla Pal and Siyan Yi

Chapter 18 **Development and differentiability of three brief interventions for risky alcohol use that include varying doses of motivational interviewing....165**
Jennifer E. Hettema, Stephanie A. Cockrell, Abigail Reeves, Karen S. Ingersoll, Paula J. Lum, Richard Saitz, Cristina M. Murray-Krezan and Valerie A. Carrejo

Chapter 19 **Barriers and facilitators affecting the implementation of substance use screening in primary care clinics: a qualitative study of patients, providers and staff....173**
Jennifer McNeely, Pritika C. Kumar, Traci Rieckmann, Erica Sedlander, Sarah Farkas, Christine Chollak, Joseph L. Kannry, Aida Vega, Eva A. Waite, Lauren A. Peccoralo, Richard N. Rosenthal, Dennis McCarty and John Rotrosen

Chapter 20 **Alcohol consumption patterns and HIV viral suppression among persons receiving HIV care....188**
R. L. Cook, Z. Zhou, N. E. Kelso-Chichetto, J. Janelle, J. P. Morano, C. Somboonwit, W. Carter, G. E. Ibanez, N. Ennis, C. L. Cook, R. A. Cohen, B. Brumback and K. Bryant

Chapter 21 **Barriers to addiction treatment among formerly incarcerated adults with substance use disorders....197**
Mandy D. Owens, Jessica A. Chen, Tracy L. Simpson, Christine Timko and Emily C. Williams

Chapter 22 **Racial/ethnic differences in the association between alcohol use and mortality among men living with HIV....208**
Kara M. Bensley, Kathleen A. McGinnis, David A. Fiellin, Adam J. Gordon, Kevin L. Kraemer, Kendall J. Bryant, E. Jennifer Edelman, Stephen Crystal, Julie R. Gaither, P. Todd Korthuis, Brandon D. L. Marshall, India J. Ornelas, K. C. Gary Chan, Julia C. Dombrowski, John C. Fortney, Amy C. Justice and Emily C. Williams

Chapter 23 ***MySafeRx:* a mobile technology platform integrating motivational coaching, adherence monitoring and electronic pill dispensing for enhancing buprenorphine/naloxone adherence during opioid use disorder treatment....219**
Zev Schuman-Olivier, Jacob T. Borodovsky, Jackson Steinkamp, Qays Munir, Kyle Butler, Mary Ann Greene, Jonah Goldblatt, Hai Yi Xie and Lisa A. Marsch

Chapter 24 **Delivery of screening and brief intervention for unhealthy alcohol use in an urban academic Federally Qualified Health Center....233**
Marcus A. Bachhuber, Megan A. O'Grady, Henry Chung, Charles J. Neighbors, Joseph DeLuca, Elenita M. D'Aloia, Arelis Diaz and Chinazo O. Cunningham

Chapter 25 **Convenience without disclosure: a formative research study of a proposed integrated methadone and antiretroviral therapy service delivery model....243**
Alexis Cooke, Haneefa Saleem, Dorothy Mushi, Jessie Mbwambo, Saria Hassan and Barrot H. Lambdin

Permissions

List of Contributors

Index

Preface

A brain disorder in which there is a compulsive engagement in rewarding stimuli despite adverse consequences is known as addiction. The main features which attract addictive stimuli include the fact that they appear to be reinforcing and intrinsically rewarding. A person addicted to such stimuli will seek repeated exposure to them as these substances generate a feeling of positivity and pleasure. Alcoholism, nicotine addiction, cocaine addiction, gambling addiction, sexual addiction and food addiction are some of the common types of drug and behavioral addictions. The risk of addiction is quite high in the age of adolescence. The topics included in this book on addiction are of utmost significance and bound to provide incredible insights to readers. It strives to provide a fair idea about this disorder to help develop a better understanding of the clinical advances related to it. A number of latest researches have been included to keep the readers up-to-date with the global concepts in the study of addiction.

The researches compiled throughout the book are authentic and of high quality, combining several disciplines and from very diverse regions from around the world. Drawing on the contributions of many researchers from diverse countries, the book's objective is to provide the readers with the latest achievements in the area of research. This book will surely be a source of knowledge to all interested and researching the field.

In the end, I would like to express my deep sense of gratitude to all the authors for meeting the set deadlines in completing and submitting their research chapters. I would also like to thank the publisher for the support offered to us throughout the course of the book. Finally, I extend my sincere thanks to my family for being a constant source of inspiration and encouragement.

Editor

Multifaceted academic detailing program to increase pharmacotherapy for alcohol use disorder: interrupted time series evaluation of effectiveness

Alex H. S. Harris[1*], Thomas Bowe[1], Hildi Hagedorn[2], Andrea Nevedal[1], Andrea K. Finlay[1], Risha Gidwani[1], Craig Rosen[1], Chad Kay[3] and Melissa Christopher[3]

Abstract

Background: Active consideration of effective medications to treat alcohol use disorder (AUD) is a consensus standard of care, yet knowledge and use of these medications are very low across diverse settings. This study evaluated the overall effectiveness a multifaceted academic detailing program to address this persistent quality problem in the US Veterans Health Administration (VHA), as well as the context and process factors that explained variation in effectiveness across sites.

Methods: An interrupted time series design, analyzed with mixed-effects segmented logistic regression, was used to evaluate changes in level and rate of change in the monthly percent of patients with a clinically documented AUD who received naltrexone, acamprosate, disulfiram, or topiramate. Using data from a 20 month post-implementation period, intervention sites (n = 37) were compared to their own 16 month pre-implementation performance and separately to the rest of VHA.

Results: From immediately pre-intervention to the end of the observation period, the percent of patients in the intervention sites with AUD who received medication increased over 3.4 % in absolute terms and 68 % in relative terms (i.e., 4.9–8.3 %). This change was significant compared to the pre-implementation period in the intervention sites and secular trends in control sites. Sites with lower pre-implementation adoption, more person hours of detailing, but fewer people detailed, had larger immediate increases in medication receipt after implementation. The average number of detailing encounters per person was associated with steeper increases in slope over time.

Conclusions: This study found empirical support for a multifaceted quality improvement strategy aimed at increasing access to and utilization of pharmacotherapy for AUD. Future studies should focus on determining how to enhance the programs effects, especially in non-responsive locations.

Keywords: Pharmacotherapy, Medication assisted treatment, Alcohol use disorder, Quality improvement, Implementation, Guideline adherence, Practice guidelines

Background

Both psychosocial and pharmacological treatments for alcohol use disorder (AUD; formerly abuse and dependence) have been found to be effective in reducing symptoms and improving functioning in diverse patient populations [1–5]. In the United States (US), 16.6 million people over 18 years of age in 2013 (7.0 %) met diagnostic criteria for AUD yet only 1.3 million (7.8 %) received any formal treatment [6]. Even within the Veterans Health Administration (VHA), the largest integrated healthcare system in the US with a well-developed system of 220

*Correspondence: Alexander.Harris2@va.gov
[1] Center for Innovation to Implementation, Health Services Research and Development, VA Palo Alto Health Care System, Menlo Park, CA, USA
Full list of author information is available at the end of the article

specialty addiction programs, the treatment rate among the roughly 400,000 patients clinically diagnosed with an AUD in fiscal year 2013 (6.8 % of all VA patients) was only 32 %. Clearly, developing and evaluating strategies to improve access to and engagement in effective treatments for AUD is of utmost importance [7].

Several medications are US Federal Drug Administration (FDA)-approved for the treatment of AUD, and/or have support of effectiveness from high-quality meta-analysis, namely naltrexone, acamprosate, disulfiram, and topiramate. These medications can be prescribed and managed in diverse clinical settings [1–3], allowing patients more options regarding the type and location of their AUD treatment, thus potentially increasing access and treatment engagement. However among both providers and patients, knowledge and use of these medications to treat AUD in the US is very low and variable [8–13]. In VHA, low and variable utilization of these medications for AUD persists even though all of them are on the national formulary and supported by VHA clinical practice guidelines and policies [14]. The VA Uniform Mental Health Services Handbook states that evidence-based pharmacotherapy is to be offered and available to all patients diagnosed with AUD if not medically contraindicated [14]. However, among the VHA patients diagnosed with AUD in FY13, only 5.8 % received evidenced-based pharmacotherapy. Even among Veterans seeking treatment in one of VHA's specialty addiction treatment programs, only 9.9 % received medication treatment for AUD [9, 15].

Not only is the overall rate of medication receipt low for patients with AUD in VHA, there is substantial facility-level variability [9, 15]. The rate of pharmacotherapy for AUD among Veterans who received SUD specialty care in FY13 ranged from 0 to 21 % across facilities. Low prescribing rates and significant variation across facilities suggests that significant gaps exist in patients' access to these medications, especially in some locations. The existence of facilitative formulary and clinical policies, as well as near real time performance monitoring [16], may be necessary but has not been sufficient to adequately improve performance on this standard of care.

To address this substantial and persistent quality gap, VHA's Office of Patient Care Services funded the Academic Detailing for Mental Health Initiatives Program that developed and executed campaigns to improve implementation of pharmacological treatment for several mental health and addictive disorders, including tobacco dependence, schizophrenia, depression, posttraumatic stress disorder, and most recently, and the focus of this study, AUD. In 2013, this quality improvement program sent clinical pharmacy specialists ("academic detailers") to clinical settings within two western VHA networks. The academic detailers strove to educate, motivate, and enable key health care providers to identify and address the spectrum of hazardous alcohol use, especially to facilitate more active consideration of pharmacological treatment options for AUD. The effectiveness of the AUD campaign of the Academic Detailing Program, and the context and process factors that might be associated with its effectiveness, have not been rigorously evaluated. Thus, the goal of the current study is to evaluate this multifaceted implementation strategy as means to increase utilization of pharmacotherapy for AUD, as well as to provide data that might inform and enhance the ongoing expansion of academic detailing programming across VHA.

Methods

The academic detailing program

The primary goal of the Academic Detailing AUD Campaign was to increase the proportion of patients with AUD who were receiving treatment with naltrexone, acamprosate, disulfiram, or topiramate. Simple academic detailing interventions have been shown to have small but significant effects on prescribing practices [17]. However the approach evaluated here was more elaborate and multifaceted than typical academic detailing or educational outreach interventions [17]. Aspects of the program were similar to an external facilitation model where barriers and problems are iteratively identified and addressed in real time [18, 19]. No firm standard existed for the intended number of detailing encounters per site. However given the positive relationship between number of educational outreach visits by pharmaceutical representatives and sales [20], multiple visits were attempted, especially in sites with persistent non-response. As such, this program was akin to a hybrid academic detailing/audit and feedback/external facilitation intervention [19, 21]. Another unique and key feature of the program was the implementation of a real-time informatics dashboard so clinicians and detailers could identify patients who might be candidates for the medications (e.g., recent diagnosis of AUD, not currently receiving medications), as well as to assess site-level performance. Audit and feedback has been shown to be more effective when baseline performance is low, when feedback is given more than once, is given verbally and in writing, and when coupled with support and a clear action plan [17], which were all features of this program.

Table 1 outlines the major activities of the program. After Identifying leadership partners and establishing buy-in (Step 1), detailers identified clinical staff with a high volume of patients with AUD (Step 2), and detailing encounters were requested with these priority clinical staff (Step 3). The goal then was to build rapport and

Table 1 Features and methods of academic detailing for mental health initiatives program

Identify leadership partners and establish buy-in: Meeting were requested and conducted with key clinical and pharmacy leadership to explain the goals and methods of the initiative, as well as address concerns and high-level barriers
Identify clinical staff with a high volume of patients with AUD in both primary care and mental health/addiction specialty care: using administrative data, the program identified staff with large numbers of AUD patients
Request detailing encounters with these priority providers, citing the previously established leadership support and enthusiasm
Build relationships with priority providers, engaging them in discussions about evidence-based medications and other practices (e.g., brief intervention for risky drinking): the goal was repeated visits to establish rapport and perceived value by the clinicians who received the resources and services
Explore barriers to prescribing the medications and applying the practices
Examine and address knowledge and beliefs about the supporting evidence
Address knowledge and misunderstandings about policies and scope of competence (e.g., belief that policy prohibits primary care clinicians from prescribing naltrexone or other AUD medications)
Identify and problem-solve structural or logistical barriers (e.g., local policy or practice, staffing medication management visits.)
Introduce the providers to additional resources and tools including patient education tools, and pocket cards with FAQs
Introduce real-time, electronic medical record-integrated audit and feedback tools to identify actionable patients
Seek a commitment from the clinician to try to increase prescribing of the medications
Monitor progress and check back periodically for additional education, barrier identification, problem solving, and feedback. Monitor clinical targets (e.g., the number of patients receiving medications for AUD) and clinician use of the informatics tools, especially the case-finding dashboards. If the targeted prescribing behavior was unaffected, the next detailing session would again explore barriers, problem solve, and motivate clinicians

engage staff in discussions about evidence-based medications and other AUD treatment options (Step 4), iteratively identify barriers (Step 5), and provide additional resources including a real-time audit and feedback and case finding tool (Steps 6 and 7). Importantly, the detailers sought a commitment from staff to try to increase use of evidence-based medications for AUD (Step 8), and continued to monitor and problem solve if needed (Step 9).

Academic detailers were recruited and selected with preference for previous training experience in mental health, board certification as pharmacotherapy specialists, post graduate residency training, and strong communication skills assessed during interview process. Due to the clinical service content of the detailing encounters, candidates were sought who had provided direct patient care as part of their previous professional experience with prescribing authority under a scope of practice. The Department of Veteran's Affairs then contracted Alosa Foundation, a nonprofit organization that develops and implements academic detailing programs to improve prescribing, to provide a basic skills course in academic detailing to the six clinical pharmacists who were selected for VA facilities in California, Nevada and the Pacific Islands. In addition to Academic Detailing Basic Skills workshop, Motivational Interviewing training, adapted for use within the context of a provider outreach visit as opposed to a clinical treatment with a patient population, was another important aspect of detailer training. Campaign specific training on AUD was conducted through virtual seminars and one 3-day face-to-face conference, in which subject matter experts assisted in structuring the AUD campaign timeline and targeted goals.

From April to December 2013, the AUD campaign of the Academic Detailing Program was implemented in two western VA networks, including over 37 medical centers and community-based outpatient clinics. Detailing sessions included predominantly in-person one-on-one sessions, in-person group sessions, and educational in-service sessions, with additional follow-up conducted by email, teleconference, and telephone. A wide variety of staff received detailing encounters including psychologists, psychiatrists, nurses, social workers, clinical pharmacists, primary physicians, clinical managers and other administrators.

Analysis of overall effectiveness

We evaluated the overall effectiveness of the program using a multi-site, interrupted time series design. The main outcome for the evaluation was the monthly proportion of patients with a clinical encounter in which AUD was documented who filled a prescription for one of the targeted medications: naltrexone, acamprosate, disulfiram, or topiramate. Intervention sites had 16 months of baseline pharmacy data prior to their first detailing contact, and were observed for 20 months thereafter. Mixed-effects segmented logistic regression [22] was used to estimate the parameters for the pre- and post-implementation segments, with random effects to account for the nesting of patients within months within sites. The first model, using the intervention sites as their own controls, compared the change in level from Month 16 in the pre-implementation period to the immediate post-implementation in Month 17 (i.e., "gap") as well as the change in slope from the pre-implementation to the post-implementation period. In the second model, we

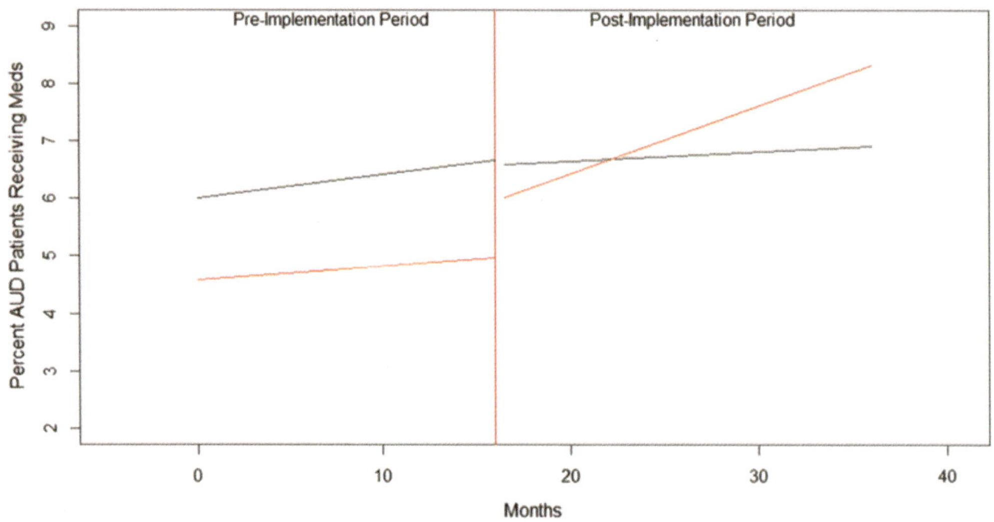

Fig. 1 Effects of academic detailing program implemented in 37 VHA sites compared to secular trend in rest of VHA. The *red* segments represent the intervention sites and the *black* segments represent the control sites

compared the pre-post gap and changes in slope in the intervention sites to non-intervention control sites to ensure that the observed effects were not due to secular trends in the rest of VHA.

Context and process factors

We then calculated and described facility-level variability in effectiveness, operationalized as the immediate pre-post implementation gaps and changes in slope. Then, we examined the context and process factors (i.e., moderators and mediators) that were associated with this variability and for which data were available from administrative sources or from Academic Detailing Program encounter logs. The main facility-level moderator examined was the pre-implementation rate of receipt of medications for AUD, calculated from VHA pharmacy data. Candidate mediators included total person-hours of detailing, total number of health care providers contacted by the program, and number of unique detailing sessions, all sourced from program encounter logs. We did not examine the effects of detailing encounter type (group vs. individual) or provider type on effectiveness due to substantial within-site variability on these factors. All candidate predictors were entered into the mixed-effect regression model described above, restricted to sites with detailing encounters, and interacted with the immediate gap and change in slope.

Results

Overall effectiveness in sites with detailing encounters

For simplicity of interpretation, we converted the mixed-effects segmented logistic regression estimates into percents and graphically represented them in Fig. 1. As represented by the red trajectory in Fig. 1, the average proportion of patients with AUD who filled a prescription for naltrexone (oral or injectable), acamprosate, disulfiram, or topiramate in the 37 intervention sites was 4.56 % at baseline. The pre-implementation slope in the intervention sites was not significantly different than zero and increased to 4.96 % by Month 16. The gap of 1.04–6.00 % between Month 16 and 17 in the intervention sites was significant ($p < .0001$). Also, the pre-to-post increase in slope in the intervention sites compared to the pre-implementation slope was significantly positive ($p < .0001$), with the proportion of patients with AUD receiving medication increasing to 8.32 % by the end of Month 36. Thus from immediately pre-intervention to the end of the observation period (Month 16–Month 36), the percent of patients with AUD who received medication increased 3.36 % in absolute terms and 67.77 % in relative terms.

Comparing medication trends in implementation and control sites

To check that these changes did not just mimic secular trends in the rest of VHA, we fitted a model that explicitly compared the four parameters in the intervention sites to the same parameters in all other VA sites. As represented by the black line in Fig. 1, at baseline in the rest of VHA, 6.01 % of patients with AUD filled a prescription for one of the medications, a proportion significantly higher than the intervention sites. The slope for the rest of VHA in the pre-intervention period was not significantly different than zero and increased to 6.67 % by the end of Month 16. The gap of −0.09 % between Month 16 and 17 in the rest of VHA to 6.58 % was slightly negative. The slope in the post-implementation period was slightly more positive than the pre-implementation period for the rest of VHA, ending at 6.90 % by the end of Month 36. Both the immediate gap and change in slope were significantly less than the intervention sites (p values <.001). Thus from Month 16 to Month 36 in the rest of VHA, the rate of medication receipt increased over 0.23 % in absolute terms and 3.45 % in relative terms.

Context and process factors associated with program effects

In addition to these overall effects, significant variability among the 37 sites in the effects of the Academic Detailing Program were found, with some sites having much bigger or smaller gaps and changes in slope than the overall average. Figure 2 shows the variation in the immediate post-implementation gaps for all 37 sites. Although the average gap was just over 1 %, it ranged from −1.69 to 2.14 %. The changes in slopes from the pre- to post-implementation period also varied, ranging from −0.55 to 0.08.

We then examined moderators and mediators that might explain variation in gaps and/or changes in slopes, as indicated by significant interaction terms in the mixed-effects segmented logistic regression. Descriptive statistics for these variables are presented in Table 2. Sites with lower pre-implementation adoption (i.e., lower

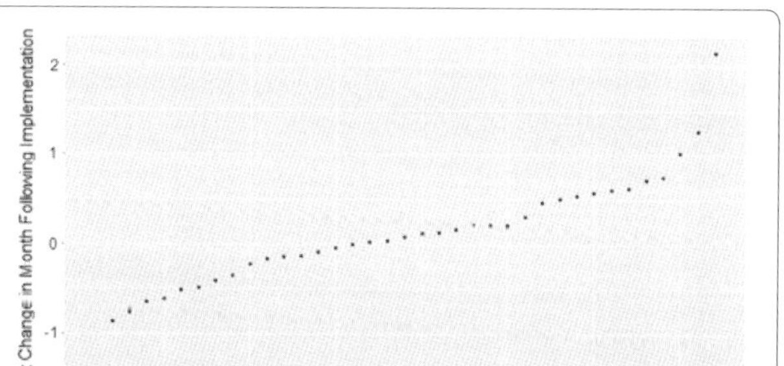

Fig. 2 Variation in percent change in patients with AUD receiving medications in month following implementation

Table 2 Descriptive statistics of site-level moderators and mediators of effectiveness

Variables	Mean (SD)	Range
Percent of AUD patients receiving medications	4.31 (2.54)	0–9.3
Person hours of detailing	26.63 (59.30)	0.15–330
Unique staff with detailing contact	31.76 (60.04)	1–325
Average encounters per detailed provider	1.12 (0.19)	1–1.8

proportion of patients receiving medications) had larger immediate increases in medication receipt after implementation (95 % confidence interval for interaction odds ratio 0.004–0.1114), as did sites with more person hours of detailing (95 % confidence interval for interaction odds ratio 1.00001–1.000187), but fewer people detailed (95 % confidence interval for interaction odds ratio 0.9904–0.9989). The average number of detailing encounters per person detailed was associated with steeper increases in slope over time (95 % confidence interval for interaction odds ratio 1.067–1.119).

Discussion

In this study, we evaluated a multifaceted academic detailing program aimed at addressing a serious and persistent problem in healthcare quality—under-utilization of medications in the treatment of AUD. Despite strong evidence of clinical effectiveness of these medications, clinical and quality managers have thus far lacked evidence-based quality improvement strategies to increase access and utilization. Using a rigorous quasi-experimental design, we found that implementation of the Academic Detailing Program for AUD was associated with an overall immediate gap up in medication receipt as well a significant increase in the slope of adoption over time. From pre-intervention to the end of the follow-up period, the rate of medication receipt in the intervention sites increased approximately 3.4 % in absolute terms and 68 % in relative terms (i.e., 4.9–8.3 %). Although the intervention sites overall had lower levels of utilization at baseline compared to the rest of VHA, levels of utilization in the intervention sites were higher by the end of the observation period. Extrapolating this effect to the entire VHA would mean that over 11,000 additional patients with AUD would receive these effective medications. To our knowledge, this is the first quality improvement strategy focused on increasing access to AUD medications to be implemented on a large scale and shown to be effective overall.

Although the Academic Detailing Program increased prescribing of medications for treatment of AUD overall, the effect varied substantially across the intervention sites. In many sites, there was no improvement or even reductions in prescription fills. In an effort to explain some of this variability, we found that initially low performing facilities tended to improve the most. This result is encouraging and instructive. Although one might argue that those with lower baseline performance were more likely to improve due to regression to the mean [23], it is common in healthcare quality efforts for high performance sites to improve more than initially low performing sites. Also, facilities that received more detailing sessions and fewer people detailed tended to have the greatest initial improvement (biggest immediate gap) while larger increases in the slope of utilization over time were experienced in facilities that had a higher average number of detailing encounters per detailed person. In general, these results support the notion that more detailing produces more positive change, and suggests that perhaps focusing on a few key prescribers up front creates an immediate bump in prescribing while broader detailing encourages sustained growth in prescribing.

Several questions are left unanswered by this investigation. First, there were many aspects of the detailing encounters for which data were unavailable, including prior knowledge level of the target clinician as well as skill and experience of the detailer. Many facilities received detailing encounters from multiple detailers making the direct examination of detailer effects difficult. Also, one aspect of detailer skill and potential impact is the ability to secure initial meetings with facility staff. We had data on completed detailing encounters but not encounter requests. These are important limitations that should be addressed in future implementations and evaluations. Second, data on use of the informatics tools was not analyzed. Qualitative interviews with detailers and detailed clinicians might have helped explain why sites varied in response to the Academic Detailing Program, and may have provided perspectives and data that could be used to refine the program. Third, the analyses were based on filled prescriptions not on written prescriptions, for which no data were available. We expect the impact of this limitation to be minimal because we have no reason to believe that reliance on outside pharmacies or the proportion of unfilled prescriptions would be different in the pre and post implementation periods. Fourth, the campaign also sought to improve rates of screening, brief intervention, and referral to specialty treatment, data for which was unavailable for evaluation. Fifth, sustainment of effects after the program stopped was not examined. Sixth, data on cost of the intervention was not collected, precluding any budget impact or other economic analyses. Finally, long-term sustainment or emergence of effects after the detailing encounters stop were not evaluated but should be investigated in future analyses.

Conclusions

Even with these limitations and caveats, this study is perhaps the first to find empirical support for a multifaceted quality improvement strategy aimed at increasing access to and utilization of effective medications in the treatment of AUD. Following the conclusion to this western VHA regional pilot for Academic Detailing for Mental Health Initiatives, in March 2015 VHA leadership requested the 21 regional networks to develop academic detailing programming to impact two other key medication safety quality improvement programs in VHA, the Opioid Safety Initiative and the Psychotropic Drug Safety Initiative. Future studies should rigorously evaluate the program's effects on other quality improvement targets, focus on determining how to enhance the program effects, especially in sites where effects are weak. It is possible that less expensive and less labor intensive strategies would be adequate in some locations while even more intensive strategies are needed elsewhere. Learning how to identify the site characteristics that might be matched to the most efficient quality improvement strategy is the overarching goal of this line of research.

Abbreviations

AUD: alcohol use disorder; US: United States; VHA: US Veterans Health Administration; FDA: US Federal Drug Administration.

Authors' contributions

AHSH conceived of the study, secured funding, supervised the analyses, and led the drafting of the manuscript. TB participated in the design of the study and performed the statistical analysis. HH, AKF, RG, CR, CK and MC participated in the design of the study provided critical input into drafting the manuscript. All authors read and approved the final manuscript.

Author details

[1] Center for Innovation to Implementation, Health Services Research and Development, VA Palo Alto Health Care System, Menlo Park, CA, USA.
[2] Center for Chronic Disease Outcomes Research, Health Services Research and Development, VA Minneapolis Health Care System, Minneapolis, MN, USA.
[3] Pharmacy Benefits Management, Academic Detailing Program, VA San Diego Health Care System, San Diego, CA, USA.

Competing interests

All authors are employees of the Veterans Health Administration. Drs. Kay and Christopher designed and are employed by the program being evaluated. Other authors are researchers independent of the program. The authors declare that they have no competing interests.

Funding

This work was supported in part by a VA HSR&D Research Career Scientist Award (RCS-14-232), the Substance Use Disorder Quality Enhancement Research Initiative (SUD QUERI), and the VA Pharmacy Benefits Management Academic Detailing Program.

References

1. Blodgett JC, Del Re AC, Maisel NC, et al. A meta-analysis of topiramate's effects for individuals with alcohol use disorders. Alcohol Clin Exp Res. 2014;38:1481–8.
2. Maisel NC, Blodgett JC, Wilbourne PL, et al. Meta-analysis of naltrexone and acamprosate for treating alcohol use disorders: when are these medications most helpful? Addiction. 2013;108:275–93.
3. Jonas DE, Amick HR, Feltner C, et al. Pharmacotherapy for adults with alcohol use disorders in outpatient settings: a systematic review and meta-analysis. JAMA. 2014;311:1889–900.
4. Magill M, Ray LA. Cognitive-behavioral treatment with adult alcohol and illicit drug users: a meta-analysis of randomized controlled trials. J Stud Alcohol Drugs. 2009;70:516–27.
5. Riper H, Andersson G, Hunter SB, et al. Treatment of comorbid alcohol use disorders and depression with cognitive–behavioural therapy and motivational interviewing: a meta-analysis. Addiction. 2014;109:394–406.

6. National Institute on Alcohol Abuse and Alcoholism. Alcohol facts and statistics. 2015. https://www.niaaa.nih.gov/alcohol-health/overview-alcohol-consumption/alcohol-facts-and-statistics
7. Ducharme LJ, Chandler RK, Harris AHS. Implementing substance abuse treatment in general medical settings: mapping the research terrain. J Subst Abuse Treat. 2016;60:110–8.
8. Harris AH, Ellerbe L, Reeder RN, et al. Pharmacotherapy for alcohol dependence: perceived treatment barriers and action strategies among Veterans Health Administration service providers. Psychol Serv. 2013;10:410–9.
9. Harris AH, Kivlahan DR, Bowe T, et al. Pharmacotherapy of alcohol use disorders in the Veterans Health Administration. Psychiatr Serv. 2010;61:392–8.
10. Mark TL, Kassed CA, Vandivort-Warren R, et al. Alcohol and opioid dependence medications: prescription trends, overall and by physician specialty. Drug Alcohol Depend. 2009;99:345–9.
11. Ducharme LJ, Knudsen HK, Roman PM. Trends in the adoption of medications for alcohol dependence. J Clin Psychopharmacol. 2006;26(Suppl. 1):S13–9.
12. Knudsen HK, Roman PM. Service delivery and pharmacotherapy for alcohol use disorder in the era of health reform: data from a national sample of treatment organizations. Subst Abus. 2016;37:230–7.
13. Rubinsky AD, Chen C, Batki SL, et al. Comparative utilization of pharmacotherapy for alcohol use disorder and other psychiatric disorders among U.S. Veterans Health Administration patients with dual diagnoses. J Psychiatr Res. 2015;69:150–7.
14. The Management of Substance Use Disorders Working Group. VA/DOD clinical practice guideline for the management of substance use disorders. Washington, DC: US Department of Veterans Affairs and Department of Defense; 2009.
15. Harris AH, Oliva E, Bowe T, et al. Pharmacotherapy of alcohol use disorders by the Veterans Health Administration: patterns of receipt and persistence. Psychiatr Serv. 2012;63:679–85.
16. Trafton JA, Greenberg G, Harris AH, et al. VHA mental health information system: applying health information technology to monitor and facilitate implementation of VHA uniform mental health services handbook requirements. Med Care. 2013;51:S29–36.
17. O'Brien MA, Rogers S, Jamtvedt G, Oxman AD, Odgaard-Jensen J, Kristoffersen DT, Forsetlund L, Bainbridge D, Freemantle N, Davis DA, et al. Educational outreach visits: effects on professional practice and health care outcomes. Cochrane Database Syst Rev. 2007;(4):CD000409.
18. Bidassie B, Williams LS, Woodward-Hagg H, et al. Key components of external facilitation in an acute stroke quality improvement collaborative in the Veterans Health Administration. Implement Sci. 2015;10:69.
19. Stetler CB, Legro MW, Rycroft-Malone J, et al. Role of "external facilitation" in implementation of research findings: a qualitative evaluation of facilitation experiences in the Veterans Health Administration. Implement Sci. 2006;1:23.
20. Schwartz TL, Kuhles DJ 2nd, Wade M, et al. Newly admitted psychiatric patient prescriptions and pharmaceutical sales visits. Ann Clin Psychiatry. 2001;13:159–62.
21. Espallargues M, Valderas JM, Alonso J. Provision of feedback on perceived health status to health care professionals: a systematic review of its impact. Med Care. 2000;38:175–86.
22. Duncan T, Duncan S. A latent growth curve modeling approach to pooled interrupted time series analysis. J Psychopathol Behav Assess. 2004;26:271–8.
23. Finney JW. Regression to the mean in substance use disorder treatment research. Addiction. 2008;103:42–52.

2

Prenatal treatment for opioid dependency: observations from a large inner-city clinic

Kelley Saia[1*], Sarah M. Bagley[2,3], Elisha M. Wachman[3], Payal P. Patel[4], Marisa D. Nadas[5] and Susan B. Brogly[6]

Abstract

Background: The objective of this study was to review changes in the prevalence of opioid use disorder in pregnancy, and to describe the prenatal care and neonatal outcomes following the implementation of buprenorphine treatment at a large US obstetrical clinic during the on-going opioid epidemic.

Methods: We conducted a retrospective cohort study of 310 women (332 pregnancies) with opioid use disorders and their neonates delivered between June 2006 and December 2010 at an obstetrical clinic in the US. Trends in patient volume, characteristics and outcomes by calendar year were assessed using the Cochran–Armitage test and linear regression.

Results: There was an almost two-fold increase in the volume of pregnant women treated annually from 2006 through 2010. Most women were treated with methadone (74%), with buprenorphine becoming more common over calendar time: 3.0% in 2006 to 41% in 2010. The mean dose of buprenorphine at delivery was: 11.4 mg in 2007, 14.1 mg in 2008, 14.1 mg in 2009, and 16.8 mg in 2010; an average increase of 2.1 mg year. There were no differences in mean methadone dose over time. From 2006 to 2010 there were increases in the prevalence of prescribed concomitant psychotropic medications and vaginal deliveries, and in the proportion of neonates treated pharmacologically for neonatal abstinence syndrome (NAS). NAS pharmacologic management also varied by calendar year with more use of neonatal morphine and clonidine in later years.

Conclusions: The number of mother–infant pairs increased significantly from 2006 to 2010 and the clinical characteristics of these patients changed over time. Our experience reflects the rising increase in opioid use disorders in pregnancy and NAS, mandating the need for expansion of comprehensive prenatal care options for these women and their children.

Background

Opioid use disorders affect a rising number of women of childbearing age [1]. From 2000 to 2009, opioid use among US pregnant women increased from 1.19 per 1000 hospital births to 5.63 per 1000 hospital births per year [2]. National attention has been given to the rising incidence of Neonatal Abstinence Syndrome (NAS) in the US, which is associated with the rise in opioid use disorders in pregnancy. NAS is a constellation of signs and symptoms of withdrawal from in utero exposure to opioids and other substances. NAS incidence increased five-fold between 2000 and 2012, currently accounting for 3% of admissions to neonatal intensive care units (NICUs) in the US [3]. Reducing the incidence of NAS begins with prevention of opioid use disorders during the childbearing years. Improving maternal and neonatal outcomes for these dyads requires expanded access to opioid treatment programs for pregnant women. Recognizing the barriers to care such as socioeconomic challenges, potential legal consequences, intimate partner violence and psychiatric comorbidities is paramount to providing effective and accessible treatment options for this population [4].

*Correspondence: kelley.saia@bmc.org
[1] Department of Obstetrics and Gynecology, Boston University School of Medicine, 85 East Concord Street, Boston, MA 02118, USA
Full list of author information is available at the end of the article

The introduction of office based prescribing of buprenorphine has increased access to opioid use disorder treatment in the US and allows for integration of opioid agonist treatment in prenatal clinic settings [5]. Historically, opioid agonist treatment with methadone was the gold standard for managing opioid use disorders in pregnant women. Based on geographic location, however, many women do not have access to a methadone treatment facility in the US [6, 7]. In addition, most obstetricians have limited training in addiction medicine or substance use disorder screening methods and are unable to provide comprehensive care for these patients [8, 9]. Even in areas where such infrastructure exists, many women are resistant to starting methadone citing the stigma of methadone treatment and the restrictions of daily dosing as the major barriers [7]. The Project Recovery-Empowerment-Social Services-Prenatal Care-Education-Community-Treatment (RESPECT), Substance Use Disorder Treatment in Pregnancy Clinic, a multidisciplinary program based at an urban, academic center was developed in response to these issues. The objectives of this study are to describe changes at our center in the prevalence of opioid use disorder in pregnancy, the delivery of prenatal care, and neonatal outcomes following the implementation of buprenorphine treatment in 2006.

Methods

Setting and participants

We conducted a retrospective cohort study of pregnant women with opioid use disorder and their neonates delivered at Boston Medical Center from June 2006—when buprenorphine treatment began in our Project RESPECT clinic—through December 2010. Project RESPECT is a multidisciplinary treatment team at Boston Medical Center consisting of three buprenorphine waivered obstetric providers, a psychiatrist, an addiction psychiatry nurse practitioner, and a licensed independent clinical social worker. Boston Medical Center is an urban safety net hospital with a labor and delivery unit, high-risk maternal fetal medicine in-patient service, level three NICU and a pediatric in-patient ward for infants with NAS. Project RESPECT operates in conjunction with local and regional methadone clinics, counseling centers, and residential treatment programs for pregnant women.

Maternal criteria for opioid agonist therapy at Project RESPECT included being 18 years of age or older, DSM IV diagnosis of substance dependence for opioids, laboratory and/or radiographic documentation of pregnancy, and voluntary consent to engage in Project RESPECT's comprehensive treatment program. All Project RESPECT patients treated with opioid agonist treatment (methadone or buprenorphine) were followed by the same specialized team. The type of opioid agonist treatment initiated was selected considering the following factors: patient choice, treatment history, disease severity and medical and psychiatric comorbidities.

Our practice protocol recommends methadone for women with more severe opioid use disorder, women with intolerance to buprenorphine, or for whom buprenorphine is medically contraindicated. In general, women for whom previous buprenorphine treatment was non-efficacious, who had a history within the last 6 months of buprenorphine diversion, who were unable to present for weekly to bi-weekly office visits, or who were unwilling to engage in independent relapse prevention counseling were offered methadone. All patients were scheduled for a prenatal care and relapse prevention visit every 1–3 weeks from initiation of care until delivery. Observed urine drug tests were done at every prenatal visit and on admission to labor and delivery. If an appointment was missed, patients were contacted and requested to come in for a urine drug test within 48 h.

Study data

Study data were obtained from electronic medical records and included maternal age, total number of prenatal visits, urine drug test results, gestational age at treatment initiation, methadone or buprenorphine dose at treatment initiation and at delivery, concomitant medication use, smoking during pregnancy, gestational age at delivery, mode of delivery, anesthesia use during delivery, infant birth weight, neonatal abstinence score using a modified Finnegan scale, amount and duration of NAS opioid treatment and length of neonatal hospital stay [10]. Neonatal treatment with opioid therapy was initiated if the neonate had three consecutive modified Finnegan scores $\geq$8 or two consecutive scores $\geq$12. Neonates delivered June 2006 through mid-January 2009 had first-line treatment with diluted tincture of opium (DTO) of 0.4 mg morphine/mL, and neonates delivered mid-January 2009 through December 2010 had first-line treatment with neonatal morphine solution. Results were converted to total morphine in equivalents over the course of the hospitalization. Morphine dosing was based on both severities of scores and neonatal birth weight. Adjunctive therapy with phenobarbital or clonidine was added for infants who continued to have scores >8 despite maximum dosing of DTO or morphine. Infants were weaned off DTO, morphine, and/or clonidine as inpatients and monitored for 24–48 h prior to discharge. Phenobarbital was weaned in the outpatient setting. This study was approved by the Boston University Medical Center Institutional Review Board.

Statistical methods

Trends in the treatment of mother–neonate pairs by calendar year were assessed using the Cochran–Armitage test for categorical variables and linear regression for continuous variables. For the linear trend model, year of birth was standardized to have a mean of zero and a standard deviation of 1 because of the small range of values relative to the mean in the original distribution. Differences in binary maternal and infant characteristics by prenatal exposure (methadone or buprenorphine) and calendar year were estimated using generalized linear models (log-link function) because the odds ratio overestimates the risk ratio given the high risk of our outcomes [11]. Linear regression was used to estimate differences in continuous outcomes. Women with >1 pregnancy were included for each pregnancy. Five women initiated therapy with buprenorphine and later were switched to methadone; these mother–neonate pairs are described, but were not included in our statistical models. One twin from each twin birth was included; analyses were run including and excluding the twin and results were unchanged. We did not account for the clustering in the small number of women (N = 20) who delivered infants from >1 pregnancy. Statistical analyses were carried out with SAS 9.3.

Results

A total of 316 pregnant opioid dependent women presented for care during the study period: 296 women had one pregnancy, 18 had two pregnancies, and two had three pregnancies; there were six sets of twins. Of the 338 pregnancies, 6 resulted in intrauterine fetal demise or still birth and the remaining were live births. The final study population included 332 mother neonate pairs from 332 pregnancies (including one twin from each of the six sets of twins) in 310 women.

The number of pregnant women with opioid use disorders rose from 2006 through 2010. There was an almost two-fold increase in the number of women treated annually from 2007 through 2010. Following the emergence of buprenorphine as a treatment option at our clinic in 2006, women treated with buprenorphine for opioid use disorder increased from 3% in 2006 to 41% in 2010. The delivery dose of buprenorphine increased on average by 2.1 mg per year from 2007 to 2010 but no such trend in the average methadone dose at delivery was found. The prevalence of prescribed concomitant psychotropic medications increased as well as the proportion of vaginal deliveries (Table 1). There was a slight decrease in the proportion of maternal urine drug tests positive for cocaine. The proportion of neonates treated pharmacologically for NAS increased over time.

There were some notable differences in maternal characteristics by opioid agonist treatment type (Table 2). Women treated with buprenorphine versus methadone were more likely to deliver in later calendar years, to have on average three more prenatal care visits, and had a 15% increased likelihood of vaginal delivery. Buprenorphine treated women had a 26% lower risk of a positive urine screen for any illicit drug after treatment initiation, 76% lower risk of a positive cocaine screen and 31% lower risk of a positive opioid screen compared to those treated with methadone.

Neonatal characteristics and NAS outcomes by calendar year are provided in Table 3. Following the changes in prenatal opioid agonist therapy at our site, the proportion of infant exposed to buprenorphine increased over time. The proportion of infants treated pharmacologically for NAS also increased from 76% in 2006 to 86% in 2010. The length of NAS treatment appears to have decreased following the replacement of DTO with morphine as a first line NAS treatment in 2009 despite a trend towards treatment starting earlier as year of birth increased. There was no discernable trend in the amount of morphine per birth weight by year of delivery. Mean gestational age at birth was stable over time and above 37 weeks, but the proportion of infants born preterm was overall high.

Discussion

We describe outcomes of pregnant women with opioid use disorders and their neonates treated at our Project RESPECT clinic from 2006 to 2010. Over the study period, the percentage of women treated with buprenorphine increased from 3 to 41%, possibly reflecting increases in patient demand, increased patient autonomy, and improved provider prescribing comfort. Buprenorphine treatment failure, defined as transition from buprenorphine to methadone during the pregnancy for non-adherence, did not show a corresponding increase. The increase in the average dose of buprenorphine prescribed over the study period may be the result of several factors including, an increase in provider prescribing comfort over time and an increase in addiction disease severity in those seeking buprenorphine treatment. Choosing the appropriate agonist medication for pregnant women with opioid use disorder is complex; multiple variables including patient preference, disease severity, psychiatric comorbidities, social supports and recovery resources must be considered.

There were important differences observed in the characteristics of women by treatment approach. Women treated with buprenorphine versus methadone attended more prenatal care visits and had fewer positive urine drug tests. In addition, these women were more likely to

Table 1 Maternal characteristics by calendar year for 332 pregnancies

Characteristic	2006 (N = 33)	2007 (N = 53)	2008 (N = 69)	2009 (N = 84)	2010 (N = 93)
Maternal age (years)	27.4 (6.0)	28.8 (5.8)	28.6 (4.7)	27.2 (4.8)	27.3 (4.7)
Gestational age at presentation for care (weeks)	18.6 (9.1)	17.0 (8.0)	18.7 (9.7)	15.3 (7.7)	16.4 (9.9)
Number of prenatal care visits	8.9 (4.9)	9.6 (4.6)	9.6 (5.0)	9.4 (4.4)	9.3 (4.3)
Initial daily dose of methadone (mg)	70.9 (35.1)	66.1 (36.4)	74.2 (49.2)	66.6 (34.0)	64.9 (29.4)
Daily dose of methadone at delivery (mg)	88.5 (36.8)	83.8 (40.4)	94.4 (52.7)	91.0 (40.8)	88.0 (35.1)
Initial daily dose of buprenorphine (mg)	–	11.6 (7.0)	10.1 (4.0)	13.2 (6.5)	12.2 (7.2)
Daily dose of buprenorphine at delivery (mg)	–	11.4 (8.4)	14.1 (6.4)	14.1 (6.1)	16.8 (8.4)
Prescribed psychiatric medications					
SSRIs	3 (9.1)	4 (7.6)	14 (20.3)	13 (15.5)	20 (21.5)
Benzodiazepines	5 (15.2)	10 (18.9)	15 (21.7)	15 (17.9)	20 (21.5)
Antipsychotics	0 (0)	4 (7.6)	4 (5.8)	4 (4.8)	7 (7.5)
Other	2 (6.1)	1 (1.9)	5 (7.3)	8 (9.5)	10 (10.8)
Smoked cigarettes	25	36	42	59	59
Hepatitis C infected	19	27	38	48	48
≥1 urine screen	31 (93.9)	50 (94.3)	69 (98.6)	79 (94.0)	88 (94.6)
≥1 positive urine screen	15 (48.4)	22 (44.0)	38 (55.9)	41 (51.9)	43 (48.9)
Urine screen positive for[a]					
Cocaine	10 (32.3)	11 (22.0)	16 (23.5)	18 (22.8)	16 (18.2)
Opioids	11 (35.5)	14 (28.0)	26 (38.2)	32 (40.5)	44 (38.6)
Benzodiazepines	1 (3.2)	4 (8.0)	9 (13.2)	8 (10.1)	3 (3.4)
Amphetamines	1 (3.2)	1 (2.0)	3 (4.4)	2 (2.5)	3 (3.4)
Vaginal delivery	16 (48.5)	27 (50.9)	38 (55.1)	53 (63.1)	62 (66.7)
Cesarean section	17 (55.5)	26 (49.1)	31 (44.9)	31 (36.9)	31 (33.3)
Anesthesia during delivery	25 (75.7)	48 (90.5)	60 (86.9)	76 (90.4)	81 (87.0)

Missing data: Initial daily dose of opioid agonist therapy, one women treated with buprenorphine in 2008, one women treated with buprenorphine in 2009, one women treated with buprenorphine in 2010, one women treated with methadone in 2006, two women treated with methadone in 2007, one woman treated with methadone in 2009; Gestational age at first prenatal visit, two women in 2006, six women in 2007, three women in 2008, five women in 2009, two women in 2010. Smoking, 6 women in 2006, 10 women in 2007, 16 women in 2008, 15 women in 2009, 18 women in 2010; Hepatitis C, 10 women in 2006, 14 women in 2007, 15 women in 2008, 17 women in 2009, 18 women in 2010. Anesthesia, 5 women in 2006, 2 women in 2007, 3 women in 2008, 3 women in 2009, 3 women in 2010

Mean ± standard deviation or number of pregnancies and percent

[a] Patients with the prescribed medication not counted as a positive test result

delivery vaginally, likely due to changes in operative delivery recommendations for hepatitis C positive women. After 2007, cesarean sections were no longer recommended to decrease vertical transmission of hepatitis C. From 2006 to 2010, our cesarean section rate decreased from 45.8 to 35%, with the largest number of buprenorphine patients delivering in the later calendar years.

Maternal severity of opioid dependence and other factors influenced our clinical prescribing, with buprenorphine typically being used in more stable pregnant women who do not need the structure of observed daily dosing [12]. Potential confounding by indication can occur in assessing the comparative outcomes of prenatal BMT versus MMT because maternal characteristics that might influence choice of prenatal treatment with BMT versus MMT likely also affect neonatal outcomes [13, 14]. Prior studies have suggested improved NAS and birth outcomes in neonates exposed to buprenorphine compared to methadone, including decreased NAS severity with shorter length of hospitalization, lower risk of NAS pharmacologic treatment, and higher gestational age at birth, birth weight, body length and head circumference [15–17]. Because of the potential for uncontrolled confounding in this and many studies published to date [18] we did not assess any causal relationships between prenatal exposure and infant outcomes. Further, the dynamic nature of clinical care in this patient population, including changes in both maternal treatment and in NAS treatment, can introduce misclassification bias in any causal assessments.

We observed changes in NAS care practices in our institution over the calendar years, including a shift from DTO to neonatal morphine solution as first-line treatment, and more clonidine use for adjunctive second-line treatment. These observed changes fit with the updated recommendations for NAS management over the past

Table 2 Maternal characteristics by prenatal opioid agonist treatment for 332 pregnancies

Characteristic	Mean and standard deviation or number and proportion		Mean difference or risk ratio and 95% CI (adjusted for year of birth)	
	Buprenorphine (N = 82)	Methadone (N = 245)	Buprenorphine and methadone (N = 5)	Buprenorphine versus methadone
Maternal age (years)	28.1 ± 5.1	27.7 ± 5.1	27.2 ± 3.3	0.76 (−0.55, 2.07)
Year of delivery[a]				
2009–2010	60 (73.2)	114 (46.5)	3 (60.0)	1.57 (1.30, 1.90)
2006–2008	22 (26.8)	131 (53.5)	2 (40.0)	1.0
Number of fetuses				
Singleton	80 (97.6)	241 (98.4)	5 (100)	–
Twin	2 (2.4)	4 (1.6)	0 (0)	
Prenatal care	82 (100)	241 (0.99)	5 (100)	–
Gestational age at presentation for care (weeks)	16.4 ± 8.9	17.2 ± 8.9	11.8 ± 8.6	−0.16 (−2.46, 2.13)
Number of prenatal care visits	11.5 ± 4.7	8.7 ± 4.3	11.6 ± 2.2	3.06 (1.92, 4.20)
Initial daily dose of opioid agonist therapy (mg)	12.0 ± 6.5	68.3 ± 37.4	12.0 ± 4.0	–
Stopped agonist therapy during pregnancy				
Yes	2 (2.4)	0 (0)	0 (0)	–
No	80 (97.6)	245 (100)	5 (100)	
Daily dose of opioid agonist therapy at delivery (mg)	15.1 ± 7.5	89.3 ± 41.7	77.0 ± 28.9	–
Smoked cigarettes	54 (65.9)	164 (66.9)	4 (80.0)	–
Hepatitis C infected	32 (39.0)	134 (54.7)	4 (80.0)	–
Prescribed SSRIs	14 (17.1)	38 (15.5)	2 (40.0)	1.01 (0.57, 1.79) 1.0
Prescribed benzodiazepines	14 (17.1)	51 (20.8)	0 (0)	0.81 (0.47, 1.39) 1.0
Prescribed antipsychotics	1 (1.2)	18 (7.4)	0 (0)	0.15 (0.02, 1.12) 1.0
Other prescribed psychiatric medications	9 (11.0)	15 (6.1)	2 (40.0)	1.60 (0.72, 3.60) 1.0
Urine screen				
≥1	78 (95.1)	233 (95.1)	5 (100)	1.02 (0.95, 1.09)
None	4 (4.9)	12 (4.9)	0 (0)	1.0
Positive urine screen				
≥1	31 (39.7)	123 (52.8)	5 (100)	0.74 (0.55, 1.01)
None	47 (60.3)	220 (47.2)	0 (0)	1.0
Cocaine urine screen				
Positive	5 (6.4)	63 (27.0)	3 (60.0)	0.24 (0.10, 0.57)
Negative	73 (93.6)	170 (73.0)	2 (40.0)	1.0
Non-prescribed opioid urine screen				
Positive	22 (28.2)	90 (38.6)	5 (100)	0.69 (0.46, 1.02)
Negative	56 (71.8)	143 (61.4)	0 (0)	1.0
Non-prescribed benzodiazepines urine screen				
Positive	7 (9.0)	18 (7.7)	0 (0)	1.27 (0.54, 2.98)
Negative	71 (91.0)	215 (92.3)	5 (100)	1.0
Non-prescribed amphetamine urine screen				
Positive	3 (3.9)	7 (3.0)	0 (0)	1.34 (0.34, 5.31)
Negative	75 (96.1)	226 (97.0)	5 (100)	1.0
Mode of delivery				
Vaginal	55 (67.1)	138 (56.3)	3 (60.0)	1.15 (0.95, 1.39)
Cesarean section	27 (32.9)	107 (43.7)	2 (40.0)	1.0

Table 2 continued

Characteristic	Mean and standard deviation or number and proportion		Mean difference or risk ratio and 95% CI (adjusted for year of birth)	
	Buprenorphine (N = 82)	Methadone (N = 245)	Buprenorphine and methadone (N = 5)	Buprenorphine versus methadone
Anesthesia during delivery				
Yes	76 (93.8)	209 (90.9)	5 (100)	1.03 (0.96, 1.11)
No	5 (6.2)	21 (9.1)	0 (0)	1.0

Missing data: Initial daily dose of opioid agonist therapy, three women treated with buprenorphine, six women treated with methadone; Gestational age at first prenatal visit, one woman treated with methadone. Number of prenatal care visits, two women treated with methadone; Smoking, 12 women treated with buprenorphine, 52 women treated with methadone, 1 woman treated with methadone and buprenorphine; Hepatitis C infection, 11 women treated with buprenorphine, 62 women treated with methadone, 1 woman treated with methadone and buprenorphine; Anesthesia, one women treated with buprenorphine, and 15 women treated with methadone

[a] Unadjusted result

Table 3 Neonatal characteristics by year of birth

Characteristic	2006 (N = 33)	2007 (N = 53)	2008 (N = 69)	2009 (N = 84)	2010 (N = 93)
Prenatal opioid agonist therapy exposure					
Methadone	32 (97.0)	48 (90.6)	51 (79.3)	62 (73.8)	52 (55.9)
Buprenorphine	1 (3.3)	5 (9.4)	16 (23.2)	22 (26.2)	38 (40.9)
Methadone and buprenorphine	0 (0)	0 (0)	2 (2.9)	0 (0)	3 (3.2)
Length of hospitalization (days)	23.2 ± 10.3	24.2 ± 12.7	24.1 ± 12.9	21.9 ± 11.1	20.8 ± 10.9
Pharmacologically treated for NAS	25 (75.8)	43 (81.1)	62 (89.9)	72 (85.7)	80 (86.0)
Age at NAS treatment Initiation (days)	2.5 ± 2.1	2.4 ± 1.9	2.9 ± 3.1	2.0 ± 1.7	1.9 ± 1.4
First-line NAS treatment					
Morphine	0 (0)	0 (0)	1 (1.6)	67 (93.1)	80 (100.0)
DTO	25 (100)	43 (100)	61 (98.4)	5 (6.9)	0 (0)
Total morphine used to treat NAS, mg per kg birth weight[a]	6.0 ± 3.7	6.7 ± 6.2	3.6 ± 3.5	8.9 ± 8.4	6.4 ± 5.4
Additional NAS treatment with Phenobarbital	9 (36.0)	9 (20.9)	10 (16.1)	23 (31.9)	18 (22.5)
Clonidine	0 (0)	0 (0)	0 (0)	2 (2.8)	8 (10.0)
Length of NAS treatment (days)	20.6 ± 9.6	20.6 ± 10.2	19.5 ± 10.1	19.2 ± 9.5	17.5 ± 7.8
Peak Finnegan score among neonates treated for NAS	13.9 ± 2.8	13.3 ± 3.5	11.9 ± 2.6	12.9 ± 3.0	11.9 ± 2.5
Gestational age at birth (weeks)	37.9 ± 1.8	38.7 ± 2.2	38.0 ± 2.5	38.2 ± 2.5	38.7 ± 2.3
Preterm birth (<37 weeks)	7 (21.2)	6 (11.3)	17 (24.6)	16 (19.1)	12 (12.9)
Birth weight (g)	2895.8 ± 373.1	2786.6 ± 728.0	2807.9 ± 599.6	2898.5 ± 652.3	2974.2 ± 580.2

Missing data: Birth weight, one neonate; Length of stay, one neonate; Total mg of morphine per kg of birth weight: one neonate; Peak Finnegan Score, twelve neonates

NAS neonatal abstinence syndrome, *DTO* diluted tincture of opium

[a] Morphine dose equivalent determined for DTO treated neonates

decade. Morphine and methadone are recommended by the American Academy of Pediatrics (AAP) as preferred agents over DTO [19, 20]. While the majority of institutions in the US use morphine, a recent single-center randomized control trial found that methadone was associated with shorter hospitalizations in comparison with morphine [21]. In addition, some institutions have started to transition infants home on methadone to complete weaning [22, 23]. Recent national trends in adjunctive medications for NAS favor clonidine as an acceptable option over phenobarbital [24, 25]. There is also a trend towards more emphasis on breastfeeding, rooming-in, and other non-pharmacologic care interventions to best manage NAS [18, 26]. Lastly, though the Finnegan scale is the current gold standard for NAS assessments, newer scales are under development [26]. Significant variability in NAS care remains and there is a need for more high quality clinical trials to best guide management.

Strengths of our study include being conducted at a single large clinic that is a leader in addiction medicine with standardized approaches for treating prenatal opioid use disorders and for assessing and treating NAS, and the largest sample size of opioid dependent mother–neonate pairs studied to date. Limitations of our study include the potential for error in chart abstraction and limited variables available clinically, especially potential confounders. Our institutional NAS clinical guidelines changed midway through the study period to use of neonatal morphine solution versus DTO as first-line therapy. Although DTO was converted to morphine equivalent dose, some differences in the pharmacology of these treatments may exist.

Conclusions

The choice of opioid agonist treatment remains a complex issue, with the overriding goal of maintaining maternal stability throughout the pregnancy and the post-partum period to improve both maternal and neonatal outcomes. Future research is needed to evaluate whether maternal addiction severity and choice of opioid agonist treatment affect neonatal outcomes and maternal long-term recovery. Accessible prenatal care combined with opioid use disorder treatment for pregnant women in the US must be adopted to address the needs of this underserved and growing population. Boston Medical Center's obstetric care and addiction medicine treatment clinic, Project RESPECT, demonstrates the feasibility of such a model in a large urban center. Reducing health care costs and improving the care for opioid-exposed newborns cannot be accomplished without parallel development and implementation of comprehensive care for opioid dependent pregnant women.

Authors' contributions

KS, SMB and EMW conceived of the study design, methods, interpretation of the results, and drafting and revising the manuscript. PPP and contributed to the initial data collection and early manuscripts revisions. SBB contributed to the study design, methods, interpretation of the results, drafting and revision of the manuscript and performed the data analysis. All authors read and approved the final manuscript.

Author details

[1] Department of Obstetrics and Gynecology, Boston University School of Medicine, 85 East Concord Street, Boston, MA 02118, USA. [2] Section of General Internal Medicine, Boston University School of Medicine, Boston, MA, USA. [3] Department of Pediatrics, Boston University School of Medicine, Boston, MA, USA. [4] Harvard Vanguard Medical Associates, Newton Wellesley Hospital, Newton, MA, USA. [5] Department of Obstetrics and Gynecology, Albert Einstein College of Medicine, Bronx, NY, USA. [6] Department of Surgery, Queen's University, Kingston, Canada.

Acknowledgements

We would like to thank Mary Beth Howard, MD; Jessica A McHugh, MD; Lindsay Miller, MD; Maureen P Sullivan, RN; Olivera Vragovic, MBA; Howard J Cabral, PhD; and Lynn Borgotta, MD, MPH for their assistance with data collection and data analysis planning. A special thanks to Shruthi Mahalingaiah, MD for her research mentorship. This publication was supported by the Boston University School of Public Health Pilot Fund (S. Brogly and K. Saia) and by the Eunice Kennedy Shriver National Institutes of Child Health and Human Development under Grant Number 1R21HD081271-01 REVISED (S. Brogly). The content is solely the responsibility of the authors and does not necessarily represent the official views of the National Institutes of Health.

Competing interests

The authors declare that they have no competing interests.

References

1. CDC. Demographic and substance use trends among heroin users- United States, 2002–2013. MMWR. 2015;64:719–25.
2. Patrick SW, Schumacher RE, Benneyworth BD, Krans EE, McAllister JM, Davis MM. Neonatal abstinence syndrome and associated health care expenditures: United States, 2000–2009. JAMA. 2012;307:1934–40.
3. Tolia VN, Patrick SW, Bennett MM, Murthy K, Sousa J, Smith PB, Clark RH, Spitzer AR. Increasing incidence of the neonatal abstinence syndrome in U.S. neonatal ICUs. N Engl J Med. 2015;372:2118–26.
4. Wendell AD. Overview and epidemiology of substance abuse in pregnancy. Clin Obstet Gynecol. 2013;56:91–6.
5. Turner L, Kruszewski SP, Alexander GC. Trends in the use of buprenorphine by office-based physicians in the United States, 2003–2013. Am J Addict. 2015;24:24–9.
6. Dick AW, Pacula RL, Gordon AJ, Sorbero M, Burns RM, Leslie D, Stein BD. Growth in buprenorphine waivers for physicians increased potential access to opioid agonist treatment, 2002–11. Health Aff (Millwood). 2015;34:1028–34.
7. Livingston JD, Milne T, Fang ML, Amari E. The effectiveness of interventions for reducing stigma related to substance use disorders: a systematic review. Addiction. 2012;107:39–50.
8. Herzig K, Huynh D, Gilbert P, Danley DW, Jackson R, Gerbert B. Comparing prenatal providers' approaches to four different risks: alcohol, tobacco, drugs, and domestic violence. Women Health. 2006;43:83–101.
9. Isaacson JH, Fleming M, Kraus M, Kahn R, Mundt M. A national survey of training in substance use disorders in residency programs. J Stud Alcohol. 2000;61:912–5.
10. Finnegan LP, Connaughton JF Jr, Kron RE, Emich JP. Neonatal abstinence syndrome: assessment and management. Addict Dis. 1975;2:141–58.
11. Spiegelman D, Hertzmark E. Easy SAS calculations for risk or prevalence ratios and differences. Am J Epidemiol. 2005;162:199–200.
12. Cicero TJ, Surratt HL, Inciardi JA, Munoz A. Relationship between therapeutic use and abuse of opioid analgesics in rural, surburban, and urban locations in the United States. Pharmacoepidemiol Drug Saf. 2007;16:827–40.
13. Brogly SB, Hahn KA, Diaz SH, Werler M. Confounding of the comparative safety of prenatal opioid agonist therapy. J Addict Res Ther. 2015;6:252.
14. Brogly SB, Saia KA, Walley AY, Du HM, Sebastiani P. Prenatal buprenorphine versus methadone exposure and neonatal outcomes: systematic review and meta-analysis. Am J Epidemiol. 2014;180:673–86.
15. Metz V, Jagsch R, Ebner N, Wurzl J, Pribasnig A, Aschauer C, Fischer G. Impact of treatment approach on maternal and neonatal outcome in pregnant opioid-maintained women. Hum Psychopharmacol. 2011;26:412–21.
16. Jones HE, Johnson RE, Jasinski DR, O'Grady KE, Chisholm CA, Choo RE, Crocetti M, Dudas R, Harrow C, Huestis MA, et al. Buprenorphine versus methadone in the treatment of pregnant opioid-dependent patients: effects on the neonatal abstinence syndrome. Drug Alcohol Depend. 2005;79:1–10.
17. Welle-Strand GK, Skurtveit S, Jones HE, Waal H, Bakstad B, Bjarko L, Ravndal E. Neonatal outcomes following in utero exposure to methadone or buprenorphine: a National Cohort Study of opioid-agonist treatment of Pregnant Women in Norway from 1996 to 2009. Drug Alcohol Depend. 2013;127:200–6.
18. Bagley SM, Wachman EM, Holland E, Brogly SB. Review of the assessment and management of neonatal abstinence syndrome. Addict Sci Clin Pract. 2014;9:19.
19. Hudak ML, Tan RC. Neonatal drug withdrawal. Pediatrics. 2012;129:e540–60.
20. Koktajlo S, Robinson CA, Presti A. Use of tincture of opium compared to oral morphine for the treatment of neonatal abstinence syndrome. J Opioid Manag. 2013;9:62–70.

21. Brown MS, Hayes MJ, Thornton LM. Methadone versus morphine for treatment of neonatal abstinence syndrome: a prospective randomized clinical trial. J Perinatol. 2015;35:278–83.
22. Lee J, Hulman S, Musci MJ, Stang E. Neonatal abstinence syndrome: influence of a combined inpatient/outpatient methadone treatment regimen on the average length of stay of a medicaid NICU population. Popul Health Manag. 2015;18:392–7.
23. Backes CH, Backes CR, Gardner D, Nankervis CA, Giannone PJ, Cordero L. Neonatal abstinence syndrome: transitioning methadone-treated infants from an inpatient to an outpatient setting. J Perinatol. 2012;32:425–30.
24. Agthe AG, Kim GR, Mathias KB, Hendrix CW, Chavez-Valdez R, Jansson L, Lewis TR, Yaster M, Gauda EB. Clonidine as an adjunct therapy to opioids for neonatal abstinence syndrome: a randomized, controlled trial. Pediatrics. 2009;123:849–56.
25. Surran B, Visintainer P, Chamberlain S, Kopcsa K, Shah B, Singh R. Efficacy of clonidine versus phenobarbital in reducing neonatal morphine sulfate therapy days for neonatal abstinence syndrome: a prospective randomized clinical trial. J Perinatol. 2013;33:954–9.
26. Holmes AV, Atwood EC, Whalen B, Beliveau J, Jarvis JD, Matulis JC, Ralston SL. Rooming-into treat neonatal abstinence syndrome: improved family-centered care at lower cost. Pediatrics. 2016;137:e20152929.

3

A qualitative study of treatment-seeking heroin users in contemporary China

Anna Lembke[1*] and Niushen Zhang[2]

Abstract

Background: Heroin has emerged as the primary drug of concern in China, with as many as three million contemporary users. Once a Chinese citizen has been identified by Chinese law enforcement as a 'drug addict', that individual is 'registered' in an official government tracking system for the rest of his or her life, independent of verified rehabilitation and recovery. Most of what is known about heroin users in China is based on studies of registered heroin users participating, often involuntarily, in government-sponsored treatment.

Methods: Using Grounded Theory Methodology, we collected and analyzed in-depth interviews of heroin users voluntarily seeking treatment at a new, non-government-sponsored, for-profit, addiction treatment hospital in Beijing, China.

Results: We identified three major themes among our participants: (1) intense social stigma towards individuals with drug addiction; (2) a desire for anonymous, confidential treatment to avoid social stigma and the loss of personal freedom that accompanies participation in government-sponsored treatment; and (3) a deep mistrust of government-sponsored treatment and a search for more effective alternatives.

Conclusion: Despite a desire for treatment, our subjects were reluctant to access government-sponsored treatment facilities because of fear of a stigmatized identity, fear of loss of personal freedom, and lack of faith in the efficacy and safety of government-sponsored treatments. Their willingness to pay cash at a new, non-government-sponsored, addiction treatment facility illustrates the lengths to which they will go to remain 'unregistered' and to discover better alternatives. That the Chinese government allows such facilities to operate outside of government surveillance suggests a new openness to alternative options to combat China's rising drug epidemic. The efficacy of these alternative options, however, remains in question.

Keywords: China, Heroin, Addiction, Treatment, Methadone, Qualitative

Background

Beginning in the mid-nineteenth century when Britain defeated the Qing government and forced legal importation of opium (the Opium Wars), opioid use began to escalate in China. By 1906, about 27 % of the adult, male population was addicted to opium [1]. Beginning in the 1950's, the newly formed Communist government launched a massive, three-year, antidrug campaign, which led to the shutdown of production sites, sentencing of drug offenders, mandatory treatment and rehabilitation of millions of drug addicted persons, and ultimately to the claim that there was a near disappearance of opioid use and drug trafficking [2]. With the establishment of the "open-door" policy in the 1980's and China's proximity to major production sources (the Golden Triangle and the Golden Crescent), illegal drug trafficking re-emerged in China [1].

Heroin is now the primary drug of concern in China, followed by amphetamine-type stimulants and tranquilizers [3]. The Chinese Ministry of Public Security 2012 Annual Report on Drug Control estimates that 1.156 million of the 1.794 million drug-dependent persons registered by the national public security system are addicted to heroin [4]. By some earlier estimates, the

*Correspondence: alembke@stanford.edu
[1] Department of Psychiatry and Behavioral Sciences, Stanford University School of Medicine, 401 Quarry Road, Stanford, CA 94306, USA
Full list of author information is available at the end of the article

actual number of heroin users, including the unregistered users, is more than twice that number [3]; and the total number of drug users in China may be as high as 7 million, with China predicted to have the most heroin users of any country in the world within 5 years [5].

To date, the Chinese government has set up three types of facilities to target the problem of drug use and addiction. They include the compulsory detoxification institutions (CDI), the rehabilitation units through labor (RUL), and the voluntary detoxification institutions (VDI) such as methadone maintenance treatment (MMT) clinics. The CDI and RUL are run by law enforcement agencies and the MMT is run by the Department of Health [6].

Currently, the regulations stipulate three levels of penalty for illicit drug use: (1) First time illicit drug users are fined and/or placed in local detention centers for up to 2 weeks; (2) regular illicit drug users and those with drug dependencies are confined to residential rehabilitation centers for periods from one to 6 months; (3) drug users who relapse after compulsory detoxification are placed in compulsory labor re-education centers for one to 3 years [6, 7]. Once an individual has been identified by law enforcement agencies as an illicit drug user, that individual is 'registered' in official government tracking systems for the rest of his or her life, independent of verified rehabilitation and recovery. Despite these measures, the number of registered drug users in China increased 19-fold between 1990 and 2009 [8].

The first MMT clinics were opened in 2004 [9] as a reaction to the failure of the strictly punitive approach that was stated in the "Regulations on Prohibition against Narcotics" from 1990 [6]. In 2004, eight MMT clinics served 1029 drug users. By the end of 2011, MMT clinics had expanded to 738 clinics serving 344,254 drug users. Now MMT reaches approximately 30 % of registered intravenous drug users in China [9]. According to a systematic review by Zhang et al., MMT services in China are closely monitored by the public security, and police raids and arrests near MMT sites are common. Furthermore, random urine testing in MMT clinics that are positive for heroin can result in immediate compulsory detention. Police arrest and detention in compulsory rehabilitation is the most common cause of drop out (22.2 %) [9].

The majority of the research on heroin users in China to date is based on studies of registered users in government treatment facilities for compulsory detoxification and rehabilitation. Findings show that most are younger than 35 years, have lower levels of education (high school or less), have a history of alcohol and tobacco use prior to drug use, have unstable jobs, and have a high likelihood of relapse [2, 6].

In this explorative, qualitative study, we collected and analyzed in-depth interviews with heroin users seeking treatment for heroin addiction at a new, voluntary, for-profit, addiction treatment facility in Beijing, China, which is government-approved but not government sponsored. Its clients are not required to disclose their identity or become registered with the government tracking system. Using Grounded Theory Methodology, we sought to capture a deeper understanding of the precipitants, experiences, and beliefs among contemporary heroin users living in China who are voluntarily seeking treatment at a non-government-sponsored treatment facility.

Methods

Research setting

All interviews were conducted at a voluntary, non-government sponsored, inpatient, addiction treatment hospital in Beijing, China, which will henceforth, pseudonymously, be called "New Hospital". We chose New Hospital as it was the only treatment facility in Beijing which granted us permission to interview patients in person. We solicited several government-sponsored treatment facilities in Beijing in the months preceding field work, but despite our efforts, we were not granted permission.

New Hospital officially opened on August 2013 as a for-profit, private, civilian-invested venture ("ming ban qi ye") as distinct from more traditional government-run institutions. Although Beijing government officials are aware of the existence of New Hospital and have sanctioned its existence, as attested to by an official document we were shown, patients at New Hospital can receive their treatment without triggering registration with government officials as an illicit drug user, a status which becomes permanently attached to the individual identification card in the national civilian database.

New Hospital has 40 inpatient beds dedicated to the treatment of drug addiction, and averages 20–40 admissions per month. The average length of stay is 1 week. Eighty percent of patients seek treatment for heroin addiction. Ten percent seek treatment for methamphetamine addiction. Ten percent seek treatment for other drug addictions, including most commonly tramadol and meperidine. In terms of the patient population at New Hospital, the majority (75 %) of patients comes from outside the Beijing area, predominantly from urban areas in the provinces of Inner Mongolia and ShanXi. Over 90 % of admitted patients are men, and most are in their 40's. The estimated percent of patient who returned at least once in the first year for a second round of treatment was approximately 40–50 %.

New Hospital has a website describing its services, but otherwise relies primarily on word-of-mouth referral from patients and providers. The advertised treatments offered at New Hospital include methadone detoxification, adjunctive psychiatric treatment including psychiatric medications, and behavioral interventions.

New Hospital does not take health insurance. Anyone who seeks admission and has the resources to pay out of pocket for the treatment can be admitted to New Hospital. Patients are expected to pay cash up front depending on the number of days they plan to stay. The average cost per day for treatment is 300 renminbi (RMB), or fifty dollars, not including meals, but can cost more or less depending on a pre-ordained algorithm that includes severity of drug use history, type of drug addiction, private vs shared room, etc. To put that in perspective, an average salary in Beijing, China is 5000 RMB per month [10], or 833 US dollars. Given that the average length of stay is 1 week, treatment at New Hospital costs on average 2100 RMB, or nearly half of the average monthly salary.

Two psychiatrists staff the unit at any given time, along with a total of eight ancillary health care providers. Providers are paid according to a fee structure that is at least partly based on the number of patients seen, and the type of care delivered. In other words, New Hospital runs on a cash-basis fee-for-service business model similar to many US hospitals.

Data collection and analysis

Approval was obtained from the Stanford Institutional Review Board (IRB) to conduct anonymous interviews with patients with addiction in China. The consent form was translated into Mandarin Chinese and approved by the Stanford IRB in both English and Mandarin. The study protocol and consent form were subsequently approved by the administration of New Hospital prior to recruitment.

In July 2014, we conducted nine, in-depth interviews of heroin users with self-identified 'heroin addiction' seeking treatment for such at New Hospital. The sample was primarily determined by opportunity and access, which serendipitously included five unregistered heroin addicted persons (55.5 % of the study sample), an otherwise difficult population to capture. The criteria for participation in the study were: (1) Seeking treatment for heroin use/addiction, and (2) willingness to undergo an in-depth interview. All patients met DSM-V criteria for an opioid use disorder, although that was not an inclusion criterion per se.

Participants were recruited by New Hospital staff on the day of the interview, by asking who might be willing to sit for an interview. A portion of potential participants declined to participate, but specific number of refusals was not obtained. In a system known to be coercive, the knowledge of refusal of participation suggests true voluntariness, which is of ethical importance. Those who agreed to participate were led to a private room separate from regular hospital rooms and corridors, to maximize privacy. Prior to initiating the interview, the interviewer reviewed the verbal consent form with the potential participant. The consent form detailed the study purpose, procedures, and potential risks. Potential participants were again informed that participation was voluntary. None refused to participate at that juncture. Consent was obtained verbally. At no point was the participant asked his/her name. Nor was the participant's name associated with the written notes at any time in the course of obtaining data, including on the verbal consent form, which did not include a signature line.

The research team consisted of the principal investigator who served as the interviewer. She was also the first reviewer for coding of the transcripts. The principal investigator is a psychiatrist and addiction medicine expert trained in qualitative interviewing skills, ethics, and safety. The interviews were conducted in Mandarin Chinese with the assistance of a skilled interpreter who had experience as a medical translator. The principal investigator asked questions in English and the interpreter translated the questions into Chinese. The interpreter then translated the participants' responses into English. The principal investigator took hand-written notes in English during the interview, which later served as transcripts for coding. The research team also consisted of an independent reviewer who also coded the transcript and analyzed the data. The independent reviewer is a neurologist trained in qualitative interviewing skills, ethics, and safety.

This study used Grounded Theory methodology [11, 12]. Grounded Theory seeks to characterize complex social phenomenon by inductive analysis of data which are gathered in an iterative process, which allows multiple potential hypotheses to emerge in the course of data collection, instead of generating hypotheses a priori. Subsequent interviews seek to challenge or confirm emerging themes. Interviews are concluded when the coders identify that emerging themes have been saturated.

This study represents a convenience sample of those individuals at New Hospital who were both willing and able to be interviewed during the time frame of the study period. Despite the small sample size (N = 9), both reviewers concurred that the sample reached saturation in terms of the types of themes that emerged from the interviews.

The in-depth interviews lasted up to 120 min. The interviewer began simply by asking participants to describe how the events of their lives led them to seek treatment at New Hospital. As per Grounded-Theory

Methodology, the interviewer sought to minimize undue influence on the natural unfolding of the autobiographical narratives. The interviewer might interject at points to clarify or explore some point the participant raised in more depth; but with intention, the content generated was initially participant-driven. Two to three interviews were conducted during the morning and analysis was performed immediately in the afternoon (the same day as the interview) by the first and second reviewer. Coding was performed by each reviewer independently. Data were broken down into smaller components and labeled by topic such as "stigma" and "forced labor camps." Qualitative coding software was not used.

After coding was completed, the two reviewers compared coding lists to understand and explain variation in the data [13]. The codes were then combined and related to one another and classified into emerging themes/concepts such as "a desire for anonymous, confidential treatment." Analysis highlighted relationships and demonstrated gaps in the existing data. For example, we wondered why individuals who were already in the government registry would value anonymous, confidential treatment, when their anonymity had already been compromised. Questions for future interviews were augmented to fill in those gaps and guide deeper exploration of the emerging theory. Theoretical saturation was reached when all of the major themes were well developed and supported by data.

When all the interviews were complete, the two independent reviewers came to consensus on the most important themes that emerged from the data. These themes constitute the results of this qualitative work (substantive theory), and are described below. Any text in quotes is a verbatim quote from a participant.

Results

Description of study sample

The sample of participants included six men and three women. Two were between the ages of 30–39 and seven were in their 40s. Four of the participants were from Inner Mongolia, one was from Beijing, three were from Tianjing, and one was from Shanxi. Only one of the participants had attended college and eight had not finished high school. Five were married, three were divorced, and one was single. Almost all (8/9) had children. Most (7/9) of the participants were either employed or self-employed. Seven reported using heroin for greater than a decade. The age of first use varied widely, from teens to 40's. Six subjects reported using heroin through inhalation (smoking, snorting, 'chasing the dragon') and three administered heroin intravenously.

Four of the subjects reported spending some time within a compulsory detoxification centers (rehabilitation unit through labor RUL), and these individuals were also registered with the government as 'illicit drug addicts'. The other five were unregistered. Only one of the participants had received treatment through an official government-sanctioned methadone maintenance clinic (MMT). All New Hospital patients reported methadone-facilitated detoxification as the mainstay of their treatment at New Hospital. All participants had co-morbid tobacco use, seven used alcohol on a regular basis, and six had used other illicit drugs at some point in their lives after trying heroin first.

Theme #1: Intense social stigma towards individuals with drug addiction

All subjects universally endorsed severe stigma towards drug-addicted persons in China. They described experiences of being ostracized and shunned, or fear of such, once their drug use became known to others. Furthermore, registered users described little hope of establishing a new, non-stigmatized, non-drug using identity, even after sustained abstinence.

> *"Chinese people look down on drug addicts. Heroin addicts have ... a lot of loneliness. People don't understand what a drug addict feels." (Male, 46 years old, never married, a registered heroin user.)*

> *"No way can I tell my husband or my daughter about my addiction. They would never be able to accept it. My daughter is 17. She's in America now. She is self-confident and has a bright future. This would destroy her." (Female, 40 years old, married, an unregistered heroin user.)*

> *"My friends don't know I'm addicted, but if they did, they would not want to have anything to do with me." (Female, 45 years old, married, an unregistered heroin user.)*

> *"As a drug addict, society abandons you. It's hard to get on the right path. People still don't treat you like a real person. Even once you've quit, you're still viewed as a drug addict and that becomes your identity. No one outside my circle of drug friends wants to associate with me, but I can't associate with my old friends or I will relapse. I want to work, but no one will hire me. I've become a total waste of a person. I feel so much regret. It has destroyed my family and my life. Addicts are people too. Not all addicts are bad people. They are good people too." (Male, 44 years old, divorced, a registered heroin user.)*

Theme #2: A desire for anonymous, confidential treatment to avoid social stigma and loss of personal freedom that accompanies participation in government-sponsored treatment

All of our unregistered subjects (5/9) endorsed choosing New Hospital because it provided an anonymous alternative to government-sponsored treatment options, allowing them to get treatment without being identified on the public registry as 'drug addict'. They viewed becoming registered, and the ensuing social stigma, as affecting not just their lives, but also their children's lives.

> *"Part of the reason I relapsed is because I don't have methadone. I thought about buying methadone from the black market, but it's too expensive -2,000 RMB for 500 ml. So, instead, I just buy heroin. I don't dare go to a methadone clinic because I don't want my name on the public record." (Male, 38 years old, married, an unregistered heroin user.)*

> *"Once you go to an MMT clinic, you're on the record, and if you don't show up, the government will come check up on you." (Female, 45 years old, married, an unregistered heroin user.)*

> *"I would not go to a methadone maintenance clinic because it would ruin my business. In China, they have a tough view of addicts and drug use is a crime. In China they don't trust addicts. Chinese people believe you can't do business with addicts." (Female, 40 years old, married, an unregistered heroin user.)*

> *"If my name gets on the public record, my children can't join the armed forces and they can't ever get a government job." (Male, 38 years old, married, an unregistered heroin user.)*

Based on the reports of registered users in our sample (4/9), the fears of unregistered users were well-founded. Some registered users described government surveillance and loss of personal privacy, even in the absence of participation in government treatment. Government authorities visited them in their homes un-announced to ask them about drug use, and sometimes demanded urine toxicology tests on the spot to assess their use. Their neighbors learned what the visits from authorities were for, and soon everyone they had contact with—neighbors, employers, remote acquaintances—were aware of their drug user status. One subject described relocating to a new town to avoid the discrimination she experienced in her home neighborhood.

Registered users chose New Hospital over government-sponsored treatments to avoid the loss of personal freedom they risked if their ongoing heroin use was detected while participating in voluntary treatment. They had each experienced China's rehabilitation units through labor (RULs) first hand, and described these places as punitive and ultimately ineffective.

> *"I spent 6 months in a forced program in Inner Mongolia. It was too horrifying. I was treated like less than an animal. I had no human rights. I can't even talk about it." (Male, 44 years old, divorced, a registered heroin user.)*

> *"In 9/2012 I was arrested for heroin and that was when my family found out about my addiction. I went to a forced detention center for seven months and it was basically like jail. There was no medicine, no methadone, no freedom. They taught us about detention center regulations and Chinese laws regarding drug use. They had us watch videos of people getting arrested for drugs. I talked to my family through a glass window. I made some friends. I got discharged early to care for aging parents, and because I wasn't having any more withdrawal. The loss of freedom made everything painful. And I swore to myself that I would never do drugs again. One month later, I relapsed." (Male, 46 years old, college graduate, never married, a registered heroin user.)*

> *"I went to a camp in Datong. I stayed for two years and three months. They made us work sometimes, but there wasn't much to do. Sometimes we made paper bags. There was no treatment in the camp, no methadone, no detox, no medical follow-up after I was discharged from the camp. I relapsed after 20 days." (Male, 41 years old, middle school graduate, divorced, a registered heroin user)*

> *"I was arrested for heroin and spent six months in a forced detention camp. It was like jail. We lived 20-30 people to a cell. If there was work, we did it, like making plastic flowers. Otherwise we would just sit there and do nothing. No medication, no treatment. I relapsed 6 months after I got out." (Female, 46 years old, divorced and remarried, a registered heroin user.)*

Theme #3: A deep mistrust of government-sponsored treatment, and a search for new, more effective alternatives

Among all of our participants, but particularly among registered users who had participated in government-sponsored addiction treatment, there was a deep sense of mistrust and futility regarding government-sponsored treatments. Many were skeptical of methadone maintenance in principle.

"I tried methadone maintenance for 6 months. But they never gave me enough. To feel better, I would have to shoot up heroin at the same time. They don't really care if you get better or not." (Male, 44 years old, married, a registered heroin user.)

"I've never been on methadone maintenance, and I won't try it. It's more addictive than heroin. Methadone must be worse than illegal drugs, otherwise why would the government control it so closely?" (Male, 41 years old, divorced, a registered heroin user)

"I am not interested in methadone maintenance. Methadone is more addictive than heroin. My boyfriend was on methadone maintenance for a while, and was using heroin at the same time, so I know it doesn't work." (Female, 46 years old, divorced, a registered heroin user.)

Subjects expressed hope that New Hospital, because it was new, might provide more effective and innovative solutions. For most, New Hospital was just one more stop in a long line of treatments, and many were returning to New Hospital a second, third, and in one case a sixth time.

"My Mom brought me here, and I came because I felt sorry for her. She hopes that since this is a new hospital, they will be able to help me. I want to stop. From my heart I do. But I've tried to kick the habit for 10 years, then one taste gets me back to the beginning again." (Male, 41 years old, divorced, a registered heroin user.)

"I came here for the psychiatric treatment they advertise on their website, along with the addiction treatment. But I haven't gotten any psychiatric treatment. There are no activities. Just a methadone taper. That's it. There is not anywhere to exercise either. Sometimes I can't sit still. I just pace in my room and in the hallway. I can't even go outside." (Male, 38 years old, married, an unregistered heroin user.)

One subject received "addiction surgery" at another private facility before coming to New Hospital, a 'surgery' we presume involved an opioid-antagonist implant.

"In 2007, I got the addiction surgery. I went to Wuhan province for the surgery. My parents made me go, and they paid for it. After the surgery, I tried shooting up heroin and I couldn't get the feeling. For the next 6 months I shot up everyday with no feeling. I did not think about stopping because I still had money. After six months, the feeling came back. I guess the surgery didn't work, so I'm here now, hoping they'll have something new and better for me."(Male, 38 years old, married, an unregistered heroin user.)

Discussion

We explore the beliefs and motivations of a subset of treatment-seeking heroin users in contemporary China; specifically, a small group of individuals willing to pay as much as half of their monthly earnings on a week's worth of treatment at New Hospital. New Hospital is a private, for-profit, non-government-sponsored, inpatient, addiction treatment setting offering methadone detoxification as the main-stay of its treatment for clients with opioid-use disorders.

In China, the existence of New Hospital, outside of government surveillance and with a regular base of customers, is remarkable given that methadone treatment is offered *for free* at government-sponsored treatment facilities throughout the country. Our data suggest that New Hospital and facilities like it have emerged in China's current addiction-treatment-landscape to serve the needs of those wanting treatment, but wishing to avoid the stigmatized identity and loss of personal freedom that comes with participating in government-sponsored treatment.

Both registered and unregistered heroin users in our study had personally experienced and/or were aware of intense social stigma directed toward heroin users in China. Our findings are consistent with several studies exploring stigma and addiction in China. In a survey study of beliefs about persons with drug addiction in China, most respondents endorsed believing that drug addiction is caused by a person's own weak will (82.0 %) and hedonistic lifestyle (81.3 %) [14]. Survey respondents furthermore expressed a strong desire to have limited or no contact with heroin users. Another study found that Chinese employers discriminate against applicants with substance use disorders [15]. According to a review by Tang and Hao, drug addiction, along with prostitution and gambling, in most government documents, is referred to as an 'ugly social phenomenon' and a personality flaw, rather than a medical disorder; and both lay persons and professionals think punishment is an important component of drug treatment [16].

According to our data, unregistered heroin users seeking treatment at New Hospital are motivated by a desire to preserve their anonymity and to avoid the social, legal, and economic consequences of becoming registered with the government as 'drug addicts'. At least one prior study of heroin users in China has identified fear of government registry as a barrier to participation in government-sponsored methadone maintenance clinics, with unregistered participants expressing a unanimous desire to avoid any treatment that might confer a status of 'illicit-drug user' with the Chinese authorities [17].

Registered users seeking treatment at New Hospital sought confidential treatment as well, to avoid the threat of imprisonment at forced detention camps, where they had experienced a demeaning loss of personal freedom, received little or no addiction treatment, and by most accounts, engaged in little labor. In 1999, about 224,000 drug-addicted individuals resided at compulsory detoxification centers and 120,000 drug-addicted individuals resided at re-education-through-labor institutes [16]. To date, there are sparse data on the living conditions and activities inside these compulsory detoxification and labor re-education centers. According to Amon et al., "These centers are neither prisons nor hospitals: individuals are held without due process protections or judicial oversight of detention. At the same time, the centers lack evidence-based drug-dependency treatment and, often, any trained health care personnel" [18].

Many of our subjects expressed a desire for new and innovative treatments as another prime motivator for seeking help at New Hospital. Whether for-profit 'rehabs' like New Hospital actually provide innovative or even effective treatment, remains to be seen. At least one participant expressed skepticism about New Hospital's mission and integrity, suggesting it may not provide what it promises, and as such, may be just one more for-profit enterprise in the burgeoning Chinese capitalistic economy, preying on the desperate and vulnerable. Regardless, the coexistence of New Hospital alongside government-sponsored treatment, implies a new openness on the part of the government to augment the current system, possibly as part of a broader campaign to curb China's rising drug problem.

China's current system of registering and imprisoning drug-addicted persons is not unique to China. Vietnam has a similar system in which addicted persons are registered and monitored using a national database. Since the 1990's, the internment of drug users in compulsory treatment centers has been a specific focus of Vietnam's drug policy. Drug users in Vietnam are reluctant to access existing treatment services, fearing police detection and detention [19].

Limitations of this study include small sample size, convenience sampling, and reliance on self-report. We do not know how many individuals who were asked to participate declined. Our findings may lack generalizability, given the small number of participants from one unique treatment setting. Also, only three out of the nine participants reported history of injection drug use, suggesting on average a less severely addicted population. According to available data, intravenous injection is the most common means of heroin use in China, with injecting drug users accounting for 59–85 % of users [9]. Other potential limitations include issues of translation between English and Mandarin, in which subtle nuances of slang terms and differences in dialects may have limited communication.

Conclusion

This qualitative study of treatment-seeking heroin users in contemporary China is intended to be exploratory and hypothesis-generating. Our data suggest directions for future research, and raise questions with policy implications, such as:

1. Would launching a public health campaign to decrease the stigma of addiction and promote addiction treatment in China increase utilization of voluntary government-sponsored addiction services?
2. Would eliminating government registration of heroin users increase utilization of voluntary government-sponsored addiction services in China, in particular, methadone maintenance clinics?
3. Would elimination of forced imprisonment when ongoing illicit heroin use is detected, increase utilization of government-sponsored addiction services in China, in particular methadone maintenance clinics?
4. Would reforming forced detention camps in China to include more actual addiction treatment lead to better outcomes, despite their compulsory nature?
5. Do private, for-profit, addiction treatment facilities like New Hospital provide a viable and effective alternative to government-sponsored treatment in China's evolving drug-treatment landscape?

Authors' contributions

AL conceived of the study, and collaborated with NZ in data collection, data analysis, and manuscript preparation. NZ collaborated with AL in data analysis and manuscript preparation. Both authors read and approved the final manuscript.

Author details

[1] Department of Psychiatry and Behavioral Sciences, Stanford University School of Medicine, 401 Quarry Road, Stanford, CA 94306, USA. [2] Department of Neurology, Stanford University School of Medicine, Stanford, CA 94306, USA.

Acknowledgements

This study was sponsored by a Stanford Center at Peking University Faculty Research Grant.

Competing interests

The authors declare that they have no competing interests.

References

1. Lu L, Wang X. Drug addiction in China. Ann N Y Acad Sci. 2008;1141:304–17. doi:10.1196/annals.1441.025.
2. Huang K, Zhang L, Liu J. Drug problems in contemporary China: a profile of Chinese drug users in a metropolitan area. Int J Drug Policy. 2011;22(2):128–32.
3. UNODC. World Drug Report. United Nations Publication, Sales No. E.12. XI.1; 2012.
4. Jiang H, Han Y, Du J, Wu F, Zhang R, Zhang H, et al. Factors associated with one year retention to methadone maintenance treatment program among patients with heroin dependence in China. Subst Abuse Treat Prev Policy [Internet]. Substance Abuse Treatment, Prevention, and Policy; 2014 Jan [cited 2014 Aug 26];9(1):11. http://www.pubmedcentral.nih.gov/articlerender.fcgi?artid=3974188&tool=pmcentrez&rendertype=abstract.
5. Kurlantzkk J. China's drug problem and looming HIV epidemic. World Policy J. 2014;19(2):70–5.
6. Du W-J, Xiang Y-T, Wang Z-M, Chi Y, Zheng Y, Luo X-N, et al. Socio-demographic and clinical characteristics of 3129 heroin users in the first methadone maintenance treatment clinic in China. Drug Alcohol Depend [Internet]. 2008 Apr 1 [cited 2014 Aug 26];94(1-3):158–64. http://www.ncbi.nlm.nih.gov/pubmed/18164146.
7. Tang YL, Zhao D, Zhao C, Cubells JF. Opiate addiction in China: current situation and treatments. Addiction. 2006;101:657–65.
8. YanPing B, ZhiMin L. Current situation and trends of drug abuse and HIV/AIDS in China. HIV Ther. 2009;3:237–40.
9. Zhang L, Chow EPF, Zhuang X, Liang Y, Wang Y, Tang C, et al. Methadone maintenance treatment participant retention and behavioural effectiveness in China: a systematic review and meta-analysis. PLoS One [Internet]. 2013 Jan [cited 2014 Aug 26];8(7):e68906. http://www.pubmedcentral.nih.gov/articlerender.fcgi?artid=3724877&tool=pmcentrez&rendertype=abstract.
10. China Briefing. Average wages in China: Determining minimum and maximum social insurance contributions [Internet]. 2013. http://www.china-briefing.com/news/2013/11/19/average-wages-in-china-determining-minimum-and-maximum-social-insurance-contributions.html.
11. Charmaz K. Constructing grounded theory: a practical guide through qualitative analysis. London: Sage Publications; 2012.
12. Lingard L, Albert M, Levinson W. Grounded theory, mixed methods, and action research. BMJ [Internet]. 2008;337:a567. http://www.ncbi.nlm.nih.gov/pubmed/18687728.
13. Sbaraini A, Carter SM, Evans R, Blinkhorn A. How to do a grounded theory study: a worked example of a study of dental practices. BMC Med Res Methodol [Internet]. BioMed Central Ltd; 2011;11(1):128. http://www.biomedcentral.com/1471-2288/11/128.
14. Luo T, Wang J, Li Y, Wang X, Tan L, Deng Q, et al. Stigmatization of people with drug dependence in China: a community-based study in Hunan province. Drug Alcohol Depend [Internet]. Elsevier Ireland Ltd; 2014 Jan 1 [cited 2014 Aug 23];134:285–9. http://www.ncbi.nlm.nih.gov/pubmed/24239068.
15. Corrigan PW, Tsang HWH, Shi K, Lam CS, Larson J. Chinese and American employers' perspectives regarding hiring people with behaviorally driven health conditions: the role of stigma. Soc Sci Med [Internet]. Elsevier Ltd; 2010 Dec [cited 2014 Aug 23];71(12):2162–9. http://www.pubmedcentral.nih.gov/articlerender.fcgi?artid=2996889&tool=pmcentrez&rendertype=abstract.
16. Tang Y-L, Hao W. Improving drug addiction treatment in China. Addiction [Internet]. Blackwell Publishing Ltd; 2007 Jul 1;102(7):1057–63. http://dx.doi.org/10.1111/j.1360-0443.2007.01849.x.
17. Lin C, Wu Z, Detels R. Opiate users' perceived barriers against attending methadone maintenance therapy: a qualitative study in China. Subst Use Misuse [Internet]. 2011 Jan [cited 2014 Aug 23];46(9):1190–8. http://www.pubmedcentral.nih.gov/articlerender.fcgi?artid=3392119&tool=pmcentrez&rendertype=abstract.
18. Amon J, Pearshouse R, Cohen J, Schleifer R. Compulsory drug detention centers in China, Cambodia, Vietnam, and Laos: health and human rights abuses. Health Hum Rights [Internet]. 2013 Jan;15(2):124–37. http://www.ncbi.nlm.nih.gov/pubmed/24421160.
19. Vuong T, Ali T, Baldwin S, Mills S. Drug Policy in Vietnam: a decade of change? Int J Drug Policy. 2012;23:319–26.

Implementation of integrated stepped care for unhealthy alcohol use in HIV clinics

E. Jennifer Edelman[1,2*], Nathan B. Hansen[2,3], Christopher J. Cutter[1], Cheryl Danton[1], Lynn E. Fiellin[1,2], Patrick G. O'Connor[1], Emily C. Williams[4,5], Stephen A. Maisto[6], Kendall J. Bryant[7] and David A. Fiellin[1,2]

Abstract

Background: Effective counseling and pharmacotherapy for unhealthy alcohol use are rarely provided in HIV treatment settings to patients. Our goal was to describe factors influencing implementation of a stepped care model to address unhealthy alcohol use in HIV clinics from the perspectives of social workers, psychologists and addiction psychiatrists.

Methods: We conducted two focus groups with Social Workers (n = 4), Psychologists (n = 2), and Addiction Psychiatrists (n = 4) involved in an ongoing randomized controlled trial evaluating the effectiveness of integrated stepped care for unhealthy alcohol use in HIV-infected patients at five Veterans Health Administration (VA) HIV clinics. Data collection and analyses were guided by the Consolidated Framework for Implementation Research (CFIR) domains, with a focus on the three domains which we considered to be most relevant: *intervention characteristics* (i.e. motivational interviewing, pharmacotherapy), the *inner setting* (i.e. HIV clinics), and *characteristics of individuals* (i.e. the providers). A multidisciplinary team used directed content analysis to identify major themes.

Results: From the providers' perspective, the major implementation themes that emerged by CFIR domain included: (1) *Intervention characteristics*: providers valued tools and processes for facilitating patient motivation for treatment of unhealthy alcohol use given their perceived lack of motivation, but expressed a desire for greater flexibility; (2) *Inner setting*: treating unhealthy alcohol use in HIV clinics was perceived by providers to be consistent with VA priorities; and (3) *Characteristics of individuals:* there was high self-efficacy to conduct the intervention, an expressed need for more consistent utilization to maintain skills, and consideration of alternative models for delivering the components of the intervention.

Conclusions: Use of the CFIR framework reveals that implementation of integrated stepped care for unhealthy alcohol use in HIV clinics is facilitated by tools to help providers enhance patient motivation or address unhealthy alcohol use among patients perceived to be unmotivated. Implementation may be facilitated by its consistency with organizational values and existing models of care and attention to optimizing provider self-efficacy and roles (i.e. approaches to treatment integration).

Keywords: HIV, Alcohol-related disorders, Qualitative methods, Diffusion of innovation

Background

Unhealthy alcohol use, defined as the spectrum of drinking including at-risk drinking and alcohol use disorders [1], is common among HIV-infected patients and associated with a range of adverse health outcomes. Unhealthy alcohol use among HIV-infected patients is associated with poor antiretroviral therapy (ART) adherence [2–8]; impaired treatment response; and decreased quality of HIV care [5, 6, 9]. In turn, individuals who stop drinking experience an improved response to HIV therapy [5, 10]. Further, unhealthy alcohol use increases the risk of important medical comorbidites, such as

*Correspondence: ejennifer.edelman@yale.edu
[1] Yale University School of Medicine, 367 Cedar Street, ESH A, New Haven, CT 06510, USA
Full list of author information is available at the end of the article

cardiovascular disease [11], liver disease [12] and malignancy [13] and is associated with sexual risk behaviors and ongoing HIV transmission [14, 15].

Integration of treatment for unhealthy alcohol use into HIV clinics

Despite the high prevalence and adverse effects of unhealthy alcohol use, few effective interventions for unhealthy alcohol use are offered in HIV clinics [16–21]. Interventions that have been shown to be effective for decreasing unhealthy alcohol use in uninfected patients, including brief interventions for at-risk drinking [22], Motivational Enhancement Therapy, and alcohol pharmacotherapies [23, 24] are not routinely provided in HIV clinics [25, 26]. One advantage of integrating the treatment of unhealthy alcohol use into HIV clinics is that it provides "one stop shopping" and limits potential losses to follow-up seen with referral to off-site treatment. However, integrated treatments are often based on screening strategies and must contend with low levels of knowledge regarding alcohol-associated health risks and motivation among non-treatment seeking individuals [27, 28]. Also, providers often neglect to discuss or recognize unhealthy alcohol use [29–32] and are underprepared to provide treatment [33]. In addition, treatments for unhealthy alcohol use are not uniformly effective, which provides a rationale for stepped care approaches. Stepped care approaches, which have been applied to chronic disease conditions (e.g. depression and hypertension), typically start with a low-intensity evidence-based intervention with increasing the intensity of treatment if patients fail to respond to initial treatment strategies [34, 35].

The innovation: integrated stepped care for unhealthy alcohol use in HIV clinics

To address a need for effective treatment models for unhealthy alcohol use among HIV-infected patients through HIV clinics, we are conducting the *Starting Ethanol Treatment in Primary care Trial (STEP Trials)*, a series of three linked multi-site randomized clinical trials designed to evaluate the implementation and effectiveness of integrated stepped care among HIV-infected patients with unhealthy alcohol use. Briefly, HIV-infected patients are recruited into one of three trials based on their alcohol use—(1) at-risk drinking [36], (2) moderate alcohol consumption in the presence of liver disease (MALD) (defined as any alcohol consumption in the past month in the presence of a FIB-4 score greater than 1.45, a validated marker of liver fibrosis [12, 37, 38], or active Hepatitis C virus infection based on serology and presence of a detectable viral load) or (3) alcohol abuse or dependence criteria [39]. Each trial compares integrated stepped care to treatment as usual.

Patients are recruited from one of five Infectious Disease Clinics within the Veterans Health Administration (VA). Patients in the stepped care arm receive evidence-based interventions of increasing intensity (or not) based on their response to initial treatments. Social workers deliver a brief intervention (the Brief Negotiated Interview [BNI]) [40–42] with a two-week telephone booster to patients with at-risk drinking or MALD; Psychologists deliver four sessions of Motivational Enhancement Therapy [43]; and Addiction Psychiatrists provide Addiction Physician Management, with an emphasis on offering pharmacotherapy. Addiction Psychiatrists were encouraged to prescribe pharmacotherapy based on what they thought was most likely to benefit the individual patient. This includes Food and Drug Administration (FDA) approved pharmacotherapies for alcohol dependence (i.e. disulfiram, naltrexone, acamprosate) and prescribing of medications with evidence of efficacy (e.g. topiramate, gabapentin).

To enhance implementation and consistency of the intervention across sites, providers received an initial training and are provided with manuals and structured encountered forms to guide each visit. Providers are also given a "Feedback Form" to review patient-specific data, including self-reported alcohol use, other substance use, level of bother by alcohol use, motivation for treatment, and biomarkers known to be impacted by alcohol [liver function, HCV status, HIV biomarkers, and VACS Index score (a validated prognostic marker of morbidity and mortality found to be responsive to levels of alcohol use)] [44–46] with the patient. Visits with providers occur within the HIV Clinic or nearby available office-space. The *STEP Trials* is occurring in the context of current VA initiatives focused on developing patient-centered medical homes, known as Patient Aligned Care Teams (PACTs), and its extensions (i.e. Primary Care-Mental Health Integration [PC-MHI] and Health Promotion and Disease Prevention [HPDP] Programs) [47, 48]. These VA programs have been developed to promote the use of multidisciplinary teams to address a range of health related issues in the context of co-located and collaborative care within primary care settings [48].

Consistent with effectiveness-implementation hybrid study designs intended to evaluate a clinical intervention while collecting data on implementation [49], we conducted the current qualitative study to examine perspectives of providers on the implementation of integrated stepped care for unhealthy alcohol use and inform implementation efforts in other HIV clinical settings. Given its suitability for examining factors impacting implementation of clinical interventions across different settings and disciplines, including addiction treatment, we used the Consolidated Framework for Implementation Research (CFIR) to guide data collection and a directed content analysis [50–54].

Methods

Study overview

After approximately 1 year of project implementation and patient care, we conducted two focus groups with Social Workers, Psychologists and Addiction Psychiatrists who were delivering stepped care to address unhealthy alcohol use in HIV clinics in the context of the *STEP Trials*. We chose qualitative methods given their appropriateness for studying complex processes with regards to patient, physician and organizational-level factors associated with implementation of evidence-based interventions [55]. We used a directed content analysis [56, 57] due to its successful use in the past to elucidate implementation efforts according to the CFIR and other implementation science constructs [58–61] (Fig. 1). The protocol was approved by Yale University's Human Investigations Committee and VA Connecticut Healthcare System's Institutional Review Board.

Study design and participants

While the VA-based healthcare system is an integrated healthcare system, including both primary HIV care and addiction treatment services within the same medical center complex, the level of direct integration of providers into HIV clinics in the context of routine clinical care (i.e. not in the context of the *STEP Trials)* differs across sites (Table 1). We recruited members of the three types of providers (i.e. Social Workers, Psychologists, and Addiction Psychiatrists) from the five participating HIV clinics who were involved with the *STEP Trials*. The focus groups were conducted as part of a national meeting whereby participants attended based on availability. None of the potential interventionists declined to participate though some were unable due to their unavailability to travel to the meeting. We chose to conduct focus groups given our expectation that the group interaction

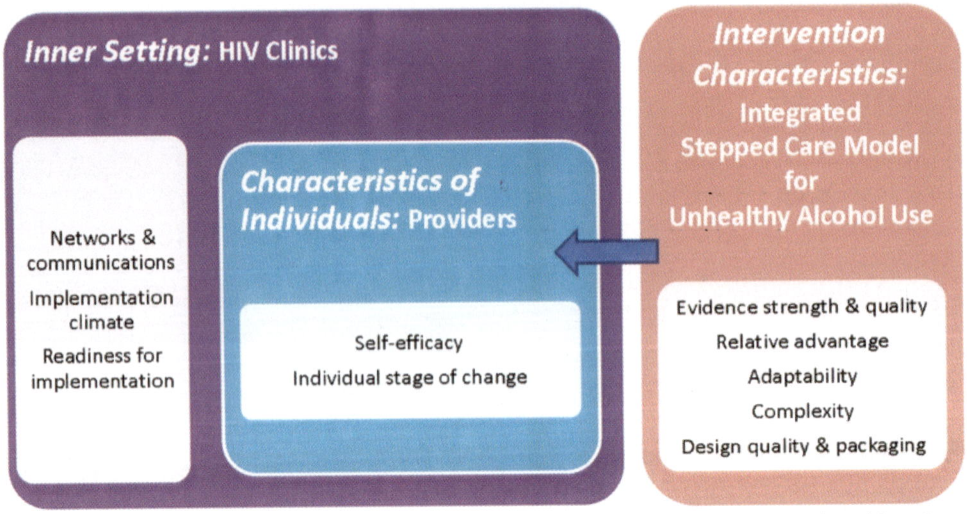

Fig. 1 Integrated stepped care for unhealthy alcohol use in HIV clinics: relevant CFIR domains and constructs*. *Adapted from Damschroder LJ, Aron DC, Keith RE, Kirsh SR, Alexander JA, Lowery JC. Fostering implementation of health services research findings into practice: A consolidated framework for advancing implementation science. CFIR Figure and Explanatory Text.

Table 1 Pre-implementation provider integration into HIV clinic and additional considerations by site

HIV clinic characteristics	Social worker	Psychologist	Addiction psychiatrist	Additional considerations
Site 1	Yes	No	No	n/a
Site 2	Yes	Yes	No	n/a
Site 3	No	Yes	No	n/a
Site 4	No	No	No	n/a
Site 5	No	No	No	Providers at geographically dispersed VA-based locations

would generate unique insights about shared experiences, while also allowing us to learn about differences across sites [55]. All providers gave verbal informed consent and the study was HIPAA compliant.

Data collection

The two focus groups were facilitated by investigators with experience conducting qualitative research [62–68]. One focus group (facilitated by EJE, DAF, NH and SM) consisted of Social Workers and Psychologists and the other (facilitated by EJE, DAF, LEF) consisted of Addiction Psychiatrists.

Focus group procedures

Based on the CFIR framework [54] and multi-disciplinary input, we used grand tour questions (i.e. open ended questions intended to stimulate discussion), and probes (i.e. prompts) to examine the perceived impact of *intervention characteristics*, *inner setting* and *characteristics of the individuals* (Fig. 1) on the delivery of integrated stepped care for unhealthy alcohol use in HIV clinics (Text Box) [69]. These CFIR domains were chosen as the focus of this investigation as they were the most directly relevant to the experiences of the providers delivering this innovative intervention and consistent with prior guidance regarding how to apply the CFIR [54, 59].

Providers were encouraged to discuss their experience of delivering integrated stepped care in the context of their usual role and not as part of a research project, per se. They were instructed that their responses would be kept confidential, would not impact their current employment or any aspect of involvement in the research. They were also invited to complete a brief demographic survey after the focus groups were completed. The focus groups were recorded, professionally transcribed, and reviewed for accuracy [55].

Text Box: Focus Group Guides: Example Grand Tour Questions with Probes

***Intervention Characteristics*: Can you tell me about your experiences with treating HIV-infected patients for their unhealthy alcohol use in the context of the *STEP Trials*?**

How does the integrated stepped care approach compare to other treatment approaches?

What made it easier?

What make it more difficult?

Does the intervention feel like something you would create? How would you change it?

***Intervention Characteristics:* How did you find the patients responded to your treatment and the integrated stepped care treatment approach, in general?**

How motivated were patients to participate?

What seemed to impact their motivation?

How could this have been improved?

***Characteristics of the Individuals:* What was your experience with delivering the intervention?**

What aspects did you find most effective?

What aspects did you find least effective?

How did it fit in with your other roles and responsibilities?

How comfortable are you in delivering this type of intervention?

What changes would you make in the training materials to increase their usability?

***Inner Setting:* Can you tell me more about how you communicated with others involved in the care of your patients with unhealthy alcohol use?**

What about social workers/psychologists/psychiatrists?

What about the patients' primary care provider?

***Inner Setting:* How important is treating unhealthy alcohol use to your supervisor? To the VA?**

Does this get measured in any way?

What kinds of resources are dedicated to this?

Do you think your supervisor would support you to do this kind of work even after the trial ends?

Describe some of the complexities in implementing this treatment model with regards to the duration, scope, disruption of other activities, number of steps.

Grand tour questions in bold; CFIR constructs noted in bold with italics

Qualitative analysis

Six individuals of our multidisciplinary team, including members not present at the focus groups and one member not previously involved in the project, applied content analysis with a deductive approach to code the transcripts [56, 57]. Team members were trained on the CFIR framework [54] in advance and used the domains and constructs as predetermined codes [52]. The transcripts were independently reviewed line by line, and elements of the CFIR domains and constructs were assigned to meaning units (i.e. transcript text) [57]. Team members met to discuss emerging ideas, resolve discrepancies and reach consensus regarding the codes. One author (EJE) then re-reviewed the transcripts to systematically apply these codes. To organize the data and facilitate retrieval, we used qualitative analysis software (AtlasTi version 6.2, Berlin, Germany). We organized the transcript text by domains and constructs and then re-reviewed the quotes for themes and illustrative text and discussed as a group. To increase the rigor of our approach, we reviewed a summary of our findings with participants to confirm that we had accurately understood and conveyed their experiences [55].

Results

Participating providers included Social Workers (n = 4), Psychologists (n = 2) and Addiction Psychiatrists (n = 4) (Table 2). We present themes and representative quotes organized by the CFIR domains and their sub-domains,

Table 2 Relevant CFIR Domains with definitions as applied to integrated stepped care for unhealthy alcohol use

Domain	Definition
I. Intervention characteristics: integrated stepped care for unhealthy alcohol use	
Evidence strength & quality	Providers' perception of the quality and validity of evidence supporting the belief that integrated stepped care for unhealthy alcohol use will lead to decreased unhealthy alcohol use
Relative advantage	Providers' perception of the advantage of implementing integrated stepped care for unhealthy alcohol use versus an alternative solution
Adaptability	The degree to which integrated stepped care for unhealthy alcohol use can be adapted, tailored, refined, or reinvented to meet local needs
Complexity	Perceived difficulty of implementation, reflected by duration, scope, radicalness, disruptiveness, centrality, and intricacy and number of steps required to implement
Design quality & packaging	Perceived excellence in how integrated stepped care for unhealthy alcohol use is bundled, presented, and assembled
II. Inner domain: HIV clinics	
Networks and communications	The nature and quality of webs of social networks and the nature and quality of formal and informal communications within VA-based HIV clinics and across providers
Implementation climate	The absorptive capacity for change, shared receptivity of involved individuals to integrated stepped care for unhealthy alcohol use and the extent to which use of it will be rewarded, supported, and expected within the VA
Tension for change	The degree to which providers perceive the current situation as intolerable or needing change
Compatibility	The degree of tangible fit between meaning and values attached to integrated stepped care for unhealthy alcohol use by involved individuals, how those align with individuals' own norms, values, and perceived risks and needs, and how this treatment model with existing workflows and systems
Relative priority	Individuals' shared perception of the importance of the implementation within the VA-based HIV clinics
Readiness for implementation	Tangible and immediate indicators of organizational commitment to its decision to implement integrated stepped care for unhealthy alcohol use
Available resources	The level of resources dedicated for implementation and on-going operations, including money, training, education, physical space, and time
Access to knowledge & information	Ease of access to digestible information and knowledge about the intervention and how to incorporate it into work tasks
III. Characteristics of individuals: providers	
Self-efficacy	Providers' belief in their own capabilities to execute courses of action to achieve implementation goals
Individual stage of change	Characterization of the phase a provider is in, as he/she progresses toward skilled, enthusiastic and sustained use of integrated stepped care for unhealthy alcohol use

Adapted from Damschroder LJ, Aron DC, Keith RE, Kirsh SR, Alexander JA, Lowery JC. Fostering implementation of health services research findings into practice: A consolidated framework for advancing implementation science. CFIR Constructs with Short Definitions.

Table 3 Provider characteristics

Characteristic	Overall (n = 9)	Social workers (n = 4)	Psychologists (n = 2)	Addiction psychiatrists (n = 3)
Age, mean (SD) in years	44 (11)	35 (8)*	54 (1)	45 (11)
Race (%)				
White	78	100	50	67
Black	11	0	50	0
Asian	11	0	0	33
Ethnicity, Hispanic (%)	11	25	0	0
Gender, Female (%)	89	100	100	67
Average number weekly patients, mean (SD)	23 (20)	20 (18)	23 (18)	29 (29)
Number HIV-infected, mean (SD)	8 (11)	15 (14)	2 (1)	2 (1)
Number with an alcohol use disorder or alcohol related problem, mean (SD)	12 (12)	5 (5)	16 (20)	17 (14)
Years in current role, mean (SD), [range]	8 (8), [1–24]	5 (7), [1–15]	6 (4), [3–9]	14 (10)

One social worker did not provide data on age and focus groups included one additional Addiction Psychiatrist who declined to complete the survey; thus these data are missing

with a focus on *intervention characteristics*, the *inner setting*, and *characteristics of the individuals*. The definitions used for each domain and sub-domain as applied to the *STEP Trials* are listed in Table 3.

Intervention Characteristics Domain: Integrated Stepped Care Model

Providers indicated that the integrated stepped care model quality, content and packaging facilitated implementation, yet believed it would benefit from adaptability with regards to content, duration and source of the intervention.

Evidence strength and quality

Social Workers and Psychologists, alike, endorsed fundamental aspects of the intervention, such as motivational interviewing, and recognized that it was evidence-based and believed it to be of high quality. For example, one provider described:

> *I come from an addiction background before coming to the Infectious Disease clinic, and my mental health background. So motivational interviewing is kind of like magic dust...*

Similarly, the Addiction Psychiatrists were familiar with strong data supporting the use of pharmacotherapy to treat alcohol use disorders as recommended within the stepped care model:

> *I was thinking about the COMBINE Study and the medical management was a very powerful intervention.. I recall from Project COMBINE that included recommendations of going to AA, but it also included me prescribing medication.*

Relative advantage

As participants were often not treatment seeking, the providers found it helpful that the intervention contained tools, such as personalized normative feedback, for promoting motivation:

> *The one where it talked about your drinking [compared to norms], in both my cases they were surprised by the results. It was palpable. You could tell. They... you know. What do you think of what I've just said in terms of, this shows there is such—this high percentile [compared to] drinking [norms] the language is–was surprising to them.*

Adaptability

Providers reported a desire for increased flexibility regarding the number of treatment sessions, as well as an ability to expand the scope of the focus to address other prevalent and important risk behaviors. On one hand, they felt that more time was needed to effectively build rapport and expressed a desire to be able to tailor the number of treatment sessions to participant needs. On the other hand, there was an expressed preference to maintain the treatment number as finite. For example, one Psychologist reported:

> *The one thing I probably would change, I think I would want more than, maybe just a little more than four sessions, for me... My guys worked, so we had to kind of shuffle around to get 'em in on off days, so committing to 4 sessions was easy. But I felt like they—you were just at that point where you're holding your kids' hips as he's bicycling without training wheels and I just let him go, and he was just taking off—Session number 4. Done. And if I only had just a 5th, maybe just a 5th session, would be the one thing that I would change... [But] I'm all for... therapy ending.*

Similarly, one Addiction Psychiatrist echoed these sentiments:

> *...you start to build a [rapport], and then, because of this session slots issue you cannot see him anymore.*

Providers were also eager to extend the intervention to address drug use in addition to alcohol use:

> *The only other thing too that I also thought about in terms of I think all of our patients, we're only focusing on alcohol use... we have like a huge crack epidemic too... So it's also interesting to me that we're only talking to them about how alcohol impacts their body, and I'm ignoring the fact... he's like, "No, I did not drink, I just smoked crack yesterday." Great. You know.*

In addition, there was a stated interest by one Social Worker to extend the focus from impact on health to HIV prevention efforts:

> *I mean, talking about the relationship between your sex practices and your substance use, talking about the relationship between lack of condom use and substance use, that's all huge in our clinic. There's a huge correlation between that. Even to asking them about, are you disclosing your sex—when they go to sex parties, there's a whole, that's a whole 'nother-... I would totally be interested in seeing how we could do best practices in the VA with prevention positives.*

Complexity

Some aspects of integrated stepped care for unhealthy alcohol use were perceived to be complex. Identifying appropriate individuals for the intervention was among the greatest challenges. Providers expressed a need for clear processes for identifying HIV-infected individuals with unhealthy alcohol use:

> *Yeah, unless you had, when they come to the clinic, you provide them with a packet of paperwork for them to fill out, and you have the AUDIT-C or whatever other screening tools you're using, I think it's going to be difficult to implement.*

Other challenges with implementation of the intervention included the time involved as well as management of the logistics. It was felt that dedicated staffing was needed to manage the logistics involved with intervention implementation. According to one Social Worker:

> *Somebody would have to be tracking to make sure that it went the right way. There's gotta be a way... in terms of tracking someone would have to be responsible for it. It might be unrealistic to think that with 1100 or 1500 person caseloads, a Social Worker would really be able to do that well. I mean, things would fall through the cracks.*

With regards to the time involved in delivering the intervention, one Social Worker reflected on the complexity of implementing the intervention with regards to time and logistics:

> *I think the word "brief" can be deceiving sometimes... I don't think that 20 min which I think was the original design was always necessarily [enough time]- I think sometimes it drags out more so to 40 something to really bring 'em around. And then the phone booster depending on, same thing, like the resource needs, can be a challenge. And in my real world I think scheduling a phone appointment, if it's not [the research coordinator] reminding me that I have to do the phone appointment, and me finding it on my Outlook is challenging, just because I have walk-in clinics.*

This contrasted with overall sentiments that the intervention required less time and effort than initially anticipated given participant flow as described by another social worker:

> *...it's not like we're seeing this huge amount of patients. But I think that when you're presenting it to people... it'd be helpful to kind of inform them of that up front... but it's not that big of a workload difference.*

Design quality and packaging

The providers reported that the intervention packaging provided useful and novel tools for facilitating alcohol-related discussions:

> *Social Worker 1: This is more structured, I didn't have readiness tools and things like that, but, which are great.*
> *Social Worker 2: I also like the feedback tool, because we don't always have like their levels right in front of us, I mean we can obviously click through the whole chart and look at all of their labs... So it puts it in a nice neat package in terms of providing them with the feedback and having all the normative data and everything else.*

These sentiments were shared by the Psychologists:

> *Psychologist 1: One, we sent them home with a sort of a homework form [and we said, bring it back]. I think that has the effect in some ways of sort of holding them accountable, when you have to write down what you've done. Write your sins down.*
> *Psychologist 2: In my experience, the feedback form was absolutely helpful, and because it allowed them to—both of them to, whether they wanted to see how much they were drinking or not, and related it to specific incidents, that allowed them to see those triggers.*

Providers felt that the initial packaging would be improved with more accurate representation of the impact on workflow. As described by one Social Worker:

> *I think you can—just by acknowledging, "you're probably already using these, and you're probably already doing this, we just want to give you a format and kind of keep track of it." Because you're not indicating that you're adding any more work on... So you're not adding on anything more on their caseloads. Especially like if you're doing it within the ID clinic, and the social workers within the clinic are already meeting with these patients. So, I think it's just acknowledging that.*

In addition to recommendations regarding how the intervention is packaged to the providers, there was a perceived need for additional patient-centered materials as it related to communicating about pharmacotherapy treatment options:

> *For some of my patients, not just in the trial, they've had prior experience with disulfiram. And they don't want to go there. And they lump all the medicines together into I'm talking to them about disulfiram. It doesn't matter what I say, it's just like the Charlie Brown, waw waw, waw waw, waw waw. They thinking in their mind, disulfiram, if I slip up I'm going to get sick and die, I can't take medication. It would be nice to have like a table or something to say, "This is this medicine, it's what it does; this is this medicine,*

this one's different"...

Inner Setting Domain: HIV Clinics

Addressing unhealthy alcohol use was compatible with norms, values, and basic assumptions of the VA, and integrated care was compatible with VA priorities (i.e. creating a medical home) but implementation seemed to be affected by networks and communication, the implementation climate and readiness for implementation.

Networks and communications

Providers reported that communication among those providers who were co-located in HIV clinics was strong and this facilitated implementation of the intervention. For example, there was fluid and ongoing communication between ID providers and Social Workers:

And the doctors refer as they're seeing patients that have the social work-related concerns, as needed.

Among providers who were not traditionally based in the clinic, however, there was an expressed need for tighter links of communication. As one Addiction Psychiatrist stated:

One thing I would like is... a local call—a local meeting—that would be very helpful too. See what's going on... It would be nice to hear what's going on.

This was also noted by the Social Workers regarding communication with the Addiction Psychiatrists:

Social Worker 1: I know we're all only a phone call away but we don't—also if you have elevators at that level where they're seeing the addiction psychiatrist, they're not necessarily having contact with us anymore, so there's not that communication on that level.
Social Worker 2: Oh yeah, we work as a team. I knock on their door, they knock on my door, no, we definitely work as a team, except, the same thing, the addiction psychiatrist is in a separate part of—you know, our building is very large.

Implementation climate

Aspects (i.e. sub-domains) of the implementation climate most impacting the implementation climate included the tension for change, compatibility, and relative priority.

Tension for change

There was a recognized need for integrated addiction services. As described by one of the Addiction Psychiatrists:

That's something if a position can be carved out... and there is a need. There is such a need. Because I get so many phone calls.

Similarly, developing effective models for treating unhealthy alcohol use were recognized as a priority among VA leadership, with a current focus on specialty settings:

I would say we'd be supported at the national level... But right now, frankly our challenge is getting—where we've been focusing our energy is getting the specialty programs to prescribe medication for alcohol dependence or use disorders. The uptake is really low, nationally.

Compatibility

The Social Worker-based intervention (i.e. the BNI and booster) was highly consistent with ongoing efforts:

It's basically what we—I mean, at least me, what I have been doing.

Social Workers who pre-implementation were embedded into the HIV clinics (see Table 1) conduct comprehensive assessments, which typically include an evaluation of alcohol use, as part of routine care promote compatibility of the intervention:

The way that we operate is, I see all of our new patients ideally like when either they're newly diagnosed [with HIV] or new to our clinic. Ideally before their initial physician's appointment, when they come in and get their initial lab work done? I see them, do a comprehensive bio-psychosocial assessment, and or provide like post-HIV diagnosis counseling, and then see them as needed from there on out, depending on what their resource needs are and psychosocial stressors. And the patients that are long established, I see them either when they come as a walk-into see me because they need something, or because the doctors think that they need to see me, or the nurse or the pharmacist or whomever in the clinic.

The structure was consistent with the PACTs:

I think it would be a great... the PACT teams all have now a social worker, a nurse. I think that would be where... And everybody's supposed to have a primary care. Should be assigned a primary care. So I think adding this [intervention] in that team, would be... you would catch the majority of people.

The intervention was also thought to be consistent with ongoing efforts to promote integrated services:

So they would be more integrated and they would work more like a team, as opposed to being a group practice of independent providers which is how most mental health clinics are now. And so they've been rolling this out for about a year or so, and part of what they've talked about is how would you integrate addiction treatment into that.

Relative priority

Addressing unhealthy alcohol use was a priority, particularly when it related to HIV-related outcomes, but one of many priorities:

But we still, like even before this study I was gonna—we used this framework. You know, when you're dealing with somebody who's, for example, you go into one of the [clinic] meetings and they're not taking their HIV meds like they're supposed to, and they're developing all this resistance and one of the identified reasons is alcohol, I call them in, talk to them and then hopefully it leads to a referral... but as our role as social workers to the clinic we'd be neglecting a lot of the other important information if we solely focused on the alcohol without addressing all of the other psychosocial stressors and concerns.

Readiness for implementation

Aspects (i.e. sub-domains) most impacting readiness for implementation included available resources and access to knowledge and information.

Available resources

In reflecting about potential providers that might be appropriate for delivering the intervention, nurses were not believed to be appropriate:

We have nurses but our nurses are really directed in nature versus like looking at a framework. This is a lot more probing, and our nurses are much more prescriptive and directive in nature. I don't know if that's across the board though.

Access to knowledge and information

There was a perceived need to raise awareness and educate important stakeholders, including patients and HIV providers alike, about pharmacotherapy. As one Addiction Psychiatrist described:

But something, I mean it makes sense—pharmaceutical companies don't just create something and publish some papers and let it go at that. In order to get people to uptake it they do proactively go out and detail. So we really shouldn't be surprised if we publish a paper and people don't uptake it either... if we could convince the ID docs to at least initiate it, to talk about naltrexone a little bit, and maybe we don't have to burden them with managing it. But if we could get them to just sell it a little better.

Other Addiction Psychiatrists also commented on their challenges with initiating pharmacotherapy to treat alcohol use disorders:

Addiction Psychiatrist 1: One guy came almost every session. Unfortunately he just said, "I like to talk to you, not like to take medicine from you."
Addiction Psychiatrist 2: I have been more successful prescribing SSRI's and [tricylics rather than acamprosate]. There's a fair bit of resistance [to pharmacotherapy]... It's like, some of—a good number of them have been in AA, so you don't need a pill—it's-anything. That resistance, I don't know—I don't need a pill to–I can do it on my own. A lot of patients, it's from the AA end. And probably some of the pressure is also from... their primary care docs or their cardiologists have never thought about naltrexone.

Characteristics of Individuals Domain: Providers (i.e. Social Workers, Psychologists and Addiction Psychiatrists)

Providers endorsed high self-efficacy regarding their implementation, but voiced a need for more consistent utilization of the intervention to maintain skills and discussed alternative models and roles for delivering the components of the intervention.

Self-efficacy

One Social Worker expressed her enthusiasm for the intervention and comfort with implementing the intervention:

I'd be seeing them anyways. And so I'm glad to know that you have educated me, and it fits. It definitely fits with what we're doing.

This provider attributed treatment success to be most related to the participants and did not attribute it to her treatment or the intervention:

I think level of engagement has something to do with it. When we talked, I—the first client that I had was just so into it that by the time the second session, he was way ahead, way ahead, and so all I could do was affirm what he was doing.

Low patient volume necessitated relearning of materials. One Psychologist stated:

And there's too much time in between [patients]. It's almost like having to relearn it every [time].

Individual stage of change

Whether HIV providers should be responsible for delivering components of the intervention (e.g. the BNI) was questioned by a Social Worker and Addiction Psychiatrist. As described by one Social Worker:

> *But if it's such a brief thing, and they already have a relationship with their physician, doesn't it make sense to have the physician do this, and then they have the MET with a social worker, I feel like most social workers that I come cross in the VA, could probably do the MET [stuff].*

One Addiction Psychiatrist also agreed that the HIV provider would be effective at delivering pharmacotherapy:

> *I think that it could also be powerful if the medication was coming from the Infectious Disease doc, the person who saved my life saying, I think it's important for your health and your management of your HIV disease, that you stop drinking, and I'm willing to work with you... I do think that there's something powerful when the doc who's saved your life says, "I think you should do something." That carries a lot of weight. As opposed to this other person I referred you to. So that would be my only suggestion. But I don't know if you could get ID docs to... I would submit that they have great motivational skills, because if they can get folks to take HIV meds, then they know how to motivate people.*

Discussion

Focusing on three CFIR domains, we examined factors impacting the implementation of a model of stepped care for unhealthy alcohol use in HIV clinics. Based on the experiences of Social Workers, Psychologists and Addiction Psychiatrists from five different clinics, several factors emerged as deserving careful consideration for future implementation efforts. First, the providers deemed patients as not typically seeking treatment, and thus materials and processes for facilitating patient motivation for treatment of their unhealthy alcohol use were key and should have greater flexibility. Second, treating unhealthy alcohol use in HIV clinics was perceived by providers to be consistent with VA priorities, which are focused on both screening for and intervening upon unhealthy alcohol use and promoting medical home models of care. Third, depending on the existing role of the provider, there was variability in the perceptions regarding the ideal model for promoting integrated care. These data represent a novel contribution to the literature as they shed light on important factors deserving consideration in implementation of a stepped care model for unhealthy alcohol use in HIV clinics and identify actionable opportunities for future implementation efforts.

Because HIV-infected patients with unhealthy alcohol use were generally not seeking treatment, an advantage of the integrated stepped care model included the tools and process which facilitated patient motivation for treatment. Prior work has demonstrated that HIV-infected patients drink to cope with negative emotions, to promote social interactions, and in response to social pressure [28]; these motivations might be a barrier to treatment. The design of the integrated stepped care model (i.e. Social Worker and Psychologist-delivered manualized counseling focused on enhancing patient motivation to change their alcohol consumption and structured, personalized feedback for patients) facilitated its implementation. While the providers found these techniques to be familiar, they found that the integrated stepped care model provided them with new techniques and materials for enhancing patient motivation, which they perceived to be a barrier to promoting treatment. Indeed, these tools may serve to reinforce motivations to decrease alcohol consumption that have been previously identified as reasons that HIV-infected patients limit their drinking (i.e. concerns about the impact of alcohol use on social functioning, lifestyle incompatibility and physical and mental functioning) [70].

Importantly, treating unhealthy alcohol use through clinic-based settings was perceived by providers to be consistent with VA priorities. Specifically, there have been extensive efforts to promote evidence-based AUDIT-C screening followed by appropriate intervention (i.e. brief intervention, specialty care) for unhealthy alcohol use across VA settings [71, 72]. In contrast, uptake of evidence-based pharmacotherapy for alcohol use disorders has been slow [73–75] despite VA guidelines supporting the use of pharmacotherapy [76]. Addiction Psychiatrists generally recognized accessible pharmacotherapy as an important treatment option for alcohol use disorders, yet reported variable success in initiating treatment. This suggests that patient and HIV provider-targeted education and marketing may be important for improving uptake among non-treatment seeking individuals in the setting of shared-decision making after consideration of all available treatment options [77].

Furthermore, providers found that the integrated stepped care model was consistent with VA priorities given recent initiatives to develop and evaluate new models for delivering screening and treatment for unhealthy alcohol use. Providers also perceived the integrated stepped care model as consistent with PACT as well as PC-MHI and HPDP initiatives, which has important implications for potential future scalability. Such models tend to promote improved communication and tighter networks and allow for flexibility in session duration and specific content, as desired by providers in this study.

While providers were consistent in their reported beliefs that the integrated stepped care model offered a high quality intervention, there were differences based on provider experience and type regarding the ideal way in which to integrate treatment of unhealthy alcohol use into HIV clinics. For example, while some Social Workers believed it was ideal for social workers to deliver the BNI, other suggested that either Infectious Disease Physicians or nurses might provide these services. Additionally, they felt they had the requisite skills and experience to provide the MET intervention. Similarly, it was suggested by Addiction Psychiatrists that Infectious Disease Physicians might be best positioned to engage patients in treatment for unhealthy alcohol use. That a tension exists regarding how to best integrate services is not surprising. On one hand, Infectious Disease and HIV-specialty trained physicians, who increasingly serve as the primary care physician for HIV-infected patients, have an existing relationship with the patient and are managing other treatments. However, prior multi-site studies indicate that HIV providers are often unaware of their patient's alcohol use and often do not discuss it, even with patients with higher levels of drinking [29, 30, 78]. Moreover, only 65 % of HIV providers reported high comfort with discussing substance use [32]. Thus, it is likely that team-based approaches as structured in the integrated stepped care model, which do not rely on HIV providers to deliver treatment for unhealthy alcohol use, are likely to be an important strategy for effectively addressing unhealthy alcohol use. This model is consistent with others developed to treat other substance use disorders (i.e. buprenorphine for opioid use disorders in HIV clinics) [79–81] and supports the integration of social workers, Psychologists and Addition Psychiatrists into HIV clinics. If effectiveness of integrated stepped care for unhealthy alcohol use in HIV clinics is demonstrated, future studies should focus on determining the optimal role of HIV providers, based on their knowledge and self-efficacy, for delivering such treatments. In addition, the extent to which such an intervention should target other health behaviors, such as drug use or sexual risk behaviors, warrants investigation.

The results of this study should be interpreted in the context of its limitations. First, the providers represented a convenience sample of individuals involved with an ongoing randomized controlled trial. Our results may not reflect the opinions of other providers involved with the randomized controlled trial or apply to other VA-based providers more generally. Second, our interview guides were not piloted in advance of our study. In retrospect, given the expressed need to address alcohol along with other drug use and HIV prevention, we would have asked Addiction Psychiatrists further about their comfort prescribing pharmacotherapy for other substances (i.e. tobacco, opioids, cocaine) using an integrated model and how they might address HIV risk behaviors and prevention. Third, these findings may not transfer universally to other HIV clinical settings, particularly settings where Psychologists and Addiction Psychiatrists are less available. The goal of the *STEP Trials* is to evaluate the effectiveness of integrated care from Psychologist and Addiction Psychiatrists, along with Social Workers. If effectiveness is demonstrated, issues of generalizability of this and the main study's findings to other HIV clinical settings will be carefully considered. Fourth, this qualitative study was conducted during the 1st year of implementation of integrated stepped care in the context of a randomized controlled trial. Whether these findings will apply at later stages is unclear; though this study does provide important insights to inform planning phases and initial implementation of integrated stepped care models. Fifth, given our small sample size, we are unable to determine whether we had reached thematic saturation. Regardless, this study provides meaningful data given its focus on implementation of a novel model of care for unhealthy alcohol use in HIV clinics based on a robust deductive approach to data analysis, which revealed consistency in findings within and across different groups of providers. Sixth, our study may have been subject to social desirability bias given the proportion of interviewers relative to interventionists; however, we felt that the diverse perspectives of the interviewers served to enhance the richness of the conversation and data collection.

Conclusions

In conclusion, our study represents an important step in identifying key considerations based upon the CFIR constructs when implementing an integrated stepped care model for unhealthy alcohol use in HIV clinics. We found that implementation of this model may be facilitated by tools to help providers enhance patient motivation, close alignment with organizational values and existing models of care, and optimization of provider self-efficacy and roles. Future efforts aimed at obtaining the perspectives of additional providers, as well as patients and HIV providers will be important for developing a comprehensive understanding of factors impacting implementation of integrated stepped care for unhealthy alcohol use in HIV clinics. In addition, consideration of alternative models involving various providers completing the primary components of the intervention, will be important for informing the development of successful interventions.

Authors' contributions

EJE participated in all aspects of this study, including writing the HIC protocol, leading the data analysis and writing the first draft of the manuscript. NBH and SAM contributed to design of the data collection tools, participated in data collection and analysis. CD contributed to the design of the data collection tools and data analysis. LEF participated in data collection. PGOC and ECW participated in data analysis. DAF participated in all aspects of this study, including conceiving the study design, leading the data collection, and revising of the manuscript. All authors made substantial contributions to the revising of the manuscript. All authors read and approved the final manuscript.

Author details

[1] Yale University School of Medicine, 367 Cedar Street, ESH A, New Haven, CT 06510, USA. [2] Center for Interdisciplinary Research On AIDS, Yale University School of Public Health, 135 College Street, New Haven, CT 06510, USA. [3] College of Public Health, University of Georgia, 131 Wright Hall, Health Sciences Campus, Athens, GA 30602, USA. [4] VA Puget Sound Health Care System, Center of Innovation for Veteran-Centered and Value-Driven Care, 1100 Olive Way, Suite 1400, Seattle, WA 98101, USA. [5] Department of Health Services, University of Washington, 1959 NE Pacific Street, Magnuson Health Sciences Center, Room H-664, Seattle, WA 98195, USA. [6] Syracuse University, 430 Huntington Hall, Syracuse, NY 13244, USA. [7] National Institute on Alcohol Abuse and Alcoholism HIV/AIDS Program, 5635 Fishers Lane, Bethesda, MD 20892-7003, USA.

Competing interests

The authors declare that they have no competing interests.

Funding

This work was generously supported by grants from the National Institute on Alcohol Abuse and Alcoholism (NIAAA) (1U01AA020795, 2K05 AA16928) and the National Institute on Drug Abuse (NIDA) (K12DA033312-02). Dr. Williams is supported by a Career Development Award from VA Health Services Research & Development (CDA 12-276) and is an investigator with the Implementation Research Institute (IRI) at the George Warren Brown School of Social Work at Washington University in St. Louis. IRI is supported through an award from the National Institute of Mental Health (R25 MH080916-01A2) and the Department of Veterans Affairs, Health Services Research & Development Service, Quality Enhancement Research Initiative (QUERI). Neither NIH nor the VA had a role in the study design; in the collection, analysis and interpretation of data; in the writing of the report; and in the decision to submit the article for publication. Dr. Kendall Bryant, a NIAAA employee and scientific collaborator on the project, participated in the analysis and interpretation of data; in the writing of the report; and in the decision to submit the article for publication.

Disclosures

Earlier versions of this work were presented as poster presentations at the 38th Annual Research Society on Alcoholism Scientific Meeting on June 24, 2015 in San Antonio, Texas and the 8th Annual Conference on the Science of Dissemination and Implementation on December 15, 2015 in Washington, D.C.

References

1. Saitz R. Clinical practice. Unhealthy alcohol use. N Engl J Med. 2005;352(6):596–607. doi:10.1056/NEJMcp042262.
2. Fabris P, Tositti G, Manfrin V, Giordani MT, Vaglia A, Cattelan AM, et al. Does alcohol intake affect highly active antiretroviral therapy (HAART) response in HIV-positive patients? J Acquir Immune Defic Syndr. 2000;25:92–3.
3. Cook RL, Sereika SM, Hunt SC, Woodward WC, Erlen JA, Conigliaro J. Problem drinking and medication adherence among persons with HIV infection. J Gen Intern Med. 2001;16:83–8.
4. Galvan FH, Bing EG, Fleishman JA, London AS, Caetano R, Burnam MA, et al. The prevalence of alcohol consumption and heavy drinking among people with HIV in the United States: results from the HIV cost and services utilization study. J Stud Alcohol. 2002;63:179–86.
5. Lucas GM, Gebo KA, Chaisson RE, Moore RD. Longitudinal assessment of the effects of drug and alcohol abuse on HIV-1 treatment outcomes in an urban clinic. Aids. 2002;16(5):767–74.
6. Samet JH, Horton NJ, Traphagen ET, Lyon SM, Freedberg KA. Alcohol consumption and HIV disease progression: are they related? Alcohol Clin Exp Res. 2003;27(5):862–7.
7. Arnsten JH, Demas PA, Grant RW, Gourevitch MN, Farzadegan H, Howard AA, et al. Impact of active drug use on antiretroviral therapy adherence and viral suppression in HIV-infected drug users. J Gen Int Med. 2002;17:377–81.
8. Williams EC, Bradley KA, Balderson BH, McClure JB, Grothaus L, McCoy K, et al. Alcohol and associated characteristics among older persons living with human immunodeficiency virus on antiretroviral therapy. Subst Abus. 2014;35(3):245–53. doi:10.1080/08897077.2014.890997.
9. Korthuis PT, Zephyrin LC, Fleishman JA, Saha S, Josephs JS, McGrath MM, et al. Health-related quality of life in HIV-infected patients: the role of substance use. AIDS Patient Care STDS. 2008;22(11):859–67.
10. Korthuis PT, Fiellin DA, McGinnis KA, Skanderson M, Justice AC, Gordon AJ, et al. Unhealthy alcohol and illicit drug use are associated with decreased quality of HIV care. J Acquir Immune Defic Syndr. 2012;61(2):171–8. doi:10.1097/QAI.0b013e31826741aa.
11. Freiberg MS, McGinnis KA, Kraemer K, Samet JH, Conigliaro J, Curtis Ellison R, et al. The association between alcohol consumption and prevalent cardiovascular diseases among HIV-infected and HIV-uninfected men. J Acquir Immune Defic Syndr. 2010;53(2):247–53. doi:10.1097/QAI.0b013e3181c6c4b7.
12. Lim JK, Tate JP, Fultz SL, Goulet JL, Conigliaro J, Bryant KJ, et al. Relationship between alcohol use categories and noninvasive markers of advanced hepatic fibrosis in HIV-infected, chronic hepatitis C virus-infected, and uninfected patients. Clin Infect Dis. 2014;. doi:10.1093/cid/ciu097.
13. McGinnis KA, Fultz SL, Skanderson M, Conigliaro J, Bryant K, Justice AC. Hepatocellular carcinoma and non-Hodgkin's lymphoma: the roles of HIV, hepatitis C infection, and alcohol abuse. J Clin Oncol. 2006;24(31):5005–9. doi:10.1200/JCO.2006.05.7984.
14. Mayer KH, Skeer MR, O'Cleirigh C, Goshe BM, Safren SA. Factors associated with amplified hiv transmission behavior among american men who have sex with men engaged in care: implications for clinical providers. Ann Behav Med. 2013;. doi:10.1007/s12160-013-9527-1.
15. Cook RL, McGinnis KA, Kraemer KL, Gordon AJ, Conigliaro J, Maisto SA, et al. Intoxication before intercourse and risky sexual behavior in male veterans with and without human immunodeficiency virus infection. Med Care. 2006;44(8 Suppl 2):S31–6. doi:10.1097/01.mlr.0000223710.35008.d9 **00005650-200608002-00005 [pii]**.
16. Lefevre F, O'Leary B, Moran M, Mossar M, Yarnold PR, Martin GJ, et al. Alcohol consumption among HIV-infected patients. J Gen Intern Med. 1995;10(8):458–60.
17. Petry NM. Alcohol use in HIV patients: what we don't know may hurt us. Int J STD AIDS. 1999;10(9):561–70.
18. Cook RL, Sereika SM, Hunt SC, Woodward WC, Erlen JA, Conigliaro J. Problem drinking and medication adherence among persons with HIV infection. J Gen Intern Med. 2001;16(2):83–8.
19. Samet JH, Cheng DM, Libman H, Nunes DP, Alperen JK, Saitz R. Alcohol consumption and HIV disease progression. J Acquir Immune Defic Syndr. 2007;46(2):194–9. doi:10.1097/QAI.0b013e318142aabb.
20. Samet JH, Horton NJ, Traphagen ET, Lyon SM, Freedberg KA. Alcohol consumption and HIV disease progression: are they related? Alcohol Clin Exp Res. 2003;27(5):862–7. doi:10.1097/01.ALC.0000065438.80967.56.
21. Samet JH, Phillips SJ, Horton NJ, Traphagen ET, Freedberg KA. Detecting alcohol problems in HIV-infected patients: use of the CAGE questionnaire. AIDS Res Hum Retroviruses. 2004;20(2):151–5. doi:10.1089/088922204773004860.
22. Jonas DE, Garbutt JC, Amick HR, Brown JM, Brownley KA, Council CL, et al. Behavioral counseling after screening for alcohol misuse in primary care: a systematic review and meta-analysis for the US preventive services task force. Ann Intern Med. 2012;. doi:10.7326/0003-4819-157-9-201211060-00544.
23. Anton RF, O'Malley SS, Ciraulo DA, Cisler RA, Couper D, Donovan DM, et al. Combined pharmacotherapies and behavioral interventions for alcohol dependence: the COMBINE study: a randomized controlled trial. JAMA. 2006;295(17):2003–17. doi:10.1001/jama.295.17.2003.

24. Jonas DE, Amick HR, Feltner C, Bobashev G, Thomas K, Wines R, et al. Pharmacotherapy for adults with alcohol use disorders in outpatient settings: a systematic review and meta-analysis. JAMA. 2014;311(18):1889–900. doi:10.1001/jama.2014.3628.
25. Brown JL, DeMartini KS, Sales JM, Swartzendruber AL, DiClemente RJ. Interventions to reduce alcohol use among HIV-infected individuals: a review and critique of the literature. Curr HIV/AIDS Rep. 2013;10(4):356–70. doi:10.1007/s11904-013-0174-8.
26. Hasin DS, Aharonovich E, O'Leary A, Greenstein E, Pavlicova M, Arunajadai S, et al. Reducing heavy drinking in HIV primary care: a randomized trial of brief intervention, with and without technological enhancement. Addiction. 2013;108(7):1230–40. doi:10.1111/add.12127.
27. Elliott JC, Aharonovich E, O'Leary A, Wainberg M, Hasin DS. Drinking motives as prospective predictors of outcome in an intervention trial with heavily drinking HIV patients. Drug Alcohol Depend. 2014;134:290–5. doi:10.1016/j.drugalcdep.2013.10.026.
28. Elliott JC, Aharonovich E, O'Leary A, Wainberg M, Hasin DS. Drinking motives among HIV primary care patients. AIDS Behav. 2014;18(7):1315–23. doi:10.1007/s10461-013-0644-4.
29. Metsch LR, Pereyra M, Colfax G, Dawson-Rose C, Cardenas G, McKirnan D, et al. HIV-positive patients' discussion of alcohol use with their HIV primary care providers. Drug Alcohol Depend. 2008;95(1–2):37–44. doi:10.1016/j.drugalcdep.2007.12.006.
30. Conigliaro J, Gordon AJ, McGinnis KA, Rabeneck L, Justice AC. How harmful is hazardous alcohol use and abuse in HIV infection: do health care providers know who is at risk? J Acquir Immune Defic Syndr. 2003;33(4):521–5.
31. Conigliaro J, Justice AC, Gordon AJ, Bryant K. Role of alcohol in determining human immunodeficiency virus (HIV)-relevant outcomes: a conceptual model to guide the implementation of evidence-based interventions into practice. Med Care. 2006;44(8 Suppl 2):S1–6. doi:10.1097/01.mlr.0000223659.36369.cf.
32. Korthuis PT, Saha S, Chander G, McCarty D, Moore RD, Cohn JA, et al. Substance use and the quality of patient-provider communication in HIV clinics. AIDS Behav. 2011;15(4):832–41. doi:10.1007/s10461-010-9779-8.
33. Montague BT, Kahler CW, Colby SM, McHugh RK, Squires D, Fitzgerald B, et al. Attitudes and training needs of new england hiv care and addiction treatment providers: opportunities for better integration of hiv and alcohol treatment services. Addict Disord Their Treat. 2015;14(1):16–28. doi:10.1097/ADT.0000000000000040.
34. van Straten A, Hill J, Richards DA, Cuijpers P. Stepped care treatment delivery for depression: a systematic review and meta-analysis. Psychol Med. 2014;45:1–16. doi:10.1017/S0033291714000701.
35. James PA, Oparil S, Carter BL, Cushman WC, Dennison-Himmelfarb C, Handler J, et al. 2014 evidence-based guideline for the management of high blood pressure in adults: report from the panel members appointed to the Eighth Joint National Committee (JNC 8). JAMA. 2014;311(5):507–20. doi:10.1001/jama.2013.284427.
36. National Institute on Alcohol Abuse and Alcoholism. What's "at-risk" or "heavy" drinking? http://rethinkingdrinking.niaaa.nih.gov/IsYourDrinkingPatternRisky/WhatsAtRiskOrHeavyDrinking.asp. Accessed 18 July 2011.
37. Sterling RK, Lissen E, Clumeck N, Sola R, Correa MC, Montaner J, et al. Development of a simple noninvasive index to predict significant fibrosis in patients with HIV/HCV coinfection. Hepatology. 2006;43(6):1317–25. doi:10.1002/hep.21178.
38. Mendeni M, Foca E, Gotti D, Ladisa N, Angarano G, Albini L, et al. Evaluation of liver fibrosis: concordance analysis between noninvasive scores (APRI and FIB-4) evolution and predictors in a cohort of HIV-infected patients without hepatitis C and B infection. Clin Infect Dis. 2011;52(9):1164–73. doi:10.1093/cid/cir071.
39. American Psychiatric Association. Diagnostic and Statistical Manual of Mental Disorders (DSM-IV), fourth edition Washington. Washington: American Psychiatric Press; 1994.
40. D'Onofrio G, Pantalon MV, Degutis LC, Fiellin DA, O'Connor PG. Development and implementation of an emergency practitioner-performed brief intervention for hazardous and harmful drinkers in the emergency department. Acad Emerg Med. 2005;12(3):249–56. doi:10.1197/j.aem.2004.10.021.
41. Pantalon MV, Martino S, Dziura J, Li FY, Owens PH, Fiellin DA, et al. Development of a scale to measure practitioner adherence to a brief intervention in the emergency department. J Subst Abuse Treat. 2012;43(4):382–8. doi:10.1016/j.jsat.2012.08.011.
42. D'Onofrio G, Fiellin DA, Pantalon MV, Chawarski MC, Owens PH, Degutis LC, et al. A brief intervention reduces hazardous and harmful drinking in emergency department patients. Ann Emerg Med. 2012;. doi:10.1016/j.annemergmed.2012.02.006.
43. Miller WR, Zweben A, DiClememte CC, Rycharik RG. Motivational enhancement therapy manual: a clinical research guide for therapists treating individuals with alcohol abuse and dependence, NIAAA Project MATCH Monograph. 1992. http://pubs.niaaa.nih.gov/publications/ProjectMatch/match02.pdf. Accessed 1 Jan 2015
44. Justice AC, McGinnis KA, Skanderson M, Chang CC, Gibert CL, Goetz MB, et al. Towards a combined prognostic index for survival in HIV infection: the role of 'non-HIV' biomarkers. HIV Med. 2010;11(2):143–51. doi:10.1111/j.1468-1293.2009.00757.x.
45. Justice AC, Modur SP, Tate JP, Althoff KN, Jacobson LP, Gebo KA, et al. Predictive accuracy of the veterans aging cohort study index for mortality with HIV infection: a North American cross cohort analysis. J Acquir Immune Defic Syndr. 2013;62(2):149–63. doi:10.1097/QAI.0b013e31827df36c.
46. Tate JP, Justice AC, Hughes MD, Bonnet F, Reiss P, Mocroft A, et al. An internationally generalizable risk index for mortality after 1 year of antiretroviral therapy. AIDS. 2013;27(4):563–72. doi:10.1097/QAD.0b013e32835b8c7f.
47. Rosland AM, Nelson K, Sun H, Dolan ED, Maynard C, Bryson C, et al. The patient-centered medical home in the Veterans Health Administration. Am J Manag Care. 2013;19(7):e263–72.
48. Kearney LK, Post EP, Zeiss A, Goldstein MG, Dundon M. The role of mental and behavioral health in the application of the patient-centered medical home in the department of veterans affairs. Transl Behav Med. 2011;1(4):624–8. doi:10.1007/s13142-011-0093-4.
49. Curran GM, Bauer M, Mittman B, Pyne JM, Stetler C. Effectiveness-implementation hybrid designs: combining elements of clinical effectiveness and implementation research to enhance public health impact. Med Care. 2012;50(3):217–26. doi:10.1097/MLR.0b013e3182408812.
50. McGovern MP, Saunders EC, Kim E. Substance abuse treatment implementation research. J Subst Abuse Treat. 2013;44(1):1–3. doi:10.1016/j.jsat.2012.09.006.
51. Green CA, McCarty D, Mertens J, Lynch FL, Hilde A, Firemark A, et al. A qualitative study of the adoption of buprenorphine for opioid addiction treatment. J Subst Abuse Treat. 2014;46(3):390–401. doi:10.1016/j.jsat.2013.09.002.
52. Hartzler B, Lash SJ, Roll JM. Contingency management in substance abuse treatment: a structured review of the evidence for its transportability. Drug Alcohol Depend. 2012;122(1–2):1–10. doi:10.1016/j.drugalcdep.2011.11.011.
53. Damschroder LJ, Hagedorn HJ. A guiding framework and approach for implementation research in substance use disorders treatment. Psychol Addict Behav. 2011;25(2):194–205. doi:10.1037/a0022284.
54. Damschroder LJ, Aron DC, Keith RE, Kirsh SR, Alexander JA, Lowery JC. Fostering implementation of health services research findings into practice: a consolidated framework for advancing implementation science. Implement Sci. 2009;4:50. doi:10.1186/1748-5908-4-50.
55. Curry LA, Nembhard IM, Bradley EH. Qualitative and mixed methods provide unique contributions to outcomes research. Circulation. 2009;119(10):1442–52.
56. Hsieh HF, Shannon SE. Three approaches to qualitative content analysis. Qual Health Res. 2005;15(9):1277–88. doi:10.1177/1049732305276687.
57. Elo S, Kyngas H. The qualitative content analysis process. J Adv Nurs. 2008;62(1):107–15. doi:10.1111/j.1365-2648.2007.04569.x.
58. Fredriksson M, Eldh A, Vengberg S, Dahlstrom T, Halford C, Wallin L, et al. Local politico-administrative perspectives on quality improvement based on national registry data in Sweden: a qualitative study using the consolidated framework for implementation research. Implement Sci. 2014;9(1):777. doi:10.1186/s13012-014-0189-6.
59. Damschroder LJ, Lowery JC. Evaluation of a large-scale weight management program using the consolidated framework for implementation research (CFIR). Implement Sci. 2013;8:51. doi:10.1186/1748-5908-8-51.
60. Murphy K, O'Connor DA, Browning CJ, French SD, Michie S, Francis JJ, et al. Understanding diagnosis and management of dementia and guideline implementation in general practice: a qualitative study

using the theoretical domains framework. Implement Sci. 2014;9:31. doi:10.1186/1748-5908-9-31.
61. Bergstrom A, Peterson S, Namusoko S, Waiswa P, Wallin L. Knowledge translation in Uganda: a qualitative study of Ugandan midwives' and managers' perceived relevance of the sub-elements of the context cornerstone in the PARIHS framework. Implement Sci. 2012;7:117. doi:10.1186/1748-5908-7-117.
62. Barry DT, Irwin KS, Jones ES, Becker WC, Tetrault JM, Sullivan LE, et al. Opioids, chronic pain, and addiction in primary care. J Pain. 2010;11(12):1442–50. doi:10.1016/j.jpain.2010.04.002.
63. Barry DT, Irwin KS, Jones ES, Becker WC, Tetrault JM, Sullivan LE, et al. Integrating buprenorphine treatment into office-based practice: a qualitative study. J Gen Intern Med. 2009;24(2):218–25. doi:10.1007/s11606-008-0881-9.
64. Hieftje K, Rosenthal MS, Camenga DR, Edelman EJ, Fiellin LE. A qualitative study to inform the development of a video game for adolescent HIV prevention. Games Health J. 2012;1(4):294–8. doi:10.1089/g4h.2012.0025.
65. Edelman EJ, Cole CA, Richardson W, Boshnack N, Jenkins H, Rosenthal MS. Opportunities for improving partner notification for HIV: results from a community-based participatory research study. AIDS Behav. 2014;. doi:10.1007/s10461-013-0692-9.
66. Maisto SA, Carey KB, Carey MP, Purnine DM, Barnes KL. Methods of changing patterns of substance use among individuals with co-occurring schizophrenia and substance use disorder. J Subst Abuse Treat. 1999;17(3):221–7.
67. Noel NE, Ogle RL, Maisto SA, Jackson LA Jr. What Do Women Want? A qualitative study of dating. Violence Against Women. 2014;. doi:10.1177/1077801214555472.
68. Fox AM, Jackson SS, Hansen NB, Gasa N, Crewe M, Sikkema KJ. In their own voices: a qualitative study of women's risk for intimate partner violence and HIV in South Africa. Violence Against Women. 2007;13(6):583–602. doi:10.1177/1077801207299209.
69. Crabtree BF, Miller WL. Doing Qualitative Research. 2nd edn. Thousand Oaks: Sage Publications; 1999.
70. Elliott JC, Aharonovich E, Hasin DS. Reasons for limiting drinking in an HIV primary care sample. Alcohol Clin Exp Res. 2014;38(6):1720–7. doi:10.1111/acer.12401.
71. Bradley KA, Williams EC, Achtmeyer CE, Volpp B, Collins BJ, Kivlahan DR. Implementation of evidence-based alcohol screening in the Veterans Health Administration. Am J Manag Care. 2006;12(10):597–606.
72. Williams EC, Rubinsky AD, Chavez LJ, Lapham GT, Rittmueller SE, Achtmeyer CE, et al. An early evaluation of implementation of brief intervention for unhealthy alcohol use in the US veterans health administration. Addiction. 2014;109(9):1472–81. doi:10.1111/add.12600.
73. Iheanacho T, Issa M, Marienfeld C, Rosenheck R. Use of naltrexone for alcohol use disorders in the Veterans' Health Administration: a national study. Drug Alcohol Depend. 2013;132(1–2):122–6. doi:10.1016/j.drugalcdep.2013.01.016.
74. Marienfeld C, Iheanacho T, Issa M, Rosenheck RA. Long-acting injectable depot naltrexone use in the Veterans' Health Administration: a national study. Addict Behav. 2014;39(2):434–8. doi:10.1016/j.addbeh.2013.05.006.
75. Del Re AC, Gordon AJ, Lembke A, Harris AH. Prescription of topiramate to treat alcohol use disorders in the veterans health administration. Addict Sci Clin Pract. 2013;8:12. doi:10.1186/1940-0640-8-12.
76. Group; TMoSUDW. VA/DoD Clinical practice guideline for management of Substance Use Disorders (SUD). In: Department of veterans affairs DoD. 2009.
77. Bradley KA, Kivlahan DR. Bringing patient-centered care to patients with alcohol use disorders. JAMA. 2014;311(18):1861–2. doi:10.1001/jama.2014.3629.
78. Korthuis PT, Josephs JS, Fleishman JA, Hellinger J, Himelhoch S, Chander G, et al. Substance abuse treatment in human immunodeficiency virus: the role of patient-provider discussions. J Subst Abuse Treat. 2008;35(3):294–303. doi:10.1016/j.jsat.2007.11.005.
79. Fiellin DA, Weiss L, Botsko M, Egan JE, Altice FL, Bazerman LB, et al. Drug treatment outcomes among HIV-infected opioid-dependent patients receiving buprenorphine/naloxone. J Acquir Immune Defic Syndr. 2011;56(Suppl 1):S33–8. doi:10.1097/QAI.0b013e3182097537.
80. Korthuis PT, Fiellin DA, Fu R, Lum PJ, Altice FL, Sohler N, et al. Improving adherence to HIV quality of care indicators in persons with opioid dependence: the role of buprenorphine. J Acquir Immune Defic Syndr. 2011;56(Suppl 1):S83–90. doi:10.1097/QAI.0b013e31820bc9a5.
81. Drainoni ML, Farrell C, Sorensen-Alawad A, Palmisano JN, Chaisson C, Walley AY. Patient perspectives of an integrated program of medical care and substance use treatment. AIDS Patient Care STDS. 2014;28(2):71–81. doi:10.1089/apc.2013.0179.

5

Emerging adults in substance misuse intervention: preintervention characteristics and responses to a motivation-enhancing program

Blair Beadnell[1*], Michele A. Crisafulli[2], Pamela A. Stafford[1] and Erin A. Casey[3]

Abstract

Background: Emerging adulthood is an age of particularly risky behavior. Substance misuse during this phase of life can be the beginning of longer-term problems, making intervention programs particularly important. This study's purposes were to identify alcohol use profile subgroups, describe the preintervention characteristics of each, and assess how many participants transitioned to lower-risk profiles during the course of the intervention.

Methods: We used latent transition analyses to categorize 1183 people court ordered to attend Prime For Life® (PFL), a motivation-enhancing program, into preintervention and postintervention profiles. We then assessed how many made transitions between these profiles during the course of the intervention.

Results: Profiles included two low-risk statuses (abstinence and light drinking) and two high-risk statuses (occasional heavy drinking and frequent heavy drinking). We found that people in profile subgroups that reflected heavier 90-day preintervention drinking were likely to transition to profiles reflecting postintervention intentions for lower-risk drinking in the subsequent 90 days. In contrast, the likelihood of transitioning from a lower-risk to a higher-risk profile was extremely low. These positive changes were found for people of both sexes and for those above versus below the legal drinking age, albeit for more women than men in the heaviest drinking group.

Conclusions: Findings showed positive changes during intervention for many emerging adult participants attending PFL. Further research is needed that include comparison conditions, as well as examine longer-term outcomes in this population.

Keywords: Prevention, Emerging adults, Latent transition analysis, Alcohol, Alcohol use disorder, Motivation-enhancing

Background

Emerging adulthood (EA), a developmental period situated between adolescence and adulthood, is a time of particular concern with substance use. Initially conceptualized by Arnett in 2000, EA is typically seen as lasting from approximately age 18–25 (though in some cases through the late twenties) [1]. The characteristics of this developmental stage include being a period of identity exploration, instability, self-focus, transition, and optimism. These elements contribute to it being a time of high risk-taking behaviors [2]. In particular, the early twenties is a period during which rates of alcohol use and related problems increase to their highest point [3–5].

Classification of drinking patterns among emerging adults

Researchers have added to knowledge on alcohol use by using methods that take into account that drinking behavior is best reflected not by any one aspect, but by a combination. While alcohol research typically examines

*Correspondence: blair.beadnell@primeforlife.org
[1] Prevention Research Institute, 841 Corporate Drive, Suite 300, Lexington, KY 40503, USA
Full list of author information is available at the end of the article

both quantity (the amount of alcohol consumed) and frequency (how often alcohol is used), these are often examined separately. However, looking at these together to see drinking patterns can more accurately determine individuals' level of risk. Accordingly, classification techniques such as cluster analysis and mixture modeling (e.g., latent class and latent transition analysis) help investigators identify subgroups with unique alcohol use profiles based on typical quantity and frequency.

In the EA population, fairly consistent subgroups representing gradations of risky drinking emerge when using these techniques. There is a common thread across studies of finding lower-risk profiles (no use and occasional low use groups) and higher-risk profiles (occasional high use and frequent high use groups). For example, Auerbach and Collins identified five groups that showed varying levels of risk among individuals 18.5–22.5 years old: no use, occasional low use, occasional high use, frequent high use, and frequent high use with heavy episodic drinking [6]. Cleveland and colleagues found four drinking patterns among college students (i.e., nondrinkers, weekend nonbingers, weekend bingers, and heavy drinkers) and among non-college 18–22 year olds (i.e., nondrinkers, weekend light drinkers, weekend risky drinkers, and daily drinkers) [7, 8]. These profiles showed predictive validity in that those with the heavier drinking profiles were more likely to show negative consequences from drinking (e.g., feeling sick, missing work, driving while impaired, and getting into fights) [8].

Using these classification techniques, sex and age emerge as important factors related to EA drinking patterns and responsiveness to intervention. In one study using growth mixture modeling to categorize intervention efficacy, older and female college students were more likely to respond favorably [9]. Similar patterns appear in research of naturally-occurring drinking trajectories (i.e., outside of the intervention context). One study found that EA women were underrepresented in categories showing continued high use or increased use with age, while overrepresented in a category of never having problematic use [10]. In terms of age, questions remain about the trajectories along which drinking evolves over the years of EA. There is evidence that a heavier drinking pattern when below the legal drinking age predicts continuation in such a pattern once the legal drinking age is reached [6]. As such, problematic drinking at younger ages may be an indicator of future problems. However, while partially predictive, drinking early in EA does not necessarily determine an individual's later status. For example, Schulenberg and Magos [10] reviewed studies showing changes in drinking trajectories can occur such that earlier heavy drinking patterns can resolve later in people's developmental trajectory. Given these indications that sex and age might play roles in EA drinking trajectories, their influence is an important topic to investigate.

Classification techniques can be useful for informing applied intervention research in two ways. One is by allowing for examination of participants' preintervention substance use patterns, as opposed to relying on individual variables. This more nuanced information about groups of participants presenting for intervention may help program design and implementation. For example, optimally effective intervention content might differ for target groups whose high-risk use is regular versus episodic, or when both patterns exist. Another way classification techniques are useful is by providing information on the clinical significance of changes made by participants. Specifically, longitudinal classification methods like latent transition analysis (LTA) allow calculation of the percentage of people making meaningful changes. These sorts of analyses are a useful supplement to traditional tests that focus on the statistical significance of average changes over time and, moreover, respond to calls for examination of the practical utility of intervention programs [11, 12]. This study capitalized on the usefulness of classification methods by examining initial changes during a motivation-enhancing (ME) intervention among EAs receiving an indicated substance use prevention program.

Motivation enhancing substance use interventions and emerging adults

Intervention methods often examined with EAs engaging in high-risk behaviors include cognitive-behavioral approaches, particularly those incorporating methods targeting motivation for change. Specifically, many indicated prevention programs incorporate principles from motivational interviewing (MI) and are thus often called motivation-enhancing (ME) approaches. Both ME and MI approaches involve a collaborative counseling style intended to strengthen commitment to change, particularly by eliciting and building on participants' already existing motivation for change [13].

Theoretically, ME interventions should be especially well-suited for EAs because they provide a framework for working with the resistance to authority and ambivalence about change that often characterize this developmental period [2]. Indeed, research has shown preliminary support for ME with EAs. Specifically, several studies have shown that interventions incorporating ME elements can decrease substance use and/or consequences among college students [14–17]. Additionally, a recent meta-analysis showed that brief ME and cognitive-behavioral interventions are both associated with improvements in alcohol consumption and consequences among young adults, although effects were attenuated to non-significance by 2-year follow-up [18].

The Transtheoretical Model (TTM) [19] provides a theoretical lens through which to view the meaning and importance of immediate gains achieved during the course of ME interventions such as the one examined in this study. The model posits that intentional behavior change involves moving through multiple stages and completing numerous cognitive and behavioral tasks along the way. ME interventions are often geared toward individuals in earlier stages of change, particularly precontemplation (where individuals have no intention of making changes) and contemplation (where they are considering but ambivalent about making changes). In such cases, a successful short-term outcome would be movement to a later stage of change, such as preparation, in which people have made a decision to change and begun preparing to do so (but have not yet necessarily made any behavioral changes). The model sees such movement as an important step in setting the stage for behavioral change. However, this does not guarantee longer-term success: meta-analyses show only moderate correlations between intentions and behavior ranging from .40 to .82 (overall $r = .53$) [20]. Nevertheless, intentions have meaning in that the TTM and other influential health behavior theories (e.g., the Theory of Reasoned Action and the Theory of Planned Behavior) see them as necessary precursors to subsequent behavior change [21, 22].

Study purpose

While ME programs are theoretically well-suited to and have shown promise with this age group, little is known about changes EAs make when participating in these approaches. This includes understanding what drinking profile subgroups exist in an intervention population, in what proportions, and whether some are more versus less likely to show improvements during the course of the ME intervention. Additionally, while potentially important given the previously mentioned findings about age and sex, little is known about whether demographic characteristics are related to preintervention profiles, and changes made during intervention.

To examine these questions, this study focused on initial change from baseline to immediately postintervention among EAs in an ME substance use intervention. We analyzed data from individuals attending Prime For Life® (PFL), a group-delivered ME indicated prevention program. Participants had all experienced negative consequences of substance use in the form of being arrested for driving while intoxicated, and all were required to complete the program to regain driving privileges. Described in more detail below, PFL focuses on encouraging the reduction of negative social, legal, occupational, and health consequences from alcohol and drug misuse. A previous data collection showed PFL to be effective in producing short-term changes in cognitive outcomes [23]. Another study showed that such changes are meaningful and translate into longer-term improvements: in an examination of driving records of PFL attendees in a 2-day version of the program, PFL participants had lower 3-year recidivism rates compared to standard care conditions [24]. In both datasets, changes occurred for emerging adults as well as the broader range of adult participants. Moreover, moderation analyses showed that improvements in cognitive outcomes (e.g., understanding tolerance, perceived risk for addiction, perceived risk for negative consequences, and problem recognition) were similar or greater for EA participants. In terms of recidivism, moderation analyses showed that PFL's lower rearrest rates occurred for 18–29 year olds in the same way as for other adults receiving PFL, although this advantage of PFL over standard care did not extend to 18–29 year olds required to receive additional substance use treatment beyond the PFL.

The present study had three specific purposes. One was to identify subgroups based on patterns of preintervention alcohol use in a sample of EAs attending a court-ordered intervention (PFL). Second, we sought to quantify the extent to which participants transitioned from previous patterns of heavy alcohol use to postintervention patterns characterized by intentions to use substances less in the future. Third, we wished to determine whether sex and being of legal drinking age were predictors of these transitions to lower alcohol use intentions.

We guided our interpretation of results based on drinking guidelines taught in PFL. Known as the 0–1–2–3 guidelines, these define the amount of drinking considered "low risk." The low-risk guidelines for alcohol were the same for both women and men, and included no more than one standard drink (defined as ½ ounce of pure alcohol at the time of this data collection) in an hour, two standard drinks daily, or three standard drinks on any day. Based on this, we considered drinking less than three drinks in a day as low risk, and four or more as high risk. Although the guidelines have additional aspects (e.g., a peak amount per week as 14 standard drinks, and abstinence for those who have already developed an alcohol use disorder) we did not have data to consider these.

Methods

Participants

Participants ($N = 1183$) came from ten states in the U.S. (Georgia, Iowa, Indiana, Kentucky, North Carolina, Montana, North Dakota, South Carolina, Tennessee, and Utah), and had been arrested for impaired driving. All were required to attend the program (either automatically or from being court-ordered) and completed it. These states use PFL for arrestees, with program completion required as a prerequisite for reinstating driving privileges. Participants received PFL from impaired driving schools or substance abuse treatment agencies in 2011 and 2012. Participants paid the program cost out of pocket, and the price varied depending on the state (states typically mandate the maximum cost agencies can charge for program attendance). Cost typically ranged from none (if public funding was available to a participant), or anywhere between $150 and $500.

Procedure

Using structured protocols and scripts, PFL instructors distributed paper and pencil questionnaires to the group at the beginning of the first session and immediately after the last session ended. Data collection methods prevented instructors from seeing participant responses. The length of time between administration of baseline and posttest questionnaires varied due to state regulations from 2 to 14 days (with the intervention being 12–20 h).

Materials and measures

The previously pilot tested questionnaires took approximately 15 min to complete. Questions asked about number of drinks in a 90 day period and provided responses ranging from "0" to "24 or more," except where otherwise noted. Questionnaires defined one standard drink following the PFL risk guidelines used at the time (12 oz of beer, 4 oz of wine, or 1.25 oz of 80-proof alcohol). In a previous psychometric evaluation, test retest reliability of items ranged from $r = .72–.94$.

Demographics

Participants reported on their sex and age. For analyses, we dichotomized age as being legal drinking age (21–25) or not (18–20).

Alcohol consumption and intentions

Items were drawn from epidemiological studies [25, 26] about the quantity and frequency of drinking. Questions regarding preintervention drinking asked about the 90 days of behavior prior to attending PFL; at posttest, the same questions were asked but about intentions for the next 90 days.

The preintervention quantity items were "In the 90 days before this program, on days when I drank, I usually had...". Participants could choose any number from 0 to 24 or more, and for analyses we created an ordinal variable of 0, 1–3, 4–6, and 7 or more. This categorization captured variation in drinking in a parsimonious way while aligning to the PFL drinking guidelines taught in the program (e.g., with the 0 and the 1–3 categories falling within what is considered low risk; and the other categories representing two levels of higher-risk drinking). Frequency items assessed frequency of drinking above the PFL guidelines using the introductory statement "In the 90 days before this program" and two items: "I drank 4–6 drinks" and "I drank 7 or more drinks." Response categories were "not at all," "less than once a week," "about once a week," "2–3 days a week," "4–6 days a week," and "most days." We categorized these as "never," "less than once a week," and "one or more times a week." Questionnaires used the same item wording and response option coding for postintervention future intentions by changing the introductory statements (e.g., "In the next 90 days, I intend to ...").

For alcohol use during the 90-day period before intervention, we used postintervention retrospective responses about drinking that occurred during those 90 days before PFL. We based this decision on previous research indicating that individuals experiencing legal issues based on their substance use and participating in court-ordered intervention report higher levels of previous use when asked following program participation than when queried about the same time period prior to the program [27, 28]. While we cannot be certain these postintervention-collected data were more accurate, we see reason to believe that it might be. Specifically, this population is subject to factors hypothesized to decrease the accuracy of self-report such as unhappiness about attending a court-ordered program, social desirability, and concerns about confidentiality given their legal entanglements [29]. We reasoned that these factors were likely to be less salient at the postintervention timepoint after participants became familiar with the instructors and program, which may have allowed for more accurate reporting.

Description of Prime For Life

PFL is a theory-based, manualized, structured, and motivation-enhancing indicated prevention program. It provides information drawn from scientific research about hazards attendant to high-risk levels of substance use focusing on the importance of personal choice in preventing future problems. Negative consequences include health and impairment problems secondary to high-risk substance use and reflect all aspects of life. Specifically, participants identify the areas of life they value and then self-assess the extent to which their substance use threatens them. PFL does not solely promote abstinence but instead provides guidelines for low-risk use based on an extensive review of the literature examining health and impairment consequences [30]. The program helps participants assess their risk for substance dependence and develop individualized plans to change behavior.

PFL is an ME-based program, and therefore emphasizes the manner in which the program is delivered. It uses three specific empirically supported practices: (1) establishing an effective partnership between instructors and participants, (2) diffusing discord, and (3) providing clear direction [13]. The progress and activities of PFL are guided by the Lifestyle Risk Reduction Model [31], the Transtheoretical Model [32], and persuasion theory [33]. PFL is typically delivered in a group format, and program length varies from 12 to 20 h depending on requirements mandated in each state. Instructors always administer the same core program components, with only the number of optional activities varying. PFL instructors complete a new instructor training conducted by PRI staff and then a self-review process after their first group; most are licensed substance abuse professionals.

Analysis strategy

We first conducted preliminary analyses (described later) to assess whether statistically significant changes occurred in which participants intended to drink less in the future than they had drank before attending the intervention. We then conducted LTA analyses in Mplus v7 guided by methods described by Collins and Lanza [34]. LTA is a statistical method for identifying subgroups, called statuses, of individuals at more than one timepoint. In addition, it estimates transition probabilities, which are the probabilities of transitioning from each Time 1 status to each Time 2 status. We treated preintervention drinking behavior and postintervention drinking intentions as two timepoints; referred here as baseline and posttest, respectively. We treated drinking variables as ordinal in the LTA and—to maximize interpretability of the results—fixed item-response probabilities to be equal across timepoints. Additionally, we specified intervention group membership as a clustering variable in multilevel aggregated analysis in order to adjust model parameters to correctly calculate standard errors [35].

As a first step, we compared models with varying numbers of statuses. We based our decisions about the optimal number of statuses by seeking a balance between statistical criteria (i.e., BIC, AIC, and entropy), parsimony, and theoretical interpretability and meaningfulness. As recommended by Collins and Lanza [34], we paid less attention to the p value for G^2 given that its distribution is not well represented by the Chi square distribution. In terms of other statistical criteria, the parametric bootstrapped likelihood ratio test is an often-used statistic that helps identify the optimal number of statuses. However, we were unable to use it because the test is not available in Mplus when using multilevel data or when there is more than one latent status variable. Thus, we instead chose to focus on the criteria described above. As a next step, we added sex and being of legal drinking age as predictors of baseline status and transition probabilities.

Results

Sample characteristics

Of the 4645 individuals who completed baseline questionnaires, 1199 met our inclusion criteria of being between 18 and 25 years old, having been arrested for impaired driving (rather than another substance use infraction such as drug possession), and having completed the PFL program. We included 1183 (98.7%) in all analyses after removing 16 with missing data (2 missing sex, 15 missing data on all drinking variables).

Most participants were male (69%) and Caucasian (81%). In terms of race/ethnicity, the rest identified as Asian (1%), Black (8%), Hispanic (5%), Native American (2%), Multiracial (3%), or "Other" (<1%). Participants ranged from 18 to 25 years old (M = 22, SD = 1.99), with 76% at or above the legal drinking age (21 or older). About three-quarters had never been married (76%). Educationally, 8% had not finished high school, 34% had completed high school or obtained a GED, 41% had attended but not completed college, 7% had a 2-year college degree, and 10% had a 4-year college or graduate degree. Of six items reflecting substance dependence symptoms experienced in the previous year (e.g., failing to meet normal expectations, drinking in the morning, trying but failing to cut down), 27% endorsed none, 39% one or two, and 34% three to six. Unfortunately, we do not have specific information on the amount of time between arrest and program enrollment; however, unpublished data from a separate PFL program evaluation suggest this varies widely (i.e., anywhere from less than 3 months to 2 years or more, with the majority being between 3 and 12 months).

Missing data

Missing data rates on variables used as indicators of status membership were low among the analysis sample of 1183 and appeared to be due to occasional skipping of items. The amount missing on any one variable ranged from 0.8 to 2.1%, with no discernable pattern. Mplus uses maximum likelihood estimation, which allowed the inclusion of participants missing some variables.

Preliminary analysis: comparison of preintervention drinking to future intentions at postintervention

Table 1 shows distributions of the drinking variables used in the LTA and comparisons of preintervention drinking to intended future drinking. Generalized Estimating Equation comparisons showed that participants intended to drink less in the future than they had in the past on

Table 1 Distributions of drinking variables used in the latent transition analysis ($N = 1183$)

Alcohol use	Preintervention drinking (previous 90 days)		Intentions at postintervention (for next 90 days)		Intentions at postintervention compared to preintervention drinking[a]	
	%	*n*	%	*n*	χ^2 ($df = 1$)	*p*
Usual daily quantity					533.60	<.001
0 drinks	13.6	159	27.3	318		
1–3	22.3	261	50.3	586		
4–6	32.8	385	15.8	184		
7–9	14.0	164	3.8	44		
≥10	17.3	204	2.8	32		
Frequency 4–6					448.34	<.001
Never	29.7	348	60.7	712		
<Once a week	33.6	393	26.4	310		
≥Once a week	36.7	430	12.9	151		
Frequency ≥7					389.30	<.001
Never	43.5	504	73.9	862		
<Once a week	30.2	350	17.9	209		
≥Once a week	26.3	304	8.2	95		

[a] Computed using Generalized Estimating Equation (GEE) analysis

each variable. In particular, many more participants reported intending to completely abstain or to drink in lower-risk amounts (1–3 drinks) than they had in the 90 days before attending the intervention.

Identification of latent statuses

Preliminary latent class analysis models showed the smallest BIC values for the three and four status models (7439.9 and 7436.4 for preintervention drinking, and 5577.3 and 5580.2 for intentions at postintervention, respectively) compared to the two and five status models at the same timepoints (7740.5 and 7466.2 for preintervention drinking, and 5746.6 and 5628.1 for intentions at postintervention, respectively). Entropy scores were acceptably high (>.80) regardless of the number of status groups. We found at both timepoints that the four status model provided the best theoretical interpretability and was the most informative.

We then proceeded to the LTA. Table 2 shows fit statistics for two through five status models. Here, the four and five status models had the lowest BIC values. Entropy values were uniformly high across models. While the five status model had the lowest AIC, we found that the additional status group did not add theoretical value and, thus, we favored the more parsimonious four status model.

Table 3 provides each status group's drinking profile. The top of Table 3 summarizes the proportion of the sample belonging to each of the four status groups for both preintervention drinking and postintervention intentions, and Fig. 1 depicts this visually. As indicated earlier, preintervention profiles represented behavior in the 90 days before intervention, and postintervention profiles represented drinking intentions for the 90 days following PFL attendance. The table orders the profiles from least drinking to greatest drinking, and we labeled the groups to indicate low versus high risk (according to the guidelines taught in the PFL program). We labeled each status group according to what the item response probabilities suggested were its preponderant characteristics. Two groups corresponded to low-risk (LR) drinking according to the PFL guidelines. The LR/no use group represented abstinence from drinking. The LR/light use group profile involved drinking, with the usual number of drinks being 1–3, relatively low probability of drinking 4–6 drinks, and no probability of drinking 7 or more drinks. The other two groups showed high risk (HR) by the usual number of drinks and frequency of binge drinking falling outside the PFL guidelines. The HR/occasional heavy use group was characterized by some probability of having a usual number of drinks within the guidelines (1–3) but a higher probability of being outside of them (4–6). Heavy drinking (4–6, and 7 or more drinks) was likely to occur fairly infrequently (less than once a week). The remaining profile, the HR/frequent heavy use status, was one with a high probability of a usual number of drinks outside the guidelines and this occurring at least once a week.

Table 4 shows the transition probabilities. In other words, each row in Table 4 shows the likelihood that

Table 2 Model fit statistics for two to five status LTA models

Number of latent statuses	−*LL*	G^2	*df*	*AIC*	*BIC*	*Entropy*	Status counts[a]	
							Preintervention drinking	Intentions at postintervention
Two	6627.1	1945.2	1985	13,292.2	13,388.7	0.89	813, 370	349, 834
Three	6239.0	1245.3	1971	12,541.9	12,704.4	0.88	302, 502, 379	708, 138, 337
Four	6102.6	958.3	1955	12,299.1	12,537.7	0.86	365, 226, 135, 457	106, 388, 443, 246
Five	6041.7	854.1	1940	12,211.4	12,536.3	0.85	235, 136, 302, 225, 285	114, 452, 180, 383, 54

[a] Status counts based on most likely group membership

Table 3 Characteristics of status groups from LTA model ($N = 1183$)

Variables	Status group			
	Low risk (LR)		High risk (HR)	
	No use	Light use	Occasional heavy use	Frequent heavy use
Proportion in each status				
Preintervention drinking (previous 90 days)	0.18	0.13	0.39	0.30
Intentions at postintervention (for next 90 days)	0.31	0.39	0.21	0.09
Item-response probabilities[a]				
Usual quantity[b]				
0	0.77	0.00	0.02	0.02
1–3	0.11	0.97	0.29	0.08
4–6	0.09	0.03	0.53	0.26
7–9	0.02	0.00	0.11	0.24
≥10	0.01	0.00	0.05	0.40
Frequency 4–6[c]				
Never	1.00	0.73	0.03	0.10
<Once a week	0.00	0.27	0.70	0.11
≥Once a week	0.00	0.00	0.27	0.79
Frequency ≥7[c]				
Never	1.00	1.00	0.30	0.03
<Once a week	0.00	0.00	0.70	0.13
≥Once a week	0.00	0.00	0.00	0.84

[a] Item-response probabilities can be thought of as the frequency distribution for each variable within that status. These were the same for both preintervention drinking and postintervention intentions (they were constrained to be equal across timepoints). We labeled each status group according to the preponderant characteristics suggested by the item-response probabilities

[b] Prior/intended usual quantity of drinks

[c] Prior/intended frequency of consuming 4–6 or ≥7 drinks

people in a particular preintervention drinking status either remained there or transitioned to a different status regarding their intentions at postintervention. People in both LR status groups typically remained in the same status postintervention. Specifically, 93 and 84% of LR/no use and LR/light use individuals, respectively, remained in the same status. Of the remaining LR/light use participants, 15% transitioned to the LR/no use status. In terms of people in HR groups, many transitioned to lower-risk statuses. For example, those in the HR/occasional heavy use status at baseline generally transitioned to the LR/no use and LR/light use statuses (22 and 47%), but infrequently to the HR/frequent heavy use status (1%). There was no single most common transition made by people in the HR/frequent heavy use status: 26% remained and another 32% transitioned to the other HR status. In other words, 58% of people in the highest-risk status at baseline continued to exhibit high-risk intentions postintervention, although they did most often show improvement to intending occasional heavy use rather than to maintain their frequent heavy use. The remaining 20 and 22% transitioned to the LR statuses.

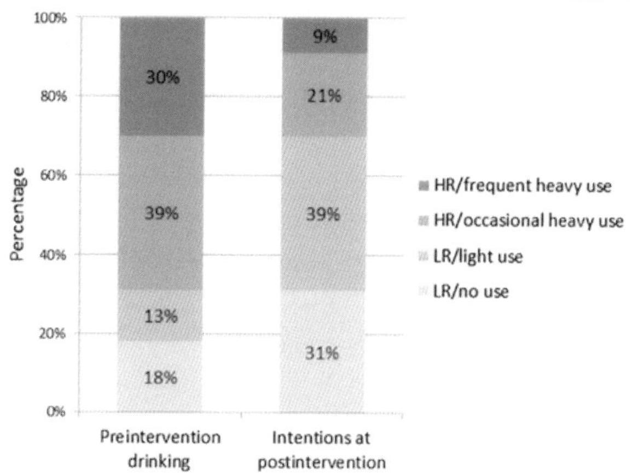

Fig. 1 Percentage in their most likely LTA statuses based on preintervention drinking and future intentions at postintervention

Prediction by sex and legal drinking age

As mentioned, sex and being of legal drinking age were included in the LTA as predictors of preintervention drinking status and transitions to statuses representing future intentions at postintervention. In multinomial logistic regression, sex was not related to preintervention status group membership. Specifically, females were not statistically significantly more likely to be in the preintervention LR/light use, HR/occasional heavy use, or HR/frequent heavy use statuses than they were to be in LR/no risk status; *odds ratios* (*OR*) $= 1.69$, 1.01, and 0.71, $p = .07$, .97, and .11; respectively. Table 5 shows the prediction of transition probabilities to relatively lower-risk statuses. Being female predicted greater likelihood of improvement in terms of transitioning from the HR/frequent heavy use status to each remaining status. For example, the table shows that women were more likely than men to transition from the HR/frequent heavy use to the LR/no use group ($OR = 3.02$). Otherwise, females and males had similar probabilities of improving. Figure 2 shows the most likely status memberships broken out by sex. This illustrates the net effects of sex on preintervention drinking status and subsequent transitions. As can be seen, while a relatively small number of participants remained in the HR/frequent heavy use status, women were particularly unlikely to do so.

Those of legal drinking age were more likely to be in the preintervention LR/light use and HR/occasional heavy use statuses compared to the LR/no use status; $OR = 3.55$ and 1.90, both $p < .01$. However, age was not associated with greater likelihood of membership in the HR/frequent heavy use status; *odds ratio* $= 1.30$, $p = .22$. As shown in Table 5, being of legal drinking age did not statistically significantly predict subsequent transitions. Figure 2 shows the net effects of age on preintervention status and subsequent transitions. Most notably, people above and below the drinking age were equally likely to be in one of the LR postintervention intentions statuses. However, those over the legal drinking age were more likely to be in the LR/light use rather than the LR/no use status.

Discussion

This study focused on the substance use patterns of emerging adults, a group particularly likely to use substances in high-risk and detrimental ways. We categorized participants with impaired driving offenses into substance use profiles reflecting their drinking in the 90 days before the start of their attendance at an indicated prevention program. We then showed transitions between these profile groups and others that were based on drinking intentions reported at postintervention for the following 90 days. Additionally, we assessed whether initial status memberships and transitions differed by sex and age group. The overall finding was that many participants attending PFL, a motivation-enhancing (ME) program, showed transitions to lower-risk profiles. This was true for people of both sexes and age groups, albeit with some variation for the heaviest drinking males compared to females.

In light of the challenges in effectively intervening with emerging adults, these are encouraging findings in terms of people during this developmental stage showing movement to increased readiness to change. The use of LTA in this study allowed us to provide more nuanced and clinically meaningful information than is sometimes

Table 4 Transition probabilities from preintervention drinking to future intentions at postintervention ($N = 1183$)

Preintervention drinking status (previous 90 days)	Intentions at postintervention status (for next 90 days)			
	Low risk (LR)		High risk (HR)	
	No use	Light use	Occasional heavy use	Frequent heavy use
LR/no use	0.93	0.03	0.02	0.02
LR/light use	0.15	0.84	0.00	0.01
HR/occasional heavy use	0.22	0.47	0.30	0.01
HR/frequent heavy use	0.20	0.22	0.32	0.26

Table 5 Odds ratios for sex and age predicting the transitioning to each lower risk status

Preintervention drinking status (previous 90 days)	Intentions at postintervention status (for next 90 days)			
	Low risk (LR)		High risk (HR)	
	No use	Light use	Occasional heavy use	Frequent heavy use
Effect of being female, compared to male				
LR/no use	–	–	–	–
LR/light use	2.65	Reference[a]	–	–
HR/occasional heavy use	0.73	1.56	Reference[a]	–
HR/frequent heavy use	3.02**	3.29**	2.78*	Reference[a]
Effect of being legal drinking age, compared to <21 years				
LR/no use	–	–	–	–
LR/light use	2.56	Reference[a]	–	–
HR/occasional heavy use	0.54	1.79	Reference[a]	–
HR/frequent heavy use	1.27	1.47	1.91	Reference[a]

* $p < .05$; ** $p < .01$

[a] Remaining in the same status group was the reference condition for each odds ratio. Said differently, each odds ratio represents the odds of switching to the lower-risk status group versus staying in the original status group

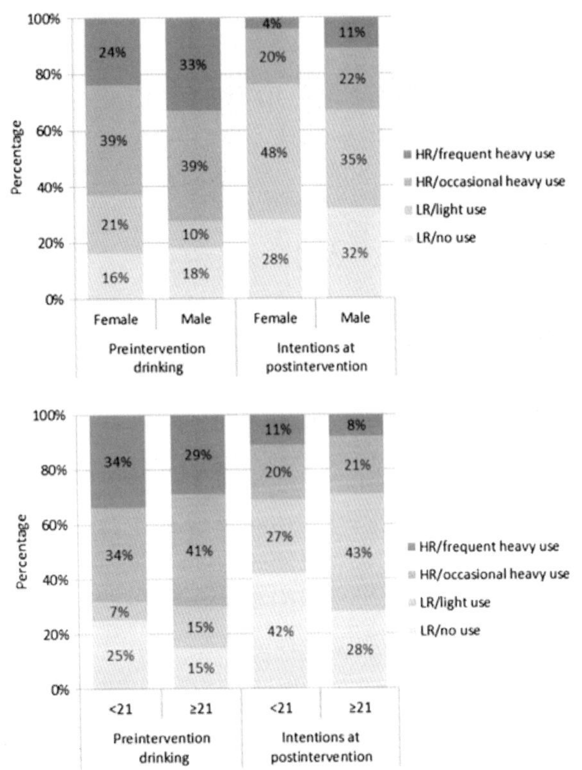

Fig. 2 Percentage in their most likely LTA statuses based on preintervention drinking and future intentions at postintervention, by sex and age

provided in traditional null hypothesis testing. Specifically, it deepens understanding of the characteristics of EAs that interventionists can expect in such contexts, who among them makes changes and in what ways, and the role demographics may play in influencing these changes in this important population.

Knowledge of drinking profiles among EAs attending interventions is of practical relevance to interventionists. For instance, it is important to understand that, even prior to intervention, EA participants exhibit drinking patterns reflecting a range of severity from abstinence to frequent heavy use. In light of prior literature on EA alcohol use, it is not surprising that occasional and frequent heavy drinkers comprised the largest percentage of the sample. Nonetheless, almost a third reported lower risk either in the form of abstinence or, at most, light drinking. It may seem odd at first that such individuals exist in a sample arrested for impaired driving, and this may come as a surprise to interventionists used to working with EAs. One explanation might be that, for some, the impaired driving was due to illicit drug use rather than drinking. However, that is an unlikely explanation given that law enforcement has not yet perfected methods for detecting drug use among drivers. More likely is that the arrest, or its legal and social consequences, provided a catalyst for some that led to behavior change, whether achieved alone or after seeking outside assistance. For individuals attending the intervention 90 days or more after their arrest, such behavior change would have already occurred before the period assessed in this study's baseline measurement and thus previous higher-risk use would not be captured.

As mentioned earlier, the Transtheoretical Model [19] provides a useful framework for understanding the implications of these findings for interventions with EAs. Postintervention statuses were based on future intentions and thus provide an indicator of readiness to change, including participant goals for that change. As such, this is conceptually consistent with the stages of change. Knowing that these status transitions occur may offer practical assistance to professionals who design or provide substance use intervention programs. Specifically, this information can guide the choices made about which intervention elements are needed, and in what circumstances, during the course of working with EAs. For example, the transition from HR/frequent use to HR/occasional use reflects an intention to change, but not an intention to move to low-risk use. In this case, there would be three primary practitioner tasks: (1) express and explore concerns about continued high-risk use while supporting client autonomy; (2) help develop plans for achieving the client's desired change in frequency of high-risk use; and (3) help create a method for the client to evaluate the plan's effectiveness in achieving long-term goals. Conversely, when clients remain in LR/no use—essentially an action or maintenance stage of change—the practitioner's task is to help them identify potential threats to their action plan and revise as needed. The difference between these two examples emphasizes the need for interventionists to avoid assuming their audience is composed largely of people actively drinking in high-risk amounts. Rather, it is important to be aware of and address the broad range of people receiving services. As a result, group-based interventions should contain content that both supports those who have already begun making changes and increases motivation for change among those who have not [36]. As always, interventionists providing individual one-on-one interventions should carefully assess current drinking patterns and match counseling goals to the appropriate stage of change [32].

Results indicate that many individuals have lower-risk intentions for their future drinking relative to their preintervention alcohol use behavior. While over two-thirds reported either occasionally or frequently drinking in high-risk amounts immediately prior to PFL, less than a third intended to do so in the 90 days immediately following intervention. Moreover, we see two specific, positive patterns in terms of the actual transitions from each preintervention drinking to postintervention intentions status. First, those in preintervention LR statuses were likely to remain in the corresponding postintervention status, with transition to a higher-risk drinking profile being extremely rare. Second, many in HR statuses transitioned to a status reflecting future intentions of lesser drinking. For example, only a quarter of participants in the worst-case profile (the HR/frequent heavy use status) remained there. The rest transitioned to a lower-risk intention status, albeit with some only moving so far as the other HR intention status (i.e., intending occasional as opposed to frequent heavy use). While a change to intending less frequent high-risk use does not obviate potential hazards, it does reduce the overall risk and reflects an important public health change when spread over a population of heavy users, who experience a disproportionate number of consequences secondary to their high-risk use.

One interpretation of these transitions is that they reflect people's preferred strategy for decreasing their risk. If so, the results suggest continuing to drink, but in lower-risk amounts, is a somewhat more popular choice for women, those of legal drinking age, and people whose previous high-risk drinking was only occasional. In contrast, men were likely to intend to lower their risk through abstinence as commonly as through light use. Similarly, those under the legal drinking age were more likely to lean towards abstinence rather than light drinking as a way of lowering risk. Interestingly, it appears that people who are frequent heavy drinkers preintervention express a range of reduction goals at postintervention. Some may prefer to occasionally drink heavily in the future while others may prefer to drink in lighter amounts or to be abstinent. Future research might explore such choices more thoroughly, including looking at what characterizes people preferring these different risk reduction strategies and how successful they are at achieving their stated goals.

A small number of participants who were in HR statuses at preintervention—both occasional and frequent heavy drinkers—remained in the corresponding status in terms of their postintervention intentions. Although we cannot know whether this study's observed transitions were caused by the intervention (since there was no comparison condition), to the extent that they were these participants appear to have responded less well. This is a reminder that decreasing alcohol-related risk may be particularly challenging among EAs, given they are in what is typically the heaviest drinking period of life. While we did not find that being of legal drinking age was associated with transition from HR statuses, women were more likely than men to transition from the HR/frequent heavy use to lower-risk statuses. Although many EA men with this preintervention drinking pattern did transition from this status, our finding suggests there may be a subgroup among them that is particularly challenging to influence. While the analyses do not provide information about what other characteristics are associated with not transitioning to lower- risk profiles, this would be a fruitful area for future research. In particular, identifying individuals unlikely to respond to a relatively brief ME indicated prevention program may provide a basis for prescreening and funneling these individuals to alternative interventions that may be more successful. For example, these may be individuals whose substance use is such that they might benefit from more intensive individual treatment. Conversely, not all heavy drinking people may need additional treatment. For some, indicated prevention appears to be enough.

Study limitations

Readers should consider this study's results in the context of its limitations. First, the data were self-reported and did not include corroboration by other means (e.g., biomarkers or collateral reports). Second, they solely reflect future intentions at postintervention, and we do not know about longer-term outcomes, including behavior. Given that intentions are known to be correlated with subsequent behavior only to a moderate extent, it is likely that a portion of individuals who intended to make positive changes later failed to do so. Since behavioral and other outcomes are unknown, future research should apply these techniques using follow-up data on actual drinking behavior. Third, the analyses included no comparison group; therefore, caution should be used in interpreting the benefits shown until replication can occur in an experimental study. Finally, we do not know the extent to which the distribution of questionnaires by instructors, the legal requirement to attend the program, or other unmeasured factors may have influenced the results.

Conclusions

These analyses provide information about an important population: emerging adults with an impaired driving arrest. Interventions with this group are not only important for public safety, but also have public health value in that some members of this group are likely to have developed—or be developing—longer-term substance use problems. Indeed, some participants did report pre-intervention problematic drinking profiles despite having experienced the negative consequence of an arrest. The results show that short-term changes can occur in this important—and sometimes hard to influence—age group during the course of ME intervention (in this case, PFL). Additionally, analyses provide clues to preferred methods of risk reduction. Future research can extend this by describing the longer-term outcomes, and can profit from this approach of categorizing individuals according to their drinking profiles.

Abbreviations

AIC: Akaike information criterion; BIC: Bayesian information criterion; EA: emerging adulthood/emerging adult; HR: high risk; LCA: latent class analysis; LR: low risk; LTA: latent transition analysis; ME: motivation-enhancing; MI: motivational interviewing; OR: odds ratio; OUI: operating a vehicle under the influence of alcohol or drugs; PFL: Prime For Life.

Authors' contributions

BB, MC, and PS conceived the study. BB coordinated the manuscript preparation; BB, MC, and PS participated in its writing; and EC provided editorial input. PS led questionnaire design, data collection, and data management. BB designed the statistical analysis, which he and EC conducted. All authors read and approved the final manuscript.

Author details

[1] Prevention Research Institute, 841 Corporate Drive, Suite 300, Lexington, KY 40503, USA. [2] University of Maryland, Baltimore County, 1000 Hilltop Circle, Baltimore, MD 21250, USA. [3] Social Work Program, University of Washington (Tacoma), 1900 Commerce Street, Box 358425, Tacoma, WA 98402, USA.

Acknowledgements

We thank Dr. David Rosengren for providing feedback about study findings and their interpretation, and for editorial contributions to the final manuscript.

Competing interests

Prevention Research Institute (PRI), the private nonprofit organization that developed and sells the Prime For Life® intervention, conducted this study. Authors Beadnell and Stafford are PRI employees, and Casey a paid PRI contractor. At the time the manuscript was prepared, Crisafulli was a PRI graduate assistant.

References

1. Arnett J. Emerging adulthood: a theory of development from the late teens through the twenties. Am Psychol. 2000;55:469–80.
2. Baer J, Peterson P. Motivational interviewing with adolescents and young adults. In: Miller W, Rollnick S, editors. Motivational interviewing: preparing people for change. New York: Guilford; 2002. p. 320–32.
3. Arnett J. The developmental context of substance use in emerging adulthood. J Drug Issues. 2005;35:235–53. doi:10.1177/002204260503500202.
4. Casswell S, Pledger M, Pratap S. Trajectories of drinking from 18 to 26 years: identification and prediction. Addiction. 2002;97:1427–37.
5. Johnston LD, O'Malley PM, Bachman JG, Schulenberg JE. Monitoring the Future National Survey results on drug use, 1975–2003 (NIH Publication No. 04-5508). Bethesda: Department of Health and Human Services. 2003. http://monitoringthefuture.org/pubs/monographs/vol2_2003.pdf. Accessed 3 Oct 2015.
6. Auerbach KA, Collins LM. A multidimensional developmental model of alcohol use during emerging adulthood. J Stud Alcohol. 2006;67(6):917–25.
7. Cleveland MJ, Lanza ST, Ray AE, Turrisi R, Mallet KA. Transitions in first-year college student drinking behaviors: does pre-college drinking moderate the effects of parent- and peer-based intervention components? Psychol Addict Behav. 2012;26(3):440–50.
8. Cleveland MJ, Mallett KA, White HR, Turrisi R, Favero S. Patterns of alcohol use and related consequences in non-college-attending emerging adults. J Stud Alcohol. 2013;74:84–93.
9. Henson JM, Pearson MR, Carey KB. Defining and characterizing differences in college alcohol intervention efficacy: a growth mixture modeling application. J Consult Clin Psychol. 2015;83:370–81.
10. Schulenberg JE, Magos JL. A developmental perspective on alcohol use and heavy drinking during adolescence and the transition to young adulthood. J Stud Alcohol. 2002;14:54–70.
11. Flay B, Biglan A, Boruch R, Castro F, Gottfredson D, Kellam S, et al. Standards of evidence: criteria for efficacy, effectiveness, and dissemination. Prev Sci. 2005;6:151–75.
12. Jacobson N, Truax P. Clinical significance: a statistical approach to defining meaningful change in psychotherapy research. J Consult Clin Psychol. 1991;59:12–9.
13. Miller W, Rollnick S. Motivational interviewing: helping people change. 3rd ed. New York: Guilford Press; 2013.
14. Cronce J, Larimer M. Individual-focused approaches to the prevention of college student drinking. Alcohol Res Health. 2011;34:210–21.
15. Hustad J, Mastroleo N, Kong L, Urwin R, Zeman S, LaSalle L, et al. The comparative effectiveness of individual and group brief motivational

interventions for mandated college students. Psychol Addict Behav. 2014;28:74–84. doi:10.1037/a0034899.
16. Larimer M, Cronce J. Identification, prevention, and treatment: a review of individual-focused strategies to reduce problematic alcohol consumption by college students. J Stud Alcohol Suppl. 2002;14:148–63.
17. Larimer M, Cronce J. Identification, prevention, and treatment revisited: individual-focused college drinking prevention strategies 1999–2006. Addict Behav. 2007;32:2439–68. doi:10.1016/j.addbeh.2007.05.006.
18. Tanner-Smith E, Lipsey M. Brief alcohol interventions for adolescents and young adults: a systematic review and meta-analysis. J Subst Abuse Treat. 2015;51:1–18. doi:10.1016/j.jsat.2014.09.001.
19. Prochaska J, DiClemente C. Stages and processes of self-change of smoking: toward an integrative model of change. J Consult Clin Psychol. 1983;51(3):390–5.
20. Sheeran P. Intention-behavior relations: a conceptual and empirical review. Eur Rev Soc Psychol. 2002;12:1–36.
21. Fishbein M, Ajzen I. Belief, attitude, intention, and behavior: an introduction to theory and research. Reading: Addison-Wesley; 1975.
22. Ajzen I. The theory of planned behavior. Organ Behav Hum Decis. 1991;50:179–211.
23. Beadnell B, Nason M, Stafford P, Rosengren D, Daugherty R. Short-term outcomes of a motivation-enhancing approach to DUI intervention. Accid Anal Prev. 2012;45:792–801.
24. Beadnell B, Crisafulli MA, Stafford PA, Rosengren DB, DiClemente CC. Operating under the influence: three year recidivism rates for a motivation-enhancing intervention versus standard care programs. Accid Anal Prev. 2015;80:48–56.
25. Greenfield T, Kerr W. Alcohol measurement methodology in epidemiology: recent advances and opportunities. Addiction. 2008;103:1082–99.
26. Greenfield T, Nayak M, Bond J, Ye Y, Midanik L. Maximum quantity consumed and alcohol-related problems: assessing the most alcohol drunk with two measures. Alcohol Clin Exp Res. 2006;30:1576–82.
27. Rosengren DB, Beadnell B, Nason M, Stafford P, Daugherty R. Reports of past alcohol and drug use following participation in a motivation enhancing intervention: implications for clinical assessment and program evaluation. Subst Abuse Treat Prev Policy. 2012;7:19.
28. Stinchfield R. Measurement, instruments, scales, and tests: reliability of adolescent self-reported pretreatment alcohol and other drug use. Subst Use Misuse. 1997;32(4):425–34.
29. Del Boca FK, Darkes J. The validity of self-reports of alcohol consumption: state of the science and challenges for research. Addiction. 2003;98:1–12.
30. Daugherty R, O'Bryan T. PRIME for life instructor manual version 8. Lexington: Prevention Research Institute; 2004.
31. Daugherty R, Leukefeld C. Risk reduction strategies to prevent alcohol and drug problems in adulthood. In: Gullotta T, Bloom M, editors. The encyclopedia of primary prevention and health promotion. New York: Kluwer Academic/Plenum Publishers; 2003. p. 1079–86.
32. DiClemente C. Addiction and change: how addictions develop and addicted people recover. New York: Guilford Press; 2003.
33. Petty R, Brinol P. Persuasion: from single to multiple metacognitive processes. Perspect Psychol Sci. 2008;3:137–47.
34. Collins LM, Lanza ST. Latent class and latent transition analysis. Hoboken: Wiley; 2010.
35. Muthén B, Satorra A. Complex sample data in structural equation modeling. Sociol Methodol. 1995;25:267–316.
36. Velasquez M, Crouch C, Stephens N, DiClemente C. Group treatment for substance use. New York: Guilford Press; 2015.

6

The association between age of onset of opioid use and comorbidity among opioid dependent patients receiving methadone maintenance therapy

Leen Naji[1†], Brittany Burns Dennis[2,3†], Monica Bawor[2], Michael Varenbut[4], Jeff Daiter[4], Carolyn Plater[4], Guillaume Pare[3], David C. Marsh[4,5], Andrew Worster[4,6], Dipika Desai[7], James MacKillop[11,12], Lehana Thabane[8,9,10] and Zainab Samaan[3,7,11,12*]

Abstract

Background: Opioid use disorder (OUD) affects approximately 21.9 million people worldwide. This study aims to determine the association between age of onset of opioid use and comorbid disorders, both physical and psychiatric, in patients receiving methadone maintenance treatment (MMT) for OUD. Understanding this association may inform clinical practice about important prognostic factors of patients on MMT, enabling clinicians to identify high-risk patients.

Methods: This study includes data collected between June 2011 and August 2016 for the Genetics of Opioid Addiction research collaborative between McMaster University and the Canadian Addiction Treatment Centers. All patients were interviewed by trained health professionals using the Mini-International Neuropsychiatric Interview and case report forms. Physical comorbidities were verified using patients' electronic medical records. A multi-variable logistic regression model was constructed to determine the strength of the association between age of onset of opioid use and the presence of physical or psychiatric comorbidity while adjusting for current age, sex, body mass index, methadone dose and smoking status.

Results: Data from 627 MMT patients with a mean age of 38.8 years (SD = 11.07) were analyzed. Individuals with an age of onset of opioid use younger than 18 years were found to be at higher odds for having a physical or psychiatric comorbid disorder compared to individuals with an age of onset of opioid use of 31 years or older (odds ratio 2.94, 95% confidence interval 1.20, 7.19, $p = 0.02$). A significant association was not found between the risk of having a comorbidity and an age of onset of opioid use between 18 and 25 years or 26 and 30 years, compared to an age of onset of opioid use of 31 years or older.

Conclusion: Our study demonstrates that the younger one begins to use opioids, the greater their chance of having a physical or psychiatric co-morbidity. Understanding the risk posed by an earlier onset of opioid use for the later development of comorbid disorders informs clinical practice about important prognostic predictors and aids in the identification of high-risk patients.

Keywords: Opioid use disorder, Risk prediction, Substance use, Methadone, Opioid substitution treatment

*Correspondence: samaanz@mcmaster.ca
†Leen Naji and Brittany Burns Dennis contributed equally to this work
[12] Department of Psychiatry and Behavioural Neuroscience, McMaster University, 100 West 5th Street, Hamilton, ON L8N 3K7, Canada
Full list of author information is available at the end of the article

Background

Opioid use disorder (OUD) is a serious health concern associated with significant morbidity and mortality [1]. It is the second most prevalent illicit drug use disorder, affecting approximately 21.9 million people worldwide [1]. Despite evidence that the prevalence of pain has remained unchanged, the rate of opioid prescriptions has nearly quadrupled since 1999 [2]. Estimates based on The National Survey on Drug Use and Health indicate that 12.5 million people in the United States alone misused opioids in 2015, in addition to the 0.8 million people who misused heroin that year [3].

Previous research demonstrates a potential predictive association between the use of opioids and the presence of comorbidities, likely secondary to a variety of factors including chronic intoxication, poor hygiene, life style habits and risk-taking behavior [4–17]. For instance, the prevalence of human immunodeficiency virus (HIV) is found to be higher among opioid users compared to non-users, as is the prevalence of infections such as hepatitis and tuberculosis [16, 18, 19]. Several studies have also linked opioid use to serious cardiac abnormalities, such as infective endocarditis, and a higher rate of epileptic seizures [5, 6, 9, 13]. Additionally, opioid use has been associated with chronic pain, liver disease and mental health comorbidities, such as depression and anxiety disorders [4, 10, 12]. While these studies do not establish causation, potential pathophysiological processes contributing to the development of these comorbidities may be hypothesized. For instance, while infectious diseases may be associated with injecting drug use and risk-taking behavior, the neurological abnormalities are likely due to the neurotoxic effects of drug use leading to cerebral lesions [15].

Understanding the association between age of onset of opioid use and the presence of physical or psychiatric comorbidity has seldom been the primary focus of previous studies. While addiction medicine clinicians may argue that pretreatment opioid use history seems logically inherent as a predictor for future health complications, there is a paucity of well-powered studies to support such claims [5, 11, 15, 17, 20]. The rare times this issue is addressed in the literature, the primary focus is often the correlation between long substance use history and neurological deficits or infectious diseases. For instance, studies have demonstrated neurological abnormalities such as epilepsy, polyneuropathy, and pressure palsy increased with the duration of opioid use disorder [15]. Additionally, some studies have found an association between the duration of heroin use and the presence of comorbidities, including HIV and hepatitis C [17, 20].

Nevertheless, no study to date has addressed nor quantified the risk between age of onset of opioid use and the presence of physical or psychiatric comorbidities. Thus, the purpose of this study is to investigate this association using data from an on-going prospective cohort study. Understanding the association between the age of onset of opioid use and the presence of comorbid disorders informs clinical practice about important prognostic factors, enabling clinicians to identify high-risk patients. The opportunity to identify these patients would allow us to monitor them more closely, provide more intensive treatment strategies as well as preventative measures to reduce the risk of them developing a disease and/or progressing in their course of illness. These findings may also help to educate the public on the risks of opioid use above and beyond the direct effects of drug use, as well as identify modifiable factors that may increase the future risk of comorbidity in patients with OUD.

Methods

This study was approved by the Hamilton Integrated Research Ethics Board (11-056). We used data collected primarily for the Genetics of Opioid Addiction (GENOA), a research collaborative between the Canadian Addiction Treatment Center (CATC, formerly known as the Ontario Addition Treatment Centre and home to the largest network of methadone clinics in North America) and McMaster University [21]. CATC clinical sites follow the same treatment strategy and are managed centrally. In order to be included in our study, participants had to be 18 years of age or older, had to provide written informed consent, and had to have been receiving methadone maintenance treatment (MMT) for OUD as defined in the Fifth Edition of the diagnostic and statistical manual of mental disorders (DSM-5) [22]. All study participants were interviewed by trained health care professionals between June 2011 and August 2016. Previously piloted case report forms were used to obtain patient data, and physical comorbidities were confirmed using patients' electronic medical records [21]. To be included, participants must have also completed the Mini-International Neuropsychiatric Interview (M.I.N.I.) at the time of inclusion into the study, which was used to determine psychiatric comorbidities [23]. For this study, 683 patients met the eligibility criteria for inclusion (Fig. 1).

Our primary outcome was the composite of a physical or psychiatric co-morbid disorder. Physical comorbidities were identified through self-report and patients' electronic medical records, and included HIV, hepatitis, liver disease, chronic pain and epilepsy, among others. Psychiatric diagnoses were ascertained based on the M.I.N.I. Patients were also required to complete a baseline questionnaire, providing details about their age of onset of opioid use, the duration of time they have been receiving

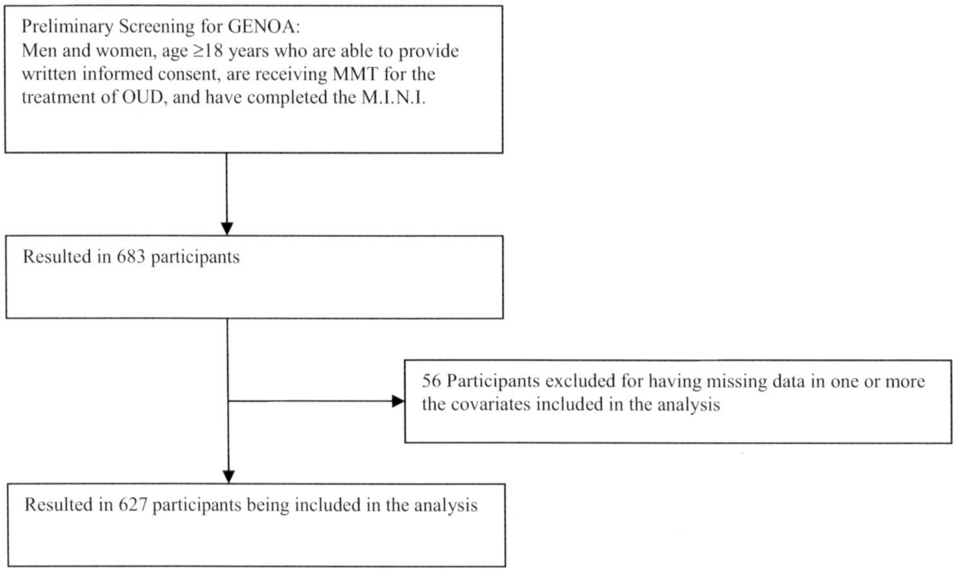

Fig. 1 GENOA: eligibility screening and inclusion flow diagram for participant selection

MMT and their current methadone dose, prescribed and non-prescribed medications, as well as illicit substance use [21].

Statistical analysis

We used descriptive statistics to summarize the participants' demographic and baseline characteristics. We expressed continuous variables using mean [standard deviation (SD)] and categorical variables using percent. We performed the primary analysis by regressing the presence of a physical or psychiatric comorbidity, as composite outcome, onto the age of onset of opioid use after categorizing age of onset of opioid use into four categories: Children: 17 years and younger (n = 119), youth: 18–25 years of age (n = 244), young adults: 26–30 years of age (n = 97), and 31 years of age and older (n = 167). We conducted the regression such that each category is compared to the reference group of 31 years of age and older. We adjusted for important potential cofounders, specifically current age, sex, methadone dose, BMI and smoking status. Older age is known to be associated with more comorbidities [24]. Additionally, the prevalence of many psychiatric disorders such as depression and physical comorbidities such as chronic pain are more prevalent in women than men [25–31]. High doses of methadone are associated with prolonged QTc intervals and arrhythmias such as Torsades de pointes [32, 33]. Smokers and obese individuals are also at heightened risk for numerous serious comorbidities, including coronary artery disease and strokes [34, 35].

We performed secondary analyses investigating the association between the age of onset of opioid use and the presence of physical or psychiatric comorbidity, separately, while still adjusting for the aforementioned covariates as in the primary analysis.

We employed Stata 13 to complete the logistic regression analyses [36]. All study data have been quality checked and entered into Research Electronic Data Capture (RedCap) database at the Population Genomics Program, Chanchlani Research Centre, McMaster University server [37].

Results

Participants' characteristics

Of the 683 participants eligible for inclusion into our study, those with missing values for one or more of the covariates analyzed were dropped from the analysis (n = 56). Therefore, we analyzed data from 627 subjects. Please refer to Fig. 1 for the participants' inclusion diagram. The mean current age of participants was 38.8 years (SD = 11.1), more than half of whom were males (54.9%) (Table 1). The mean age of onset of opioid use was 25.6 years (SD = 8.8). The majority of participants (86.3%) had at least one comorbid physical or psychiatric disorder. Most (68.3%) participants were found to have at least one comorbid physical disorder, with chronic pain and hepatitis being the most common comorbidities (40.2 and 22.5% of participants, respectively). Additionally, 57.7% of participants were diagnosed with a psychiatric disorder, the majority of which constituted an anxiety disorder (33.8% of participants).

Table 1 Baseline participant characteristics (total N = 627)

	Mean (SD)	Median (IQR)
Participant characteristic		
Current age (years)	38.8 (11.1)	37.0 (19.0)
Methadone dose (mg/day)	77.24 (46.10)	70.00 (55.00)
Age of onset of opioid use (years)	25.6 (8.8)	24.0 (13.0)
BMI (kg/m^2)	27.92 (8.88)	26.03 (7.76)
	Percentage of total (N)	
Female	45.1 (283)	
Current smoking	84.5 (530)	
Participants with ≥1 comorbidity	86.3 (541)	
Participants with physical comorbidity[a]	68.3 (428)	
Participants with psychiatric comorbidity[b]	57.7 (362)	
Age of onset of opioid use categories		
17 years and younger	19.0 (119)	
18–25 years	38.9 (244)	
26–30 years	15.5 (97)	
31 years and older	26.6 (167)	

[a] The physical comorbidities comprising the composite outcome included chronic pain (n = 252), epilepsy (n = 16), hepatitis (n = 141), liver disease (n = 31), HIV (n = 3), pulmonary disorders such as asthma and chronic obstructive pulmonary disorder (n = 52), diabetes mellitus type I or type II (n = 33), cardiovascular history including hypertension or cardiomyopathy (n = 33), arthritis (n = 25), inflammatory bowel disease (n = 6), endocrine disorders including hypothyroidism and hyperthyroidism (n = 15), cancer (n = 6), renal disorders (n = 5), neurological disorders including neuropathies and multiple sclerosis (n = 20), endometriosis (n = 7), dermatological disorders including eczema and psoriasis (n = 2), inactive TB (n = 2), and syphilis (n = 1)

[b] The psychiatric comorbidities comprising the composite outcome included mood disorders such as depression and mania (n = 87), anxiety disorders such as generalized anxiety and obsessive compulsive disorder (n = 212), substance use disorders other than opioids (n = 83), psychotic disorders (n = 24), eating disorders (n = 4), antisocial personality disorder (n = 144)

Primary outcome

We determined the strength of the association between age of onset of opioid use and the presence of physical or psychiatric comorbidity using a multi-variable logistic regression model. A summary of our results is provided in Table 2. Younger age of onset was significantly correlated to the presence of a physical or psychiatric comorbidity, when adjusting for current age, sex, BMI, methadone dose and smoking status (Table 2). These results indicate that the risk of comorbidity is highest in those who started using opioids before 18 years of age, as they were almost three-fold more likely of to have a physical or psychiatric comorbidity compared to those who began using opioids at the age of 31 and older (odds ratio (OR) 2.94, 95% confidence interval (CI) 1.20, 7.19, $p = 0.02$). As expected, current age was also found to be significantly associated with physical or psychiatric comorbidity, implying that older individuals are at higher risk for the presence of a comorbidity (OR 1.05, 95% CI 1.02, 1.08, $p < 0.01$). Finally, women were more likely to have a physical or psychiatric comorbidity than men (OR 1.70, 95% CI 1.04, 2.75, $p = 0.03$).

Table 2 Multivariable logistic regression analysis: the presence of physical or psychiatric comorbidity (N = 627)

	Odds ratio, (95% confidence interval)	*p* value
Covariates		
Current age (years)	1.05 (1.02, 1.08)	<0.01*
Sex	1.70 (1.04, 2.75)	0.03
BMI	1.02 (0.99, 1.06)	0.19
Methadone dose (mg/day)	1.00 (1.00, 1.01)	0.77
Smoking status	1.56 (0.85, 2.88)	0.15
Age of onset of opioid use categories (in reference to 31 years and older)		
17 years old and younger	2.94 (1.20, 7.19)	0.02
18–25 years	1.71 (0.83, 3.51)	0.14
26–30 years	2.05 (0.89, 4.74)	0.09

56 eligible participants were excluded from the multi-variable regression analysis for having missing values for one or more of the covariates of interest. As such, 167, 97, 244 and 119 patients from the 31 years and older, 26–30 years, 18–25 years, and 17 years and younger subgroups were included in the analysis, respectively

* <0.01 = 0.002

Of note, our secondary analyses revealed that an age of onset of opioid use of younger than 18 years of age was significantly associated with an increased risk of having both a physical (OR 2.39, 95% CI 1.18, 4.85, $p = 0.02$) and psychiatric (OR 1.97, 95% CI 1.14, 3.40, $p = 0.02$) comorbidity, compared to those who began using opioids after the age of 30.

Discussion

Our study revealed that within a sample of patients receiving MMT for OUD, there exists a significant association between the age of onset of opioid use and the presence of one or more psychiatric or physical comorbidity, including but not limited to anxiety disorder, chronic pain, liver disease, epilepsy, HIV and hepatitis. In other words, our study demonstrates that within this population, the younger one begins to use opioids, the greater their chance of having a physical or psychiatric co-morbidity.

If an earlier age of onset of opioid use is assumed to implicate a longer duration of substance use, the findings of our present study would be in accordance with the limited available literature investigating the association between duration of opioid use and the presence of a physical comorbidity [5, 11, 15, 17]. These investigations have found a positive association between duration of opioid use and the presence of neurological abnormalities or an HCV positive status [5, 11, 15, 17].

Additionally, our study is the first to quantify the association between the odds of having comorbidity and the age of onset of opioid use. Our results demonstrate that an age of onset of opioid use younger than 18 years of age is significantly associated with an increased likelihood of having a psychiatric comorbidity, compared to an age of onset beyond 30. Though we cannot claim causality due to the cross-sectional design of this study, the association between psychiatric comorbidity and a younger age of onset of opioid use may be explained by the fact that adolescence represents a period of time in which the brain is subject to critical neurochemical and functional changes, as well as maturing behavior and cognition [38]. Psychosocial and environmental factors, including drug use, are thought to interfere with this stage of development and may ultimately impact mental health [39]. Additionally, there exists a body of evidence that supports the presence of a positive correlation between drug use, including opioids, and psychiatric comorbidities other than substance use disorder [40–42].

Moreover, our study found that women with OUD were more likely than men to have a physical or psychiatric comorbidity. This is consistent with previously published literature which has found that women are more severely affected by the deleterious effects of drug use on physical and mental health [26, 29]. This may be explained by the fact many psychiatric disorders, including major depression and generalized anxiety disorder, are more prevalent in women than men in the general population [25, 27, 28]. As well, a study by Grella et al. [28] has found that this difference in prevalence is accentuated in patients with OUD. Moreover, chronic pain, which is the most prevalent physical comorbidity included in our composite outcome, is also more commonly found in women than in men in the general population [30, 31].

This study adds to the field of addiction by addressing age of onset of opioid use as a risk factor for concurrent physical ailments and psychiatric disorders in patients with OUD on MMT. Several factors render our study unique amongst the available literature on this topic, allowing us to draw more reliable conclusions from our findings. This study included a large sample size of a clinical population receiving standardized MMT across multiple different sites. Second, our investigation obtained an older sample of participants, where the mean age of participants was 38.8 years. This is in contrast to the available literature, which primarily focuses on opioid users in their mid-twenties [5, 11, 14, 15, 17]. Studying an older age group provides us with the opportunity to gain a better understanding of the risks associated with a longer duration of opioid use, as well as a better chance of identifying physical and psychiatric comorbidities that may not be captured in a younger cohort.

Limitations

There are specific limitations of studying OUD, one being the multifaceted nature of addiction itself. There are numerous ways in which confounding can inevitably influence the results obtained during this study. OUD involves a complex network of variables all of which unavoidably modify individual patient health outcomes. It is important to note that this study has taken time to outline the most important confounders and adjust for them, however the complex social conditions which surround each individual patient can as might be expected, be construed as a primary contributor to their health outcome. We acknowledge that these exposures investigated in this study are only a piece of the larger network of factors that impact OUD patients' health outcomes.

Additionally, the cross sectional nature of this study is a factor that may compromise the quality of the evidence obtained. We are unable to establish a temporal relationship between the age of onset of opioid use and the presence of comorbid disorders. An inception cohort study design would be ideal to establish the age of onset of opioid use and ensuring all participants were free of physical and psychiatric comorbidity at baseline. However, following patients from the onset of opioid use onto the development of addiction may prove both unethical and unfeasible given the need for early intervention if addiction is suspected and the potential high attrition rate.

Finally, our comorbidity outcome was dichotomized which may take away from the magnitude of the burden of certain diseases. Now that we have established that an association does exist, we encourage future research to investigate the association between age of onset of opioid use and 10-year mortality risk or quality of life, using surrogate outcomes such as the Charlson Comorbidity Index [43].

Conclusion

Our study identified a significant association between age of onset of opioid use and the presence of a physical or psychiatric comorbidity in patients receiving MMT for OUD. Specifically, a younger age of onset was found to be associated with an increased likelihood of having a physical and/or psychiatric comorbidity. The results of this study may serve to enhance therapeutic guidelines for patients receiving MMT by identifying high-risk patient groups and addressing them accordingly. The opportunity to identify these patients would allow us to monitor them more closely, provide more intensive treatment strategies as well as implement preventative measures to reduce the risk of them developing a disease and/or progressing in their course of illness.

Abbreviations

MMT: methadone maintenance therapy; OUD: opioid use disorder; HIV: human immunodeficiency virus; GENOA: Genetics of Opioid Addiction; CATC: Canadian Addiction Treatment Center; DSM-5: diagnostic and statistical manual of mental disorders; M.I.N.I.: Mini-International Neuropsychiatric Interview; RedCap: Research Electronic Data Capture.

Authors' contributions

Conceived and designed the experiments: LN, BBD, LT, ZS. Analyzed the data: BBD, MB, LN, ZS. Wrote the first draft of the manuscript: LN, BBD, MB, ZS. Contributed to the writing of the final manuscript, made critical revisions and approved the final results and conclusions: LN, BBD, MB, MV, JD, CP, GP, DCM, AW, DD, JM, LT, ZS. All authors reviewed and approved of the final manuscript.

Author details

[1] Michael Degroote School of Medicine, McMaster University, Hamilton, Canada. [2] St. George's University of London, London, UK. [3] Department of Clinical Epidemiology and Biostatistics, McMaster University, Hamilton, Canada. [4] Canadian Addiction Treatment Centres, Richmond Hill, Canada. [5] Northern Ontario School of Medicine, Sudbury, ON, Canada. [6] Department of Medicine, Hamilton General Hospital, Hamilton, Canada. [7] Population Genomic Program, Chanchalani Research Centre, McMaster University, Hamilton, Canada. [8] Departments of Pediatrics and Anesthesia, McMaster University, Hamilton, Canada. [9] Centre for Evaluation of Medicine, St Joseph's Healthcare, Hamilton, Canada. [10] Biostatistics Unit, Father Sean O'Sullivan Research Centre, St Joseph's Healthcare, Hamilton, Canada. [11] Peter Boris Centre for Addictions Research, Hamilton, Canada. [12] Department of Psychiatry and Behavioural Neuroscience, McMaster University, 100 West 5th Street, Hamilton, ON L8N 3K7, Canada.

Acknowledgements

We sincerely appreciate the effort contributed by several parties in the completion of this Project. First, this project would not have been possible without the great collaboration cemented between GENOA and the CATC network of clinical sites. We would like to sincerely thank all the participants from the GENOA and CATC facilities who generously donated their time, information and samples, without them this study would not be possible. We would also like to extend our earnest appreciation to the GENOA and CATC clinical staff for all their great efforts in patient recruitment and data collection. We would like to thank Jacqueline Hudson for her great dedication as the research assistant on the GENOA team. Finally, we would like to thank the McMaster University undergraduate team of students, including Sindoora Iyer, Anuja Bhalerao, Herman Bami and Andrew Kamphuis, who contributed a great deal of time in helping with data entry and quality control.

Competing interests

The authors declare that they have no competing interests.

Funding

This work was funded by the Canadian Institutes for Health Research (CIHR) Drug Safety and Effectiveness Network grant (Grant Number: 126639). Brittany B. Dennis and Monica Bawor are supported by the Intersections of Mental Health Perspectives in Addiction Research Training fellowship, supported by CIHR and the British Columbia Centre of Excellence for Women's Health. This work was also supported by the Peter Boris Centre for Addiction Research and Chanchlani Research Centre. The funders had no role in the design or execution of the study, collection or analysis of the data, and preparation or review of the manuscript.

References

1. UN Office on Drugs and Crime (UNODC). World Drug Report 2010 (United Nations, Publication, Sales No. E.10.XI.13). http://www.unodc.org/documents/wdr/WDR_2010/World_Drug_Report_2010_lo-res.pdf. Accessed 20 Dec 2016.
2. Center for Disease Control and Prevention: Opioid Basics. Understanding the epidemic. http://www.cdc.gov/drugoverdose/epidemic/ (2016). Accessed 20 Dec 2016.
3. Center for Behavioral Health Statistics and Quality. 2015 National Survey on Drug Use and Health: Detailed Tables. Rockville: Substance Abuse and Mental Health Services Administration; 2016.
4. Amari E, Rehm J, Goldner E, Fischer B. Nonmedical prescription opioid use and mental health and pain comorbidities: a narrative review. Can J Psychiatry Revue canadienne de psychiatrie. 2011;56(8):495–502.
5. Basu D, Banerjee A, Harish T, Mattoo SK. Disproportionately high rate of epileptic seizure in patients abusing dextropropoxyphene. Am J Addict Am Acad Psychiatr Alcohol Addict. 2009;18(5):417–21.
6. Chong E, Poh KK, Shen L, Yeh IB, Chai P. Infective endocarditis secondary to intravenous Subutex abuse. Singapore Med J. 2009;50(1):34–42.
7. Cicero TJ, Surratt HL, Kurtz S, Ellis MS, Inciardi JA. Patterns of prescription opioid abuse and comorbidity in an aging treatment population. J Subst Abuse Treat. 2012;42(1):87–94.
8. Ghate SR, Haroutiunian S, Winslow R, McAdam-Marx C. Cost and comorbidities associated with opioid abuse in managed care and Medicaid patients in the United Stated: a comparison of two recently published studies. J Pain Palliat Care Pharmacother. 2010;24(3):251–8.
9. Ho RC, Ho EC, Tan CH, Mak A. Pulmonary hypertension in first episode infective endocarditis among intravenous buprenorphine users: case report. Am J Drug Alcohol Abuse. 2009;35(3):199–202.
10. Jensen-Dahm C, Gasse C, Astrup A, Mortensen PB, Waldemar G. Frequent use of opioids in patients with dementia and nursing home residents—a study of the entire elderly population of Denmark. Alzheimer's Dement J Alzheimer's Assoc. 2014;11(6):691–9.
11. Jovanovic-Cupic V, Martinovic Z, Nesic N. Seizures associated with intoxication and abuse of tramadol. Clin Toxicol. 2006;44(2):143–6.
12. Kobus AM, Smith DH, Morasco BJ, et al. Correlates of higher-dose opioid medication use for low back pain in primary care. J Pain Official J Am Pain Soc. 2012;13(11):1131–8.
13. Manninen PH. Opioids and seizures. Can J Anaesth Journal canadien d'anesthesie. 1997;44(5 Pt 1):463–6.
14. Mattoo SK, Singh SM, Bhardwaj R, Kumar S, Basu D, Kulhara P. Prevalence and correlates of epileptic seizure in substance-abusing subjects. Psychiatry Clin Neurosci. 2009;63(4):580–2.
15. Paur R, Wallner C, Hermann P, Stollberger C, Finsterer J. Neurological abnormalities in opiate addicts with and without substitution therapy. Am J Drug Alcohol Abuse. 2012;38(3):239–45.
16. Zhang L, Zhang D, Chen W, Zou X, Ling L. High prevalence of HIV, HCV and tuberculosis and associated risk behaviours among new entrants of methadone maintenance treatment clinics in Guangdong Province, China. PLoS ONE. 2013;8(10):e76931.
17. Roux P, Fugon L, Jones JD, Comer SD. Hepatitis C infection in non-treatment-seeking heroin users: the burden of cocaine injection. Am J Addict Am Acad Psychiatr Alcohol Addict. 2013;22(6):613–8.
18. Klepser ME, Klepser TB. Drug treatment of HIV-related opportunistic infections. Drugs. 1997;53(1):40–73.
19. Sulkowski MS, Mast EE, Seeff LB, Thomas DL. Hepatitis C virus infection as an opportunistic disease in persons infected with human immunodeficiency virus. Clin Infect Dis. 2000;30(Suppl 1):S77–84.
20. Han B, Gfroerer JC, Colliver JD. Associations between duration of illicit drug use and health conditions: results from the 2005–2007 national surveys on drug use and health. Ann Epidemiol. 2010;20(4):289–97.
21. Samaan Z, Bawor M, Dennis BB, et al. Genetic influence on methadone treatment outcomes in patients undergoing methadone maintenance treatment for opioid addiction: a pilot study. Neuropsychiatr Dis Treat. 2014;10:1503–8.
22. Association AP. Diagnostic and statistical manual of mental disorders. 5th ed. Arlington: VAPPO; 2013.

23. Sheehan DV, Lecrubier Y, Sheehan KH, et al. The Mini-International Neuropsychiatric Interview (M.I.N.I.): the development and validation of a structured diagnostic psychiatric interview for DSM-IV and ICD-10. J Clin Psychiatry. 1998;59(Suppl 20):22–3.
24. Piccirillo JF, Vlahiotis A, Barrett LB, Flood KL, Spitznagel EL, Steyerberg EW. The changing prevalence of comorbidity across the age spectrum. Crit Rev Oncol Hematol. 2008;67(2):124–32.
25. Grant BF, Weissman MM. Gender and the prevalence of psychiatric disorders. In: Narrow WE, First MB, Sirovatk M, Regier DA, editors. Age and gender considerations in psychiatric diagnosis: a research agenda for DSM-V. Arlington: American Psychiatric Association; 2007. p. 31–45.
26. Center for Disease Control and Prevention. Prescription painkiller overdoses: a growing epidemic, especially among women. http://www.cdc.gov/vitalsigns/prescriptionpainkilleroverdoses/index.html (2013). Accessed 21 Dec 2016.
27. World Health Organization. Gender and women's mental health. http://www.who.int/mental_health/prevention/genderwomen/en/ (2016). Accessed 21 Dec 2016.
28. Grella CE, Karno MP, Warda US, Niv N, Moore AA. Gender and comorbidity among individuals with opioid use disorders in the NESARC study. Addict Behav. 2009;34(6–7):498–504.
29. Hernandez-Avila CA, Rounsaville BJ, Kranzler HR. Opioid-, cannabis- and alcohol-dependent women show more rapid progression to substance abuse treatment. Drug Alcohol Depend. 2004;74(3):265–72.
30. Johannes CB, Le TK, Zhou X, Johnston JA, Dworkin RH. The prevalence of chronic pain in United States adults: results of an Internet-based survey. J Pain. 2010;11(11):1230–9.
31. van Hecke O, Torrance N, Smith BH. Chronic pain epidemiology and its clinical relevance. Br J Anaesth. 2013;111(1):13–8.
32. Krantz MJ, Lewkowiez L, Hays H, Woodroffe MA, Robertson AD, Mehler PS. Torsade de pointes associated with very-high-dose methadone. Ann Intern Med. 2002;137(6):501–4.
33. Kreek MJ, Borg L, Ducat E, Ray B. Pharmacotherapy in the treatment of addiction: methadone. J Addict Dis. 2010;29(2):200–16.
34. Center for Disease Control and Prevention: Fact Sheets. Health effects of cigarette smoking. http://www.cdc.gov/tobacco/data_statistics/fact_sheets/health_effects/effects_cig_smoking/ (2016). Accessed 20 Dec 2016.
35. Center for Disease Control and Prevention: Fact Sheets. Adult obesity causes and consequences. http://www.cdc.gov/obesity/adult/causes.html (2016). Accessed 20 Dec 2016.
36. StataCorp. Stata statistical software: release 13. TSL: College Station; 2013.
37. Harris PATR, Thielke R, Payne J, Gonzalez N, Conde JG. Research electronic data capture (REDCap)—a metadata-driven methodology and workflow process for providing translational research informatics support. J Biomed Inform. 2009;42(2):377–81.
38. Gomes FV, Rincon-Cortes M, Grace AA. Adolescence as a period of vulnerability and intervention in schizophrenia: insights from the MAM model. Neurosci Biobehav Rev. 2016;70:260–70.
39. Paus T, Keshavan M, Giedd JN. Why do many psychiatric disorders emerge during adolescence? Nat Rev Neurosci. 2008;9(12):947–57.
40. Kessler RC, Nelson CB, McGonagle KA, Edlund MJ, Frank RG, Leaf PJ. The epidemiology of co-occurring addictive and mental disorders: implications for prevention and service utilization. Am J Orthopsychiatry. 1996;66(1):17–31.
41. Ross HE, Glaser FB, Germanson T. The prevalence of psychiatric disorders in patients with alcohol and other drug problems. Arch Gen Psychiatry. 1988;45(11):1023–31.
42. Vivek K, Dalal P, Trivedi J, Pankaj K. A study of psychiatric comorbidity in opioid dependence. Delhi Psychiatry J. 2010;13(1):86–8.
43. Charlson ME, Pompei P, Ales KL, MacKenzie CR. A new method of classifying prognostic comorbidity in longitudinal studies: development and validation. J Chronic Dis. 1987;40(5):373–83.

Feasibility of a computer-assisted social network motivational interviewing intervention for substance use and HIV risk behaviors for housing first residents

Karen Chan Osilla*, David P. Kennedy, Sarah B. Hunter and Ervant Maksabedian

Abstract

Background: Social networks play positive and negative roles in the lives of homeless people influencing their alcohol and/or other drug (AOD) and HIV risk behaviors.

Methods: We developed a four-session computer-assisted social network motivational interviewing intervention for homeless adults transitioning into housing. We examined the acceptability of the intervention among staff and residents at an organization that provides permanent supportive housing through iterative rounds of beta testing. Staff were 3 men and 3 women who were residential support staff (i.e., case managers and administrators). Residents were 8 men (7 African American, 1 Hispanic) and 3 women (2 African American, 1 Hispanic) who had histories of AOD and HIV risk behaviors. We conducted a focus group with staff who gave input on how to improve the delivery of the intervention to enhance understanding and receptivity among new residents. We conducted semi-structured qualitative interviews and collected self-report satisfaction data from residents.

Results: Three themes emerged over the course of the resident interviews. Residents reported that the intervention was helpful in discussing their social network, that seeing the visualizations was more impactful than just talking about their network, and that the intervention prompted thoughts about changing their AOD use and HIV risk networks.

Conclusions: This study is the first of its kind that has developed, with input from Housing First staff and residents, a motivational interviewing intervention that targets both the structure and composition of one's social network. These results suggest that providing visual network feedback with a guided motivational interviewing discussion is a promising approach to supporting network change.

ClinicalTrials.gov Identifier NCT02140359

Keywords: Social network intervention, HIV risk behaviors, Data visualization, Alcohol and other drug use, Homelessness, Housing First, Motivational interviewing, EgoWeb

Background

Substance use disorders and HIV infection are interrelated public health problems facing the homeless. An estimated 30–50 % of homeless adults experience alcohol and/or drug (AOD) use disorders [1, 2], and homeless persons have been found to have rates of HIV infection 3–9 times greater than those with stable housing [3]. While AOD use is a leading cause of homelessness, AOD use is exacerbated by the stress of being homeless and exposure to other people who use AODs [2, 4, 5].

Social networks play positive and negative roles in the lives of homeless people [6–8]. Social networks—naturally occurring groups of people—can influence an individual's health and behaviors through social comparison,

*Correspondence: karenc@rand.org
RAND Corporation, 1776 Main Street, PO Box 2138, Santa Monica, CA 90407-2138, USA

social sanctions and rewards, flows of information, support and resources, stress reduction, and socialization [9–12]. In the context of AOD and HIV risk behaviors, social networks can increase AOD use and HIV risk among those who are homeless, but also facilitate entry into AOD recovery programs and other healthy lifestyle changes [2, 4, 5, 13–16]. Continuous, recent homelessness is associated with the amount of AOD and HIV risk behaviors in social networks while total time spent homeless over a lifetime is associated with less dense and more disconnected networks (e.g., more isolated network members) [17]. Another study found that homeless individuals with co-occurring mental illness and substance use disorders experienced shrinking social networks, which reduced interactions with people who influenced them to use AOD, but also increased their social isolation and reduced their access to positive social resources, such as social support [14]. Thus, developing interventions that focus on social networks may assist individuals in supporting healthy behaviors.

Many social network interventions that target health improvement and behavior change utilize network analysis to identify techniques for spreading an intervention's impact throughout a group [18, 19]. Common techniques include identifying key individuals or sets of individuals (e.g., those most central to the network, those most popular) to spread the intervention or modifying links among members of a group to make the intervention spread much more efficiently [19]. Other social network intervention approaches that target AOD behavior change primarily promote modifications to network composition (i.e., the quality and type of individuals in a network; removing substance users from the network) [20–28]. These interventions do not address the *structure* of social networks (i.e., relationship between network members; "Do people in your network interact with each other? How often have these two people interacted?").

Addressing changes in network structure may be particularly important to homeless individuals transitioning into housing. Removing someone who drinks from a network is much easier if the person is disconnected from the rest of the network compared to someone who is highly interconnected. How these people are connected to each other (e.g., Are their new neighbors connected to their high-risk street contacts?) may impact how well they are able to negotiate this change. An intervention that focuses on both network composition (e.g., people they interact with that use AODs) and structure (e.g., people in one's network who could meet one another to form a new support group) may help individuals make informed choices about their social interactions. To our knowledge, there are no interventions that take into account both compositional and structural characteristics of social networks targeting homeless individuals transitioning to housing.

The style in which network information is conveyed may be as important as the content itself. Motivational interviewing (MI) is a conversational style that is often used by facilitators conducting interventions that target AOD and risk behaviors. A facilitator that uses MI is collaborative and nonjudgmental, and focuses on strengthening the client's own motivation and commitment to change [29]. The four processes of MI emphasize client engagement (establishing a helpful relationship, understanding barriers and reasons to change), focusing (identifying change area, and setting an agenda), evocation (eliciting the client's motivation to change and building their self-efficacy), and planning (developing a commitment to change and formulating an action plan). We are aware of one recently developed MI intervention enhanced with a social network component that found that female adolescents who received the intervention had fewer AOD and HIV risk behaviors compared to those who did not receive the intervention at 1 month follow-up [27]. In this intervention, about 5 min were spent describing each of the network members the teens named and their association with substance use risk and support/encouragement. To our knowledge, visualizations were not presented, the intervention was developed for and tested with a limited sample of participants (i.e., female adolescents), and did not address network structure.

The current intervention extends this previous work by developing a computer-assisted social network intervention for homeless adults transitioning into housing. The intervention is computer or tablet-assisted so that a facilitator can collect personal network information from the participant, show visualizations of their social network immediately afterwards, and discuss potential areas of change using MI. The current paper describes the acceptability (likes/dislikes, ease of use, and helpfulness) of the intervention among residential support staff and formerly homeless people with histories of AOD and HIV risk behaviors.

Methods

Setting

This study was conducted in collaboration with Skid Row Housing Trust (SRHT), one of the largest Housing First providers in Los Angeles County. SRHT manages 22 buildings with over 1700 individual units, many of which provide housing plus support to residents (i.e., permanent supportive housing). Housing First programs provide housing without requiring AOD abstinence for new residents [30–32]. Studies have demonstrated that HF residents have similar [33] or improved [32, 34] AOD outcomes after 1–2 years compared to residents who receive AOD treatment first, and reduced health service expenses compared to those on waiting lists [35]. The current Housing First program provides permanent supportive housing (PSH), which are housing units that are supported by the U.S. Department of Housing and Urban Development (HUD). To be eligible for a PSH unit, an individual must meet the definition of chronic homelessness (i.e., an individual with a disabling condition who has been continuously homeless for a year or more, or has had at least 4 episodes of homelessness in the past 3 years).

Participants and procedures

Overview

We conducted a 4-step iterative process to develop and evaluate the acceptability of the intervention. First, we conducted a focus group with staff (n = 6) to show them a draft of our intervention and discuss how residents might respond. Second, we role-played a first session with long-term residents (n = 6) who had resided in PSH for more than 1 year, and then conducted a focus group with these long-term residents to ascertain their acceptability of the session. Third, long-term residents and case managers nominated new residents (n = 5) with current AOD concerns, and we conducted a first session with each of them who provided us feedback on the acceptability of the intervention. Finally, a subset of these new residents (n = 3) then returned for a second session and provided feedback again. We revised the intervention iteratively between each step and obtained feedback on successive versions of the intervention.

Staff focus group

First, we recruited six residential support staff who were case managers, program managers, and administrators at SRHT. These staff members were nominated by the organization's Resident Services Director for their diverse experience in assisting individuals entering permanent supportive housing. Participants were 3 men (2 Caucasian, 1 Hispanic) and 3 women (1 Caucasian, 1 African American, 1 Hispanic). Prior to beta-testing the intervention with residents, we developed a draft of the intervention to obtain staff feedback. The goals of the focus group were to discuss the logistics of the intervention process and obtain feedback about how they thought residents would respond to the intervention. We described the structure and content of the intervention including how the intervention visualizations would look, the intervention schedule, and how we would use tablets to deliver the intervention. We then role-played a mock intervention session, reviewed each of the intervention visualizations for feedback, and explored if the wording or visualizations were difficult to understand or may present problems if used in an intervention session with a resident. We requested their feedback on the language, structure, and presentation. Staff spoke from their professional capacity and verbally consented to the group discussion, which was audio taped and later transcribed.

Resident data collection

After the staff focus group session, we then conducted 3 rounds of beta testing (1 round with long-term residents and 2 rounds with new residents). First, we conducted individual interviews and then a focus group with long-term residents (n = 6) who had resided in SRHT for more than 1 year and residents with less PSH experience. These long-term residents were also peer advocates (i.e., employed by the housing provider to provide support to other residents) and had close contact with many new SRHT residents, and had past experience transitioning to PSH from homelessness. These residents completed a consent-to-contact form that allowed research staff to contact them by phone to schedule an in-person session. Long-term residents included 5 African American men and 1 Hispanic woman. All six long-term residents agreed to participate. At their session, each resident was asked to do three things. First, each resident participated in a role-play with one of the research staff members. Then, each resident was asked to role-play a new resident with risky AOD use and/or sexual risk behaviors while the research staff member facilitated one intervention session. After the session, the resident was asked to provide feedback about their experience. Finally, we conducted a focus group with all the long-term residents to gather collective feedback including the strengths and weaknesses of the intervention, and their perception of the acceptability and feasibility of the intervention for use with new residents. Participants were paid $25 for their participation.

We then revised the intervention by incorporating feedback from the long-term residents and conducted two rounds of individual interviews with new residents (n = 5) who had recently entered housing (< 6 months). These residents were nominated by long-term residents and case managers because of their previous or current AOD and/or HIV risk behaviors. All new residents that were nominated expressed interest by completing a consent-to-contact form. Participants included 3 men (2 African American, 1 Hispanic) and 2 women (2 African American). In the first round of beta-testing, we conducted the first intervention session with 5 participants, interviewed each participant after the session, and then asked them to complete a satisfaction survey. These sessions lasted between 45 and 60 min. After receiving this round of feedback, we revised the intervention, and then conducted a second intervention session with 3 of the 5 participants (we were unable to schedule the remaining 2 within our timeframe). Afterwards, we also conducted a debriefing interview with each participant and asked them to complete the satisfaction survey. A total of 3 facilitators led the Motivational Network Intervention (MNI) sessions with these residents, and the debriefing interviews were led by a different person by phone or in-person. The main purpose of this last round of beta-testing was to test the technology linking the sessions (e.g., if goals generated from the first session displayed correctly in the second session). All interviews were audio taped and followed a written protocol of open-ended questions. Participants were paid $25 per session, for a total of up to $50 for two sessions. All procedures were approved by the researchers' Institutional Review Board.

Intervention conceptual framework

The proposed Motivational Network Intervention (MNI) is grounded in social network theories (complex systems and social capital theories) and theories central to the MI approach [36]. The MNI targets social network structure and composition and how these are related to high-risk behaviors, such as AOD use and HIV risk behavior. Complex systems and social capital theories as applied to social networks assume that a set of social relationships between individuals in a group has emergent properties that would not be apparent in an examination of the individual parts of a larger social system [37–39] and that this system can produce positive or negative impacts on behavior [40]. These theories also suggest that changes made in one area of the system may have effects that flow throughout the rest of the system and that approaches to change should consider the potential impact on the whole system [39]. The theory of self-determination emphasizes individual autonomy and innate capacity for growth and change [41, 42]. Self-efficacy theory indicates that people with more confidence in their ability to change their behavior are more likely to change [43]. These theories are consistent with the style of MI that focuses on emphasizing an individual's autonomy and building intrinsic motivation [29]. Together, these theories suggest that an intervention that presents residents with personalized network information using a MI style may empower them to change their social environment leading to changes in their behaviors.

Intervention

Ultimately, we developed a computer-assisted intervention and a facilitator's guidebook that assists facilitators in delivering the intervention content in concert with the computer or tablet-assisted material. Consistent with the MI approach, the intervention was designed to accommodate individuals at varying levels of readiness to change including those who were not ready to change their risk behaviors and those who were ready. The MNI consists of 4 total sessions where each session is spaced about 2 weeks apart. We decided to develop a 4-session intervention to allow residents enough time to engage in network change strategies and for residents to see changes in their social networks between sessions. After developing the intervention, we beta-tested only the first two sessions with participants because the content of all the sessions was nearly identical and we primarily wanted to evaluate the content and see how repeated sessions (e.g., discussing the visualizations in sessions 1 and 2) affected the participant. The technology successfully worked during our last round of beta-testing and we did not receive any new suggestions for changing the intervention content, so we decided to stop our beta-testing. We also reasoned that following a client across the 4 sessions was more appropriate for our pilot study where we intend on evaluating the efficacy of the intervention.

Each MNI session lasted approximately 30 min and consisted of two parts: (1) A network interview with closed-ended network questions that covered the time period since their last interview (e.g., about 2 weeks) and, (2) a discussion of network visualizations facilitated by using MI. Structured network interview questions were open-ended to generate names of people in their network (e.g., "List 10 people you have interacted with in the past 2 weeks"), network composition (e.g., "How likely will (Alter 1) use alcohol or drugs in the next 2 weeks?" "Did you ever drink more alcohol than you wanted with (Alter 1)?"), and network structure questions (e.g., "Does (Alter 1) know (Alter 2)?"). Answers to these questions provided raw data to generate network visualizations. One advantage to the electronic interface was that questions could be skipped for any alters who were mentioned in previous interviews to avoid re-asking for information that does not change between interviews. For all alters named, facilitators asked participants a series of questions rating their recent relationship with the alter. For example, questions included how often they interacted, AOD use with the alter, sexual relations with the alter, and their supportive or negative interactions with the alters.

Once all network questions were asked and answered, facilitators led a discussion with the participant about the participant's social network in a MI style. They showed the participant a series of 4 network visualizations customized for the participant. The content of these visualizations were identical across the 4 sessions, but the "look" of the visualizations could change at each session depending on how much the participant's network

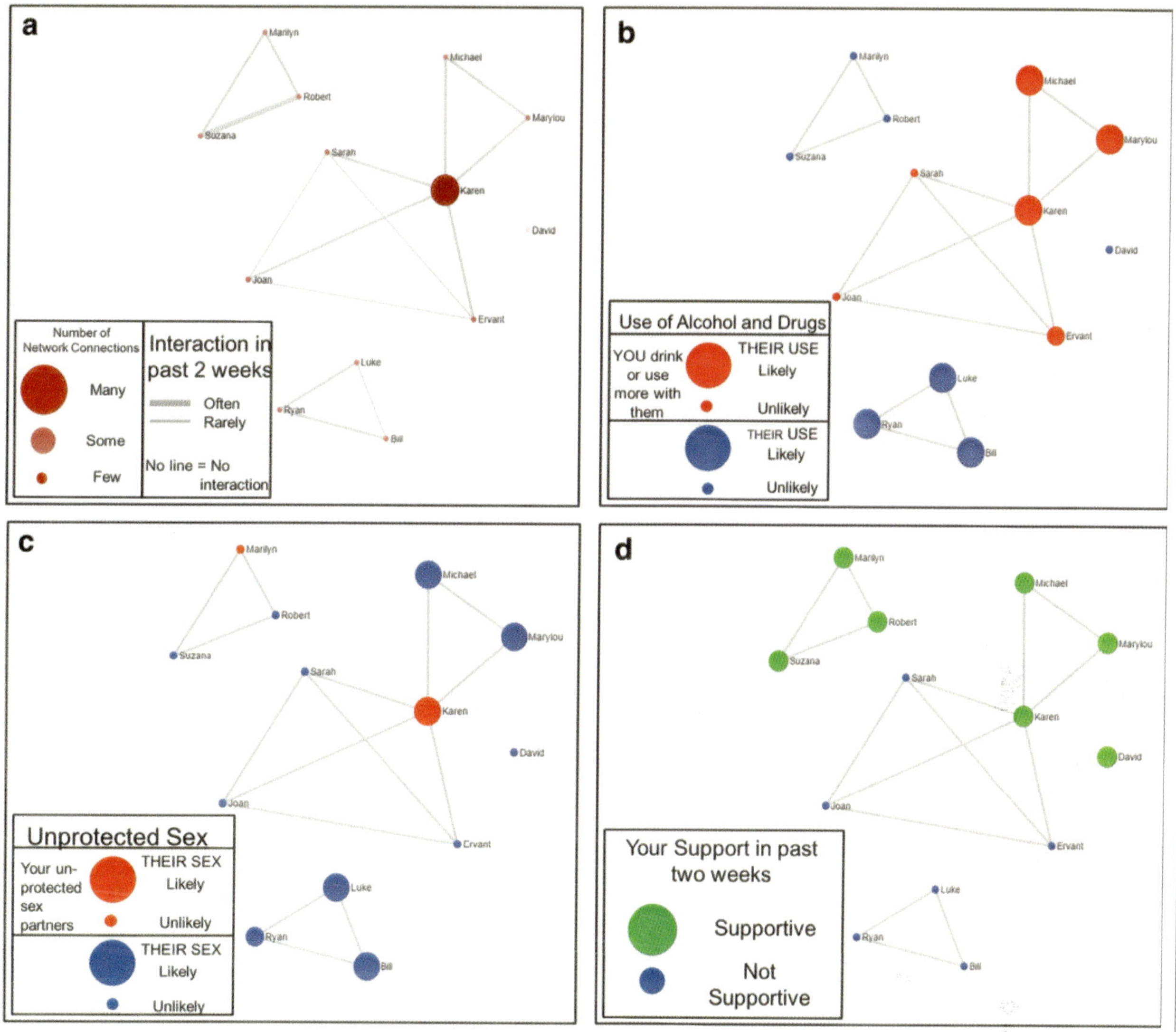

Fig. 1 Example figures from hypothetical MNI session. Network contacts are represented by *circles* (graph "nodes") and *lines* between nodes represent network contacts who interacted with each other in the past 2 weeks. The layout of the nodes, generated with the Fruchterman–Reingold force-directed placement algorithm highlights structural characteristics of the network, such as isolates (completely disconnected nodes) and components (a set of nodes tied together but disconnected from other nodes). The structural layout is consistent across the 4 diagrams. The figure in the *upper left* (**a**) uses node color and size, and line thickness to highlight other characteristics of the network structure, including the centrality of network actors (depicted by larger and darker nodes) and stronger relationship ties between actors (highlighted with *thicker lines*). The other figures use node size and color to highlight network composition. The figure in the *upper right* (**b**) highlights the likelihood of AOD use by network members with size (larger = likely, smaller = unlikely) and increased resident use when with network member by color (*red* drink or use more drugs with, and *blue* typical use). The figure in the *lower left* (**c**) highlights perceived risky sex by network members with node size (larger = likely, smaller = unlikely) and unprotected sex with network members with color (*red* had unprotected sex with, and *blue* did not have unprotected sex with). The figure in the *lower right hand* (**d**) depicts supportive network members with size and color (*large and green* supportive, *small and blue* not supportive)

changed. Figure 1 depicts examples of the 4 visualizations for a hypothetical intervention participant. Network contacts are represented by circles (nodes) and lines between nodes represent network contacts who interacted with each other in the past 2 weeks. The network display uses a "spring embedding" visualization algorithm [44], which renders the array of connections among the nodes in two dimensional space, placing people who know each other and have similar ties to other network members close together, and people who do not further apart. The distribution of these nodes and lines highlights structural features of the network such as isolates (completely disconnected nodes) and components (a set of nodes tied together but disconnected from other nodes).

The diagram labeled (a) indicates the names of people that the participant reports interacting with in the past 2 weeks and highlights structural features of the social network by node size, color, and line thickness. The larger nodes signify the people that the participant reports know a lot of other people in the network (i.e. "degree centrality" [45, 46]), while the thicker lines between nodes denote the people that the participant reports have interacted frequently with each other. The 3 remaining visualizations in Fig. 1 represent the same network while highlighting different compositional characteristics using different node colors and sizes. The diagram labeled (b) highlights AOD use in the network with larger nodes highlighting people who are likely to use AOD in the next 2 weeks, and red nodes showing people the participant reports using AOD with in the past 2 weeks. The diagram labeled (c) uses node size to highlight the people who the participant reports are likely to have unprotected sex in the next 2 weeks (bigger nodes) and node color to denote who the participant reports having unprotected sex with (red nodes). The final visualization labeled (d) depicts network contacts whom the respondent rated as supportive with larger, green nodes (vs. smaller, blue nodes).

As each network diagram is displayed and discussed, the intervention facilitators explored the pros and cons of participants' current social network composition and structure, and discussed their readiness, willingness and confidence to change risky aspects about their networks (e.g., "Tell me which of these people affect your drinking the most. What do you think about them?"). Facilitators also looked for opportunities to encourage discussion of strategies for positive behavior change. For example, if the participant has few supportive people in their network, the intervention facilitator can ask the participant, "Is there someone you haven't named who you would like to interact with more? What are some steps you can take to interact with that person in the next 2 weeks?" In addition, facilitators asked participants to rate how willing they were to change their AOD use and sexual behaviors (on a scale from 1 to 10 where "1" is not willing and "10" is very willing) when they discussed these respective network visualizations. The electronic tool included a large text box on each visualization screen and a node-level note annotation interface for recording statements from participants about making positive behavioral changes during the discussions. After discussion of the 4 visualizations, participants were asked to list some goals related to their AOD use or sexual behaviors that they would try to achieve over the next 2 weeks before their next session. As stated earlier, the four sessions were nearly identical with two exceptions. First, session 1 did not include a review of the previous session's graph. Second, session 4 included additional questions regarding future goals with their AOD and sexual risk behaviors, and how to prevent relapse if they have changed.

Measures

Interview protocol

To assess acceptability of the intervention among staff and residents, we asked about two main categories: Likes/dislikes and helpfulness in changing AOD and HIV risk behaviors to the target population of new PSH residents. To assess likes and dislikes, we asked participants about their general thoughts about the session (e.g., "What did you like/dislike? What did you think of the visualizations?"), how easy or difficult they perceived the questions to answer (e.g., "What was it like talking about the 10 or 15 people in your life right now and how it's been going?"). To assess helpfulness, we asked how the intervention might impact residents with AOD and HIV risk behaviors (e.g., "How do you think new residents will react to getting this information? How does this information affect your social network?"). Staff were also asked about the logistics of delivering the intervention (timing, frequency, and mode).

Satisfaction survey

After each interview, new resident participants ($n = 5$) completed a 20-item self-report satisfaction survey that asked about four areas. These included 6 questions about their overall impressions (e.g., "The different activities we did in the session were helpful."), 4 questions about the social network visualizations (e.g., "How helpful was the network picture highlighting alcohol and drug use?"), 4 questions about how the intervention might affect new residents (e.g., "I feel that the things I did in the session will help new residents to make the changes that they want."), and 6 questions about the facilitator (e.g., "The facilitator valued my opinion."). Participants were asked to rate each item on a 5-point Likert scale, with a higher score representing higher acceptability and satisfaction. Similar satisfaction questions have been used in prior research [47–49]. The 3 resident participants who completed a second intervention session were also asked to complete another round of the satisfaction survey.

Analyses

Qualitative analyses

The qualitative procedures and analyses for the staff focus group and resident interview were adapted from previous studies with this population and type of intervention [5, 48–56]. First, all audiotaped interviews were transcribed. Second, the written transcripts from the interviews were imported into the qualitative analysis software Dedoose

[57] for analytic purposes. Third, 3 researchers (KCO, DPK, and EM) independently reviewed the transcripts in Dedoose to identify, characterize, and categorize the key themes. The purpose of this review was to identify, label, and group together key points that spoke to what participants liked or disliked about the intervention and whether they found the intervention helpful in thinking about reducing AOD and HIV risk behaviors. Following grounded theory analyses [58], key points with similar concepts were grouped together into a category if said several times by different participants over time (e.g., comments that the visualizations were insightful). The 3 coders then tagged quotes illustrating each theme. Classic content analysis was used to identify quotes that fit each of the themes (e.g., visualizations were impactful) [59, 60]. After initial coding, team members reviewed the entire list of tagged quote excerpts, identified and discussed disagreements with initial coding, and then came to a consensus on a final set of themes. A final summary description of each theme was written into a codebook.

Quantitative analyses

We conducted descriptive analyses of the satisfaction data examining how participants rated the quality and their satisfaction with the session, social network visualizations, and facilitator. We also conducted descriptive analyses examining how participants thought the MNI would impact new residents.

Results

Staff focus group

Our staff focus group yielded three main findings regarding the language, structure, and presentation of the intervention. First, staff recommended we change certain wording (e.g., say "unprotected sex" instead of "risky sex"; query about oral sex in additional to vaginal and anal sex) to enhance resident understanding and engagement. Second, staff had mixed reactions about when we should start the intervention. Some recommended starting the first session 4 weeks or more after residents enter housing instead of within 2 weeks because they were worried that residents would not be honest about their risk behaviors, while other staff thought it may be easier to recruit clients to the study early on when they were motivated to enter housing. They recommended we clearly outline our rules about confidentiality to encourage honest reporting. Finally, staff had several positive comments about the visualizations stating they liked the colors of the nodes and the sizes of the circles to distinguish different people in their network. They stated that the visualizations may lower any defensiveness naturally engendered when discussing their substance use and sexual risk behaviors. They also recommended that we use computers versus tablets to deliver the intervention because the visualizations may be easier to see on a larger monitor. They recommended bigger fonts and surface area to see the intervention visualizations and the need to have a backup if internet connectivity was not available. Finally, staff recommended that we beta-test our intervention with long-term residents who were also peer advocates in addition to new residents because of their relevant experiences.

Residents

We group the themes from both the long-term residents and new residents together because their feedback was similar. The three themes that emerged were that the intervention was helpful in discussing their social network, that seeing the visualizations was more impactful than just talking about their network, and that the intervention prompted thoughts about changing their AOD use and HIV risk networks. Each theme is described below. Table 1 elaborates on each theme by providing additional participant quotes.

The first theme that participants frequently mentioned was how helpful the intervention was in discussing and examining the people currently in their lives. For example, one respondent said, "It made me think about who is in my life...who I interact with" and "It kind of shows you who you need to be with and who you don't need to be with." Some commented on how this insight helped them understand their own behaviors. For example, "I also see what I gravitate to more...which is good, because I can see what I'm doing."

There were some negative comments in the early stages of the beta testing regarding the number of alters and type of alters that participants were being asked to name. As a result, we changed the instructions to add flexibility to the number of alters that participants are asked to name, as the participants indicated it may be challenging for some residents to generate 20 people that they had interacted with in the past 2 weeks and others suggested that 10 names might be too few to identify important relationships. Also, participants expressed concern that the instructions were too ambiguous and that they may name children that would not be relevant to their AOD and HIV risk behavior. For example, one participant said, "because if I had named ten other different people, you would have got a totally different read, a totally different understanding. So I guess that's why I was kind of confused because I didn't know what direction you was going, what basically you were trying to find out, what were you trying to find out about?" Therefore, we modified the instructions so that participants were prompted to mention at least 10 adults (up to 15) that they had interacted with in the past 2 weeks.

Table 1 Themes from resident interviews

Theme	Participant quotes
Intervention was helpful in examining their social network	I thought it was awesome
	It was helpful to me also to stay motivated and stay positive
	It showed me the connection that one must have in order to stay focused. You can be connected to an awesome network, people that's moving forward…and also you can be connected to a network that's dying. So it is a network whether it's good or bad…it's just which one you choose to be connected to
	It helps you see who really around you is helping you, who is your support system, and how do you feel about your support system, and whether or not you're going to change your daily behavior and/or interactions
Seeing the visualizations is more impactful than just talking about their network	Well, actually I see my support system. Visually I can see it. It's different between thinking it and all that, but seeing it lets me know that this is correct
	It makes you see the pattern of your own life, and you visualize it, you know what I mean, it's not just in your mind
	With a case manager you set goals, but this is better. It shows... your activities. You know, I can see who's bad for me and who's not bad for me
	Seeing it is different than just somebody telling you or talking about it. Seeing it makes it easier to understand
Intervention prompted thoughts about changing their AOD use and HIV risk networks	I need to not be up in their face, I need them not to be up in mine, because if I could stop smoking cocaine, I know I could slow down on my drinking. But it's the environment that I be around, the environment that I be around, the people that be in my circle, and I be in their circle, I need to change that
	So as far as not drinking, I haven't been going to see my friends who drink. And I've been meeting new friends, and hoping, you know, like non-drinking, and if I go for information, I call individuals that are in AA. I'm getting closer to that also
	If I surround myself with people that have my old mentality, it's just going to keep me trapped in my same situation bringing me no type of change. So if I expand my surroundings, expand the people that I deal with, and cut out people that I know that I shouldn't be dealing with, or that aren't really beneficial to me

Second, when asked about their feedback about the visualizations, the majority of participants felt that *seeing* their networks was much different and more beneficial than merely talking about the people in their life. For example, one participant stated, "it's easy to talk about, but when I see who I should be with, who I shouldn't be with, it's a different issue, so it makes more sense", and another participant stated that they realized after seeing the visualization that "this [social network] circle is not going to work for me. You know, hearing about it is one thing, but seeing it is another." Some participants also commented that the visualizations were easy to understand. One participant stated, "it's a concrete way to see the big green circles are good, the big red ones are bad" and another participant stated, "The big circle I know for a fact there's unprotected sex there". Overall, the participants appeared to understand the purpose of using the visualizations to talk about social network change.

Finally, some residents who completed two sessions discussed how the session information helped them explore changes to their networks and/or their AOD or sexual risk behaviors. For example, one participant stated: "it showed me which ones I should be with, in case I need to, you know, if I'm trying to stop smoking, stop drinking, stop drugs, it kind of shows you who you need to be with and who you don't need to be with". Another participant stated, "I see sobriety in the smallest circles, I see social [drinkers] in the medium circles...and then I see loss of control in the larger circles, and that's why the [larger circles are] falling away from my network." While we cannot conclude whether these changes were a result of the intervention itself, participants who reported change to their AOD and HIV risk behaviors consistently noted changes to their social networks. One participant talked about his network composition and how he "cut a lot of people out" and added "replacements" for the AOD-using individuals so that he could build a stronger support system. Another participant used the visualizations of her network structure to build her self-efficacy when stating, "…and by looking at having unprotected sex, how if a couple more lines would have been more connected, I would have been a little more scared, because I don't know who's sleeping with who. So two more lines and I'd have to run to the clinic."

Satisfaction survey

Participants rated the sessions very highly as ratings were between a 4 (agree) and 5 (strongly agree; 1-5 Likert scale) in all 4 domains. Participants were highly satisfied with the overall session. On average, they agreed or strongly agreed that they had left the session with a specific goal in mind about changing their AOD use habits, as well as their social networks, and had found the session activities helpful. Participants also highly rated the social network visualizations, reporting they agreed or strongly agreed that the pictures showing their interaction, social support, alcohol and drug use, and sex and condom use were helpful. They also agreed or strongly agreed that the facilitators were well trained, valued and respected the respondent's opinions, and were helpful throughout the session. Finally, participants also thought the session would positively impact new residents.

Discussion

Delivering a motivational social network intervention for individuals transitioning into Housing First programs was found to be both acceptable to staff and residents of these programs. An intervention that focuses on an individual's social network appears especially important during this period, and for this population given findings that suggest that homeless individuals may have relatively small social networks with limited social support [14], and recent data that suggests risk behaviors such as AOD use and unprotected sex, may increase as one transitions from homelessness to supportive housing [16].

Findings from this study suggest that providing network visualizations based on a social network interview coupled with a guided discussion using a MI approach is perceived as both helpful and understandable. More specifically, staff gave input on how to improve the delivery of the intervention to enhance understanding and receptivity among new residents. Staff thought that the intervention would provide support to residents in making positive behavioral changes while transitioning from homelessness to supportive housing. In addition, resident participants overwhelmingly agreed that they thought being able to view their social network helped them better understand their personal relationships and its impact on their own behavior. Moreover, resident participants who engaged in more than one beta testing session reported that they had made behavioral changes as a result of the previous social network discussion. These results suggest that providing network visualizations with a guided MI discussion is a promising approach to supporting behavioral change.

Although the intervention tested in this study was specifically designed for homeless individuals transitioning into Housing First programs, we believe that a social network intervention that uses a MI approach could be helpful to other populations that need support for making a behavioral change. Presenting information about the structure and composition of one's network prompts individuals to consider how people in their lives and the relationships among those people are relevant to their future behavior. MI, a therapeutic style that is especially helpful for resolving ambivalence about one's behavior, has demonstrated effectiveness in reducing problematic behaviors, such as heavy drinking [61, 62]. Pairing a social network intervention with MI is a novel way in which to address how personal relationships may enhance or detract one from making healthy decisions. The intervention materials and techniques developed in this study are not specific to the homeless or Housing First programs and may be appropriate for testing in other settings.

The results presented herein represent the first phase of a clinical trial planning grant. More specifically, the findings are from iterative beta testing of the computer-assisted intervention with participants that are similar to the target population (i.e., individuals that are formerly homeless individuals as they transition to permanent supportive housing). Conducting beta testing as part of the initial intervention development is consistent with expert guidance on behavioral therapy research [63]. Next steps in the research of this intervention follow these guidelines, that is, a small pilot study where recruitment of a sample of homeless individuals that are transitioning to permanent supportive housing will be randomly assigned to receive the intervention or usual case management to explore the potential efficacy of the intervention. This pilot study [64] will be used to plan for a larger clinical trial if preliminary evidence of the intervention's efficacy is established.

Limitations

Our study has several limitations. The results presented herein are from a small purposive sample of Housing First staff and residents. The sample size is appropriate for beta testing where the goal is to collect in-depth feedback from potential users about the format of the intervention and their understanding of it. However, the study design does not allow us to make any inferential claims regarding the effectiveness of the intervention. Our findings were highly consistent across participants and therefore we saw little value in increasing the sample size. Also of note, some of the data were from a small sample of formerly homeless individuals living in project-based housing in a metropolitan area. It is possible that staff from different supportive housing programs and formerly homeless individuals living in other parts of the country (e.g., rural settings) or housing conditions (i.e., scattered sites) would have perceived the intervention differently. We acknowledge that the resident participants were living in project-based housing near large homeless encampments (i.e., Skid Row) which may make the transition to housing especially challenging and hence the need for an intervention that focuses on one's social network more relevant. The beta testing met our goals of refining the intervention in preparation for a pilot study.

Conclusions

In sum, this study is the first of its kind that has developed, with input from Housing First staff and residents, a motivational interviewing intervention that targets both the structure and composition of one's social network. The purpose of the intervention is to reduce AOD and HIV risk behaviors among those transitioning to permanent supportive housing. Previous research suggests that this transition may serve as a critical time to intervene to prevent future risk. Our results show that the intervention was perceived as acceptable by staff and residents. More research is needed with a larger sample and longer time frame to explore the potential effectiveness of the intervention in reducing AOD and HIV risk behaviors.

Authors' contributions

DPK is the PI and has overall responsibility for the intervention programming in EgoWeb, data collection, analyses, and reporting. KCO has overall responsibility of the intervention development and facilitation. DPK and EM conducted literature searches and provided summaries of previous research studies. All authors contributed to the intervention adaptation and data collection. All authors were involved in developing and editing of the manuscript and have given final approval of the version to be published. All authors read and approved the final manuscript.

Acknowledgements

This work is supported by the National Institute on Drug Abuse (NIDA) Grant R34 DA034855 (PI: David P. Kennedy). The content is solely the responsibility of the authors and does not necessarily represent the official views of NIDA or the National Institutes of Health. The authors would like to thank all of the participating staff and residents at Skid Row Housing Trust, Marylou Gilbert, and Michael Bennett without whom this research would not be possible. The authors express appreciation to David Zhang for programming of the electronic software development of EgoWeb.

Competing interests

The authors declare that they have no competing interests.

References

1. Booth BM, Sullivan G, Koegel P, Burnam A. Vulnerability factors for homelessness associated with substance dependence in a community sample of homeless adults. Am J Drug Alcohol Abuse. 2002;28(3):429–52.
2. Rhoades H, Wenzel SL, Golinelli D, Tucker JS, Kennedy DP, Green HD, et al. The social context of homeless men's substance use. Drug Alcohol Depend. 2011;118(2–3):320–5.
3. Beijer U, Wolf A, Fazel S. Prevalence of tuberculosis, hepatitis C virus, and HIV in homeless people: a systematic review and meta-analysis. Lancet Infect Dis. 2012;12(11):859–70.
4. Tucker JS, Kennedy D, Ryan G, Wenzel SL, Golinelli D, Zazzali J. Homeless women's personal networks: implications for understanding risk behavior. Hum Org. 2009;68(2):129–40.
5. Wenzel SL, Green HD, Tucker JS, Golinelli D, Kennedy DP, Ryan G, et al. The social context of homeless women's alcohol and drug use. Drug Alcohol Depend. 2009;105(1–2):16–23.
6. Reitzes DC, Crimmins TJ, Yarbrough J, Parker J. Social support and social network ties among the homeless in a downtown Atlanta park. J Community Psychol. 2011;39(3):274–91.
7. Stablein T. Helping friends and the homeless milieu: social capital and the utility of street peers. J Contemp Ethnogr. 2011;40(3):290–317.
8. Wolch JR, Rahimian A, Koegel P. Daily and periodic mobility patterns of the urban homeless. Prof Geogr. 1993;45(2):159–69.
9. Fisher JD. Possible effects of reference group-based social influence on AIDS risk behavior and AIDS prevention. Am Psychol. 1988;43(11):914–20.
10. Latkin C, Mandell W, Oziemkowska M, Celentano D, Vlahov D, Ensminger M, et al. Using social network analysis to study patterns of drug use among urban drug users at high risk for HIV/AIDS. Drug Alcohol Depend. 1995;38(1):1–9.
11. Smith KP, Christakis NA. Social networks and health. Annu Rev Sociol. 2008;34:405–29.
12. Berkman LF, Glass T, Brissette I, Seeman TE. From social integration to health: Durkheim in the new millennium. Soc Sci Med. 2000;51(6):843–57.
13. Padgett DK, Henwood B, Abrams C, Drake RE. Social relationships among persons who have experienced serious mental illness, substance abuse, and homelessness: implications for recovery. Am J Orthopsychiatry. 2008;78(3):333–9.
14. Hawkins RL, Abrams C. Disappearing acts: the social networks of formerly homeless individuals with co-occurring disorders. Soc Sci Med. 2007;65(10):2031–42.
15. Hwang SW, Kirst MJ, Chiu S, Tolomiczenko G, Kiss A, Cowan L, et al. Multidimensional social support and the health of homeless individuals. J Urban Health Bull N Y Acad Med. 2009;86(5):791–803.
16. Henwood BF, Rhoades H, Hsu H-T, Couture J, Rice E, Wenzel SL. Changes in social networks and HIV risk behaviors among homeless adults transitioning into permanent supportive housing: a mixed methods pilot study. J Mixed Methods Res. 2015;28:2015.
17. Green HD, Tucker JS, Golinelli D, Wenzel SL. Social networks, time homeless, and social support: a study of men on Skid Row. Netw Sci. 2013;1(03):305–20.
18. Carrington PJ, Scott J, Wasserman S. Models and methods in social network analysis. Cambridge, New York: Cambridge University Press; 2005.
19. Valente TW. Network Interventions. Science. 2012;337(6090):49–53.
20. Copello A, Orford J, Hodgson R, Tober G, Barrett C, Team UR. Social behaviour and network therapy—basic principles and early experiences. Addict Behav. 2002;27(3):345–66.
21. Bond J, Kaskutas LA, Weisner C. The persistent influence of social networks and alcoholics anonymous on abstinence. J Stud Alcohol. 2003;64(4):579–88.
22. Litt MD, Kadden RM, Kabela-Cormier E, Petry N. Changing network support for drinking: initial findings from the network support project. J Consult Clin Psychol. 2007;75(4):542–55.
23. Litt MD, Kadden RM, Kabela-Cormier E, Petry NM. Changing network support for drinking: network support project 2-year follow-up. J Consult Clin Psychol. 2009;77(2):229–42.
24. Groh DR, Jason LA, Keys CB. Social network variables in alcoholics anonymous: a literature review. Clin Psychol Rev. 2008;28(3):430–50.
25. Kelly JF, Stout RL, Magill M, Tonigan JS. The role of alcoholics anonymous in mobilizing adaptive social network changes: a prospective lagged mediational analysis. Drug Alcohol Depend. 2011;114(2–3):119–26.
26. Kaskutas LA, Bond J, Humphreys K. Social networks as mediators of the effect of Alcoholics Anonymous. Addiction. 2002;97(7):891–900.
27. Mason M, Pate P, Drapkin M, Sozinho K. Motivational interviewing integrated with social network counseling for female adolescents: a randomized pilot study in urban primary care. J Subst Abuse Treat. 2011;41(2):148–55.
28. Mason M, Light J, Campbell L, Keyser-Marcus L, Crewe S, Way T, et al. Peer network counseling with urban adolescents: a randomized controlled trial with moderate substance users. J Subst Abuse Treat. 2015;58:16–24.
29. Miller WR, Rollnick S. Motivational interviewing: helping people change. 3rd ed. New York: Guilford Press; 2013.
30. Kertesz SG, Crouch K, Milby JB, Cusimano RE, Schumacher JE. Housing first for homeless persons with active addiction: are we overreaching? Milbank Q. 2009;87(2):495–534.
31. Padgett DK. There's no place like (a) home: ontological security among persons with serious mental illness in the United States. Soc Sci Med. 2007;64(9):1925–36.
32. Padgett DK, Stanhope V, Henwood BF, Stefancic A. Substance use outcomes among homeless clients with serious mental illness: comparing housing first with treatment first programs. Community Ment Health J. 2011;47(2):227–32.

33. Padgett DK, Gulcur L, Tsemberis S. Housing first services for people who are homeless with co-occurring serious mental illness and substance abuse. Res Soc Work Pract. 2006;16(1):74–83.
34. Tsemberis S, Kent D, Respress C. Housing stability and recovery among chronically homeless persons with co-occuring disorders in Washington, DC. Am J Public Health. 2012;102(1):13–6.
35. Larimer ME, Malone DK, Garner MD, Atkins DC, Burlingham B, Lonczak HS, et al. Health care and public service use and costs before and after provision of housing for chronically homeless persons with severe alcohol problems. JAMA. 2009;301(13):1349–57.
36. Miller WR, Rose GS. Toward a theory of motivational interviewing. Am Psychol. 2009;64(6):527–37.
37. Newman MEJ. Complex systems: a survey. Am J Phys. 2011;79(8):800–10.
38. Wasserman S, Faust K. Social network analysis: methods and applications. New York: Cambridge University Press; 1994.
39. Monge PR, Contractor NS. Theories of communication networks. New York: Oxford University Press; 2003.
40. Coleman JS. Social capital in the creation of human-capital. Am J Sociol. 1988;94:S95–120.
41. Deci EL, Ryan RM. Intrinsic motivation and self-determination in human behavior. New York: Plenum; 1985.
42. Markland D, Ryan RM, Tobin VJ, Rollnick S. Motivational interviewing and self-determination theory. J Soc Clin Psychol. 2005;24(6):811–31.
43. Bandura A. Self-efficacy: the exercise of control. New York: Freeman; 1997.
44. Freeman LC. Visualizing social networks. J Soc Struct. 2000;1(1). https://www.cmu.edu/joss/content/articles/volume1/Freeman.html. Accessed 1 Oct 2014.
45. Freeman LC. Centrality in social networks conceptual clarification. Soc Netw. 1979;1(3):215–39.
46. McCarty C. Structure in personal networks. J Soc Struct. [Internet]. 2002; 3(1). http://www.cmu.edu/joss/content/articles/volume3/McCarty.html.
47. Marlatt GA, Baer JS, Kivlahan DR, Dimeff LA, Larimer ME, Quigley LA, et al. Screening and brief intervention for high-risk college student drinkers: results from a 2-year follow-up assessment. J Consult Clin Psychol. 1998;66(4):604–15.
48. D'Amico EJ, Osilla KC, Hunter SB. Developing a group motivational interviewing intervention for adolescents at-risk for developing an alcohol or drug use disorder. Alcohol Treat Q. 2010;28(4):417–36.
49. Osilla KC, Zellmer SP, Larimer ME, Neighbors C, Marlatt GA. A brief intervention for at-risk drinking in an employee assistance program. J Stud Alcohol Drugs. 2008;69(1):14–20.
50. Osilla KC, dela Cruz E, Miles JN, Zellmer S, Watkins K, Larimer ME, et al. Exploring productivity outcomes from a brief intervention for at-risk drinking in an employee assistance program. Addict Behav. 2010;35(3):194–200.
51. Osilla KC, Hepner KA, Munoz RF, Woo S, Watkins K. Developing an integrated treatment for substance use and depression using cognitive-behavioral therapy. J Subst Abuse Treat. 2009;37(4):412–20.
52. Stern SA, Meredith LS, Gholson J, Gore P, D'Amico EJ. Project CHAT: a brief motivational substance abuse intervention for teens in primary care. J Subst Abuse Treat. 2007;32(2):153–65.
53. Osilla KC, D'Amico EJ, Díaz-Fuentes CM, Lara M, Watkins KE. Multicultural web-based motivational interviewing for clients with a first-time DUI offense. Cult Divers Ethn Minor Psychol. 2012;18(2):192–202.
54. Brown RA, Kennedy DP, Tucker JS, Wenzel S, Golinelli D, Wertheimer S, et al. Sex and relationships on the street: how homeless men judge partner risk on Skid Row. AIDS Behav. 2011;16(3):774–84.
55. Osilla KC, D'Amico EJ, Díaz-Fuentes CM, Lara M, Watkins KE. Multicultural web-based motivational interviewing for clients with a first-time DUI offense. Cult Divers Ethn Minor Psychol. 2012;18(2):192–202.
56. Rana Y, Brown RA, Kennedy DP, Ryan GW, Stern S, Tucker JS. Understanding condom use decision making among homeless youth using event-level data. J Sex Res. 2014;52(9):1–11.
57. SocioCultural Research Consultants LLC. Dedoose. 5.0. 11, web application for managing, analyzing, and presenting qualitative and mixed method research data. Los Angeles, CA; 2014. http://www.dedoose.com/.
58. Strauss AC, Corbin J. Basics of qualitative research: techniques and procedures for developing grounded theory. Thousand Oaks: Sage Publications, Inc.; 1998.
59. Krippendorf K. Content analysis: an introduction to its methodology. Beverly Hills: Sage Publications; 1980.
60. Weber RP. Basic content analysis. Newbury Park: Sage Publications, Inc.; 1990.
61. Lundahl BW, Kunz C, Brownell C, Tollefson D, Burke BL. A meta-analysis of motivational interviewing: twenty-five years of empirical studies. Res Soc Work Pract. 2010;20(2):137–60.
62. Moyer A, Finney JW, Swearingen CE, Vergun P. Brief interventions for alcohol problems: a meta-analytic review of controlled investigations in treatment-seeking and non-treatment-seeking populations. Addiction. 2002;97(3):279–92.
63. Rounsaville BJ, Carroll KM, Onken LS. A stage model of behavioral therapies research: getting started and moving on from stage I. Clin Psychol Sci Pract. 2001;8(2):133–42.
64. Kennedy DP, Hunter SB, Osilla KC, Maksabedian E, Golinelli D, Tucker JS. A computer-assisted motivational social network intervention to reduce alcohol, drug and HIV risk behaviors among Housing First residents. Addict Sci Clin Pract. 2016;11(4):1–13.

8

Seek, test, treat: substance-using women in the HIV treatment cascade in South Africa

Wendee M. Wechsberg[1,2,3,4*], Charles van der Horst[5], Jacqueline Ndirangu[6], Irene A. Doherty[7], Tracy Kline[8], Felicia A. Browne[1], Jennifer M. Belus[9], Robin Nance[10] and William A. Zule[1]

Abstract

Background: Women in South Africa who use alcohol and other drugs face multiple barriers to HIV care. These barriers make it difficult for women to progress through each step in the HIV treatment cascade from diagnosis to treatment initiation and adherence. This paper examines correlates of HIV status, newly diagnosed HIV status, and use of antiretroviral therapy (ART).

Methods: Outreach workers recruited sexually active Black African women who used substances in Pretoria as part of a U.S. National Institutes of Health-funded geographically clustered randomized trial examining the effect of an intervention to reduce alcohol and drug use as well as sexual risk behaviors. To address the question of interest in the current investigation, cross-sectional baseline data were used. At study enrollment, all participants (N = 641) completed an interview, and underwent rapid HIV testing and biological drug screening. Those who tested positive for HIV and were eligible for ART were asked about their barriers to initiating or adhering to ART. Bivariate and multivariable logistic regression analyses were conducted to determine correlates of HIV status, newly diagnosed HIV, and ART use.

Results: At enrollment, 55% of participants tested positive for HIV, and 36% of these women were newly diagnosed. In multivariable analyses of the entire sample, women who had completed 10th grade were less likely to be living with HIV (OR 0.69; CI 0.48, 0.99) and those from the inner city were more likely to be living with HIV (OR 1.83; CI 1.26, 2.67). Among HIV-positive participants, women were less likely to be newly diagnosed if they had ever been in substance abuse treatment (OR 0.15; CI 0.03, 0.69) or used a condom at last sex (OR 0.58; CI 0.34, 0.98) and more likely to be newly diagnosed if they were physically assaulted in the past year (OR 1.97; CI 1.01, 3.84). Among women eligible for ART, fewer were likely to be on treatment (by self-report) if they had a positive urine test for opiates or cocaine (OR 0.27; CI 0.09, 0.80).

Conclusions: These results, although cross-sectional, provide some guidance for provincial authorities to address barriers to HIV care for sexually active, substance-using vulnerable women in Pretoria. Targeting the inner city with prevention campaigns, expanding and improving substance abuse treatment programs, linking clients with simultaneous HIV testing and treatment, and targeting women who have experienced sexual assault and violence may help the government achieve the UNAIDS 90-90-90 treatment target.

Clinical Trials.gov NCT01497405 registered on December 1, 2011.

Keywords: Sexually-active women, Alcohol and other drug use, Treatment cascade

*Correspondence: wmw@rti.org
[1] Substance Use, Gender and Applied Research, RTI International, 3040 East Cornwallis Road, Research Triangle Park, NC 27709-2194, USA
Full list of author information is available at the end of the article

Background

Despite progress in reducing HIV incidence, approximately 2 million people were newly infected worldwide in 2015 [1]. Biomedical approaches such as HIV treatment as prevention offer hope for reducing transmission even when condom use is low. In a study of HIV-discordant couples, antiretroviral therapy (ART) reduced HIV transmission by 93% [2]. The results of this study combined with findings from two ecological studies [3, 4] and several modeling studies [5] suggest that high rates of HIV testing and treatment could end the HIV epidemic. These findings led UNAIDS to establish the "90-90-90" treatment goals whereby 90% of all people infected with HIV will know their status, 90% of those diagnosed with HIV will receive ART, and 90% of those on ART will achieve undetectable HIV viral loads by 2020 [6].

However, achieving the 90-90-90 goals in key populations, such as people who use drugs, will require intensive efforts to find them, test them for HIV, link them to ART, and retain them in treatment [7]. To achieve the 90-90-90 goals in a country like South Africa, this approach—labeled "seek, test, treat, and retain" (STTR) [8]—will require expanding STTR efforts among people who use alcohol and other drugs, female sex workers, and men who have sex with men [9, 10].

With AIDS being the leading cause of death among women of childbearing age globally [11], it is critical to increase testing among women at high risk of HIV and link those who test positive for HIV to ART. Focusing STTR efforts on women in this group has the potential to reduce AIDS-related deaths among them. Treating HIV-positive women also reduces onward transmission of HIV to men who in turn transmit it to other women, which is a primary objective of STTR efforts. Moreover, treating HIV-positive women may help break the cycle in places like sub-Saharan Africa where two-thirds of new infections among 15–24-year-olds occurred among women in 2015 [1].

Alcohol and other drug use can interfere with STTR efforts at each step in the HIV treatment cascade [9]. Use of alcohol and other drugs may also reduce pre-exposure prophylaxis (PrEP) uptake and adherence [12]. Additionally, alcohol and other drug use exacerbates existing social and structural barriers to HIV testing and HIV-related services [13] and adversely affects health-seeking behavior and health care utilization [14, 15]. In South Africa where there are more people living with HIV than anywhere else in the world, alcohol and drug use is a growing problem, particularly in urban areas. Alcohol and marijuana use are most common, although the use of heroin, cocaine, Mandrax (methaqualone) and methamphetamine have increased significantly with injecting drug use also on the rise [16]. Therefore, it is especially pertinent to the South African context to examine both alcohol and specific drug use as predictors of progress through the HIV treatment cascade. In this paper, we hypothesized that recent alcohol and other drug use would be negatively associated with forward progress through the HIV treatment cascade. More specifically, we propose to determine predictors of current HIV status, newly diagnosed HIV cases and ART use. Each of these stages is important in reaching the 90-90-90 treatment goals.

Methods

Procedure overview

The paper presents analyses of cross-sectional baseline data collected from women who were recruited by outreach workers in Pretoria, South Africa. The complete protocol for the study was published in an open-access journal [17]. Briefly, the intervention study focuses on reducing HIV risk behaviors (e.g., alcohol or drug use, unprotected sex) in high-risk women; it also focuses on improving adherence to the Test, Treat, and Retain elements of the HIV cascade for HIV-positive women.

Sample and eligibility

To participate in the study, women had to meet the following eligibility criteria: (1) self-identify as female; (2) be Black African; (3) be aged 15 or older (15–17-year-olds had to demonstrate tacit emancipation, which shows their capacity as a minor to act without parental consent[1]) [18]; (4) report using alcohol or other drugs at least weekly during the past 90 days; (5) report unprotected vaginal sex with a male partner in the past 6 months; (6) speak English, Sesotho, Tswana, or Zulu; (7) consent to HIV rapid testing (blood), drug testing (urine), and alcohol breathalyzer; (8) provide written and verbal assent/consent to participate; and (9) provide verifiable locator information for the Pretoria area and plan to stay in the area for the next 12 months.

Recruitment

A total of 641 women enrolled in the study between May 2012 and September 2014. All of the outreach workers for the study were trained on community outreach techniques for approaching women in public places and

[1] According to South African law, adolescents under 18, the age of majority, can provide consent unassisted as long as they can provide evidence of tacit emancipation. Tacit emancipation occurs when the capacity of a minor to act without parental consent is 'enlarged' to encompass certain key areas that will enable him or her to be viewed by the law as a major. The prime consideration is the degree of financial independence that the minor has achieved. In this respect, ownership of a business or an occupation that brings in a salary is key. Residence outside the parental home is regarded as further proof of emancipation.

discreetly screening them for eligibility. Outreach workers received additional training on procedures specific to this study such as how to schedule appointments and transport women safely to the field site for enrollment and data collection. Given the differences in living conditions, access to drugs, and population density across the greater Pretoria area, we differentiated where women were recruited—either within the inner city (i.e., the Central Business District) or outside the inner city. Women recruited from the inner-city often spent time in transient forms of shelter or workplace establishments such as abandoned houses or street corners.

Outreach workers conducted eligibility screening and scheduled intake appointments for those who were eligible and interested. The appointments, conducted at the study's field site, included the following activities: rescreening for eligibility, informed consent, a computer-assisted personal interview, a finger stick of blood for rapid HIV testing, collection of a urine sample for pregnancy testing and drug screening, and a breathalyzer test for recent alcohol use. Participants received toiletries worth R100 (at the time of the study, $1 US equaled approximately 10 South African Rand) for their time and reimbursement for travel.

Self-report measures

The primary data collection instrument—the Pretoria Risk Behavior Assessment (PRBA)—included sections on sociodemographic characteristics, alcohol and other drug use, substance abuse treatment, sexual behavior, violence perpetration and victimization, and physical and mental health. In a previous study in Pretoria, the PRBA demonstrated high reliability and validity [19].

Sex risk

Three measures of sex risk were included: the number of sex acts (anal and vaginal) without a condom in the past 30 days; condom use at last sex; and engaging in sex work or trading sex for drugs, money, food, clothing, shelter, or any other goods in the past 6 months.

Alcohol and other drug use

Measures included use of marijuana, cocaine (includes powder cocaine and crack), heroin by itself, and Nyaope (heroin mixed with marijuana). For each substance, participants were asked if they had ever used it (i.e., lifetime use). Participants who reported lifetime use were asked the number of days they had used the substance in the past 30 days. We recoded these variables into any use of each drug in the past 30 days. We used the Alcohol Use Disorders Identification Test (AUDIT) to assess problem drinking using a cut-point of 20, which indicates probable alcohol dependence and a need for alcohol treatment [20].

Victimization

The PRBA included the following ordered items to measure physical and sexual abuse:

- Has anyone ever physically hurt you (i.e., someone hurt you by striking or beating you to the point that you had bruises, cuts, or broken bones)?
  - When was the last time you were physically hurt?
- Has anyone ever pressured you or forced you to participate in sexual acts against your will?
  - When was the last time you were pressured or forced to participate in sexual acts against your will?

The analyses used derived variables for physical abuse and for sexual abuse in the past year.

Mental and physical health

We used the Mental Health scale from Version 2 of the SF-36 Health Survey [21] to assess participants' mental health and the Vitality scale to assess physical health. Raw scores were computed and transformed according to instructions in the manual. Specifically, scale scores were transformed using the following formula: [(Actual raw score − lowest possible raw score)/(possible raw score range)] × 100. Higher scores on the Mental Health and Vitality scales are associated with better functioning. Our focus in this paper was to identify factors that distinguish among women in the sample at each step in the HIV treatment cascade. Therefore, we did not compare SF-36 scale scores in the sample to scores in the broader population in South Africa.

Antiretroviral therapy (ART)

To assess current ART status, the questionnaire asked participants who reported ever testing positive for HIV the following questions: "Have you ever taken any ARV medications? Are you taking any ARV medications now?"

Barriers to HIV treatment initiation and retention

We assessed barriers to HIV treatment initiation, retention in treatment, and adherence to HIV medication with the question: "Why have you stopped or not taken ARV (*anti-HIV*) medications, either now or in the past?" A list of response options followed the question along with instructions to "check all that apply." Participants also had the option to respond "other" and specify an unlisted response. The research team collapsed the responses into the themes.

Biological tests

Alcohol and other drug use

A breathalyzer was used to assess recent alcohol use. Participants provided a urine sample for drug testing. A multipanel drug test was used to assess marijuana (THC), cocaine, ecstasy (MDMA), and opiate use (Homemed Multi drug 5-Panel Dipcard).

HIV status

All participants were tested for HIV at baseline regardless of self-report. Testing was done by collecting a blood sample from a finger stick and performing two parallel rapid HIV tests (First Response® HIV 1-2.0 or ABON®-Alere HIV 1/2/O Tri-line HIV Rapid Test and iCARE One Step HIV [1&2] Whole Blood/Serum/Plasma Test). If one test was positive and the other test was either indeterminate or negative, then a confirmatory test was performed (Alere Determine™ HIV-1/2). A participant was classified as HIV positive if any two of the tests were reactive.

Housing

We captured differences in level of disadvantage by asking participants whether they lived in an informal settlement. In South Africa, most informal settlements are made up of a collection of shacks that have not been formally approved by the government. Some informal settlements may exist for years and have hundreds of thousands of residents.

Recruitment area

Women were differentiated based on location of recruitment because the city of Pretoria consists of varying levels of disparity. Women were classified as having been recruited from the inner city versus outside the inner city. The inner city indicates that women were recruited from within the Central Business District and often were found in transient forms of shelter or near drug-dealing establishments such as abandoned houses or high drug traffic street corners.

Historical factors

The recruitment period for this study overlapped with the South African government's campaign to increase HIV testing and treatment. Therefore, we included month of recruitment in our models to assess the campaign's success in reaching our population and as a potential confounder.

Statistical analysis

We used multivariable logistic regression analyses to test hypotheses regarding associations between independent variables of interest (e.g., alcohol, drug use, sex work) and HIV status, newly diagnosed with HIV, and being on ART. The analysis examining correlates of HIV status included all women in the study (n = 641). The analysis examining correlates of newly diagnosed HIV included all HIV-positive women (n = 354) whereas the analysis examining factors associated with ART use included only HIV-positive women who were eligible for ART (n = 156). Bivariate analyses examined the associations between dependent variables and each covariate. Covariates that were statistically significant at $p < .05$ in bivariate analysis were included in the multivariable model. When two highly correlated independent variables were both significantly associated with an outcome in bivariate analyses, we included only one of them in the multivariable model based on substantive and theoretical considerations. In the ART model, we excluded one variable (ever in substance abuse treatment) from the multivariable model because of small cell sizes. Analyses were performed in SPSS version 23 (IBM Corp.; Armonk, NY).

Results

Of the 1012 women screened for eligibility, 772 (76%) met all of the eligibility criteria. Most (86%) of the women who were ineligible did not meet the criterion of self-reported alcohol or other drug use at least once a week over the previous 90 days. Among eligible women, 83% (641/772) enrolled into the study. Women who declined to participate and those who enrolled into the study were similar with respect to age, language, and having a main sex partner; 53% of women who declined to participate reported sex work compared with 43% of women who enrolled in the study ($p = .01$).

Only three women reported ever injecting illicit drugs. Self-reported use of heroin—either alone or mixed with marijuana (Nyaope)—and biological test results for opiates were similar (17 vs. 18%, $p > .05$). Slightly more women reported marijuana use in the past 30 days than had a positive drug screen result (38 vs. 31%, $p > .05$). Significantly fewer women reported using cocaine in the past 30 days than tested positive for it (12 vs. 14%, $p < .05$). However, despite the statistical significance, even these results were quite similar.

HIV testing and prevalence ("seek and test")

During their baseline interview, 90% of the participants reported having been tested for HIV previously. At enrollment in the study, 55% (n = 354) of women had a positive test result for HIV. Table 1 displays characteristics of the participants stratified by HIV status as well as results from the bivariate and multivariable analyses. In Fig. 1, we present the study participants reached along the treatment cascade of seek, test and treat being only baseline data. In multivariable analyses, being older, engaging in sex work, being recruited in the inner city, and living in an informal settlement were associated with increased odds of testing positive for HIV, whereas more education had a protective effect.

Table 1 Correlates of HIV among high-risk women in Pretoria, South Africa

Variable	HIV status		Bivariate logistic regression	Multivariable logistic regression
	Negative	Positive		
Sociodemographic characteristic	(n = 287)	(n = 354)	OR (95% CI)	OR (95% CI)
Age in years, mean (SD)	29.0 (8.5)	31.5 (7.0)	1.04 (1.02, 1.07)***	1.03 (1.01, 1.05)**
% education ≥10th grade	70.4	56.5	0.55 (0.39, 0.76)***	0.69 (0.48, 0.98)*
% unemployed	82.7	87.7	1.49 (0.93, 2.38)	
% married or living as married	46.7	52.5	1.26 (0.93, 1.73)	
% ever had a family member with HIV/AIDS	59.1	64.9	1.28 (0.93, 1.76)	
% ever incarcerated (lifetime)	29.7	39.5	1.55 (1.11, 2.15)**	1.10 (0.76, 1.59)
% ever in substance abuse treatment (lifetime)	7.0	5.6	0.80 (0.42, 1.52)	
Urine drug screen and breathalyzer results				
% marijuana (THC) positive	31.4	31.4	1.0 (0.71, 1.40)	
% opiate positive	19.2	16.9	0.86 (0.57, 1.29)	
% cocaine positive	15.7	13.3	0.82 (0.53, 1.28)	
% opiate or cocaine positive	21.3	20.3	0.95 (0.64, 1.39)	
% alcohol (breathalyzer) positive	12.9	15.3	1.22 (0.77, 1.91)	
Mean breathalyzer score for women with a positive alcohol test (SD)	0.08 (0.11)	0.08 (0.11)	1.69 (0.03, 82.96)	
Self-report alcohol and drug use past 30 days				
% alcohol	84.7	88.7	1.42 (0.90, 2.25)	
% marijuana	28.6	30.5	1.01 (0.78, 1.55)	
% cocaine (rock)	13.2	10.5	0.76 (0.47, 1.24)	
% heroin and marijuana mixed (Nyaope)	18.8	15.3	0.78 (0.51, 1.17)	
Self-report Alcohol Use Disorders Identification Tests (AUDIT) score ≥20	26.5	34.2	1.44 (1.02, 2.03)*	1.43 (0.99, 2.07)
Sex risk behaviors				
% used a condom at last sex	28.5	43.3	1.92 (1.37, 2.68)***	1.45 (0.97, 2.16)
# times unprotected sex past 30 days, mean (SD)	8.6 (12.9)	8.9 (14.2)	1.00 (0.99, 1.01)	
Sex work past 6 months	26.8	45.2	2.25 (1.61, 3.14)***	1.47 (0.98, 2.22)
Victimization				
% physically assaulted past year	9.1	13.3	1.54 (0.93, 2.55)	
% sexually assaulted past year	5.2	7.3	1.44 (0.75, 2.77)	
SF-36 mental health and vitality scales				
Mental health scale score, mean (SD)[a]	65.1 (19.2)	64.3 (19)	1.00 (0.99, 1.01)	
Vitality scale score, mean (SD)[a]	34.2 (18.3)	35.7 (17.2)	1.00 (1.00, 1.01)	
Contextual factors				
% recruited from inner city[b]	24.4	40.4	2.1 (1.49, 2.96)***	1.90 (1.30, 2.78)**
Century month recruited[c], mean (SD)	150.7 (8.5)	150.3 (8.7)	0.99 (0.98, 1.01)	
% living in informal settlement[d]	30.3	38.4	1.43 (1.03, 2.00)*	1.49 (1.04, 2.14)*

* $p < .05$; ** $p < .01$; *** $p < .001$

[a] SF-36 Mental Health and Vitality scales

Transformed scale = [(Actual raw score − lowest possible raw score)/(possible raw score range)] × 100

[b] The reference group is recruited from outside the inner city

[c] Century month (CM). January 2001 = 1. The project recruited from May 2012 (CM = 136) to September 2014 (CM = 164). South Africa was in the midst of scaling up HIV testing and treatment during this period

[d] The reference group is not living in an informal settlement

Newly diagnosed with HIV

Among the 354 women who tested positive for HIV, 36% (n = 126) were newly diagnosed. Of these, 27% reported never receiving an HIV test. Among those who had been tested, the median number of months since their most recent HIV test was 23. Table 2 displays the results

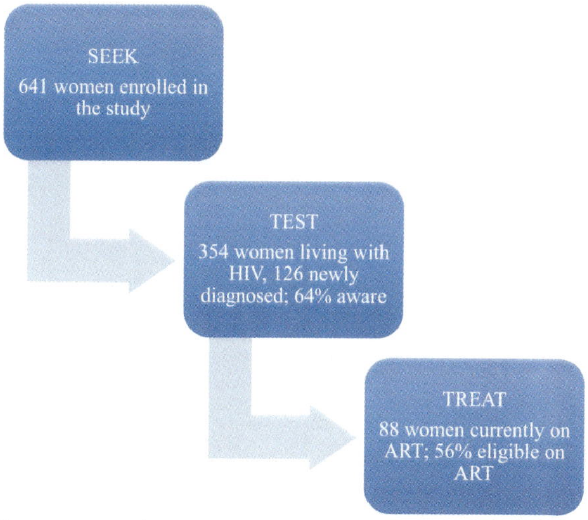

Fig. 1 HIV cascade for women recruited for the study

related to being newly diagnosed with HIV. More specifically, the multivariable analysis shows that being older, having a history of substance abuse treatment, and using a condom at last sex were associated with decreased odds of being newly diagnosed with HIV, whereas physical assault in the past 12 months was associated with increased odds of being newly diagnosed.

Treat

Among the 228 women who reported during their baseline interview that they knew they were living with HIV, 72 of these women reported that they were not eligible for ART because their CD4 count was too high. Of the 156 women who were eligible for ART, 88 (56%) reported being on ART. The analyses of factors associated with being on ART exclude the 72 women who were not eligible for it (see Table 3). In multivariable analyses, older age and later month enrolled in the project were significantly associated with increased odds of being on ART, whereas having a positive urine drug screen for either opiates or cocaine metabolites was associated with significantly decreased odds of being on ART. In additional analyses to clarify the association between a history of substance abuse treatment and not being on ART, we found that 80% of women with a history of substance abuse treatment tested positive for opiates or cocaine.

Barriers to treatment initiation and retention

When this study began recruiting, South Africa offered ART only to patients whose CD4 cell count was below 350 cells/ml. By the time recruitment ended, the government had raised the threshold for starting ART to 500 cells/ml. Tying eligibility for ART to CD4 cell count means many women were not eligible for ART.

Among participants who were eligible for ART, the primary barriers to ART initiation and retention were structural factors such as the clinic not providing ART, and individual factors, such as missing appointments (Table 4). Personal beliefs and perceived need for ART remain problematic.

Discussion

With 55% of the sample testing positive for HIV, this study demonstrates the feasibility of using community outreach to find (*seek*) women at high risk for HIV and *test* them. Women's biological susceptibility [22] combined with social determinants such as economic dependence and inequitable gender norms contribute to the high prevalence and incidence of HIV among women in developing countries [23, 24]. To prevent new infections among women in these settings, STTR efforts will need to include the men who are infecting women in addition to women. However, the most direct way to prevent women in these settings from acquiring HIV may be to offer them PrEP [25]. Contrary to our hypothesis, there was no relationship between testing positive for alcohol or other drugs and testing positive for HIV in this sample. This may be due the fact that all women in the study had to report use of alcohol and other drugs.

Similar to HIV status, there was no association between recent drug and alcohol use and being newly diagnosed with HIV in this sample, which may be explained by the high rates of HIV testing in the sample. Although 90% of the entire sample and 95% of women who tested positive for HIV reported a previous HIV test, 36% of women with a positive test were unaware of their status. Among the 92 newly diagnosed women who reported a previous HIV test, the median number of months since their most recent test was 23. To achieve the goal of 90% of HIV-positive women in this population knowing their HIV status, more women need to be tested, and they must be tested more frequently—preferably at least once a year and more frequently, if symptomatic. Because almost all of these women likely acquired HIV through sex with men, increases in HIV testing and treatment among women must be accompanied by similar increases among men to reduce incidence. Unfortunately, efforts to test and treat Black African men in South Africa have been less successful [26, 27].

During their baseline interview, only 56% of the 156 women who were aware of their HIV status and eligible for ART reported receiving it. In the multivariable model, the significant association between being recruited later in the project and being on ART suggests that the South African government's efforts to increase HIV testing and treatment are beginning to work. Nevertheless, much more work remains to be done before South Africa will achieve the 90-90-90 goals.

Table 2 Correlates of newly diagnosed HIV among HIV-positive women in Pretoria, South Africa

Variable	Previously diagnosed	Newly diagnosed	Bivariate logistic regression	Multivariable logistic regression
Sociodemographic characteristic	**n = 228**	**n = 126**	**OR (95% CI)**	**OR (95% CI)**
Age in years, mean (SD)	32.7 (6.9)	29.1 (7.0)	0.92 (0.89, 0.95)***	0.91 (0.88, 0.95)***
% education ≥10th grade	57.5	54.8	1.11 (0.71, 1.75)	
% unemployed	89.1	85.3	0.71 (0.36, 1.41)	
% married or living as married	54.4	49.2	0.81 (0.53, 1.26)	
% ever had a family member with HIV/AIDS	66.1	62.7	0.86 (0.55, 1.36)	
% ever incarcerated (lifetime)	40.8	37.3	0.86 (0.55, 1.35)	
% ever in substance abuse treatment (lifetime)	7.9	1.6	0.19 (0.04, 0.82)*	0.15 (0.03, 0.69)*
Urine drug screen and breathalyzer results				
% marijuana (THC) positive	33.3	27.8	0.77 (0.48, 1.24)	
% opiate positive	17.1	16.7	0.97 (0.54, 1.73)	
% cocaine positive	14.0	11.9	0.83 (0.43, 1.6)	
% opiate or cocaine positive	20.2	20.6	1.03 (0.60, 1.76)	
% alcohol (breathalyzer) positive	16.3	13.5	0.80 (0.43, 1.49)	
Sex risk behaviors				
% used a condom at last sex	48.9	33.3	0.52 (0.33, 0.82)**	0.58 (0.34, 0.98)**
# times unprotected sex past 30 days, mean (SD)	8.2 (12.9)	10.2 (16.3)	1.01 (0.99, 1.02)	
% engaged in sex work past 6 months	50.0	36.5	0.58 (0.37, 0.90)*	0.83 (0.49, 1.40)
Victimization				
% physically assaulted past year	10.5	18.3	1.90 (1.02, 3.52)*	1.97 (1.01, 3.84)*
% sexually assaulted past year	6.6	8.7	1.36 (0.60, 3.05)	
SF-36 mental health and vitality scales				
Mental health scale score, mean (SD)[a]	58.4 (14.4)	59.0 (15.8)	1.00 (0.99, 1.02)	
Vitality scale score, mean (SD)[b]	36.6 (16.9)	33.9 (17.7)	0.99 (0.98, 1.00)	
Contextual factors				
% recruited from inner city[b]	40.4	40.5	1.01 (0.65, 1.57)	
Century month recruited[c], mean (SD)	150.3 (8.9)	150.3 (8.4)	1.00 (0.97, 1.02)	
% living in informal settlement[d]	36.4	42.1	1.27 (0.81, 1.98)	

* $p < .05$; ** $p < .01$; *** $p < .001$

[a] SF-36 Mental Health and Vitality scales

Transformed scale = [(Actual raw score − lowest possible raw score)/(possible raw score range)] × 100

[b] The reference group is recruited from outside the inner city

[c] Century month (CM). January 2001 = 1. The project recruited from May 2012 (CM = 136) to September 2014 (CM = 164). South Africa was in the midst of scaling up HIV testing and treatment during this period

[d] The reference group is not living in an informal settlement

In contrast to the other steps in the HIV cascade, recent drug use was associated with not being on ART among women who already knew they were living with HIV. Women who had a urine drug screen result positive for cocaine or opiate metabolites were only about 25% as likely to report being on ART compared with women who tested negative. This finding is consistent with previous studies that reported heavy drug use interfered with ART initiation and retention [28]. In addition, the association between being older and being on ART may be due to older women who have been infected longer becoming symptomatic, thus leading them to seek treatment.

Findings from this paper highlight the urgent need for additional resources to increase access to treatment for substance use disorders. Studies have shown that integrating the continuum of care with substance use and HIV treatment programs can decrease alcohol and drug use and offer better overall health outcomes among patients living with HIV [29, 30]. Providing greater access to treatment for substance use disorders and co-locating health departments that offer ART and substance use treatment has the potential to increase ART initiation and retention.

In January 2015, South Africa began implementing the 2013 World Health Organization recommendation

Table 3 Factors associated with ART use among women who knew they were living with HIV and were eligible for ART

Variable	Not on ART	Currently on ART	Bivariate logistic regression	Multivariable logistic regression
Sociodemographic characteristic	**n = 68**	**n = 88**	**OR (95% CI)**	**OR (95% CI)**
Age in years, mean (SD)	30.7 (7.0)	35.9 (6.5)	1.13 (1.07, 1.19)***	1.08 (1.02, 1.15)**
% education ≥10th grade	60.3	53.4	0.92 (0.48, 1.78)	
% unemployed	86.0	86.7	1.07 (0.38, 2.96)	
% married or living as married	52.9	60.2	1.35 (0.71, 2.55)	
% family member with HIV/AIDS	59.7	79.5	2.62 (1.29, 5.35)**	2.09 (0.90, 4.82)
% ever incarcerated (lifetime)	51.5	28.4	0.37 (0.19, 0.73)**	
% ever in substance abuse treatment (lifetime)	16.2	1.1	0.06 (0.01, 0.47)**	
Urine drug screen and breathalyzer results				
% marijuana (THC) positive	50.0	19.3	0.24 (0.12, 0.49)***	
% opiate positive	30.9	4.5	0.11 (0.03, 0.33)***	
% cocaine positive	25.0	4.5	0.14 (0.05, 0.45)**	
% opiate or cocaine positive	35.3	6.8	0.13 (0.05, 0.35)***	0.27 (0.09, 0.80)*
% alcohol (breathalyzer) positive	14.7	15.9	1.10 (0.45, 2.65)	
Sex risk behaviors				
% used a condom at last sex	49.2	39.8	0.68 (0.36, 1.30)	
# times unprotected sex past 30 days, mean (SD)	10.3 (18.7)	7.5 (9.4)	0.99 (0.96, 1.01)	
% engaged in sex work past 6 months	58.8	38.6	0.44 (0.23, 0.84)*	
Victimization				
% physically assaulted past year	13.2	8.0	0.57 (0.20, 1.61)	
% sexually assaulted past year	11.8	4.5	0.36 (0.10, 1.24)	
SF-36 mental health and vitality scales				
Mental health scale score, mean (SD)[a]	56.1 (13.5)	60.6 (14.0)	1.02 (1.00, 1.05)*	1.02 (1.00, 1.04)
Vitality scale score, mean (SD)[b]	42.2 (18.8)	33.4 (14.4)	0.97 (0.95, 0.99)*	
Contextual factors				
% recruited from inner city[b]	54.4	26.1	0.30 (0.15, 0.58)***	
Century month recruited[c], mean (SD)	147.0 (8.8)	153.6 (8.3)	1.09 (1.05, 1.13)***	1.06 (1.01, 1.11)*
% living in informal settlement[d]	32.4	38.6	1.32 (0.68, 2.56)	

* $p < .05$; ** $p < .01$; *** $p < .001$

[a] SF-36 Mental Health and Vitality scales

Transformed scale = [(Actual raw score − lowest possible raw score)/(possible raw score range)] × 100

[b] The reference group is recruited from outside the inner city

[c] Century month (CM). January 2001 = 1. The project recruited from May 2012 (CM = 136) to September 2014 (CM = 164). South Africa was in the midst of scaling up HIV testing and treatment during this period

[d] The reference group is not living in an informal settlement

Table 4 Barriers to obtaining or adhering to ART

Theme	Specific items[a]	N	%
Missed appointments	Missed staging appointment, did not attend wellness appointment	24	35.3
Structural factors	Change in clinic, clinic not providing ART, lack of transportation, no identification card, no food, no place to store pills	23	33.8
Personal beliefs about ART and own readiness	Fear of side effects, fear to commit to daily dose, no need for ART, not feeling "ready," too much trouble to pick up	16	23.5
In the process of obtaining ART	Pending CD4 results, need to schedule appointment, currently attending wellness appointment	10	14.7
Other medical issues and difficulties with dosage	Only took when pregnant, getting tuberculosis treatment, need alcohol and other drug treatment first, did not follow dosage, kept missing dosage	7	10.3
Interpersonal influence	Stigma, not disclosed HIV status, boyfriend	5	7.4

[a] Not mutually exclusive

to start ART at a CD4 count of 500 instead of 350 [31]. While this change removes a barrier to ART for women with CD4 counts between 350 and 500, as of 2016, South Africa had not committed sufficient resources to implement the recommendation fully. The individual and structural barriers to ART reported in this study were similar to those reported in previous studies [32] that have interfered with achieving the 90-90-90 goals. Although the new WHO guidelines recommends providing ART to everyone regardless of CD4, and the South Africa Minister of Health announced support for these recommendations, each Province in South Africa will have to come to terms with on the ground barriers to meeting these needs [33].

Our results could be used to inform future efforts to reduce barriers to testing as well as efforts to increase treatment access and adherence to achieve the 90-90-90 target. The independent association between older age and HIV infection highlights the importance of offering prevention interventions, particularly when testing younger women. Given some of the staffing constraints in health clinics, efforts in Pretoria should focus on the inner city because women recruited from the inner city were nearly twice as likely to test positive for HIV as women recruited from other areas of Pretoria. Clearly, women who have been sexually assaulted or experienced violence should routinely be offered HIV testing. Offering substance abuse treatment at the same site where ART is offered could increase adherence to ART and help address the complex issues of substance use. Free transportation to clinics or mobile treatment vans with directly observed therapy would help as well. The positive associations between being engaged in sex work and being recruited from the inner city or living in an informal settlement provide additional support for testing sex workers and women in both contexts who use alcohol or other drugs.

Limitations

As with all cross-sectional studies, caution should be used in drawing causal inferences from associations in the multivariable models. Additionally, the study relies primarily on self-report data, which is susceptible to recall errors and socially desirable responses that may reduce the reliability and validity of the results. However, the original Risk Behavior Assessment demonstrated adequate reliability and validity [34]. Additionally, interviewers underwent intensive training and monitoring to minimize eliciting socially desirable responses and used calendars to assist participants with recall. Caution should be used in extrapolating these findings to other populations and to women in other geographic locations.

Conclusions

South Africa faces enormous challenges to achieving the UNAIDS 90-90-90 goals for HIV testing, treatment, and viral suppression. The country will need to expand the scope and increase the frequency of HIV testing among sex workers and other women who use alcohol or other drugs.

The finding that HIV-positive women recruited later in the study were more likely to be on ART than women recruited earlier suggests that South Africa is making progress in scaling up ART. Nevertheless, only 44% of women who met the current eligibility criteria for ART self-reported they were on it, and that figure drops to 30% under the new World Health Organization guidelines to treat everyone regardless of their CD4 count. South Africa faces enormous challenges just to treat 90% of people who are aware of their HIV status. The high HIV incidence rates among women suggest that for HIV treatment as prevention to be successful, STTR efforts will need to be scaled up among the men who are infecting them as well as among women.

Abbreviations

ART: antiretroviral therapy; ARV: antiretroviral; CI: confidence interval; CM: century month; HIV: human immunodeficiency virus; IRB: Institutional Review Board; MDMA: 3,4-methylenedioxy-methamphetamine; OR: odds ratio; PRBA: Pretoria Risk Behavior Assessment; PrEP: pre-exposure prophylaxis; SD: standard deviation; STTR: seek, test, treat, and retain; THC: tetrahydrocannabinol.

Authors' contributions

WMW is PI, conceived the study, and completed the final manuscript. CVH is Co-I, assisted with the original design of the study, and contributed to the final draft. JN managed the field operations and contributed to the writing. TK was responsible for the instrument and data quality. ID conducted initial analysis and along with JB contributed to writing the first drafts. FAB and RN contributed to the final draft. WAZ is Co-I, helped conceive the study, and conducted analyses and writing. All authors read and approved the final manuscript.

Author details

[1] Substance Use, Gender and Applied Research, RTI International, 3040 East Cornwallis Road, Research Triangle Park, NC 27709-2194, USA. [2] Health Policy and Management, UNC Gillings School of Global Public Health, Chapel Hill, NC, USA. [3] Department of Psychology, North Carolina State University, Raleigh, NC, USA. [4] Psychiatry and Behavioral Sciences, Duke University School of Medicine, Durham, NC, USA. [5] School of Medicine, University of North Carolina, Chapel Hill, NC, USA. [6] Substance Use, Gender and Applied Research, RTI International, Pretoria, South Africa. [7] UCB Biosciences, Raleigh, NC, USA. [8] Statistics and Epidemiology, RTI International, 3040 East Cornwallis Road, Research Triangle Park, NC 27709-2194, USA. [9] Psychology Department, University of North Carolina, Chapel Hill, NC, USA. [10] Biostatistics, School of Public Health, University of Washington, 1410 NE Campus Parkway, Seattle, WA, USA.

Acknowledgements

The content is solely the responsibility of the authors and does not necessarily represent the official views of the National Institutes of Health. We wish to thank Sharon Barrell for her editorial assistance.

Competing interests

The authors declare that they have no competing interests.

Funding
Research reported in this publication was supported by the National Institutes of Health, National Institute on Drug Abuse under award R01DA032061.

References

1. UN Women. Facts and figures: HIV and AIDS. 6/2016 edn. New York, NY: UN Women; 2016.
2. Cohen MS, Chen YQ, McCauley M, Gamble T, Hosseinipour MC, Kumarasamy N, Hakim JG, Kumwenda J, Grinsztejn B, Pilotto JH, et al. Antiretroviral therapy for the prevention of HIV-1 transmission. N Engl J Med. 2016;375(9):830–9.
3. Das M, Chu PL, Santos GM, Scheer S, Vittinghoff E, McFarland W, Colfax GN. Decreases in community viral load are accompanied by reductions in new HIV infections in San Francisco. PLoS ONE. 2010;5(6):e11068.
4. Wood E, Kerr T, Marshall BD, Li K, Zhang R, Hogg RS, Harrigan PR, Montaner JS. Longitudinal community plasma HIV-1 RNA concentrations and incidence of HIV-1 among injecting drug users: prospective cohort study. BMJ. 2009;338:b1649.
5. Eaton JW, Johnson LF, Salomon JA, Barnighausen T, Bendavid E, Bershteyn A, Bloom DE, Cambiano V, Fraser C, Hontelez JA, et al. HIV treatment as prevention: systematic comparison of mathematical models of the potential impact of antiretroviral therapy on HIV incidence in South Africa. PLoS Med. 2012;9(7):e1001245.
6. UNAIDS: 90-90-90-An ambitious treatment target to help end the AIDS epidemic. Geneva: UNAIDS; 2014.
7. Hull MW, Wu Z, Montaner JS. Optimizing the engagement of care cascade: a critical step to maximize the impact of HIV treatment as prevention. Curr Opin HIV AIDS. 2012;7(6):579–86.
8. Volkow ND, Baler RD, Normand JL. The unrealized potential of addiction science in curbing the HIV epidemic. Curr HIV Res. 2011;9(6):393–5.
9. Vagenas P, Azar MM, Copenhaver MM, Springer SA, Molina PE, Altice FL. The impact of alcohol use and related disorders on the HIV Continuum of care: a systematic review: alcohol and the HIV continuum of care. Curr HIV/AIDS Rep. 2015;12(4):421–36.
10. Williams B, Wood R, Dukay V, Delva W, Ginsburg D, Hargrove J, Stander M, Sheneberger R, Montaner J, Welte A. Treatment as prevention: preparing the way. J Int AIDS Soc. 2011;14(Suppl 1):S6.
11. WHO: Women's health In: Fact Sheet No. 334. World Health Organization; 2013. http://www.who.int/mediacentre/factsheets/fs334/en/.
12. Haberer JE, Baeten JM, Campbell J, Wangisi J, Katabira E, Ronald A, Tumwesigye E, Psaros C, Safren SA, Ware NC, et al. Adherence to antiretroviral prophylaxis for HIV prevention: a substudy cohort within a clinical trial of serodiscordant couples in East Africa. PLoS Med. 2013;10(9):e1001511.
13. Wechsberg WM, Wu LT, Zule WA, Parry CD, Browne FA, Luseno WK, Kline T, Gentry A. Substance abuse, treatment needs and access among female sex workers and non-sex workers in Pretoria, South Africa. Subst Abuse Treat Prev Policy. 2009;4:11.
14. Rumptz MH, Tobias C, Rajabiun S, Bradford J, Cabral H, Young R, Cunningham WE. Factors associated with engaging socially marginalized HIV-positive persons in primary care. AIDS Patient Care STDS. 2007;21(Suppl 1):S30–9.
15. Tobias CR, Cunningham W, Cabral HD, Cunningham CO, Eldred L, Naar-King S, Bradford J, Sohler NL, Wong MD, Drainoni ML. Living with HIV but without medical care: barriers to engagement. AIDS Patient Care STDS. 2007;21(6):426–34.
16. Dada S, Erasmus J, Burnhams NH, Parry C, Bhana A, Timol F, Fourie D, Kitshoff D, Nel E, Weimann R. Monitoring alcohol, tobacco and other drug abuse trends in South Africa (July 1996–June 2015): Phase 38. In: SACENDU Research Brief, vol. 18; 2015.
17. Wechsberg WM, Zule WA, Ndirangu J, Kline TL, Rodman NF, Doherty IA, Novak SP, van der Horst CM. The biobehavioral Women's Health CoOp in Pretoria, South Africa: study protocol for a cluster-randomized design. BMC Public Health. 1074;2014:14.
18. Cairncross v De Vos (1876) 6 Buch 5; Steenkamp v Kampfer 1914 CPD 877; Venter v De Burghersdorp Stores 1915 CPD 252; Pleat v Van Staden 1921 OPD 91; Ambaker v African Meat Co 1927 CPD 326; Ochberg v Ochberg's Estate 1941 CPD 15; Ahmed v Coovadia 1944 TPD 364; Dickens v Daley 1956 1 All SA 329 (N); 1956 2 All SA 197 (N); 1956 2 SA 11 (N); Grand Prix Motors WP (Pty) Ltd v Swart 1976 3 All SA 480 (C); 1976 3 SA 221 (C); Heaton The South African Law of Persons (3 ed) (2008) 115 et seq; Van Heerden, Cockrell and Keightley (eds) Boberg's Law of Persons and the Family (2 ed) (1999) 474; Van der Vyver and Joubert Persone- en Familiereg 131 et seq; Steyn 1927 SALJ 313; Spiro Parent and Child 249 et seq; De Wet and Van Wyk Kontraktereg en Handelsreg 64–66.
19. Wechsberg WM, Zule WA, Luseno WK, Kline TL, Browne FA, Novak SP, Ellerson RM. Effectiveness of an adapted evidence-based woman-focused intervention for sex workers and non-sex workers: the Women's Health Coop in South Africa. J Drug Issues. 2011;41(2):233–52.
20 Babor TF, Higgins-Biddle JC, Saunders JB, Monteiro MG. The Alcohol Use Disorders Identification Test: guidelines for use in primary care. vol. WHO/MSD/MSB/01.6a. Geneva: World Health Organization Department of Mental Health and Substance Dependence; 2001.
21 Ware JE, Kosinski M, Dewey JE. How to score version 2 of the SF-36. Lincoln, RI: Quality Metric Incorporated; 2000.
22 Padian NS, Shiboski SC, Jewell NP. Female-to-male transmission of human immunodeficiency virus. JAMA. 1991;266(12):1664–7.
23 Gupta GR, Ogden J, Warner A. Moving forward on women's gender-related HIV vulnerability: the good news, the bad news and what to do about it. Glob Public Health. 2011;6(Suppl 3):S370–82.
24 Stoebenau K, Heise L, Wamoyi J, Bobrova N. Revisiting the understanding of "transactional sex" in sub-Saharan Africa: a review and synthesis of the literature. Soc Sci Med. 2016;168:186–97.
25 Murnane PM, Celum C, Mugo N, Campbell JD, Donnell D, Bukusi E, Mujugira A, Tappero J, Kahle EM, Thomas KK, et al. Efficacy of preexposure prophylaxis for HIV-1 prevention among high-risk heterosexuals: subgroup analyses from a randomized trial. Aids. 2013;27(13):2155–60.
26 Doherty IA, Myers B, Zule WA, Minnis AM, Kline TL, Parry CD, Wechsberg WM. Seek, test and disclose: knowledge of HIV testing and serostatus among high-risk couples in a South African township. Sex Transm Infect. 2016;92(1):5–11.
27 Maughan-Brown B, Lloyd N, Bor J, Venkataramani AS: Changes in self-reported HIV testing during South Africa's 2010/2011 national testing campaign: gains and shortfalls. J Int AIDS Soc. 2016;19(1).
28 Dombrowski JC, Simoni JM, Katz DA, Golden MR. Barriers to HIV care and treatment among participants in a public health HIV care relinkage program. AIDS Patient Care STDs. 2015;29(5):279–87.
29 Proeschold-Bell RJ, Heine A, Pence BW, McAdam K, Quinlivan EB. A cross-site, comparative effectiveness study of an integrated HIV and substance use treatment program. AIDS Patient Care STDS. 2010;24(10):651–8.
30 Lombard F, Proescholdbell RJ, Cooper K, Musselwhite L, Quinlivan EB. Adaptations across clinical sites of an integrated treatment model for persons with HIV and substance abuse. AIDS Patient Care STDS. 2009;23(8):631–8.
31 Department of Health. National consolidated guidelines for the prevention of mother-to-child transmission of HIV (PMTCT) and the management of HIV in children, adolescents and adults. Pretoria: Department of Health; 2014.
32 Kagee A, Remien R, Berkman A, Hoffman S, Campos L, Swartz L. Structural barriers to ART adherence in Southern Africa: challenges and potential ways forward. Glob Public Health. 2011;6(1):83–97.
33 UNAIDS: South Africa takes bold step to provide HIV treatment for all. Geneva: UNAIDS; 2016.
34 Needle R, Fisher DG, Weatherby N, Chitwood D, Brown B, Cesari H, Booth R, Williams ML, Watters J, Andersen M. Reliability of self-reported HIV risk behaviors of drug users. Psychol Addict Behav. 1995;9(4):242.

Health evaluation and referral assistant: a randomized controlled trial to improve smoking cessation among emergency department patients

Edwin D. Boudreaux[1*], Beau Abar[2], Brianna Haskins[3], Brigitte Bauman[4] and Grant Grissom[5]

Abstract

Background: Computer technologies hold promise for implementing tobacco screening, brief intervention, and referral to treatment (SBIRT). This study aims to evaluate a computerized tobacco SBIRT system called the Health Evaluation and Referral Assistant (HERA).

Methods: Smokers (n = 421) presenting to an emergency department were randomly assigned to the HERA or a minimal-treatment Control and were followed for 3 months. Analyses compared smoking cessation treatment provider contact, treatment initiation, treatment completion, and smoking behavior across condition using univariable comparisons, generalized estimating equations (GEE), and post hoc Chi square analyses.

Results: HERA participants were more likely to initiate contact with a treatment provider but did not differ on treatment initiation, quit attempts, or sustained abstinence. Subanalyses revealed HERA participants who accepted a faxed referral were more likely to initiate treatment but were not more likely to stop smoking.

Conclusions: The HERA promoted initial contact with a smoking cessation provider and the faxed referral further promoted treatment initiation, but it did not lead to improved abstinence.

Trial registration: ClinicalTrials.gov number NCT01153373

Keywords: Tobacco, Brief intervention, Emergency medicine, Facilitated referral, Tobacco treatment, Tobacco screening

Background

Each year tobacco use kills 430,000 Americans for an average of over 5 million years of potential life lost annually [1–4]. Smoking cessation is a cost-effective disease prevention strategy that has shown immediate and substantive health benefits in those who successfully quit [3]. While much attention has focused on primary care as a setting to promote smoking cessation, hospital emergency departments (EDs) are uniquely positioned for tobacco intervention efforts as well. The prevalence of tobacco use among ED patients exceeds the national average [2, 5, 6], with a 2014 study reporting an overall prevalence of more than double the national average [5]. Furthermore, disadvantaged and underserved populations, such as minority patients, underinsured, and low income households, rely disproportionately upon EDs for primary care services [7]. With over 130 million visits annually, ED originated tobacco control efforts have the potential for substantial impact on public health by effecting change in hard to reach populations [7, 8].

This potential was recognized by the Robert Wood Johnson Foundation which recommended implementation of routine screening, brief intervention, and referral to treatment (SBIRT) for tobacco in the ED setting,

*Correspondence: Edwin.Boudreaux@umassmed.edu
[1] Departments of Emergency Medicine, Psychiatry, and Quantitative Health Sciences, University of Massachusetts Medical School, LA-189, 55 Lake Avenue North, Worcester, MA 01655, USA
Full list of author information is available at the end of the article

and strongly encouraged research to develop tobacco interventions specific to the needs of EDs [7]. Additionally, a joint statement by the American College of Emergency Physicians and the Emergency Nurses Association recommended that ED healthcare providers universally screen and counsel tobacco users seeking care in the ED. They proposed using a brief Ask, Advise, Refer model, which consists of Asking about tobacco use, Advising patients to quit, and Referring patients to specialized treatment for tobacco use [2, 3]. The Ask, Advise, Refer model has since been adopted by researchers in their work to refine an effective ED-appropriate strategy for tobacco SBIRT [9, 10].

While much literature supports the utility of tobacco SBIRT for the ED population [2–7, 9–11], questions still remain regarding the most effective and appropriate SBIRT protocol. Factors likely to impede clinician intervention include competing time demands, lack of specialized behavioral health training, and a mission centered on acute rather than chronic medical care [6–8]. To maximize successful implementation, procedures should be convenient, brief, require minimum specialized training, and focus on connecting patients to outpatient resources after the ED visit. Traditional strategies typically do not meet all of these requirements and result in inconsistent adoption [12]. Behavioral intervention technology advancement has allowed for the development of computer-assisted SBIRT models which aim to reduce interruptions in clinical care and reduce clinician burden without sacrificing effectiveness [8].

The objective of this study was to test a new web-based program to facilitate tobacco SBIRT called the Health Evaluation and Referral Assistant (HERA). The HERA was patterned after face-to-face SBIRT models and is self-administered by patients on a computer during their medical visit. This study tested the hypotheses that the HERA would result in greater outpatient smoking cessation treatment initiation and increased smoking cessation over three months post-visit as compared with a minimal intervention control condition.

Methods

A full description of the HERA development and RCT methods were previously reported [12, 13]. Although the HERA assesses for and refers patients to treatment for tobacco, alcohol, and illicit drug use, only results pertaining to tobacco are reported in this paper. Subsequent papers will address the other substance classes. This clinical trial was registered with ClinicalTrials.gov as the Dynamic Assessment and Referral System (ClinicalTrials.gov Identifier: NCT01153373).

HERA

Assessment The HERA uses the two-item Heavy Smoking Index (HSI) to assess nicotine dependence [14]. Age of first smoking cigarettes regularly, use of other forms of tobacco, such as cigars or smokeless tobacco, and readiness to change were also assessed. Participants who expressed interest in quitting were asked when they would like to quit (within the next 30 days, Within the next 6 months, more than 6 months from now), and if they would like help connecting with a smoking cessation counselor or treatment program (Yes, No).

A checklist of psychiatric diagnoses was used to document psychiatric history [none, anxiety or panic attacks or post-traumatic stress disorder (PTSD), depression or bipolar disorder, schizophrenia or schizoaffective disorder, anorexia or bulimia, attention deficit disorder (ADD, ADHD), other]. Participants were also screened for depression using the Patient Health Questionaire-2 (PHQ-2) [15].

Report generator Two reports using the assessment data were produced, and are described in detail by Boudreaux et al. [12, 13]. The Healthcare Provider Report is a summary of the assessment and was reviewed by the patient's treating physician. The Patient Feedback Report consisted of three sections: (1) the Face Sheet, which included an overview and tailored tobacco referral list, (2) the Patient Assessment Summary, which provided personally tailored feedback related to the patient's tobacco use, and (3) the Motivation Toolkit, which consisted of several worksheets rooted in motivational interviewing [16] and the transtheoretical model [17].

Referral generator The referral generator draws upon a library of smoking cessation treatment services maintained by Polaris Health Directions, Inc. The library is used to generate personally tailored referral lists containing free and fee-for-service treatment options, including free state quitlines, and to send dynamic referrals. A dynamic referral is a faxed referral to a "best match" facility based on the individual's ZIP code, insurance, and desire for telephone or in-person treatment. If accepted by the patient, the dynamic referral was faxed by the HERA and included a brief assessment summary and the patient's contact information. The participating services agreed to contact the individual within 48 h of receiving the referral to perform an initial evaluation and explore treatment options.

Procedure

Patients were enrolled from four EDs (see Table 1) during 8 AM to 7 PM, with shifts representing all days of the week. Research assistants (RAs) approached consecutive adult patients at their bedside. All patients who smoked

Table 1 Site characteristics

Type	Annual volume	Location	Race/ ethnicity
Academic, urban	90,733	Worcester, MA	W 82 %, H 11 %, B 4 %
Community, urban	47,364	Worcester, MA	W 74 %, H 14 %, B 9 %
Community, suburban	23,217	Marlboro, MA	W 80 %, H 15 %, B 3 %, U 2 %
Academic, urban	59,482	Camden, NJ	W 35 %, H 20 %, B 45 %

W white, non-Hispanic, *H* Hispanic, *B* black, *U* unknown, *MA* Massachusetts, *NJ* New Jersey

within the past 30 days and 18 years or older were considered. Patients with risky alcohol use or illicit drug use, including those who currently demonstrate tobacco dependence, were enrolled into the larger trial and examined separately due to the overarching goal of intervening on the most salient/emergent substance-related concerns. The current paper focuses only on tobacco users who did not abuse alcohol or use drugs. Exclusion criteria included severe illness or distress, cognitive insufficiency, in state custody or restraints, being held involuntarily, and language barriers. Patients were enrolled regardless of whether they were admitted or discharged; the study components, including baseline and intervention, were completed prior to leaving the ED. Participants were randomized to either the intervention or control condition by a random number generator from the Java programming language standard library embedded within the HERA. Immediately following discharge/transfer from the ED, the enrolling RA completed a short interview with the participant, either in person before he or she left the ED or by phone within 48 h (post-visit interview). A trained RA unaffiliated with the performance sites contacted all participants by telephone at 4 and 12 weeks following the ED visit to assess tobacco treatment initiation and to re-assess tobacco use. Biological verification of abstinence was not obtained. The study was approved by the Institutional Review Boards for all performance sites. All participants gave their informed consent and signed a written consent form prior to their inclusion in the study.

Study conditions

Intervention and control conditions were treated the same in all respects related to study procedures. Those in the intervention condition (HERA) (1) were offered a dynamic referral, (2) their treating physician was given the Healthcare Provider Report, and (3) the patient was given the Patient Feedback Report, which included a personally tailored referral list. Those assigned to the minimal intervention control condition (Control) completed the HERA assessment but were not offered the dynamic referral, and the reports were not made available to either the healthcare provider or the patient. However, Control group patients did receive a standardized, printed list of local smoking cessation treatment providers and included the toll-free tobacco quitline 1-800-QUIT-NOW.

Blinding

The RA performing the outcome assessments was partially blinded. Because the HERA is heavily focused on the referral process, and different patients received different types of referrals, the follow-up questions were keyed to the referral type received at baseline (printed list vs. dynamic referral) to avoid confusion. Despite blinding efforts, the nature of the questions revealed some information about the group assignment if the participant had accepted a dynamic referral. For example, only patients who chose a dynamic referral were asked whether they had been contacted by a smoking cessation counselor.

Measures

HERA The HERA assessment was described under methods/assessment module.

Post-visit interview Immediately following discharge/transfer from the ED, the enrolling RA completed a short interview to ascertain if the treating clinicians provided tobacco counseling, education materials, or referrals for tobacco treatment. Chart review was not used because of unreliability associated with documenting tasks such as counseling.

Follow-up assessment All participants were asked if they had made initial contact with a smoking cessation counselor or treatment program (treatment contact), completed an initial assessment (treatment initiation), attended any additional treatment sessions beyond the initial assessment (treatment engagement), and completed treatment (treatment completion). Any of these milestones could have occurred in person or by telephone. The RA interviewed the participant by phone to assess a self-reported quit attempt defined as intentional abstinence for 24 h, efforts to decrease tobacco use, the HSI, and sustained abstinence since the ED visit.

Data analyses

In addition to univariable comparisons, the primary analysis consisted of a series of generalized estimating equation (GEE) analyses comparing the control and intervention conditions on outcomes of interest (tobacco treatment provider contact, treatment initiation, tobacco use) during the 4 and 12 week follow-up. When GEE models were statistically significant, post hoc Chi square analyses were used to provide greater context for the observed findings. These models were unconditional (i.e., included no covariates) due to random assignment equating groups on potential confounding characteristics. A series of planned Chi square analyses were also performed for outcome data available at a single time point (e.g., ED counseling, treatment completion).

Analyses were supplemented by examining differences across individuals in the control condition versus those in the intervention condition that accepted a dynamic referral and those in the intervention (dynamic referral) condition that declined a dynamic referral (tailored list only). These supplemental models included baseline HSI and readiness to quit as covariates to account for preexisting differences between individuals who accept a referral and those who do not. All GEE models were performed first using multiple imputation with 20 datasets to account for missing data at each of the follow-ups. These models were then recapitulated under intention-to-treat principles (i.e., non-retained participants provided with the least favorable outcome), and the patterns of statistical significance of primary predictors and covariates were identical. Observed frequencies were presented in each table, with the percentages representing intention-to-treat values. An alpha level of 0.05 was used to indicate statistical significance for all comparisons, and all analyses were performed using SPSS 22 (IBM, 2012).

Results

Preliminary analysis

Of 600 tobacco users who met eligibility criteria and who did not demonstrate risky alcohol and/or drug use, 427 individuals were enrolled (see Fig. 1). Those enrolled were not statistically different across demographics and enrollment site to those who were not enrolled, except enrolled individuals were slightly younger ($M = 39.5$ years; SD $= 12.3$) than non-enrolled individuals ($M = 43.0$ years; SD $= 14.3$), $t\ (598) = 2.52$, $p = 0.01$. Of the 427 participants enrolled, 215 were assigned to the control condition and 212 to the intervention. Six were eliminated due to either having been deceased before the follow-up assessment was complete or withdrawal from the study because of duplicate enrollment, resulting in an analyzed sample of 421 participants (211 Control, 210 HERA). At baseline, there were no differences between the two conditions on demographics, mental health diagnoses, HSI, pack years, or readiness to change (p values >0.10) (Table 2).

Of the 421 analyzed participants, 412 (98 %) completed the post-visit interview, 314 (75 %) completed the one-month follow-up, and 295 (70 %) completed the three-month follow-up (see Fig. 1). There were no differences between retained individuals and those lost to follow-up on intervention condition, most demographic characteristics, baseline HSI score, pack years, or readiness to change (p values >0.05); however, retained participants were slightly older ($M = 39.8$ years; SD $= 12.3$) than those lost to follow-up ($M = 37.0$ years; SD $= 11.7$), $t\ (419) = 2.18$, $p = 0.03$.

Comparisons on outcomes of interest

Specialized smoking cessation treatment Initial contact between participants and a smoking cessation treatment provider was significantly more common in the intervention condition than the control condition (odds ratio $= 2.69$; see Table 3), with significant differences observed at each follow-up [1 month $\chi^2\ (1) = 8.16$, $p = 0.004$; 3 months $\chi^2\ (1) = 11.65$, $p = 0.001$]. Although treatment initiation, treatment engagement, and treatment completion rates were higher in the intervention condition compared to the control, these differences did not reach statistical significance (p values >0.05). Among the participants in the HERA, 72 (34 %) accepted a dynamic referral.

Tobacco use Quit attempts, efforts to reduce smoking, HSI, and sustained abstinence at both follow-up periods were not statistically different across intervention and control conditions (see Table 3).

Physician behavior Clinician counseling, provision of educational materials, and provision of referrals, beyond those provided as part of the study protocol, were not statistically different across intervention and control conditions (see Table 3).

Exploring the effect of dynamic referrals Supplemental GEE analyses demonstrated large differences across groups on treatment contact. Using dummy codes (control condition as the reference), results indicated that experimental participants who accepted a dynamic referral made contact with a provider a much greater rate than control individuals (odds ratio $= 11.89$, 95 % CI 6.70–21.09, $p < 0.001$; see Table 4). Effects on treatment initiation were of relatively similar magnitude, with much higher rates of initiation among experimental participants who accepted a dynamic referral and control participants (odds ratio $= 4.41$, 95 % CI 2.11–9.21, $p < 0.001$). There were no differences in treatment initiation between experimental individuals who did not accept a dynamic referral and control individuals (odds ratio $= 0.52$, 95 % CI 0.18–1.49, $p = 0.22$). The differences in treatment initiation between experimental participants who accepted a dynamic referral and control participants remained significant (p values <0.05) when accounting for baseline readiness to change and baseline HSI in post hoc GEE models (see Table 5).

There was also a significant effect of group membership on engagement in cessation treatment, $\chi^2\ (1) = 6.60$,

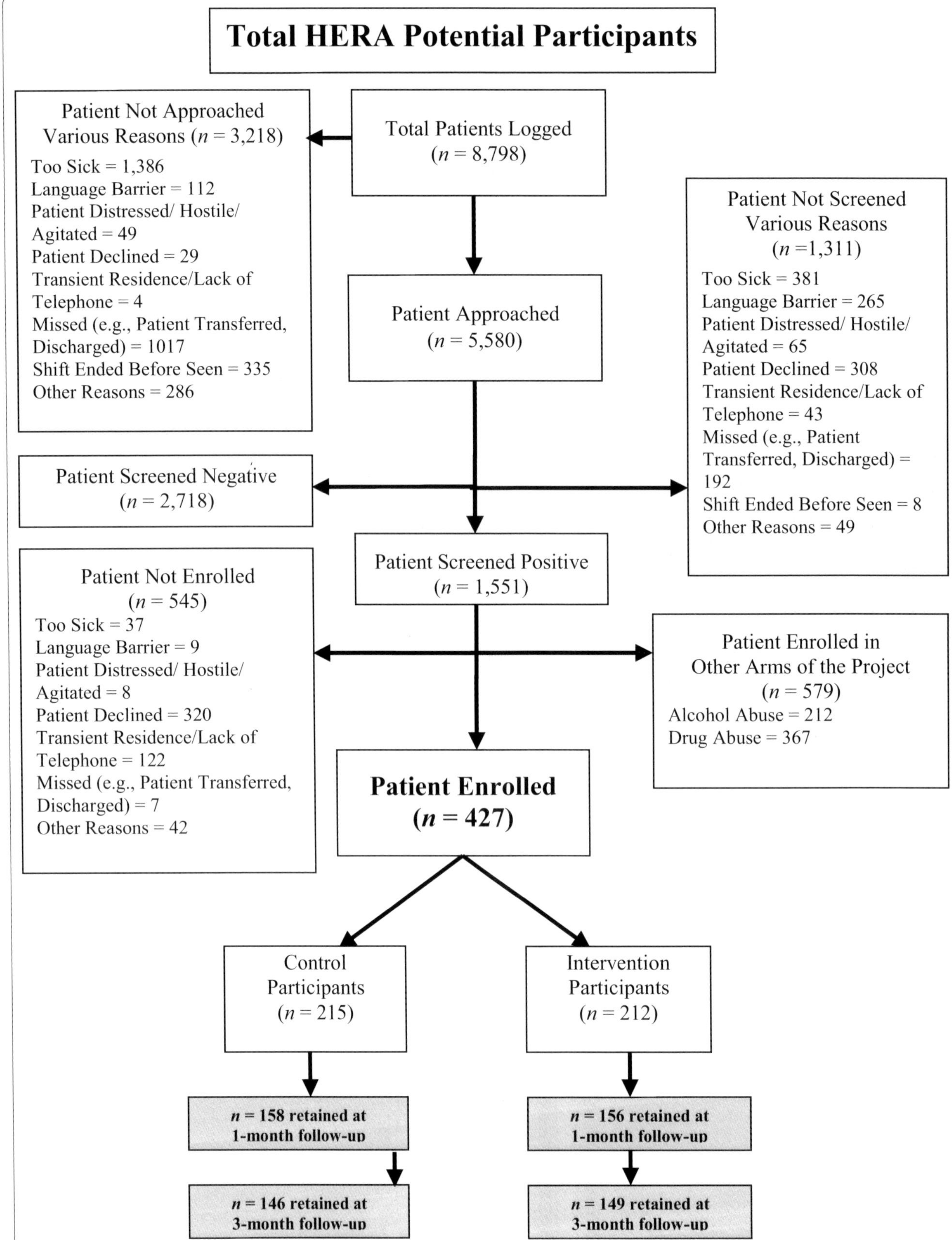

Fig. 1 Enrollment flow for the HERA RCT—tobacco

Table 2 Demographic characteristics of the analyzed sample

	Frequency	%	Mean	Standard deviation
Participant sex				
Male	150	35.6 %		
Female	271	64.4 %		
Participant age			39.0	12.2
Data collection site				
Cooper University Hospital (NJ)	233	55.3 %		
UMass University Hospital (MA)	178	42.3 %		
UMass Memorial Hospital (MA)	4	1.0 %		
Marlborough Hospital (MA)	6	1.4 %		
Race				
White	291	69.1 %		
Black	114	27.1 %		
Other/undocumented	16	3.8 %		
Ethnicity				
Non-hispanic/Latino	339	80.5 %		
Hispanic/Latino	67	15.9 %		
Not documented	15	3.6 %		
Insurance status[a]				
Private insurance	80	19.0 %		
Medicaid	127	30.2 %		
State financed insurance—non-medicaid	78	18.5 %		
Medicare	69	16.4 %		
Other kind of insurance not listed	27	6.4 %		
No insurance	73	17.3 %		
PHQ-2			1.7	1.7
Any mental health diagnosis	240	57.0 %		
Anxiety/panic attacks/PTSD	158	37.5 %		
Depression/bipolar disorder	150	35.6 %		
Schizophrenia/schizoaffective disorder	12	2.9 %		
Anorexia/bulimia	4	1.0 %		
ADD/ADHD	29	6.9 %		
Other mental health diagnosis	17	4.0 %		
Baseline HSI score			2.5	1.4
Pack years			18.2	14.9
Other tobacco used in past 30 days				
Cigars	14	3.3 %		
Smokeless tobacco (Dip, Snuff, Chew)	2	0.5 %		
Experimental condition				
Intervention	210	49.9 %		
Control	211	50.1 %		
Referral[b]				
Tailored, printed list of providers (only)	138	65.7 %		
Dynamic referral accepted	72	34.3 %		

Risky alcohol and illicit drug users were excluded from the tobacco sample; they were enrolled and randomized into the alcohol and drug use samples, to be reported separately

[a] Insurance status categories are not mutually exclusive (i.e. participants can have multiple types of insurance)

[b] Only participants in the intervention condition. All patients in the intervention group received the tailored, printed list of providers by default. Dynamic referral consists of a faxed referral with a brief tobacco use summary to a tobacco treatment provider matched to the individual based on location of residence and preference for telephone vs. in-person treatment. All patients in the intervention group received the tailored, printed list of providers by default

Table 3 Comparisons between intervention and control conditions

	Intervention ($n = 210$)	Control ($n = 211$)
ED clinician (MD/RN) counseling[a]		
MD/RN asked about tobacco use	172 (81.9 %)	165 (78.2 %)
MD/RN counseled participant to quit	73 (34.8 %)	68 (32.2 %)
Received educational materials	8 (3.8 %)	14 (6.6 %)
Received a smoking cessation referral	5 (2.4 %)	11 (5.2 %)
Outpatient smoking cessation treatment		
Contact with tobacco treatment provider GEE odds ratio = 2.69 (95 % CI 1.65–4.39), $p < 0.001$		
Contact at 1 month	35 (16.7 %)	16 (7.6 %)
Contact at 3 months	48 (22.9 %)	27 (12.8 %)
Initiated treatment (evaluated by tobacco treatment provider) GEE odds ratio = 1.69 (95 % CI 0.86–3.31), $p = 0.13$		
Treatment initiation at 1 month	10 (4.8 %)	8 (3.8 %)
Treatment initiation at 3 months	21 (10.0 %)	14 (6.6 %)
Treatment engagement at either time	8 (3.8 %)	7 (3.3 %)
Treatment completion	7 (3.3 %)	6 (2.8 %)
Smoking behavior		
Used tobacco (since ED visit) GEE odds ratio = 0.98 (95 % CI 0.62–1.55), $p = 0.93$		
Abstinent for first month (since visit)	13 (6.2 %)	19 (9.0 %)
Abstinent for 3 months (since visit)	8 (3.8 %)	9 (4.3 %)
At least one quit attempt at 1 month	68 (32.4 %)	72 (34.1 %)
At least one quit attempt at 3 months	105 (50.0 %)	118 (55.9 %)
Attempted to reduce use at 1 month	125 (59.5 %)	122 (57.8 %)
Attempted to reduce use at 3 months	150 (71.4 %)	154 (73.0 %)

All percentages and analyses use the ITT principal of worst outcome for missing values

[a] ED clinician behavior assessment included behaviors over and above the materials provided as part of the research study. All patients in both groups had tobacco assessed as part of the study and received a referral list. The control group received a pre-printed list, while the intervention group received a personally tailored list, as well as a dynamic referral if desired

$p = 0.037$ (see Table 4). While engagement was relatively infrequent across all groups, the rate of engagement for those accepting a dynamic referral was more than double the rate observed in the control condition (8.3 vs. 3.3 %; see Table 4). This effect, however, was no longer significant when baseline readiness to change tobacco use and HSI were included as covariates (odds ratio control vs. tailored list only = 0.78, 95 % CI 0.19–3.18, $p = 0.73$; odds ratio control vs. dynamic referral = 1.83, 95 % CI 0.58–5.76, $p = 0.30$). There were no effects of group membership on tobacco cessation (see Tables 4 and 5).

Discussion

Providing tobacco interventions in the ED is important because many patients treated in EDs do not receive care anywhere else, which makes this setting important for comprehensive public health efforts to improve tobacco cessation [18]. However, there are unique barriers that make incorporating interventions into routine clinical care difficult, including competing priorities, time demands, acute care scope of practice, and a lack of clinician training related to smoking cessation interventions. As a result, technology facilitated interventions may be a particularly good fit. The results of this clinical trial studying a novel, single administration, stand-alone computerized intervention were mixed. Overall, the results suggested that the HERA may improve the critical step of initiating contact with an outpatient smoking cessation treatment provider after the ED visit, with the dynamic referral further promoting the next step of treatment initiation, but these effects do not translate into continued engagement in treatment or changes in smoking behavior over the 3 months following the ED visit. The low engagement rates of the HERA are consistent with rates from a similar study by Willet et al. to investigate the utility of faxed referrals to promote engagement with tobacco quitlines [19].

Factors that may have affected the HERA's impact upon treatment and smoking cessation include lack of supportive efforts by ED staff, the low intensity of the HERA intervention, and barriers to patient follow through after contact with a smoking cessation treatment provider. It was deployed largely as a stand-alone intervention, because the practical realities of current ED practice suggested this would be the model most likely to be used in the ED environment. Although the clinicians who received the Healthcare Provider Report were educated on how to interpret the findings, and it could have prompted them to provide counseling to the patient, they were not specifically trained or mandated to provide counseling or any additional intervention materials. The analyses showed that, in fact, the intervention group did not receive any additional counseling or smoking cessation materials from their treating clinicians. A study of ED-based multicomponent intervention for tobacco use by Bernstein et al. [20] found that patients who received enhanced care in a variety of forms, including clinician counseling, nicotine patches, and follow-up phone call, were more likely to be abstinent at 3 months than those receiving standard referral. Greater clinician involvement may be needed to increase abstinence.

The HERA was a one-time interaction designed to be brief out of sensitivity to the time demands in the ED. This could have adversely affected its clinical impact. Future technology interventions may need to incorporate more powerful motivational interventions, such as interactive multi-media content, and longitudinal interaction after the ED visit. Longitudinal computerized interventions that provide personalized feedback reports over time have demonstrated evidence of effectiveness

Table 4 Comparisons across intervention, tailored list only; intervention, dynamic referral; and control conditions

	Intervention-provider list (*n* = 138)	Intervention-dynamic referral (*n* = 72)	Control (*n* = 211)
Outpatient smoking cessation treatment			
Contact with tobacco treatment provider			
Contact at 1 month	3 (2.0 %)	32 (44.4 %)	16 (7.6 %)
Contact at 3 months	6 (4.3 %)	42 (58.3 %)	27 (12.8 %)
Initiated treatment (evaluated by tobacco treatment provider)			
Treatment initiation at 1 month	2 (1.4 %)	8 (11.1 %)	8 (3.8 %)
Treatment initiation at 3 months	3 (2.2 %)	18 (25.0 %)	14 (6.6 %)
Treatment engagement, either time	2 (1.4 %)	6 (8.3 %)	7 (3.3 %)
Treatment completion	2 (1.4 %)	5 (6.9 %)	6 (2.8 %)
Tobacco cessation			
Abstinent for first month (since visit)	10 (7.2 %)	3 (4.2 %)	19 (9.0 %)
Abstinent for 3 months (since visit)	6 (4.3 %)	2 (2.8 %)	9 (4.3 %)
At least one quit attempt at 1 month	47 (34.1 %)	21 (29.2 %)	72 (34.1 %)
At least one quit attempt at 3 months	72 (52.2 %)	33 (45.8 %)	118 (55.9 %)
Attempted to reduce use at 1 month	80 (58.0 %)	45 (62.5 %)	122 (57.8 %)
Attempted to reduce use at 3 months	98 (71.0 %)	52 (72.2 %)	154 (73.0 %)

Table 5 Follow-up GEE results with covariates

	Predictor	Odds ratio (95 % CI)	*p* value
Treatment contact	Heavy Smoking Index	1.13 (0.90–1.140)	0.29
	Readiness to quit	1.21 (0.84–1.75)	0.30
	Intervention (list) vs. control	0.61 (0.27–1.41)	0.25
	Intervention (DR) vs. control	10.96 (6.12–19.61)	<0.001
Treatment initiation	Heavy Smoking Index	1.16 (0.85–1.59)	0.34
	Readiness to quit	1.60 (0.87–2.94)	0.13
	Intervention (list) vs. control	0.61 (0.20–1.85)	0.38
	Intervention (DR) vs. control	3.74 (1.79–7.81)	<0.001
Abstinence	Heavy Smoking Index	0.90 (0.74–1.08)	0.26
	Readiness to quit	1.10 (0.83–1.45)	0.51
	Intervention (list) vs. control	1.06 (0.61–1.86)	0.82
	Intervention (DR) vs. control	0.82 (0.36–1.85)	0.62

DR dynamic referral

in several well-controlled trials, such as the Tobacco Expert System [21–23]. Blending the report generating and dynamic referral capabilities of the HERA with the longitudinal support and monitoring of systems like the Tobacco Expert System may represent the next evolution in technology facilitated tobacco interventions.

The HERA may not have promoted treatment initiation and engagement because other insurmountable barriers might have been present. For example, even for an indi vidual who is highly motivated and successfully connects with a smoking cessation treatment provider, attending in-person counseling sessions can be impossible if he or she does not have transportation, has young children but no access to childcare, or works during hours when the services are available [7]. Moreover, some smoking cessation services charge a fee, which may have been prohibitive for some patients. Individuals were offered a toll-free telephone counseling option through the tobacco quitline 1-800-QUIT-NOW to help address cost and inconvenience barriers, but this may not have been sufficient to account for all barriers

Limitations

Several limitations affect interpretation of the findings. The study did not use biochemical validation of smoking abstinence. The impact on interpretation is likely to be minimal, because a treatment effect on smoking status was not observed. A minimal treatment control group was used, rather than true treatment as usual. The assessment and resource list may have acted as an intervention and artificially inflated treatment contact and behavior change compared to true treatment as usual. The study enrolled ED patients, which have been shown to change their smoking behavior after the ED visit naturalistically, especially when they perceived their visit to be smoking-related [7, 24–26]. It is particularly difficult to extend an intervention effect beyond this natural change motivator of the visit itself. Costs associated with the treatment services may have been a barrier to treatment initiation and engagement, but were partially mitigated by the inclusion of free treatment options in addition to the fee-for-service selections. Furthermore, some evidence suggests cost does influence follow-up with smoking cessation treatment referrals [27]. The study was also limited because participants were not questioned about why they failed to initiate or remain engaged with treatment after receiving the referral, and such barriers should be explored in future studies of this or similar systems. By focusing solely on tobacco users who do not abuse alcohol and/or drugs, the generalizability of our findings is somewhat limited. Future research should seek to examine the efficacy of automated referral generation systems for tobacco cessation among all tobacco users. Finally, the study follow-up period was limited to 3 months because of the restrictions associated with the NIH SBIR/STTR funding mechanism.

Conclusion

The HERA helps to satisfy clinical practice mandates to Ask, Advise, and Refer tobacco users in the ED setting and was effective at promoting initial contact with a tobacco treatment provider. The dynamic referral option further promoted treatment initiation. However, the HERA, when deployed as a stand-alone intervention, did not lead to sustained post-visit tobacco treatment engagement or changes in smoking behavior within 3 months after the ED visit. The results raise the question of whether the Ask, Advise, and Refer method is adequate for all populations, particularly those discouraged by, or unable to pay, fees associated with treatment services or those with a lack of access to healthcare, which were represented by this study. The study highlights the importance of developing and studying interventions that work in conjunction with tobacco treatment linkage strategies.

Abbreviations

SBIRT: screening, brief intervention, and referral to treatment; HERA: health evaluation and referral assistant; GEE: generalized estimating equation; ED: emergency department; RCT: randomized controlled trial; HSI: Heavy Smoking Index; RA: research assistant.

Authors' contributions

EDB participated in the study design, oversaw study completion, assisted in data interpretation, and oversaw manuscript preparation. BA completed the data analyses, assisted in data interpretation, and assisted in manuscript preparation. BH assisted in manuscript preparation. BB assisted in study design, study completion, and manuscript preparation. GG assisted in study design, study completion, and manuscript preparation. All authors read and approved the final manuscript.

Author details

[1] Departments of Emergency Medicine, Psychiatry, and Quantitative Health Sciences, University of Massachusetts Medical School, LA-189, 55 Lake Avenue North, Worcester, MA 01655, USA. [2] Departments of Emergency Medicine, Psychiatry, and Public Health Sciences, University of Rochester Medical Center, Rochester, NY, USA. [3] Department of Emergency Medicine, University of Massachusetts Medical School, Worcester, MA, USA. [4] Department of Emergency Medicine, Cooper Medical School of Rowan University, Camden, NJ, USA. [5] Polaris Health Directions, Inc, Langhorne, PA, USA.

Acknowledgements

Funding

This study was funded by a Small Business Technology Transfer grant from the National Institutes of Health (R42DA021455) to Polaris Health Directions, Inc. An agreement related to technology used in this study exists between the University of Massachusetts Medical School and Polaris Health Directions. Dr. Boudreaux is an employee of the University of Massachusetts Medical School and receives consulting income from Polaris Health Directions. In addition, if the aforementioned technology should be licensed and result in licensing-related income, Dr. Boudreaux would receive a share under the University's allocation policy to inventors. Dr. Grissom is an employee of Polaris Health Directions. Dr. Abar, Dr. Baumann, and Ms. Haskins have no conflicts to disclose.

The prototype of the HERA was called the Dynamic Assessment and Referral System for Substance Abuse (DARSSA). The name was changed to reflect our long-term plans to expand the system to provide SBIRT for other non-substance problems, like depression and interpersonal violence.

Competing interests

Edwin D. Boudreaux is an employee of the University of Massachusetts Medical Center and receives consulting income and licensing revenue from Polaris Health Directions. Grant Grissom is the President of Polaris Health Directions. Polaris Health Directions, Inc, intends to market HERA for financial gain. An intellectual property and licensing agreement exists between the University of Massachusetts Medical School and Polaris Health Directions. Beau Abar, Brianna Haskins, and Brigitte Bauman declare that they have no competing interests.

References

1. Centers for disease control and prevention. Smoking-attributable mortality, years of potential life lost, and productivity losses—United States, 2000–2004. MMWR. 2008;57:1226–8.
2. Bernstein SL, Boudreaux ED, Cydulka RK, Rhodes KV, Lettman NA, Almeida SL, et al. American College of Emergency Physicians Task Force on Smoking Cessation. Tobacco control interventions in the emergency department: a joint statement of emergency medicine organizations. J Emerg Nurs. 2006;32(5):370–81.
3. Anders ME, Sheffer CE, Barone CP, Holmes TM, Simpson DD, Duncan AM. Emergency department-initiated tobacco dependence treatment. Am J Health Behav. 2011;35(5):546–56.
4. Centers for disease control and prevention. Smoking is the leading preventable cause of death in the United States. 2014. http://www.cdc.gov/tobacco/data_statistics/fact_sheets/health_effects/effects_cig_smoking/. Accessed 17 April 2015.
5. Sanjuan PM, Rice SL, Witkiewitz K, Mandler RN, Crandall C, Bogenschutz MP. Alcohol, tobacco, and drug use among emergency department patients. Drug Alcohol Depend. 2014;138:32–8.
6. Cunningham RM, Bernstein SL, Walton M, Broderick K, Vaca FE, Woolard R, et al. Alcohol, tobacco, and other drugs: future directions for screening and intervention in the emergency department. Acad Emerg Med. 2009;16:1078–88.
7. Boudreaux ED, Baumann BM, Perry J, Marks D, Francies S, Camargo CA, et al. Emergency department initiated treatments for tobacco (EDITT): a pilot study. Ann Behav Med. 2008;36(3):314–25.
8. Murphy MK, Bijur PE, Rosenbloom D, Bernstein SL, Gallagher EJ. Feasibility of a computer-assisted alcohol SBIRT program in an urban emergency department: patient and research staff perspectives. Addict Sci Clin Pract. 2013;8(1):1–10.
9. Bernstein SL, Boudreaux ED, Cabral L, Cydulka RK, Schwegman D, Larkin GL, et al. Efficacy of a brief intervention to improve emergency physicians' smoking cessation counseling skills, knowledge, and attitudes. Subst Abus. 2009;30(2):158–81.

10. Bernstein SL, Boudreaux ED, Cabral L, Cydulka RK, Schwegman D, Larkin GL, et al. Nicotine dependence, motivation to quit, and diagnosis among adult emergency department patients who smoke: a national survey. Nicotine Tob Res. 2008;10(8):1277–82.
11. Greenberg MR, Weinstock M, Fenimore DG, Siezega GM. Emergency department tobacco cessation program: staff participation and intervention success among patients. J Am Osteopath Assoc. 2008;108(8):391–6.
12. Boudreaux ED, Bedek KL, Gilles D, Baumann BM, Hollenberg S, Lord SA, et al. The dynamic assessment and referral system for substance abuse (DARSSA): development, functionality, and end-user satisfaction. Drug Alcohol Depend. 2009;99(1):37–46.
13. Boudreaux ED, Abar B, Baumann BM, Grissom G. A randomized clinical trial of the health evaluation and referral assistant (HERA): research methods. Contemp Clin Trials. 2013;35(2):87–96.
14. Heatherton TF, Kozlowski LT, Frecker RC, Rickert W, Robinson J. Measuring the heaviness of smoking: using self-reported time to the first cigarette of the day and number of cigarettes smoked per day. Br J Addict. 1989;84:791–800.
15. Kroenke K, Spitzer RL, Williams JB. The patient health questionnaire-2: validity of a two-item depression screener. Med Care. 2003;41(11):1284–92.
16. Miller WR, Rollnic S, Moyers TB. Motivational interviewing: helping people change. New York: Guilford Press; 2013.
17. Prochaska JO, DiClemente CC, Norcross JC. In search of how people change. Applications to addictive behaviors. Am Psychol. 1992;47(9):1102–14.
18. Bernstein SL, Bernstein E, Boudreaux ED, Babcock-Irvin C, Mello MJ, Kapur AK, et al. Public health considerations in knowledge translation in the emergency department. Acad Emerg Med. 2007;14(11):1036–41.
19. Willett JG, Hood NE, Burns EK, Swetlick JL, Wilson SM, Lang DA, et al. Clincial faxed referrals to a tobacco quitline: reach, enrollment, and participant characteristics. Am J Prev Med. 2009;36(4):337–40.
20. Bernstein SL, Bijur P, Cooperman N, Jearld S, Arnsten JH, Moadel A, et al. Efficacy of an emergency department-based multicomponent intervention for smokers with substance use disorders. J Subst Abuse Treat. 2013;44(1):139–42.
21. Velicer WF, Prochaska JO, Bellis JM, DiClemente CC, Rossi JS, Fava JL, et al. An expert system intervention for smoking cessation. Addict Behav. 1993;18(3):269–90.
22. Prochaska JO, Velicer WF, Fava JL, Rossi JS, Tsoh JY. Evaluating a population-based recruitment approach and a stage-based expert system intervention for smoking cessation. Addict Behav. 2001;26(4):583–602.
23. Prochaska JO, Velicer WF, Fava JL, Ruggiero L, Laforge RG, Rossi JS, et al. Counselor and stimulus control enhancements of a stage-matched expert system intervention for smokers in a managed care setting. Prev Med. 2001;32(1):23–32.
24. Boudreaux ED, Abar B, O'Hea EL, Sullivan AF, Cydulka R, Bernstein SL, et al. Cognitive and affective predictors of smoking after a sentinel health event. Psychol Health Med. 2014;19(4):402–9.
25. Boudreaux ED, Baumann BM, Camargo CA Jr, O'Hea EL, Ziedonis DM. Changes in smoking associated with an acute health event: theoretical and practical implications. Ann Behav Med. 2007;33:189–99.
26. Bock BC, Becker BM, Niaura RS, Partridge R, Fava JL, Trask P. Smoking cessation among patients in an emergency chest pain observation unit: outcomes of the chest pain smoking study (CPSS). Nicotine Tob Res. 2008;10(10):1523–31.
27. Ozhathil DK, Abar B, Baumann BM, Camargo CA Jr, Ziedonis D, Boudreaux ED. The effect of removing cost as a barrier to treatment initiation with outpatient tobacco dependence clinics among emergency department patients. Acad Emerg Med. 2011;18(6):662–4.

10

How do people with mood and anxiety disorders perceive and interpret the Drinking Motives Questionnaire? A think-aloud study in a clinical setting

Christina Nehlin[1,2*], Margareta Wennberg[2] and Caisa Öster[1,2]

Abstract

Background: Research has identified drinking motives as the final common pathway to alcohol use, and associations between specific drinking motives and drinking patterns have consistently been demonstrated. Data on drinking motives can be used for research, in the planning of prevention strategies and for treatment purposes. The Drinking Motives Questionnaire-Revised (DMQ-R) has become the most used measure of drinking motives. So far, the questionnaire has not been investigated with qualitative methods. The aim of this study was to investigate acceptability, accuracy and usability of the DMQ-R among persons receiving outpatient psychiatric care by studying how responders perceive and interpret the questionnaire.

Method: A cognitive interviewing technique, the think-aloud method, was used to collect data from 16 non-alcohol dependent patients seeking outpatient psychiatric care (12 women, 4 men). To analyse data, Qualitative Content Analysis was applied in which themes were formed from data only and not from predetermined areas of interest.

Results: Overall, acceptability of the DMQ-R was high although answers were sometimes given with low accuracy. Responders pointed out that they perceived the questionnaire as non-confrontational and exhaustive. Further, the DMQ-R seemed to launch processes of self-reflection.

Conclusions: Taken together, the results suggest a support for the use of DMQ-R also in the group of psychiatric outpatients. Still, when interpreting the DMQ-R, a certain insecurity of the exactness of answers should be considered. The graphic design should be particularly clear in this group of patients.

Keywords: Questionnaires, Drinking motives, DMQ-R, Think-aloud method, Psychiatric care

Background

Drinking motives have drawn increasing interest because of their role in the development of alcohol-related problems. Research has identified drinking motives as the final common pathway to alcohol use [1, 2]. Associations between specific drinking motives and drinking patterns have consistently been demonstrated (e.g. [3–5]). For example, emotionally oriented motives are more often associated to high levels of drinking and to negative consequences [6]. Data on drinking motives may be useful for research purposes, when planning of prevention strategies and for tailoring of treatment.

The Drinking Motives Questionnaire-Revised (DMQ-R) [1] is a self-report questionnaire to assess the relative frequency of four separate motives for drinking. The questionnaire was developed in 1994 for use in college student populations. It has become the most used measure of drinking motives; the original study by Cooper [1] has been cited over 1000 times (Scopus, November 2017). Most studies using the DMQ-R have focused on students and young adults. In recent years,

*Correspondence: christina.nehlin.gordh@neuro.uu.se
[1] Department of Neuroscience, Psychiatry, Uppsala University, UAS ing 10, 75185 Uppsala, Sweden
Full list of author information is available at the end of the article

the DMQ-R has been applied also in studies in the general population [7, 8]. Although the questionnaire was developed for non-clinical samples, it has recently been used in studies of persons with alcohol use problems [3, 9]. Further, in a recent study our group could confirm the four-factor structure of the Swedish version of the DMQ-R in a group of adults seeking outpatient psychiatric care [10].

To evaluate the performance of a questionnaire, direct study of the question-and answer process is recommended [11, 12]. Still, only a small number of studies have investigated how respondents in health care settings interpret questions and statements and what their thoughts are when doing so [13–16]. Results from those studies indicate that, although well validated with standard psychometric methods, questionnaires are not always perceived as intended: responders may interpret questions in unexpected ways and have difficulties understanding them [13]. To our knowledge, no such studies have been performed in a psychiatric setting.

The DMQ-R has not been investigated with qualitative methods. To extend the knowledge about the psychometric properties, the usability and utility of the DMQ-R in different settings, a project called "Motives for drinking" was initiated (for previous reports, see [3, 10]). This study is a part of that project, aiming to further investigate the benefits and shortcomings of the questionnaire by studying how respondents perceive and interpret the questionnaire. The specific aim of this study was to provide qualitative knowledge of acceptability, accuracy and usability of the DMQ-R among persons receiving outpatient psychiatric care by studying how responders perceive and interpret the questionnaire.

Method

Setting and participants

Data were collected among patients visiting a psychiatric outpatient clinic for mood and anxiety disorders at a university hospital in Sweden. The hospital's procedure includes referring those patients who have a substance use disorder or psychosis as a main diagnosis to separate specialist clinics and those patients did not take part in this study. In the eligible group of patients with mood and anxiety disorders, co-morbidity with personality disorders or ADHD/autism spectrum disorders may occur, but no patient was diagnosed with any substance use disorder. The only criterion for inclusion was having consumed alcohol during the last 12 months. All staff at the outpatient unit were asked to inform and invite their patients to participate in the study. No compensation was offered. The project was approved by the Ethical Review Board of Uppsala University (Reg. No. 2015/434).

The Drinking Motives Questionnaire-Revised (DMQ-R)

The Drinking Motives Questionnaire-Revised (DMQ-R) [1] measures four types of drinking motives: enhancement, coping, conformity and social. Drinking to increase positive mood reflects an internal, positive-reinforcement *Enhancement* motive for alcohol consumption (e.g. drinking to feel high). Drinking to reduce negative affect reflects an internal, negative-reinforcement *Coping* motive (e.g. drinking to forget problems). Alcohol consumption to avoid negative social consequences reflects an external, negative-reinforcement *Conformity* motive (e.g. drinking to fit in with others). Drinking in order to obtain social rewards reflects an external, positive-reinforcement *Social* motive (e.g. drinking to celebrate with friends).

The DMQ-R consists of 20 items, five per dimension. Participants rated the frequency of drinking for each item on an ordinal scale with six response categories (1 = never, 2 = almost never, 3 = some of the time, 4 = about half of the time, 5 = most of the time, 6 = almost always). To avoid space-demanding iterations, all items were not fully written out. The questionnaire and its graphic design is presented in Additional file 1.

Data collection

The think-aloud method was used to collect data. This method, also known as protocol analysis, was introduced in the field of psychology in the 1980s as a way to understand elementary cognitive processes as they unfold over time [11, 17]. To provide information about their thought processes, respondents are asked to "think aloud" while completing a task [17]. The researcher assumes a non-active position in the room and only interferes to remind respondents to keep thinking aloud. The think-aloud method has been used to investigate self-report questionnaires and is also recommended for cognitive pre-testing of survey questions [11–16, 18]. Findings can be used to refine measures or highlight areas for consideration when applying them [19].

Participants in this study were offered oral and written information by their ordinary caregiver and those who chose to participate were scheduled for a session with one of the researchers MW or CN. The information pointed out that the study focused on the thoughts while answering a questionnaire rather than on the actual answers. At the session, participants were informed again and signed a consent form. They were instructed to think aloud: to say whatever came into their mind while responding to the questionnaire. They were informed that they could be reminded to keep talking, and that questions about items would not be answered by the researcher. If participants remained silent for 5–7 s when completing the DMQ-R, they were asked what they were thinking about. In case verbalized thoughts were unclear, participants were asked to explain more explicitly. At the end of the session, participants were asked what they thought of filling out the questionnaire and what its pros and cons were. They were also asked if they thought something was missing. All sessions were recorded with MP3-players and transcribed verbatim.

Data analysis

To analyse the think-aloud data, the researchers conducted Qualitative Content Analysis using an inductive approach [20]. Themes were identified and analysed inductively, i.e. themes were formed from data only and not from predetermined areas of interest.

The transcripts were read several times by authors CN and MW separately. Meaning units—words and sentences of interest for the aims of the study—were coded. Following a joint discussion, codes were sorted into themes. The material was re-read by both authors CN and MW and themes were used to sort the codes. The analysis continued until all themes were deemed to be clearly defined and distinct from one another. All authors discussed the coding of data until consensus was achieved and themes were perceived as describing the content concisely. In addition to being researchers, all authors have extensive experience in the field of psychiatric care and/or substance use treatment.

Results

Of the 16 individuals included, 12 were women and four were men None of them was diagnosed with an alcohol use disorder but all had consumed alcohol during the past 12 months. All those approached except for one patient consented to take part. Ages ranged from 26 to 67; mean age (SD) was 45.2 (10.9), median was 46.5 years. All participants were diagnosed with a mood or anxiety disorder (ICD-10 F30-48 [21]) as a main diagnosis. The interview sessions were between 3:43 and 29:33 min long with a median length of 10:39 min. All interviews were included in the analysis.

The results are presented under the three identified themes with verbatim quotes to illustrate the findings. The themes are *Interpretation of the questionnaire, Experiences rather than motives* and *Self-reflection.*

Theme: interpretation of the questionnaire

In all, 88 verbalizations concerned the interpretation of the questionnaire: the graphic design (43 comments), the formulation of questions (31 comments) and the lack of suitable response options (14 comments). The graphic design was initially confusing to some participants, a subject that generated 16 verbalizations.

> *How often do you drink...here, I am probably not supposed to fill in on the dotted lines, but in the box... [reads the response options]. So this is some kind of headline to this section... (#5, male 49 yrs)*

The fact that questions could be posed repeatedly in similar forms produced 17 comments.

Although participants generally understood the questions, some words and terms were perceived as equivocal. In all, 31 verbalizations concerned interpretations of the questions. The concept "how often" was sometimes difficult to quantify. It was associated with consumption level and not with comparisons to other times the person had consumed alcohol. Ten verbalizations were noted on this subject.

> *'Some of the times,' that's very relative. To me, 'soon' is within ten minutes. I have a friend, he thinks 'soon' is within an hour. It's just about the same with 'some of the times.' (#9, female 36 yrs)*

Another concept that was perceived equivocally was getting high (Item no. 9: "How often do you drink to get high?") One participant interpreted "to get high" as "to be intoxicated" or "really drunk". Another interpreted the wording as "slightly affected by alcohol". Still another participant contemplated:

> *...it depends on what you mean by 'high.' To get high, that's to be sort of upbeat to me. But I mostly want to calm down, so no... (#4, female 38 yrs)*

The participants sometimes had difficulty relating to the situation described in the question.

> *...because it makes social gatherings more fun. It depends on the context...if I go out after work with some colleagues, maybe we'll drink wine together. But other times it's a family gathering and I may as well drink cola...What should I put here? This was really difficult. (#13, female 49 yrs)*

Participants were eager to fulfil their task, but in all 14 verbalizations indicated difficulty finding a suitable response option. Instead, they chose a rough estimate.

> *...to celebrate...well, no...I put 'almost never,' it is... it is mostly because I want to move on from the question and I don't want to leave the questionnaire incomplete. (#10, female 53 yrs)*

Theme: experiences rather than motives

When participants reflected on the questions it was common to refer to practical experiences, situations the person had been in. Those experiences – rather than the motive for drinking—seemed to guide the response. This theme gathered 29 verbalizations.

> *...because it gives you a pleasant feeling. Yes, to me it does, it makes me calmer. Because it makes you feel more self-confident...yes, that is common. (#4, female 38 yrs)*
> *...because it gives you a pleasant feeling. If you drink moderately, yes. But if you drink too much, absolutely not. I get really sick from it. (#2, female 34 yrs)*

Theme: self-reflection

The questions led some of the participants to reflect on their alcohol use and motives. This was spontaneously commented on six times.

> *You really start reflecting on your drinking. Something happens to you when you're asked these questions. [...] You really confront yourself with these questions, and I think that might be a good thing. It could be a kind of an opening to your understanding that this isn't good, maybe. (#13, female 49 yrs)*
> *I think these questions are...they make it difficult to lie. It's easier to lie if you are asked how much, how many beers did you drink. (#8, male 35 yrs)*

Additional observations

Participants who were insecure about how to reply often chose the alternative "Some of the times".

> *"To get high. [long pause]. Hm. I don't really know. But maybe we can say "Some of the times". (#2, female 34 yrs)*

The participants that ruled out conformity motives did so particularly decisively.

> *Because your friends pressure you to drink...Never! I drink when I decide to. And if I don't feel like drinking when somebody offers me a drink, I just say no thanks. (#11, male 44 yrs)*

Some participants commented that they found the questionnaire non-confrontational and exhaustive.

> *I think...they were good questions, they were neutral. Not moralistic... they don't ask how often you drink, and so on. And they were comprehensive, I can say. They approach the question of why you drink from all kinds of angles. (#15, female 55 yrs)*

Others pointed out that it covered important areas that no one had asked them about before.

Five responders commented that an important drinking motive was that alcohol tastes good and goes well with food. One person felt a response option was missing for questions about which she was uncertain.

Discussion

This is the first study to report qualitative data from thought processes of persons responding to the DMQ-R. In our study, we were able to find out more about interpretations and reasoning among the psychiatric outpatients. Information collected using the think-aloud method would have been difficult to collect with fixed response options or by asking participants retrospective questions.

The acceptability of the questionnaire was generally high; it was well understood by the participants. However, there were many comments concerning similarities among the questions and the iterations seemed to create some vexation and insecurity. Thus, a shorter version may be to prefer. In a previous study with patients seeking psychiatric care, we found psychometric properties of the short form DMQ-R SF to be valid and even with a slightly better model fit than the DMQ-R [20]. The results of this study add to the preference for the use of the short form of DMQ-R.

A large number of verbalizations pertained to the questionnaire itself: its graphic design, the formulation of questions and the lack of suitable response options. Some respondents perceived the graphic design used in our study as confusing. For simplification, the questions were not fully written out. One patient broke off the interview after 4:30 min, as he felt his symptoms produced an uncomfortably stressful situation. Two other participants mentioned their ADHD symptoms as a possible explanation for their difficulties understanding the questionnaire. When addressing patients in psychiatric care there may be a certain need for explicitness, as their psychiatric condition may create cognitive disturbances.

The verbalizations concerning difficulties finding an apt response option indicate that some tentativeness is needed when interpreting the results of the questionnaire. The option "Some of the time" was often chosen when responders were insecure about how to reply. The responses "Some of the time" may thus represent low accuracy.

Before giving a response, many participants considered the effects alcohol has on them rather than their motives for drinking. It was clear that they were referring to their experiences and the consequences of drinking. In cognitive psychological theory, the frequently cited "Question-and answer model" (e.g. [11].) suggests that respondents must complete four actions to be able to answer a question: they must comprehend the question, retrieve the necessary information from long-term memory, make a judgement about the information needed to answer the question, and respond to the question. Thus, the thought process that leads to an answer include considering previous experiences and that became evident in the think-aloud interviews. Therefore, we do not deem this reasoning to reduce the validity of the questionnaire.

It is noteworthy that respondents spontaneously commented that the questionnaire made them start reflecting on their alcohol use. Although such verbalizations were quite rare during the interviews, considering the nature of those comments, it is likely that the questions on the DMQ-R may launch a self-reflection process. Because alcohol use even at moderate levels may impact the course of a psychiatric disorder and the treatment effects [22, 23], such processes may help prevent possible exacerbations due to alcohol. Furthermore, participants in this study perceived the questionnaire as non-confrontational and felt that it covered important areas that no one had asked them about before.

The comments concerning the graphic design generated the major share of comments. This serves as a reminder that a clear and comprehensible design is of importance, in particular in the psychiatric setting. However, design issues are easily resolved. It is more problematic that respondents differed in the interpretation of questions and situations described. Previous psychometric tests of DMQ-R have pointed out variations in item factor loadings in groups of adults as well as adolescents [8, 24, 25]. For example, in some studies item no. 9 ("...to get high") yielded a lower factor loading than other enhancement items among adults. Item no. 17 (..."because it's fun") produced a low factor loading in the enhancement motive among European students [26]. These inconsistencies may illustrate the fact that questionnaires do not pinpoint a precise measure of people's views and feelings. The result of a self-report questionnaire as reported in numbers and decimals may lead the interpreter into thinking that it is an exact measure of the responder's thoughts and beliefs. In this as well as in previous studies, findings suggest that questionnaires can be understood in unforeseen ways and that responses may be given with less accuracy than expected. We recommend caregivers as well as researchers to take this into consideration when evaluating results obtained by self-report questionnaires. Keeping this in mind, results from this as well as previous studies still suggest that the DMQ-R is of value for research, prevention and treatment purposes in patients with mood and anxiety disorders.

There are some issues to consider with respect to strengths and measures used to strengthen the weaknesses of the present study. The main strength of this study is that it investigates the questionnaire from the respondent's perspective. It was conducted in a clinical setting and used a cognitive method, previously not used with DMQ-R, to examine how people understand and interpret the questionnaire.

One potential weakness is the interview setting with a researcher present in the room that may have created bias; given that the subject is alcohol, social desirability may have played a role. Still, because of the non-confrontational nature of the questions we believe that risk was small. Further, it is possible that the think-aloud method may have increased the responders' critical attitude to questions in a way that differs from a normal response situation.

As with all research with qualitative analysis, there must be measures to strengthen the neutrality of the coder, which otherwise may affect the interpretations. Nevertheless, interpretation involves a balancing act between adding a perspective to the phenomenon under study and not assigning meaning to the text that is not there. The co-authors reduced that risk via a sound data analysis process with alternative coding and discussions of the data. Further, although the coders were experienced in psychiatric care and/or substance use treatment they were not members of the staff and had not met the participants before, which minimized the influence of pre-existing assumptions.

This type of study design gives a good understanding of perceptions in a group of individuals, but it is not possible to generalize the results from the study in a quantitative manner. Instead, description of context, process of analysis and appropriate quotations can inform and enhance readers' understandings of how the findings can be transferred to other settings or groups.

The number of participants was relatively small, however qualitative research is often based on small sample sizes where understanding of experiences and perceptions is the subject. Nevertheless, a larger sample could have made it possible to include participants of different ages, different diagnoses and different experiences of alcohol.

Conclusions

The results suggest a support for the use of DMQ-R in outpatients in psychiatric care for research, prevention and treatment purposes. Still, when interpreting the DMQ-R, a certain insecurity of the exactness of answers should be considered. The graphic design should be particularly clear in this group of patients.

Authors' contributions

CN and CÖ designed the study. MW and CN collected the data. All authors took part in analysing the data. CN prepared the draft of the manuscript. All authors read and approved the final manuscript.

Author details
[1] Department of Neuroscience, Psychiatry, Uppsala University, UAS ing 10, 75185 Uppsala, Sweden. [2] Division of Psychiatry, Uppsala University Hospital, UAS ing 10, 75185 Uppsala, Sweden.

Acknowledgements
Not applicable.

Competing interests
The authors declare that they have no competing interests.

Consent for publication
All necessary consent for publication has been met.

Funding
The study was supported financially by the Nasvell Fund for Psychiatric Research. The supporting fund has had no role in the design of the study or collection, analysis, or interpretation of data or in writing the manuscript.

References

1. Cooper M. Motivations for alcohol use among adolescents: development and validation of a four-factor model. Psychol Assess. 1994;6(2):117–28.
2. Cox WM, Klinger E. A motivational model of alcohol use. J Abnorm Psychol. 1988;97(2):168–80.
3. Hammarberg A, Oster C, Nehlin C. Drinking motives of adult patients seeking treatment for problematic alcohol use. J Addict Dis. 2017;36(2):127–35.
4. Kuntsche E, Gabhainn SN, Roberts C, Windlin B, Vieno A, Bendtsen P, Hublet A, Tynjala J, Valimaa R, Dankulincova Z, et al. Drinking motives and links to alcohol use in 13 European countries. J Stud Alcohol Drugs. 2014;75(3):428–37.
5. Kuntsche E, Stewart SH, Cooper ML. How stable is the motive-alcohol use link? A cross-national validation of the Drinking Motives Questionnaire Revised among adolescents from Switzerland, Canada, and the United States. J Stud Alcohol Drugs. 2008;69(3):388–96.
6. Kuntsche E, Knibbe R, Gmel G, Engels R. Why do young people drink? A review of drinking motives. Clin Psychol Rev. 2005;25(7):841–61.
7. Cheng H, Phillips M, Zhang Y, Wang Z. Psychometric properties of the Drinking Motives Questionnaire-Revised among community-dwelling current drinkers in the Ningxia autonomous region of China. Drug Alcohol Rev. 2016;35(4):433–41.
8. Crutzen R, Kuntsche E. Validation of the four-dimensional structure of drinking motives among adults. Eur Addict Res. 2013;19(4):222–6.
9. Mezquita L, Stewart SH, Ibanez MI, Ruiperez MA, Villa H, Moya J, Ortet G. Drinking motives in clinical and general populations. Eur Addict Res. 2011;17(5):250–61.
10. Oster C, Arinell H, Nehlin C. The Drinking Motives Questionnaire among Swedish psychiatric patients: an exploration of the four-factor structure. Drug Alcohol Rev. 2017;36(3):400–7.
11. Collins D. Pretesting survey instruments: an overview of cognitive methods. Qual Life Res Int J Qual Life Asp Treat Care Rehabil. 2003;12(3):229–38.
12. Streiner D, Norman G. Health measurement scales. A practical guide to their development and use. New York: Oxford University Press; 2008.
13. Hauge CH, Jacobs-Knight J, Jensen JL, Burgess KM, Puumala SE, Wilton G, Hanson JD. Establishing survey validity and reliability for American Indians through "think aloud" and test-retest methods. Qual Health Res. 2015;25(6):820–30.
14. Murtagh FE, Addington-Hall JM, Higginson IJ. The value of cognitive interviewing techniques in palliative care research. Palliat Med. 2007;21(2):87–93.
15. van Oort L, Schröder C, French DP. What do people think about when they answer the Brief Illness Perception Questionnaire? A 'think-aloud' study. Br J Health Psychol. 2011;16:231–45.
16. Westerman MJ, Hak T, Sprangers MA, Groen HJ, van der Wal G, The AM. Listen to their answers! Response behaviour in the measurement of physical and role functioning. Qual Life Res Int J Qual Life Asp Treat Care Rehabil. 2008;17(4):549–58.
17. Van Someren M, Barnard Y, Sandberg J. The think aloud method. London: Academic Press; 1994.
18. French DP, Cooke R, McLean N, Williams M, Sutton S. What do people think about when they answer theory of planned behaviour questionnaires? A 'think aloud' study. J Health Psychol. 2007;12(4):672–87.
19. Kaklamanou D, Armitage CJ, Jones CR. A further look into compensatory health beliefs: a think aloud study. Br J Health Psychol. 2013;18(1):139–54.
20. Graneheim UH, Lundman B. Qualitative content analysis in nursing research: concepts, procedures and measures to achieve trustworthiness. Nurse Educ Today. 2004;24(2):105–12.
21. http://www.who.int/classifications/icd/icdonlineversions/en/.
22. Castaneda R, Sussman N, Levy R, O'Malley M, Westreich L. A review of the effects of moderate alcohol intake on psychiatric and sleep disorders. Recent Dev Alcohol. 1998;14:197–226.
23. Castaneda R, Sussman N, Westreich L, Levy R, O'Malley M. A review of the effects of moderate alcohol intake on the treatment of anxiety and mood disorders. J Clin Psychiatry. 1996;57(5):207–12.
24. Gilson K, Bryant C, Bei B, Komiti A, Jackson H, Judd F. Validation of the Drinking Motives Questionnaire (DMQ) ini older adults. Addict Behav. 2013;38(5):2196–202.
25. Hauck-Filho N, Teixeira MA, Cooper ML. Confirmatory factor analysis of the Brazilian version of the Drinking Motives Questionnaire-Revised (DMQ-R). Addict Behav. 2012;37(4):524–7.
26. Nemeth S. The role of motivational components of alcohol use among youth in different settings and cultures. Budapest: Eötvös Loránd University of Science; 2011.

11

Comparison of DSM-IV and DSM-5 criteria for alcohol use disorders in VA primary care patients with frequent heavy drinking

Traci Takahashi[4,6*], Gwen Lapham[1,3], Laura J. Chavez[1,11,10], Amy K. Lee[3], Emily C. Williams[1,5], Julie E. Richards[3,5], Diane Greenberg[8,9], Anna Rubinsky[1,2,7], Douglas Berger[4,6], Eric J. Hawkins[1,2,8], Joseph O. Merrill[6] and Katharine A. Bradley[1,2,3,5,6]

Abstract

Background: Criteria for alcohol use disorders (AUD) in the Diagnostic and Statistical Manual of Mental Disorders, 5th edition (DSM-5) were intended to result in a similar prevalence of AUD as DSM-IV. We evaluated the prevalence of AUD using DSM-5 and DSM-IV criteria, and compared characteristics of patients who met criteria for: neither DSM-5 nor DSM-IV AUD, DSM-5 alone, DSM-IV alone, or both, among Veterans Administration (VA) outpatients in the Considering Healthier drinking Options In primary CarE (CHOICE) trial.

Methods: VA primary care patients who reported frequent heavy drinking and enrolled in the CHOICE trial were interviewed at baseline using the DSM-IV Mini International Neuropsychiatric Interview for AUD, as well as questions about socio-demographics, mental health, alcohol craving, and substance use. We compared characteristics across 4 mutually exclusive groups based on DSM-5 and DSM-IV criteria.

Results: Of 304 participants, 13.8% met criteria for neither DSM-5 nor DSM-IV AUD; 12.8% met criteria for DSM-5 alone, and 73.0% met criteria for both DSM-IV and DSM-5. Only 1 patient (0.3%) met criteria for DSM-IV AUD alone. Patients meeting both DSM-5 and DSM-IV criteria had more negative drinking consequences, mental health symptoms and self-reported readiness to change compared with those meeting DSM-5 criteria alone or neither DSM-5 nor DSM-IV criteria.

Conclusions: In this sample of primary care patients with frequent heavy drinking, DSM-5 identified 13% more patients with AUD than DSM-IV. This group had a lower mental health symptom burden and less self-reported readiness to change compared to those meeting criteria for both DSM-IV and DSM-5 AUD.

Trial Registration ClinicalTrials.gov NCT01400581. 2011 February 17

Keywords: Alcohol use disorder, Binge drinking, DSM-IV, DSM-5, Alcohol

Background

The Diagnostic and Statistical Manual of Mental Disorders, 5th edition (DSM-5) criteria for alcohol use disorders (AUD), released in 2013 [1], represent a significant departure from previous criteria. For the previous 20 years, since the 4th edition of the DSM (DSM-IV), alcohol dependence and abuse had been considered mutually exclusive diagnoses that together made up alcohol use disorders [2]. The diagnosis of these distinct disorders was based on "a maladaptive pattern of alcohol use leading to clinically significant impairment or distress" as

*Correspondence: Traci.Takahashi@va.gov
[4] Department of Veterans Affairs Puget Sound Health Care System, General Medicine Services, 1660 South Columbian Way (S-152), Seattle, WA 98108, USA
Full list of author information is available at the end of the article

manifested by separate criteria, with DSM-IV dependence requiring at least 3 of 7 criteria and DSM-IV alcohol abuse requiring exclusion of DSM-IV dependence and at least 1 of 4 separate criteria (Fig. 1). In part because of recent studies calling into question the hierarchical distinction between abuse and dependence [3–5], DSM-5 replaces these two diagnoses with a single spectrum of AUD with a continuum of severity. Removal of "abuse" from DSM-5 may also serve to reduce the stigma and negative judgment associated with such terminology [6]. The DSM-5 includes 11 criteria: 10 of the 11 combined DSM-IV abuse and dependence criteria (excluding legal problems) and a new criterion for craving (Fig. 1) [7]. DSM-5 further specifies AUD severity as mild, moderate or severe based on the number of diagnostic criteria endorsed, with at least 2 of 11 criteria required for a diagnosis (mild = 2–3, moderate = 4–5, severe ≥6). DSM-5 AUD was designed to reduce the number of "diagnostic orphans" that occurred with DSM-IV, whereby patients with 1 or 2 dependence criteria (and no abuse criteria) did not meet diagnostic criteria for abuse or dependence [8, 9]. Diagnostic orphans have an increased risk of developing a DSM-IV alcohol use disorder compared to those with no AUD symptoms in certain populations [e.g. young adults] and are therefore an important group to identify [10]. However, those who had DSM-IV abuse based on 1 criterion will not meet criteria for DSM-5 AUD [11]. The design of the DSM-5 AUD criteria is such that all people who met criteria for DSM-IV dependence but only some people with DSM-IV abuse will have an AUD based on DSM-5 criteria, while additional patients with only 2 symptoms of dependence will meet criteria.

DSM-5 criteria were intended to result in an overall prevalence of AUD similar to the prevalence of AUD determined from DSM-IV criteria [8]. A recent review found 12 studies that compared the prevalence of AUD based on DSM-IV and DSM-5 criteria [12]. Seven of the studies showed an increase in prevalence of AUD based on DSM-5 compared to DSM-IV, and the authors of the review concluded that DSM-5 "inflated" rates of AUD [12]. However, only one of the studies reviewed included a medical sample—patients seeking care in an emergency department. In contrast, the prevalence of AUD using DSM-5 criteria was found to be lower compared to DSM-IV criteria among high-risk Swiss young men [13] and in a large cross-national sample from the World Health Organization's World Mental Health Survey Initiative [14]. None of these studies were restricted to primary care patients and clinical samples could differ (e.g. have more severe AUD) which could decrease the impact of the shift from DSM-IV to DSM-5.

Even if a difference in the prevalence of DSM-IV and DSM-5 AUD is not observed in other settings, patients identified by the two diagnostic criteria could have different demographic or clinical profiles. Little research has focused on demographic and clinical differences between patients who meet DSM-IV and DSM-5 criteria for AUD in clinical settings. Both the change in number of diagnostic criteria required, and the change from "legal problems" to "craving," could result in differences in the

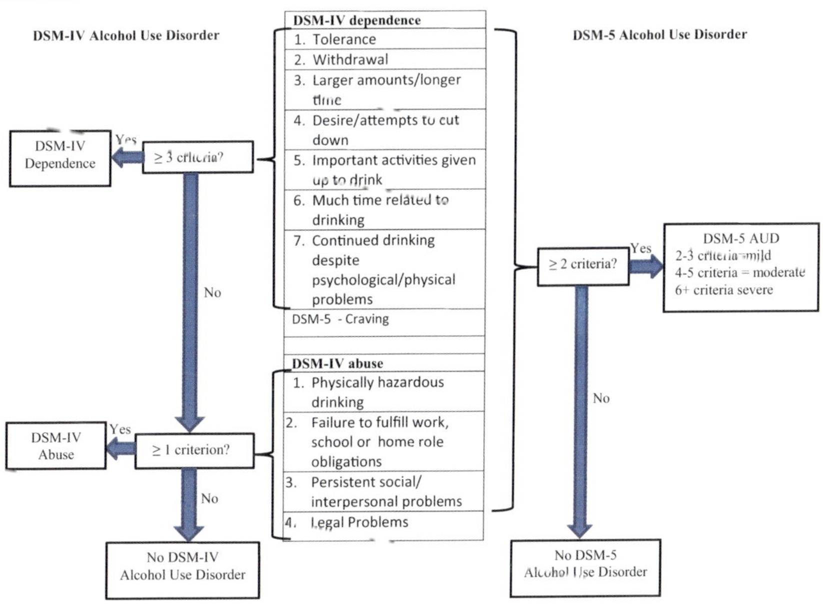

Fig. 1 DSM-IV and DSM-5 alcohol use disorder criteria (AUD)

clinical characteristics of the populations of patients diagnosed with DSM-5 AUD and DSM-IV AUD.

The purpose of the present study was to compare the characteristics of patients diagnosed with AUD according to DSM-IV and DSM-5 criteria in a clinical sample of US Veterans who received general medical care (e.g. "primary care") in Veterans Affairs (VA) clinics and reported frequent heavy drinking and were recruited into a trial of alcohol-related care management. We first describe the prevalence of DSM-IV and DSM-5 AUD, and categorize patients into four mutually exclusive groups: those who met criteria for: (1) neither DSM-IV nor DSM-5 AUD; (2) DSM-IV AUD alone; (3) DSM-5 AUD alone; or (4) both DSM-IV and DSM-5 AUD. We then compare sociodemographic characteristics, alcohol and drug related problem severity, mental health comorbidity, and readiness to change drinking across the four mutually exclusive diagnostic groups.

Methods

The Considering Healthier Drinking Options in primary CarE (aka "CHOICE") trial was a randomized controlled trial of a 12 months nurse-led care management intervention for patients with frequent heavy drinking who were receiving medical care in a general practice clinic for US Veterans of military service. Analyses presented here are from the baseline interviews (December 2011–September 2014) that assessed both DSM-IV and DSM-5 alcohol use disorders. The study was approved by both the VA Puget Sound and the Group Health Institutional Review Boards.

Study sample and setting

The CHOICE trial was conducted at three VA primary care clinics (Seattle, Tacoma, and Mount Vernon, Washington). Patients were considered potentially eligible if they were 21–75 years old and had a positive alcohol screen documented at the time of a VA outpatient visit (Alcohol Use Disorders Identification Test Consumption questionnaire [AUDIT-C] score ≥4 points for women and ≥5 for men). These cut-offs were chosen to maximize the positive predictive value for AUD. [15] In addition, providers could refer patients and flyers were posted so patients could self-refer to the study. Potentially eligible and referred patients were contacted by telephone and determined to be eligible if they reported drinking at levels that exceeded National Institute on Alcohol Abuse and Alcoholism (NIAAA) daily drinking limits on a phone screen—4 drinks (women) or 5 drinks (men), hereafter "binge"—at least twice a week on average, or once a week on average if they also reported they had ever been in alcohol treatment or attended Alcoholics Anonymous [16]. This was used as a proxy screen for AUD for the CHOICE trial because, due to stigma [17], AUD are long known to be under-diagnosed clinically [18]. Patients were excluded if—based on either chart review or telephone screening—they had cognitive impairment, did not speak English, were acutely unstable medically or psychiatrically, had less than 1 year life expectancy, were a VA employee, were enrolled in another VA intervention study, had been in alcohol treatment in the previous 90 days (including medications for AUD, but not Alcoholics Anonymous or 12 step meetings), were planning on becoming pregnant or currently pregnant, had no contact with their primary care team in the last year, or were not planning to continue care at VA Puget Sound facilities in the next year. Eligible patients provided written informed consent at a baseline enrollment visit, followed by repeat assessment of eligibility and self- and interviewer-administered questionnaires.

Measures

DSM-IV and DSM-5 alcohol use disorders (AUD) diagnoses

The Mini-International Neuropsychiatric Interview (MINI), a brief interviewer-administered diagnostic interview, was used to assess past-year AUD. The DSM-IV MINI includes 7 questions assessing dependence criteria in the past 12 months and then—if patients report 0–2 symptoms and therefore do not meet criteria for DSM-IV dependence—they are asked 4 questions to assess DSM-IV alcohol abuse criteria. This skip pattern minimizes questionnaire burden.

Although the final DSM-5 criteria for AUD were not published at the time the CHOICE trial began, the addition of a craving criterion was expected. All CHOICE trial participants were therefore also asked the following question about craving, after the DSM-IV MINI: "Was there ever a time in your life when you often had such a strong desire to drink that you couldn't stop yourself from taking a drink or found it difficult to think of anything else?" from the National Epidemiologic Survey on Alcohol and Related Conditions (NESARC) [19]. Of note, the question's timeframe of "ever" was inadvertently not changed to the "past year" for use in our measure of past year DSM-5 AUD, and the prevalence of lifetime craving is likely greater than past year craving.

Patients were categorized as having past year DSM-IV AUD using standard DSM-IV criteria: 3 or more criteria for alcohol dependence or 1 or more criteria for alcohol abuse for those who did not meet alcohol dependence criteria. Patients were categorized as having a DSM-5 AUD if they met 2 or more of the 11 DSM-5 criteria (Fig. 1). The severity of DSM-5 AUD is not reported because it may be under-estimated in patients who met DSM-IV dependence criteria, because they were not asked the 3 DSM-IV abuse questions included in the 11 DSM-5 criteria for AUD.

Socio-demographics, smoking, mental health symptoms and drug use disorders

Interviewers assessed demographic characteristics including gender, race, marital status, education and income, as well as whether patients smoked tobacco every day, some days or not at all. Patients also completed the following self-administered screening questionnaires: the 9-item Patient Health Questionnaire (PHQ-9; ≥10 points positive screen for depression), the 7-item Generalized Anxiety Disorder Screen (GAD-7; ≥10 points positive screen), and the Post-Traumatic Stress Disorder (PTSD) Checklist (PCL-C; ≥50 points positive screen). Interviewers also administered the panic disorder and drug use disorders (DUD) modules of the DSM-IV MINI. A count measure of the number of mental health and drug use conditions was constructed by summing the total number of positive screens or diagnoses (depression, generalized anxiety, PTSD, panic, and DUD).

Negative alcohol-related consequences, treatment history, and readiness to change

The Short Inventory of Problems (SIP) was used to assess each of 15 negative consequences due to drinking in the past 3 months and ever in the patient's lifetime [20–23]. The number of adverse alcohol-related consequences were summed as a measure of the total number of reported negative consequences in the past 3 months and ever. We used this descriptive measure because it reflected the number of symptoms, rather than the total SIP score which is more abstract because it takes into account both the number of negative consequences and severity. Interviewers also assessed prior treatment utilization by asking: "Have you ever gone anywhere or seen anyone for a reason that was related in any way to your drinking: a physician, counselor, Alcoholics Anonymous, or any other community agency or professional?" with 3 response options: No; Yes, prior to the past year; and Yes, during the past year [24]. Three 10-point Likert scale readiness "rulers," [25, 26] adapted from a previous primary care trial [27], were used to assess readiness to change, the importance of change, and confidence in the ability to change. For example, response options for the question "How important is it to you right now to change your drinking?" included 0 = "I don't drink; does not apply;" 1–3 = "not important;" 4–6 = "somewhat important;" and 7–10 = "very important." For this analysis, responses were dichotomized as: somewhat or ready to change (4–10) versus not (1–3); somewhat or very important to change (4–10) versus not (1–3); and somewhat or very confident in ability to change (4–10) versus not (1–3).

Analyses

We describe the socio-demographic and clinical characteristics of patients who enrolled in the CHOICE study and the prevalence of DSM-IV and DSM-5 AUD. We then categorize patients into 4 mutually exclusive groups: (1) those meeting neither DSM-IV nor DSM-5 criteria for AUD; (2) those meeting criteria for DSM-IV AUD alone; (3) those meeting criteria for DSM-5 AUD alone; and (4) those meeting criteria for both DSM-IV and DSM-5 AUD.

Finally, we describe the socio-demographic and clinical characteristics, including smoking, mental health and drug use comorbidity, negative consequences due to drinking and alcohol treatment history, across the 4 groups. The potential impact of asking about lifetime craving (instead of past year) was addressed in sensitivity analyses that omitted the craving question and used only 10 criteria for DSM-5 AUD. These analyses used the same threshold of two or more criteria to diagnose DSM-5 AUD.

In order to evaluate differences in characteristics across the mutually exclusive diagnostic groups—neither DSM-IV nor DSM-5 AUD, DSM-5 AUD alone, and both DSM-IV and DSM-5 AUD—three post hoc statistical tests were conducted using 3 aggregate outcome measures to avoid multiple statistical comparisons. The three outcomes for these post hoc analyses were: 1) number of mental health or drug use conditions (out of 5 possible); 2) number of negative alcohol-related consequences in the past-3 months on the SIP (out of 15 possible); and 3) an indicator of whether or not patients reported feeling "somewhat" to "ready" to change (versus not ready). Three generalized linear models were constructed, one for each of the 3 aggregate outcomes, with the categorical variable for the remaining DSM-IV and/or DSM-5 AUD groups as the independent variable, using the group with neither DSM-IV nor DSM-5 AUD as the referent. The outcomes (number of events; binary indicator) were assumed to have a binomial distribution, with the denominator equal to the number of possible events, and a logistic link was used. An overall post-estimation Wald test then evaluated whether the categorical variable for the mutually exclusive diagnostic groups was significant (defined as $p < 0.05$). With the exception of four missing responses for the PTSD Checklist, there were no other missing data.

Results

Characteristics of study sample of patients

Most of the 304 study participants were male (90.5%) and a majority (60.9%) were at least 50 years old (Table 1). Almost one half (45.4%) screened positive for depression (PHQ-9 ≥ 10), nearly one-third (30.3%) screened positive

Table 1 Characteristics of study population: VA primary care patients enrolled in the CHOICE trial (n = 304)

	n	(%)
Female	29	(9.5)
Age categories		
21–34	54	(17.8)
35–49	65	(21.4)
50–64	131	(43.1)
65+	54	(17.8)
Patient-reported race		
Native American	25	(8.2)
Asian	2	(0.7)
Native Hawaiian/Pacific Islander	5	(1.6)
Black	39	(12.8)
White	206	(67.8)
Multiracial	22	(7.2)
Other	5	(1.6)
Hispanic/Latino	21	(6.9)
Marital status		
Never married	56	(18.4)
Married/partnered	136	(44.7)
Separated	13	(4.3)
Divorced	91	(29.9)
Widowed	7	(2.3)
Refused/unknown	1	(0.3)
Education		
High school/GED or less	65	(21.4)
Some college/tech school	170	(55.9)
College or post graduate	69	(22.7)
Income		
<$15,000	49	(16.1)
$15,000-59,999	158	(52.0)
≥$60,000	95	(31.3)
Refused/Unknown	2	(0.7)
Smokes tobacco currently	134	(44.1)
Depression screen positive (PHQ-9 ≥ 10)	138	(45.4)
Generalized anxiety screen positive (GAD-7 ≥ 10)	92	(30.3)
PTSD screen positive (PCL-C ≥ 50)[a]	91	(30.3)
DSM-IV panic disorder– current (MINI)	29	(9.5)
DSM-IV drug use disorders past year (MINI)	57	(18.8)

[a] Four patients did not complete the PCL

for generalized anxiety (GAD ≥ 10) and the same proportion (30.3%) screened positive for PTSD (PCL ≥ 50). About one in 10 (9.5%) had symptoms consistent with DSM-IV panic disorder, while nearly one-fifth (18.8%) met criteria for a past year DSM-IV drug use disorder.

Prevalence of DSM-IV and DSM-5 alcohol use disorders

Overall, 85.9% of patients met criteria for DSM-5 AUD, whereas 73.3% met criteria for DSM-IV AUD. Of those with DSM-IV AUD, 81% met criteria for dependence and 19% for abuse alone. Table 2 shows the number of patients in each of the 4 mutually exclusive diagnostic groups: 13.8% met neither DSM-IV nor DSM-5 criteria for AUD; 0.3% met criteria for DSM-IV AUD alone, 12.8% met criteria for DSM-5 AUD alone, and 73.0% met criteria for both DSM-IV and DSM-5 AUD. The lone patient meeting criteria for DSM-IV AUD alone endorsed alcohol use despite social/interpersonal problems (1 of the 4 DSM-IV abuse criteria). Of note, in sensitivity analyses, 32 of 39 (82%) patients who met criteria for DSM-5 AUD alone still met DSM-5 criteria using only 10 DSM-5 criteria (craving question omitted because it asked about a time frame "ever" rather than past year).

Comparison of the 4 groups based on DSM-IV and DSM-5 criteria for AUD

Sociodemographic Characteristics

Comparison of sociodemographic characteristics across the 4 diagnostic groups—neither DSM-IV nor DSM-5 AUD, DSM-IV AUD alone, DSM-5 AUD alone, or both—suggested differences in age, race, marital status, and income (Table 3a). Because only 1 patient met criteria for DSM-IV alone, we compare the other 3 groups in the description of the remainder of results. Compared to patients with both DSM-IV and DSM-5 AUD, patients meeting neither DSM-IV nor DSM-5 AUD were more likely to be age 65 or more, and more likely to report white race, being married, and higher incomes (Table 3a).

Smoking, mental health symptoms and drug use disorders

Those with DSM-5 AUD alone appeared to have rates of smoking, mental health symptoms, and drug use disorders that tended to be higher than those who met criteria for neither DSM-IV nor DSM-5 AUD but lower than those who met criteria for both DSM-IV and DSM-5 (Table 3b).

Alcohol-related negative consequences

Table 3b shows the mean frequency for each consequence due to drinking in the past 3 months as reported on the SIP. For patients who met criteria for neither DSM-IV nor DSM-5 AUD, DSM-5 alone, and both DSM-IV and DSM-5 AUD, the mean number of alcohol-related negative consequences in the past 3 months was 1.0 (SD 0.3), 2.5 (SD 0.4), and 6.8 (SD 0.3) respectively. The mean number of lifetime negative consequences due to drinking for patients who met criteria for neither DSM-IV nor DSM-5 AUD, DSM-5 alone, and both DSM-IV and DSM-5 AUD, was 4.2 (SD 0.5), 6.7 (SD 0.5), and 10.1 (SD 0.3) respectively. The prevalence of having never

Table 2 Comparison of DSM-IV and DSM-5 alcohol use disorder

	DSM-5 diagnosis					
	No		Yes		Total	
	n	(%)	n	(%)	n	(%)
DSM-IV diagnosis						
No	42	(97.7)	39	(14.9)	81	(26.6)
Yes	1	(2.3)	222	(86.1)	223	(73.3)
Total	43	(14.1)[a]	261	(85.9)[a]	304	(100.0)

[a] Designates row percentages (the remainder of percentages in this table are column percentages)

sought help due to drinking among those with neither DSM-IV nor DSM-5 AUD, DSM-5 AUD alone, and both DSM-IV and DSM-5 AUD, was 78.6%, 53.8% and 36.5%, respectively.

Readiness to change and confidence in ability to change

As shown in Table 3b, the readiness to change drinking for patients who met criteria for neither DSM-IV nor DSM-5 AUD, DSM-5 alone, and both DSM-IV and DSM-5 AUD, was 40.5%, 61.5% and 74.3% respectively. While 80.2% of patients who met criteria for both DSM-IV and DSM-5 AUD reported that change was somewhat or very important, 61.5% of those with DSM-5 AUD alone and 35.7% of those who met neither DSM-IV nor DSM-5 criteria for AUD reported change was somewhat or very important. However, patients who met both DSM-IV and DSM-5 criteria were least likely to report being somewhat or very confident in their ability to change (77.0%), while those who met DSM-5 criteria alone and those who met neither DSM-IV nor DSM-5 criteria for AUD appeared to have similar rates of reporting being somewhat or very confident in their ability to change (92.9 and 89.7% respectively).

Post-hoc analyses

Because descriptive analyses suggested that patients who met criteria for DSM-5 alone may differ on the burden of negative consequences due to drinking, mental health and drug use conditions, and readiness to change from patients meeting criteria for neither DSM-IV nor DSM-5 AUD, or both DSM-IV and DSM-5 AUD, we performed post hoc statistical tests to evaluate whether differences across the mutually exclusive diagnostic groups were statistically significant. For the purposes of these post hoc analyses, the diagnostic group that included the lone subject who met DSM-IV criteria for AUD alone, was excluded resulting in a 3-way comparison. These analyses revealed that all three measures differed significantly across the 3 groups ($p < 0.001$) (Table 3b).

Discussion

In this sample of VA primary care patients at high risk for AUD due to frequent binge drinking, DSM-5 AUD criteria identified about 13% more patients with AUD than DSM-IV criteria. Almost three quarters of patients met both DSM-IV and DSM-5 criteria for AUD and 14% met criteria for neither, but only one patient out of 304 met criteria for DSM-IV AUD but not DSM-5 AUD. Moreover, in this sample of primary care patients recruited for a trial of care management for patients at high risk for AUD, there were marked differences in the clinical characteristics across the four groups. Those who met both DSM-IV and DSM-5 AUD criteria not only had more negative consequences due to drinking, but also more mental health and drug use symptoms and greater reported readiness to change compared with those who met either DSM-IV or DSM-5 AUD alone, and those who met neither DSM-IV nor DSM-5 criteria for AUD.

A unique strength of this study is that it compared DSM-IV and DSM-5 criteria in a clinical sample of heavy drinkers. This is an important population to study because it is these patients in whom assessments for AUD are used clinically. It is not possible to determine the extent to which the higher prevalence of AUD using DSM-5 criteria (85.9%) compared to DSM-IV criteria (73.3%) is due to the specific characteristics of the sample we studied—primary care patients who reported frequent binge drinking—or if this result would be found in more general clinical populations. However, this study's finding that a sizable group of patients (13%) met criteria for DSM-5 AUD alone is consistent with 7 of 12 recent studies comparing the prevalence of AUD based on DSM-IV and DSM-5 criteria in mostly non-clinical settings [12]. The fact that only one patient met criteria for DSM-IV AUD alone might be somewhat surprising. One might have expected more than 1 patient with frequent binge drinking to meet the DSM-IV AUD criteria with just 1 DSM-IV abuse criterion or 2 DSM-IV criteria that included legal consequences, which was excluded from DSM-5. However, drinking 5 or more drinks on an occasion is strongly associated with AUD symptoms

Table 3 Sociodemographic, Smoking, Mental Health and Substance Use Characteristics of Patients Meeting Criteria for Neither DSM-IV nor DSM-5 AUD, DSM-IV AUD alone, DSM-5 AUD alone, or Both

	Neither DSM-IV nor DSM-5 n = 42		DSM-IV AUD alone n = 1		DSM-5 AUD alone n = 39		Both DSM-IV & DSM-5 AUD n = 222	
(a)								
Female	5	(11.9)	0	(0.0)	4	(10.3)	20	(9.0)
Age categories								
21–34	4	(9.5)	0	(0.0)	5	(12.8)	45	(20.3)
35–49	7	(16.7)	1	(100.0)	10	(25.6)	47	(21.2)
50–64	13	(31.0)	0	(0.0)	13	(33.3)	105	(47.3)
65+	18	(42.9)	0	(0.0)	11	(28.2)	25	(11.3)
Patient-reported race								
Native American	1	(2.4)	0	(0.0)	5	(12.8)	19	(8.6)
Asian	0	(0.0)	0	(0.0)	0	(0.0)	2	(0.9)
Native Hawaiian/Pacific Islander	1	(2.4)	0	(0.0)	0	(0.0)	4	(1.8)
Black	3	(7.1)	1	(100.0)	6	(15.4)	29	(13.1)
White	36	(85.7)	0	(0.0)	28	(71.8)	142	(64.0)
Multiracial	1	(2.4)	0	(0.0)	0	(0.0)	21	(9.5)
Other	0	(0.0)	0	(0.0)	0	(0.0)	5	(2.3)
Hispanic/Latino	3	(7.1)	0	(0.0)	2	(5.1)	16	(7.2)
Marital status								
Never married	7	(16.7)	0	(0.0)	8	(20.5)	41	(18.5)
Married/partnered	22	(52.4)	0	(0.0)	18	(46.2)	96	(43.2)
Separated	1	(2.4)	0	(0.0)	2	(5.1)	10	(4.5)
Divorced	10	(23.8)	1	(100.0)	9	(23.1)	71	(32.0)
Widowed	2	(4.8)	0	(0.0)	2	(5.1)	3	(1.4)
Refused/unknown	0	(0.0)	0	(0.0)	0	(0.0)	1	(0.5)
Education								
High school/GED or less	9	(21.4)	0	(0.0)	9	(23.1)	47	(21.2)
Some college/tech school	20	(47.6)	1	(100.0)	20	(51.3)	129	(58.1)
College or post graduate	13	(31.0)	0	(0.0)	10	(25.6)	46	(20.7)
Income								
<$15,000	3	(7.1)	1	(100.0)	5	(12.8)	40	(18.0)
$15,000–59,999	20	(47.7)	0	(0.0)	22	(56.4)	116	(52.3)
≥$60,000	18	(42.9)	0	(0.0)	12	(30.8)	65	(29.3)
Refused/unknown	1	(2.4)	0	(0.0)	0	(0.0)	1	(0.5)
(b)								
Smokes currently	11	(26.2)	1	(100.0)	15	(38.5)	107	(48.2)
Depression symptoms (PHQ-9 ≥ 10)	3	(7.1)	0	(0.0)	5	(12.8)	130	(58.6)
Generalized anxiety symptoms (GAD-7 ≥ 10)	4	(9.5)	0	(0.0)	0	(0.0)	88	(39.7)
DSM-IV panic disorder—current (MINI)	1	(2.4)	0	(0.0)	6	(15.4)	84	(38.4)
DSM-IV drug use disorders past year (MINI)	2	(4.8)	0	(0.0)	1	(2.6)	26	(11.7)
Count of mental health and drug use conditions*, mean (SD)**	0	(0.0)	0	(0.0)	2	(5.1)	55	(24.8)
Negative alcohol-related consequences*	0.2	(0.1)	0	(0.0)	0.4	(0.1)	1.7	(0.1)
Negative alcohol-related consequences								
Short Inventory of Problems (SIP)—past 3 months, mean (SD)**	1.0	(0.3)	1	n/a	2.5	(0.4)	6.8	(0.3)
Short inventory of problems (SIP)—lifetime, mean (SD)	4.2	(0.5)	5	n/a	6.7	(0.5)	10.1	(0.3)
Never seen anyone/gone anywhere for drinking-related reason?	33	(78.6)	0	(0.0)	21	(53.8)	81	(36.5)
Somewhat or ready to change**	17	(40.5)	0	(0.0)	24	(61.5)	165	(74.3)
Somewhat or very Important to change	15	(35.7)	0	(0.0)	24	(61.5)	178	(80.2)

Table 3 continued

	Neither DSM-IV nor DSM-5 n = 42		DSM-IV AUD alone n = 1		DSM-5 AUD alone n = 39		Both DSM-IV & DSM-5 AUD n = 222	
Somewhat or very confident in ability to change	39	(92.9)	1	(100.0)	35	(89.7)	171	(77.0)

* Sum of the total number of positive screens for depression, generalized anxiety, PTSD, panic, and DUD

** Wald test p < 0.0

[3], and thus restriction of our sample to frequent binge drinking could account for this finding. Further research is needed on other clinical samples of patients with frequent binge drinking to understand if this unexpected finding was unique to our study sample.

Patients meeting criteria for both DSM-IV and DSM-5 AUD had relatively high rates of mental health symptoms, drug use disorders, and recent negative consequences due to drinking. Moreover, almost three quarters of these patients who met both DSM-IV and DSM-5 criteria were somewhat or very interested in changing their drinking. In contrast, patients who met criteria for DSM-5 AUD alone, who by definition met criteria for mild DSM-5 AUD, tended to report fewer negative consequences due to drinking, less tobacco use and drug use disorders, and fewer symptoms of anxiety and depression. This is an expected finding since DSM-5 was designed to better capture less severe forms of AUD and to have dimensionality such that participants with fewer DSM criteria have a milder AUD [8–10]. Further, patients who met criteria for DSM-5 AUD alone had less readiness to change compared to patients who met both DSM-IV and DSM-5 criteria, despite having similar demographic characteristics. This association between alcohol-related symptom burden and readiness to change has been previously described [28], but the finding that DSM-5 identifies more of these patients with milder alcohol-related symptoms who report less readiness to change may have clinical implications for primary care. Given the lower burden of mental health symptoms reported by patients with DSM-5 AUD alone, and their greater confidence in their ability to change their drinking, patients meeting DSM-5 criteria alone may be more likely to respond to brief opportunistic interventions in primary care compared to those who meet criteria for both DSM-IV and DSM-5 AUD. On the other hand, these patients tended to report less treatment-seeking and placing less importance on changing their drinking than those meeting both DSM-IV and DSM-5 AUD criteria and they were less likely to report that they were ready to change. These characteristics may make patients meeting criteria for DSM-5 alone more successful at self-change, but more challenging to engage in opportunistic primary care interventions—like the CHOICE trial intervention–which seek to engage patients repeatedly over time and/or interest them in medications for AUD [29, 30]. Future research will be needed to assess whether the effectiveness of the CHOICE intervention differed for those who met criteria for DSM-5 AUD alone vs both DSM-IV and DSM-5 AUD.

In this sample of primary care patients who reported frequent binge drinking and enrolled in a trial, 14% did not meet criteria for DSM-IV or DSM-5 AUD. To our knowledge, little research has focused on this group. These patients had similar rates of mental health co-morbidity compared to those with an AUD based on DSM-5 criteria alone. However, they tended to be older and reported a mean of 4 of 15 negative consequences due to drinking in their lifetimes, suggesting that they may have had prior AUD now in remission. Patients with frequent binge drinking who do not meet DSM criteria for AUD *on average* respond to opportunistic brief interventions [31], but little is known about whether older patients who have previously experienced negative consequences due to drinking and may have AUD in remission respond to brief interventions. Future research is also needed to evaluate whether alcohol medications can decrease drinking and future negative consequences related to drinking for this group.

This study has several important limitations. First, the study sample reflects VA primary care patients with frequent binge drinking who were willing to enroll in a trial in which they would be offered alcohol-related services, limiting generalizability. The prevalence of AUD based on DSM-IV and DSM-5 is likely to be markedly lower in general primary care populations, and may differ in younger and non-research populations. It is also possible that those patients meeting criteria for DSM-IV AUD alone (1 DSM-IV abuse criterion or 2 DSM-IV criteria including legal consequences) were less likely to participate in a research study on alcohol and therefore were not represented in our sample. For example, this could disproportionately impact racial minorities who may be more likely to have legal consequences of drinking [32], but less likely to participate in trials. The recruited sample was also 90% men, who tend have higher rates of AUD than women, and the sample had a relatively high prevalence of mental health symptoms and drug use disorders.

Several limitations of this study's measures should also be noted. The DSM-IV skip pattern limited our ability to measure DSM-5 AUD severity in those with DSM-IV alcohol dependence, because the interview skip pattern that did not assess the 4 questions about abuse in patients with dependence. In addition, we used a craving question with a lifetime timeframe. However, sensitivity analyses determined that the impact of the "ever" time frame of the craving question had minimal impact on our findings (Additional file 1, Additional file 2). This descriptive study also lacked a priori hypotheses about differences across the four mutually exclusive groups and did not have power to test multiple comparisons. Additional studies of the prevalence and severity of DSM-5 AUD and associated mental health comorbidity and readiness to change in primary care patients with frequent binge drinking will be important (Additional file 3).

Conclusions

Despite the above limitations, these findings may be pertinent to patients with frequent binge drinking in the VA, the largest integrated health system in the US with over 900 clinical sites nationwide. As above, this is also the first study to compare DSM-IV and DSM-5 criteria in a primary care population to our knowledge. Additionally, primary care patients with frequent binge drinking are an important clinical sample in which to study DSM diagnostic criteria. Most brief alcohol screens assess frequent or recent heavy drinking and a follow-up diagnostic assessment for AUD can aid treatment decisions (i.e. brief intervention vs. medication) [33]. Further, results of this study highlight the spectrum and complexity of patients with frequent binge drinking who might be open to receiving alcohol-related care in their primary care clinic.

In sum, in this study of VA primary care patients with frequent binge drinking, 13% of patients met DSM-5 AUD criteria but did not meet DSM-IV AUD criteria. These patients appeared to have fewer negative consequences due to drinking and less other substance use and mental health comorbidity, than patients who met criteria for both DSM-IV and DSM-5 AUD. If findings are corroborated by future primary care studies, developing and testing optimal approaches to managing these primary care patients with less complex AUD may be important.

Abbreviations

AUD: alcohol use disorders; DSM-IV: the diagnostic and statistical manual of mental disorders, 4th edition; DSM-5: the diagnostic and statistical manual of mental disorders, 5th edition; VA: veterans affairs; CHOICE: considering healthier drinking options in primary CarE; AUDIT-C: alcohol use disorders identification test consumption questionnaire; NESARC: national epidemiologic survey on alcohol and related conditions; NIAAA: national institute on alcohol abuse and alcoholism; MINI: mini-international neuropsychiatric interview; PHQ-9: 9-item patient health questionnaire; GAD: generalized anxiety disorder screen; PCL-C: post-traumatic stress disorder checklist; PTSD: post-traumatic stress disorder; DUD: drug use disorder; SIP: short inventory of problems; SD: standard deviation.

Authors' contributions

KB obtained funding and devised the concept for the CHOICE trial, along with Coinvestigators including EW, DG, EH, JM. Data coding and analyses were conducted by AR, LC, and GL. All co-authors interpreted the data regarding DSM-IV and DSM-5 AUD prevalence, patient characteristics, and their association with AUD groups. TT and KB designed the concept for the paper and were major contributors in drafting the manuscript, but all co-authors contributed to several major revisions. All authors read and approved the final manuscript.

Author details

[1] Health Services Research and Development (HSR&D), Seattle Center of Innovation for Veteran-Centered and Value-Driven Care, 1660 S. Columbian Way, Seattle, WA 98108, USA. [2] Center of Excellence in Substance Abuse Treatment and Education (CESATE), Veterans Affairs (VA) Puget Sound Health Care System, S-123-PCC, 1660 S. Columbian Way, Seattle, WA 98108, USA. [3] Kaiser Permanente Washington Health Research Institute, 1730 Minor Avenue, Ste. 1600, Seattle, WA 98101, USA. [4] Department of Veterans Affairs Puget Sound Health Care System, General Medicine Services, 1660 South Columbian Way (S-152), Seattle, WA 98108, USA. [5] Department of Health Services, University of Washington, 1959 Pacific Street, Seattle, WA 98195, USA. [6] Department of Medicine, University of Washington, 1959 NE Pacific Street, Seattle, WA 98195, USA. [7] The Kidney Health Research Collaborative, San Francisco and San Francisco VA Medical Center, University of California, 4150 Clement Street (111A1), San Francisco, CA 94121, USA. [8] Psychiatry and Behavioral Sciences, University of Washington, Seattle, WA, USA. [9] Department of Veterans Affairs Puget Sound Health Care System, Mental Health Service, 1660 South Columbian Way (S-152), Seattle, WA 98108, USA. [10] Division of Health Services Management and Policy, College of Public Health, The Ohio State University, Columbus, OH, USA. [11] Center for Innovation in Pediatric Practice, Nationwide Children's Hospital, Columbus, OH, USA.

Acknowledgements

The authors would like to thank the patients who participated in the CHOICE trial, and their primary care providers, as well as VA clinical leaders, in primary care, integrated mental health, mental health specialty clinics, psychiatric emergency services, laboratory services, pharmacy and addictions treatment, who supported this trial. The authors are indebted to Rachel Thomas, Erika Holden, and Selin Caka for their critical roles enrolling and interviewing patients at baseline, to Chester Pabiniak and Malia Oliver for all data management, to the Group Health Survey Research Group for conducting follow-up interviews, to Thomas Wickizer, Ph.D., Paul Cornia, MD, and Peter Roy-Byrne, MD for serving on our Data Safety Monitoring Board and to Raymond Anton, MD and David Oslin, MD for their valuable consultation at the study start. The views expressed in this paper are those of the authors and do not necessarily reflect the position or policy of the National Institute of Health, Department of Veterans Affairs or the United States Government.

Competing interests

The authors declare that they have no competing interests.

Funding

This work was supported by National Institute of Alcohol Abuse and Alcoholism award number AA018702; Health Services Research & Development (HSR&D) Center of Innovation for Veteran-Centered Value-Driven Care (COIN) Veterans Affairs (VA) Puget Sound Health Care System, Seattle, WA and VA Puget Sound Center of Excellence for Substance Abuse Treatment & Education and General Internal Medicine Service. Dr. Bradley is supported by a mid-career mentoring award from the National Institute on Alcohol Abuse and Alcoholism (K24-AA022128). Dr. Williams is supported by a Career Development Award from VA Health Services Research & Development (CDA 12-276).

References

1. American Psychiatric Association. Diagnostic and statistical manual of mental disorders. 5th ed. Washington, DC: American Psychiatric Association; 2013.
2. American Psychiatric Association. Diagnostic and statistical manual of mental disorders. 4th ed. Washington, DC: American Psychiatric Association; 1994.
3. Saha TD, Chou SP, Grant BF. Toward an alcohol use disorder continuum using item response theory: results from the National Epidemiologic Survey on Alcohol and Related Conditions. Psychol Med. 2006;36:931–41.
4. Proudfoot H, Baillie AJ, Teesson M. The structure of alcohol dependence in the community. Drug Alcohol Depend. 2006;81:21–6.
5. Harford TC, Yi HY, Faden VB, Chen CM. The dimensionality of DSM-IV alcohol use disorders among adolescent and adult drinkers and symptom patterns by age, gender, and race/ethnicity. Alcohol Clin Exp Res. 2009;33:868–78.
6. Kelly JF, Wakeman SE, Saitz R. Stop talking dirty: clinicians, language, and quality of care for the leading cause of preventable death in the United States. Am J Med. 2015;128:8–9.
7. Hasin D. Truth (validity) and use despite consequences: the DSM-5 substance use disorder unidimensional syndrome. Addiction. 2014;109:1781–2.
8. Hasin DS, O'Brien CP, Auriacombe M, Borges G, Bucholz K, Budney A, Compton WM, Crowley T, Ling W, Petry NM, et al. DSM-5 criteria for substance use disorders: recommendations and rationale. Am J Psychiatry. 2013;170:834–51.
9. Peer K, Rennert L, Lynch KG, Farrer L, Gelernter J, Kranzler HR. Prevalence of DSM-IV and DSM-5 alcohol, cocaine, opioid, and cannabis use disorders in a largely substance dependent sample. Drug Alcohol Depend. 2013;127:215–9.
10. Harford TC, Yi HY, Grant BF. The five-year diagnostic utility of "diagnostic orphans" for alcohol use disorders in a national sample of young adults. J Stud Alcohol Drugs. 2010;71:410–7.
11. Caetano R, Baruah J, Chartier KG. Ten-year trends (1992 to 2002) in sociodemographic predictors and indicators of alcohol abuse and dependence among whites, blacks, and Hispanics in the United States. Alcohol Clin Exp Res. 2011;35:1458–66.
12. Bartoli F, Carra G, Crocamo C, Clerici M. From DSM-IV to DSM-5 alcohol use disorder: an overview of epidemiological data. Addict Behav. 2015;41:46–50.
13. Mohler-Kuo M, Landolt MA, Maier T, Meidert U, Schonbucher V, Schnyder U. Child sexual abuse revisited: a population-based cross-sectional study among Swiss adolescents. J Adolesc Health. 2014;54(304–311):e301.
14. Slade T, Chiu WT, Glantz M, Kessler RC, Lago L, Sampson N, Al-Hamzawi A, Florescu S, Moskalewicz J, Murphy S, et al. A cross-national examination of differences in classification of lifetime alcohol use disorder between DSM-IV and DSM-5: findings from the world mental health survey. Alcohol Clin Exp Res. 2016;40:1728–36.
15. Bradley KA, DeBenedetti AF, Volk RJ, Williams EC, Frank D, Kivlahan DR. AUDIT-C as a brief screen for alcohol misuse in primary care. Alcohol Clin Exp Res. 2007;31:1208–17.
16. Bradley KA, Kivlahan DR, Zhou XH, Sporleder JL, Epler AJ, McCormick KA, Merrill JO, McDonell MB, Fihn SD. Using alcohol screening results and treatment history to assess the severity of at-risk drinking in Veterans Affairs primary care patients. Alcohol Clin Exp Res. 2004;28:448–55.
17. Keyes KM, Hatzenbuehler ML, McLaughlin KA, Link B, Olfson M, Grant BF, Hasin D. Stigma and treatment for alcohol disorders in the United States. Am J Epidemiol. 2010;172:1364–72.
18. Coulehan JL, Zettler-Segal M, Block M, McClelland M, Schulberg HC. Recognition of alcoholism and substance abuse in primary care patients. Arch Intern Med. 1987;147:349–52.
19. Agrawal A, Heath AC, Lynskey MT. DSM-IV to DSM-5: the impact of proposed revisions on diagnosis of alcohol use disorders. Addiction. 2011;106:1935–43.
20. Miller WR, Tonigan JS, Longabaugh R. The drinker inventory of consequences (DrInC): An instrument for assessing adverse consequences of alcohol abuse. Bethesda: U.S. Department of Health and Human Services; 1995.
21. Forcehimes AA, Tonigan JS, Miller WR, Kenna GA, Baer JS. Psychometrics of the drinker inventory of consequences (DrInC). Addict Behav. 2007;32:1699–704.
22. Kenna GA, Longabaugh R, Gogineni A, Woolard RH, Nirenberg TD, Becker B, Minugh PA, Carty K, Clifford PR, Karolczuk K. Can the short index of problems (SIP) be improved? Validity and reliability of the three-month SIP in an emergency department sample. J Stud Alcohol. 2005;66:433–7.
23. Allensworth-Davies D, Cheng DM, Smith PC, Samet JH, Saitz R. The short inventory of problems-modified for drug use (SIP-DU): validity in a primary care sample. Am J Addict. 2012;21:257–62.
24. Cohen E, Feinn R, Arias A, Kranzler HR. Alcohol treatment utilization: findings from the National Epidemiologic Survey on Alcohol and Related Conditions. Drug Alcohol Depend. 2007;86:214–21.
25. Miller WR, Rollnick S. Motivational interviewing: preparing people for change. 2nd ed. New York: The Guilford Press; 2002.
26. Heather N, Smailes D, Cassidy P. Development of a readiness ruler for use with alcohol brief interventions. Drug Alcohol Depend. 2008;98:235–40.
27. Saitz R, Cheng DM, Winter M, Kim TW, Meli SM, Allensworth-Davies D, Lloyd-Travaglini CA, Samet JH. Chronic care management for dependence on alcohol and other drugs: the AHEAD randomized trial. JAMA. 2013;310:1156–67.
28. Williams EC, Kivlahan DR, Saitz R, Merrill JO, Achtmeyer CE, McCormick KA, Bradley KA. Readiness to change in primary care patients who screened positive for alcohol misuse. Ann Fam Med. 2006;4:213–20.
29. Jonas D, Amick H, Feltner C, Bobashev G, Thomas K, Wines R, Kim M, Shanahan E, Gass C, Rowe C, Garbutt J. Pharmacotherapy for adults with alcohol-use disorders in outpatient settings: a systematic review and meta-analysis. JAMA. 2014;311:1889–900.
30. Kranzler HR, Covault J, Feinn R, Armeli S, Tennen H, Arias AJ, Gelernter J, Pond T, Oncken C, Kampman KM. Topiramate treatment for heavy drinkers: moderation by a GRIK1 polymorphism. Am J Psychiatry. 2014;171:445–52.
31. Jonas DE, Garbutt JC, Amick HR, Brown JM, Brownley KA, Council CL, Viera AJ, Wilkins TM, Schwartz CJ, Richmond EM, et al. Behavioral counseling after screening for alcohol misuse in primary care: a systematic review and meta-analysis for the U.S. Preventive Services Task Force. Ann Intern Med. 2012;157:645–54.
32. Keyes KM, Liu XC, Cerda M. The role of race/ethnicity in alcohol-attributable injury in the United States. Epidemiol Rev. 2012;34:89–102.
33. Oslin DW, Lynch KG, Maisto SA, Lantinga LJ, McKay JR, Possemato K, Ingram E, Wierzbicki M. A randomized clinical trial of alcohol care management delivered in Department of Veterans Affairs primary care clinics versus specialty addiction treatment. J Gen Intern Med. 2014;29:162–8.

12

Physician versus non-physician delivery of alcohol screening, brief intervention and referral to treatment in adult primary care

Jennifer R. Mertens[1*], Felicia W. Chi[2], Constance M. Weisner[2,3], Derek D. Satre[2,3], Thekla B. Ross[2], Steve Allen[2], David Pating[4], Cynthia I. Campbell[2], Yun Wendy Lu[2] and Stacy A. Sterling[2]

Abstract

Background: Unhealthy alcohol use is a major contributor to the global burden of disease and injury. The US Preventive Services Task Force has recommended alcohol screening and intervention in general medical settings since 2004. Yet less than one in six US adults report health care professionals discussing alcohol with them. Little is known about methods for increasing implementation; different staffing models may be related to implementation effectiveness. This implementation trial compared delivery of alcohol screening, brief intervention and referral to specialty treatment (SBIRT) by physicians versus non-physician providers receiving training, technical assistance, and feedback reports.

Methods: The study was a cluster randomized implementation trial (ADVISe [Alcohol Drinking as a Vital Sign]). Within a private, integrated health care system, 54 adult primary care clinics were stratified by medical center and randomly assigned in blocked groups of three to SBIRT by physicians (PCP arm) versus non-physician providers and medical assistants (NPP and MA arm), versus usual care (Control arm). NIH-recommended screening questions were added to the electronic health record (EHR) to facilitate SBIRT. We examined screening and brief intervention and referral rates by arm. We also examined patient-, physician-, and system-level factors affecting screening rates and, among those who screened positive, rates of brief intervention and referral to treatment.

Results: Screening rates were highest in the NPP and MA arm (51 %); followed by the PCP arm (9 %) and the Control arm (3.5 %). Screening increased over the 12 months after training in the NPP and MA arm but remained stable in the PCP arm. The PCP arm had higher brief intervention and referral rates (44 %) among patients screening positive than either the NPP and MA arm (3.4 %) or the Control arm (2.7 %). Higher ratio of MAs to physicians was related to higher screening rates in the NPP and MA arm and longer appointment times to screening and intervention rates in the PCP arm.

Conclusion: Findings suggest that time frames longer than 12 months may be required for full SBIRT implementation. Screening by MAs with intervention and referral by physicians as needed can be a feasible model for increasing the implementation of this critical and under-utilized preventive health service within currently predominant primary care models.

*Correspondence: MertensJenniferR@gmail.com
[1] Kaiser Permanente Northern California, 1800 Harrison, Oakland, CA 94612, USA
Full list of author information is available at the end of the article

Trial registration: Clinical Trials NCT01135654
Keywords: Alcohol screening, Brief intervention for alcohol misuse, Primary care, Unhealthy alcohol use, Cluster randomized trial, Implementation

Background

Unhealthy alcohol use is a major contributor to the global burden of disease and injury [1, 2] and accounts for one in ten deaths of US adults aged 20–64 [3]. Screening and brief intervention to address non-dependent unhealthy alcohol use within primary care is effective [4–6] and recommended in national practice guidelines (including the U.S. Preventive Services Task Force (USPSTF) [7], the U.S. National Institute on Alcohol Abuse and Alcoholism's (NIAAA) Clinician's Guide "Helping Patients Who Drink Too Much" [8], and Canada's College of Family Physicians Guideline [9]), but is seldom delivered in health care settings. Fewer than one in six Americans report being asked about or discussing their drinking with a health professional [10], and screening is rarely conducted in US primary care settings [11] outside the Veteran's Affairs Health System (VA) [12]. Since efforts to implement alcohol Screening and Brief Intervention (for non-dependent unhealthy use, such as binge drinking with no current adverse consequences [13]) and Referral to Treatment (for alcohol dependence) (SBIRT) have fallen short [14], the field has called for more SBIRT implementation research [15–17]. This is particularly timely given important new environmental factors, such as the alcohol screening and brief counseling performance measures developed and approved by American Medical Association's Physician Consortium for Performance Improvement, the Affordable Care Act's provisions for substance use services, the Mental Health Parity and Addiction Equity Act, and Medicare reimbursement codes for SBIRT [18].

Studies of SBIRT implementation within primary care settings have found implementation difficult [19–21] and have typically focused on delivery of SBIRT by physicians. A European study of a tailored, multi-faceted improvement program for physician-delivered SBIRT [20] found little change in screening and intervention behavior at 12 months. Implementation of SBIRT delivery by primary care physicians, including brief advice, has been difficult to achieve even with financial incentives provided [19].

Non-physician provision of SBIRT may also be considered as a viable approach. Babor and colleagues found higher implementation rates by non-physicians and similar effectiveness to physician-delivered screening and brief intervention [22, 23]. Moreover, use of non-physician providers to conduct behavioral and disease management interventions is increasingly being considered as an appropriate and cost-effective alternative to physician delivery, and has been found to be acceptable to patients [24–29]. There is evidence that primary care teams involving nurses or health educators for behavioral interventions have higher rates of preventive screenings, such as colorectal cancer screening [30].

The Alcohol Drinking as a Vital Sign (ADVISe) study is a cluster, randomized trial in 54 adult primary care clinics within 11 Kaiser Permanente Northern California (KPNC) medical centers. It compares implementation of primary care physician (PCP)-delivered to non-physician provider-delivered SBIRT, and to usual care. In the non-physician provider-delivered arm, medical assistants (MAs) screen and clinical health educators, behavioral medicine specialists or registered nurses deliver brief intervention and referral to treatment (NPP and MA arm). The outcomes examined are screening rates and rates of brief intervention and referral to treatment (BI/RT) among those who screened positive. Cluster randomization of clinics prevented contamination between clinicians, and also was necessary because training and quality improvement is generally conducted at the clinic level. Because there is some variation in practice and leadership across the organization by medical center [31] and consistent with prior research on physician versus non-physician SBIRT implementation [22], we present findings overall and by medical center. Based on prior research showing that non-physicians can increase implementation of preventive and behavioral interventions, and findings that the most common barriers to SBIRT delivery in primary care are limited physician time and competing priorities [28, 32–35], we hypothesized that the NPP & MA arm would have higher rates of screening and BI/RT than the PCP arm.

To inform implementation strategies, we also examine how, within each intervention arm (PCP and NPP and MA), patient, physician, and system-level factors may be associated with SBIRT implementation as the literature suggests that such factors influence implementation [36, 37]. Prior research suggests that critical factors within these domains include provider training, time constraints [28, 32, 35], lack of treatment referral resources [38], systems issues such as staff workloads, patient demographic and clinical characteristics, and integration of screening into the electronic health record (EHR) [36, 39–41]. Thus, we examined how implementation outcomes were related to patient factors including demographic characteristics and medical and psychiatric problems [42], physician factors including training, demographics and specialty [28, 43, 44], and system factors [22, 45] including office visit length, the ratio of support staff to physicians, and co-location of specialty alcohol and drug (AOD) services [46].

Due to the naturalistic design of the current study we did not measure provider attitudes. However, recent research from a large European implementation trial [47, 48] suggests that providers' role security with and commitment to addressing alcohol misuse are cross-sectionally related to reports of addressing alcohol misuse [47]. Yet, neither role security nor therapeutic commitment were prospectively related to screening or intervention [48].

To better understand the system context, we surveyed physician leaders within the study sites to understand alcohol screening practices and policies within the internal setting prior to the training and implementation processes. We hold constant a key factor found to be a salient influence on provider performance of care services—an EHR screening tool [49] made available in all three study arms. EHR use is growing steadily, both domestically [50, 51] and in many developed [52] and developing [53, 54] countries, increasing opportunities to incorporate such tools broadly. The findings on physician versus non-physician implementation and factors related to implementation within each delivery model can inform delivery and implementation of alcohol SBIRT and similar USPSTF-recommended behavioral care services [46] in primary care settings.

Methods

Setting

KPNC is a private, integrated health care delivery system covering 15 counties and serving 3.8 million members, [55] and KP covers 40 % of the insured population in California [56] with AOD services provided internally. The membership reflects the population of the region [57, 58], with more than 40 % of adult members being non-white or Hispanic, nearly 30 % with only a high school or lower level of education, and 44 % with annual incomes less than $65,000. KPNC's and the University of California San Francisco's institutional review boards approved the study.

Randomization, sample and intervention

The unit of randomization was clinic. Eleven medical centers (of 47 in KPNC) were chosen to represent both urban and suburban locations and various clinic sizes. Fifty-four primary care clinics were in the 11 KPNC medical centers, located in Fairfield, Napa, Redwood City, San Francisco, San Jose, Santa Clara, Santa Rosa, South Sacramento, South San Francisco, Vacaville, and Vallejo. The 54 clinics were stratified by medical center and randomly assigned (parallel-group design) in blocked groups of three to SBIRT by physicians (PCP arm) versus non-physician providers and medical assistants (NPP and MA arm) versus usual care (Control arm), with 18 clinics in each of the three arms.

There were 204 physicians in the PCP clinics, 189 in the NPP and MA clinics, and 163 in the Control arm clinics. We excluded two physicians in the PCP arm who used an earlier version of the screening tool (see methods below for screening tool details). In the year following the date at which each clinic had started the study (ranging from September 22, 2010 to November 24, 2010), a total of 218,667 unique patients had visits to the PCP arm physicians, 223,147 to the NPP and MA arm physicians, and 197,799 to the Control arm physicians (Fig. 1). Consistent with other studies [41, 59, 60], and because screening and interventions were intended to be part of usual care, we used KPNC's EHR and other administrative data to examine patient and provider data and did not recruit individual providers or patients.

Screening tools

The evidence-based [61] screening tool from the NIAAA Clinician's Guide [8] was added to the adult primary care EHR with an automated clinical reminder at each adult (ages 18+) patient visit. It included the NIAAA single question screener "How many times in the past year have you had 5 or more drinks in a day" (for men aged 18–65, and "4 or more drinks" for women and individuals aged 66 and older) [8, 61]. Providers and MAs were instructed to use a laminated chart (distributed to exam rooms in the intervention arms) during screening to show patients various alcoholic beverage types and their standard drink sizes. Per the NIAAA Guide and prior studies, if a patient's response was positive to the single question (i.e., >0 times exceeding the daily low-risk limit), the patient is considered an unhealthy drinker. Thus, for responses >0 times to this question, the tool prompted additional questions to assess use exceeding the NIAAA weekly low-risk limit ("On average, how many days a week do you have an alcoholic drink?" and "On a typical drinking day, how many drinks do you have?"), plus a validated two-question screener for alcohol use disorders ("In the past year, have you sometimes been under the influence of alcohol in situations where you could have caused an accident or gotten hurt?" and "Have there often been times when you had a lot more to drink than you intended to have?"; an affirmative response to either is considered a positive screening result) [62]. The EHR contained fields for recording whether a BI or RT was performed.

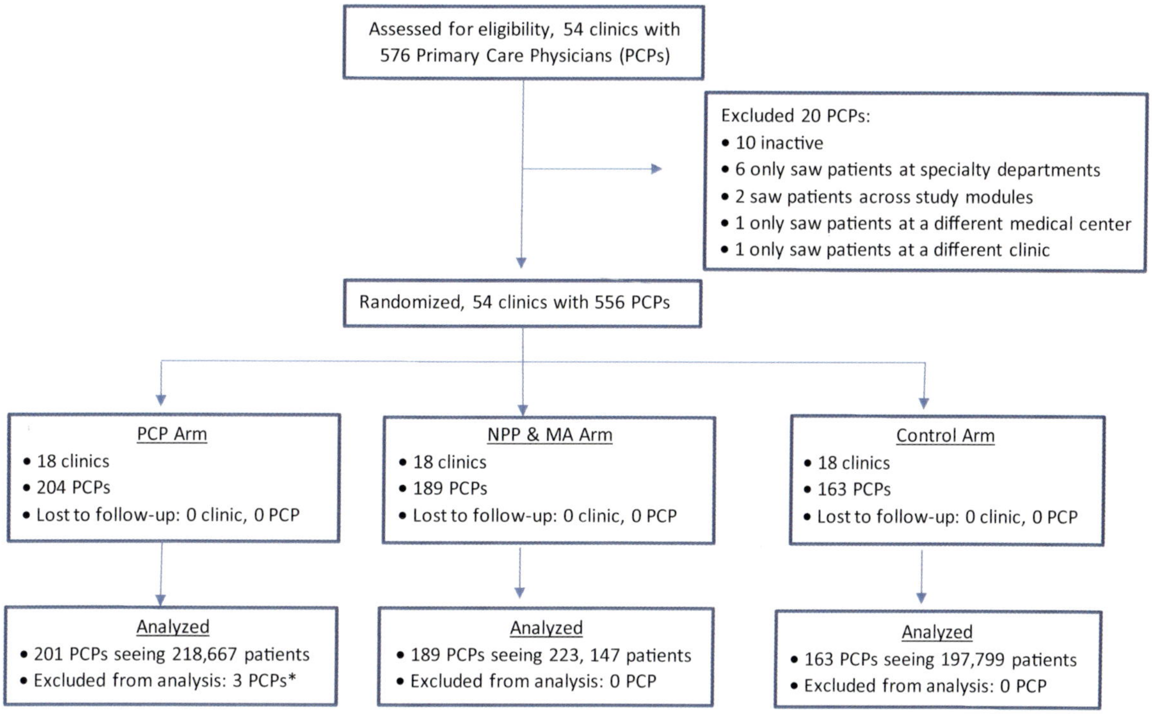

* Excluded 2 PCPs who recorded screening only in pilot/testing data table and 1 PCP who transferred to NPP & MA arm during Year 1

Fig. 1 Flow diagram of participating clinics, physicians and patients through phases of the trial

Intervention

In both PCP and NPP and MA arms, providers were trained to deliver the same intervention, drawn from the NIAAA Guide. Patients who screened positive on the alcohol use disorders risk questions would be referred to AOD treatment for further assessment and possible treatment. Patients who screened positive on the unhealthy drinking questions but negative for alcohol use disorder risk would receive brief intervention consisting of providers stating their concern and advising them to cut back to low risk limits or abstain, as outlined in the NIAAA Guide [8]. Further, providers were trained in brief motivational intervention, and to: (1) incorporate salient medical conditions if possible (e.g., "drinking above these limits can worsen your hypertension and insomnia"), and (2) ask patients how ready they were to make the recommended changes, and (3) assist in goal-setting to reduce or stop drinking if the patient was willing. Patients were given the NIAAA publication "Tips for Cutting Down on Drinking" [63].

PCP arm

Physicians were trained to conduct all aspects of SBIRT.

NPP and MA arm

MAs were trained to ask the screening question, and non-physician providers were trained to ask the questions about weekly drinking and the two alcohol disorder screening questions and to conduct BI/RT. Chiefs of medicine and administrative managers at each site determined which type of non-physician provider would be trained to provide BI/RT. In Medical Centers 1, 6, 10, and 11, clinical health educators were trained; in Medical Centers 2, 3, 4, 5, and 9, behavioral medicine specialists (clinical psychologists or licensed clinical social workers) were trained; and in Medical Centers 7 and 8, registered nurses were trained. MAs roles include escorting patients to exam rooms, collecting and recording (in the EHR) health screening data, including blood pressure and smoking. They are required to have completed a vocational medical assisting training program and are supervised by nurse managers.

Control arm

Patients received usual care. Providers and MAs had access to the same EHR resources as in the intervention arms and physicians were invited to a 30-min webinar information session on the EHR evidence-based screening tool. Prior to the study, alcohol screening was not part of the organizational workflow. There was no defined screening or intervention policy or standardized workflow for either physicians or non-physicians to address unhealthy alcohol use in the Control arm. In the Control arm webinar information session, the screening tool was described as evidence-based but additional details (such as sensitivity and specificity) were not provided. The NIAAA daily and weekly low-risk limits were given. No information or training were given on BI/RT in the Control condition.

Training

Training the trainers

Intervention training was adapted from the Alcohol Clinical Training (ACT) curriculum [64]. Trainers (internists, psychiatrists, psychologists, and social workers) attended one 4-h session on SBIRT and another 2-h session covering the KPNC-specific components including the EHR tool and referral information.

Training physicians and non-physician providers

PCP arm physicians and NPP and MA arm non-physician providers were given a 2-h training. The curriculum and duration of training were equivalent across arms; the trainings differed only in instruction about the workflow (with the NPP and MA arm including instruction about the handoff to the non-physician provider). In the NPP and MA arm, physicians were also included in the first hour of the training to learn about the importance and effectiveness of SBIRT and the workflow. The first hour included the NIAAA low-risk drinking limits [8], the USPSTF recommendations, the prevalence of unhealthy alcohol use in primary care in KPNC, evidence of the adverse health effects of unhealthy alcohol use, and effectiveness/cost-effectiveness of specialty treatment for alcohol, screening procedures and the screening tool (including sensitivity and specificity for identifying unhealthy alcohol use and a demonstration of the EHR screening tool); and an overview of the basics of the BI/RT and how to code for interventions/referrals. The second hour covered the BI/RT in more depth, including brief motivational interviewing, video case studies, and role-play practice. It also included a brief presentation by an AOD clinician about how to refer and assessment and treatment services offered at the local AOD clinic.

Each clinic also received in-person technical assistance 3 months after training. Trainers reviewed the clinics' quality feedback reports on screening, intervention, and referral rates; and addressed questions and challenges. At 6 months, clinics received a 30-min "booster" training. All physicians in the PCP arm were included in the booster training. In the NPP and MA arm, physicians, NPPs and MAs were included.

MA training

In the NPP and MA arm, MAs were trained for one hour by registered nurses. The training included information about the health impact of unhealthy alcohol use, the effectiveness of SBIRT, the evidence-based screening questions and their ability to identify unhealthy alcohol use. MAs were provided with a demonstration of the EHR screening tool. They were given training on how to ask the screening questions in the EHR, which they practiced through role-play. The trainers also addressed "normalizing" alcohol screening and intervention (e.g., comparing with smoking and exercise) as integral to routine primary care services.

Training participation

In the PCP arm, 90 % of physicians attended training. In the NPP and MA arm, 100 % of non-physician providers, 85 % of MAs, and 80 % of physicians attended. For physicians who missed training, online, on-demand training was available. For MAs who missed training, their managers and senior peers provided training using the training materials. Brief videos on the EHR tool use were available to all on the EHR information and support intranet site. In the Control arm, a half-hour webinar session on use of the EHR screening tool was available on-demand via the KPNC intranet following the live session.

Quality feedback reports

In the PCP and NPP and MA arms, quarterly reports were emailed to each clinic presenting their average screening and BI/RT rates and the names of the top five performing clinics within each arm with their mean rates.

Leadership engagement

The CEO of The Permanente Medical Group (which employs the organization's physicians) endorsed the project via a video introduction to the study training in which he discussed the links between unhealthy alcohol use and common health conditions and how SBIRT can benefit patients with unhealthy alcohol use. The Chair of the Chiefs of Adult Primary Care Medicine and the previous Chair (who retired a few months into the study) were both supportive and volunteered their clinics—"modeling" behavior for other Chiefs and physician colleagues. In the NPP and MA arm, clinic managers (to whom the MAs report) generally directed the MAs to use the screening tool, and it was generally seen as part of the MAs' responsibilities. In each medical center, the physician chiefs of medicine (to whom the physicians report) agreed to having their sites used for the project and generally encouraged (but did not mandate) the use of SBIRT by physicians and non-physician providers.

Incentives

Incentives to conduct SBIRT were limited to clinic recognition in the quality feedback reports (see "quality feedback reports" above) for high performing clinics. There were no financial incentives for any staff or providers to conduct screening, brief intervention, or referral to treatment.

Data sources and measures

Primary care leader survey

We conducted an online survey of the Chiefs of Adult Primary Care in each medical center and the Physician Leader of each clinic, to understand practices and policies related to alcohol screening and intervention prior to the training. The response rate among the 62 physicians was 73 %. Participants were offered a $50 gift card. The survey also asked the allocated office visit length in the clinic which was used to calculate average visit time for each medical center.

EHR and administrative databases

The EHR was used to extract patient age, gender, and medical comorbidities. In the year prior to each patient's index screening visit, we identified presence of a psychiatric diagnosis (i.e., psychoses, neurotic, personality and other psychiatric disorders, excluding AOD disorders) and presence of an other chronic disease diagnosis (yes/no) (i.e., Arthritis, Hypertension, Chronic Pain, Diabetes Mellitus, Asthma, Ischemic Heart Disease, Congestive Heart Failure, Stroke/Cerebrovascular Accident, Epilepsy, Parkinson's Disease, End-Stage Renal Disease, HIV, Osteoporosis, Chronic Obstructive Pulmonary Disease (COPD) (ICD-9 codes available upon request). Physician race/ethnicity, gender, age, and MD specialty (Internal Medicine, Family Medicine or other) as well as the ratio of MAs to PCPs in each clinic were drawn from the administrative databases.

For each patient in the sample (i.e., who had one or more visits to a study physician in the study year), screening (1 if screened/else 0) was measured as having been asked the single-item screener as recorded in the EHR tool on any visit to the provider within the study year. If occurring in multiple visits within 1 year, the index screening visit was defined as the first visit. BI/RT was measured as having a visit in which an intervention or referral was recorded during or within 45 days of the screening visit for those who screened positive at the screening visit. We allowed a 45-day window because providers were trained to schedule a follow-up visit for the BI/RT within 6 weeks if unable to complete during the screening visit. We examined the EHR tool (containing fields for providers to record interventions and referrals) and also the diagnostic "V-code" for "Counseling, Alcohol Prevention" as indication of brief intervention or referral (as per the training). We also reported the BI and RT rates, separately, for each arm.

Other data collection

Co-location of primary care and specialty AOD clinics was measured by examining medical center maps and confirming with local staff. Anonymous questionnaires gathered at booster sessions asked providers and MAs the average amount of time spent on screening and asked providers the average total amount of time spent on BI/RT. To inform quantitative results, provider and staff feedback on the implementation and workflow challenges at the booster sessions was documented as part of data collection, and qualitative interviews with staff and providers at each study clinic were conducted.

Analyses

Analyses were performed using SAS version 9.3 (SAS Institute Inc., Cary, NC, USA) and Stata version 10.1 (StataCorp, College Station, TX, USA). Physician survey results were examined descriptively. We calculated average monthly and annual screening rates for each medical center by study arm, and examined differences in screening rates between study arms using z statistics for comparisons of proportions. We also examined the number and percent screened for the best month over the 12 months after study start, which is the highest screening rate that each entity attained. Similarly, screening rates of BI/RT performed among those screened positive were calculated for each medical center and overall by study arm, and differences examined using Chi square tests. We also report a population-based BI/RT rate [65] by arm—this figure is the proportion of patients of all those with visits at the primary care clinics who received the intervention (regardless of being screened or not).

Within each intervention arm, multilevel logistic regression models were fitted to examine associations between patient-, physician- and system-level factors and screening and BI/RT implementation outcomes while accounting for clustering within physician and within clinic correlation of patient outcomes. Patient characteristics included age (18–24, 25–44, 45–59, and 60+), gender, and comorbid psychiatric and chronic conditions. Physician characteristics included age, gender, race/ethnicity, years serving the health plan, and specialty. System characteristics included co-location of primary care and AOD clinics, ratio of MAs to PCPs at the primary care clinic, average allocated office visit length, and number of physicians trained. For each outcome, we first fitted a series of multilevel univariate models to examine each predictor individually. All predictors associated with the outcome at $p < 0.10$ for either intervention arm were successively included in the multilevel models, with categories in the same direction being collapsed for some predictors to avoid extreme Odds Ratios (ORs) and 95 % Confidence Intervals (CIs) due to empty or small cells (for example, PCP race/ethnicity categories were collapsed to Non-White and White). Generalized Linear Latent and Mixed Models (GLLAMM) were used for multilevel analyses. We examined physician characteristics as predictors only in the PCP arm because SBIRT delivery in the NPP & MA arm was contingent on an entire team rather than an individual. No adjustments were made for multiple comparison [66].

Results

Screening practices prior to study implementation

In the survey of primary care leaders (N = 45) prior to the training, 88 % reported no policies or requirements to ask patients about alcohol. Those with policies indicated no consistent evidence-based screening methods.

Screening rates and proportion screened positive

Table 1 shows the average number of unique visits, screens per month, average percent of patients screened and the number and percent screened for the best month over the 12 months after study start in each medical center and overall. For average percent screened, the NPP and MA arm (50.9 %) was higher ($p < 0.0001$) than both the PCP arm (9.2 %) and the Control arm (3.5 %); and the PCP arm higher ($p < 0.0001$) than Control. Exceptions were three medical centers (1, 3, and 11) in which rates were higher in the Control than the PCP arm. A similar pattern was found for the best screening rate. The NPP and MA arm had higher rates (60.1 %) than either the PCP (10.7 %) or Control arm (6.0 %), and the PCP arm had higher rates than the Control arm ($p < 0.0001$), with higher rates in the Control than PCP arm for Medical Centers 1, 3, and 11. Some movement of MAs from the NPP and MA arm to other arms occurred in these medical centers; in some sites MAs covered duties for absent MAs in other clinics.

Figure 2 presents monthly average screening rates by arm across the 12 study months. NPP and MA arm rates increased from 38 % in month one to 60 % the final two months. PCP arm rates fluctuated between 8 and 10 % over time, and the Control arm had a small uptick from 2 to 6 %.

Of patients who were screened in the 12 months, the proportion screened positive for unhealthy drinking was 9.7 % in the PCP arm, 10.8 % in the NPP and MA arm, and 9.9 % in the Control arm.

Intervention and referral rates among those screened positive for unhealthy alcohol use

Table 2 presents numbers and percentages of patients with positive screens who received BI/RT. The PCP arm had higher ($p < 0.0001$) BI/RT rates (44.4 %) than either the NPP & MA arm (3.4 %) or the Control arm (2.7 %); this pattern differed only for medical center 5 (with no difference between PCP and NPP and MA arms) and medical center 9 (NPP and MA arm had higher rates than PCP arm, $p < 0.0001$). Generally, BI/RT rates did not differ between NPP and MA and Control arms with the exceptions of medical center 5 with a slightly higher NPP and MA arm rate ($p < 0.01$) and medical center 8 with a slightly higher Control arm rate ($p < 0.05$). The percent of patients who received RT (not shown) was 9.8, 0.6 and 0.2 % of those screening positive in the PCP, NPP and MA and Control arms, respectively. We also examined the proportion of all patients with primary care visits (regardless of screening) who received the BI/RT. We found that 0.63, 0.24 and 0.02 % of patients seen in the PCP, NPP and MA, and Control arms, respectively, received the BI/RT (not shown).

Post-hoc analysis for medical center 9 found that a few physicians in the NPP and MA arm delivered BI/RT themselves to their few patients screening positive; these physicians were responsible for the vast majority of BI/RTs delivered in this clinic. Post-hoc analysis comparing subtype of non-physician provider found no clinically significant difference; rates of BI/RT for behavioral medicine specialists, clinical health educators, and nurses was 4.0, 3.3, and 2.9 %, respectively (not shown).

Predictors of screening

Table 3 presents results of the multilevel models predicting screening in each of the intervention arms. Younger patients were less likely to be screened than patients over 60 years old in both arms. In both arms, women were less likely, and patients with psychiatric diagnoses and chronic medical conditions were more likely, to be screened.

In the PCP arm, we examined physician-level factors associated with screening. Older physicians were less likely, and female physicians more likely, to screen than their counterparts. Non-White physicians had four times higher odds of screening than White physicians (OR = 4.20, 95 % CI 3.99, 4.42). Each year of employment in the health plan was associated with a 30 % increase in odds of screening (OR = 1.30, 95 % CI 1.29, 1.30). Physicians with Family Practice or other specialties were far more likely to screen than Internal Medicine physicians.

Regarding system characteristics, lower odds of screening were associated with co-located primary care and AOD clinics in the PCP arm. A higher ratio of MAs vs.

Table 1 Screening rates by treatment arms in first year

	Average unique visits per month			Average screens per month			Average % screened			p value	Best month N screened			Best month % screened			p value
	PCP	NPP & MA	Control	PCP	NPP & MA	Control	PCP	NPP & MA	Control		PCP	NPP &MA	Control	PCP	NPP & MA	Control	
Medical center																	
1	1464	2797	2928	41	1107	148	2.80	39.56	5.07	a,b,c	161	1505	391	11.47	46.88	13.81	a,b',c
2	1088	1424	1392	51	824	24	4.67	57.84	1.73	a,b,c	102	1039	68	9.31	66.65	5.00	a, b,c
3	925	748	1779	58	197	403	6.28	26.33	22.64	a,b,c	126	467	697	13.15	55.12	35.49	a,b,c
4	4318	4536	1639	552	2952	4	12.77	65.29	0.26	a,b,c	861	3681	23	19.79	71.71	1.18	a,b,c
5	1569	884	1717	509	411	107	32.43	46.51	6.22	a,b,c	635	723	235	37.90	64.21	14.61	a,b,c
6	3124	7668	3372	177	3705	29	5.68	48.32	0.85	a,b,c	332	5644	63	10.15	74.68	2.02	a,b,c
7	3336	2452	1898	339	225	6	10.17	9.16	0.33	a,b,c	980	636	25	26.04	29.42	1.49	a,b,c'
8	3866	4067	5686	565	2778	167	14.62	68.32	2.94	a,b,c	964	3355	350	28.41	75.48	5.81	a,b,c
9	5117	955	2531	405	142	8	7.92	14.86	0.33	a,b,c	608	254	41	12.36	31.59	1.76	a,b,c
10	4297	5034	6031	345	1827	79	8.03	56.17	1.32	a,b,c	637	3938	195	15.07	73.16	3.39	a,b,c
11	6635	3715	3125	239	2223	138	3.60	59.85	4.41	a,b,c	355	2586	443	5.04	70.78	15.08	a,b,c
All	35,519	34,167	31935	3280	17397	1113	9.23	50.92	3.49	a,b,c	3,729	20,445	1918	10.68	60.07	6.04	a,b,c

Differences in screening rates between each of the two intervention arms vs. Control arm as well as between the two intervention arms were examined by hand calculating z statistics for comparisons of two proportions

[a] $p<0.0001$, NPP & MA vs. Control; [b]$p<0.0001$, PCP vs. Control; [b']$p<0.05$, PCP vs. Control; [c]$p<0.0001$, NPP & MA vs. PCP; [c']$p<0.01$, NPP & MA vs. PCP

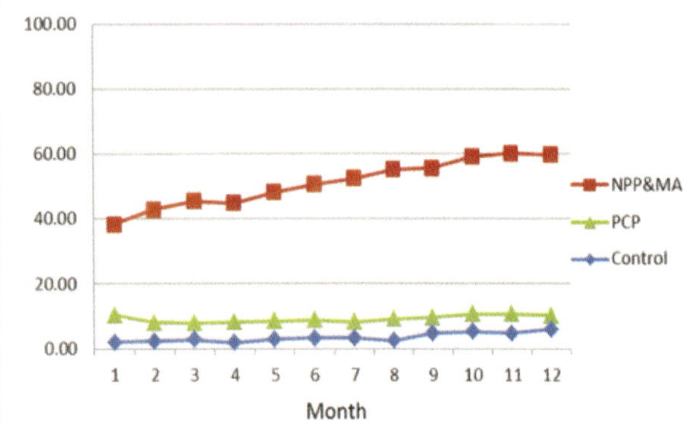

Fig. 2 Average screening rates by month for NPP and MA arm, PCP arm and control arm

physicians was associated with lower odds of screening for the PCP arm, but higher odds for the NPP and MA arm. Longer visit time was related to a higher likelihood of screening in both arms. In the PCP arm, having more physicians trained was related to a lower odds of screening. In the NPP and MA arm, all non-physician providers were trained, so we excluded this variable from the NPP and MA analysis.

Predictors of brief intervention and referral among those screened positive for unhealthy alcohol use

Table 4 presents multilevel models of BI/RT among those screened positive in the intervention arms. Females were less likely to receive BI/RT in both. In the NPP and MA arm, patients with psychiatric or chronic conditions were more likely to receive BI/RT and those aged 45–59 years had higher odds than those aged 60 and older.

Older physicians were less likely, while those who had worked at the organization longer were more likely, to provide BI/RT. On the other hand, Non-White physicians were less likely to provide BI/RT than were White physicians. Gender and specialty did not predict BI/RT delivery.

In the PCP arm, a higher ratio of MAs vs. physicians and having more physicians trained on SBIRT was associated with lower odds of BI/RT. Longer visit time was related to higher BI/RT rates. No significant associations between rates of BI/RT and system-level factors were found in the NPP and MA arm.

Discussion

Pre-implementation SBIRT practices

Consistent with research suggesting a widespread lack of SBIRT implementation [10], systematic alcohol screening was not conducted as part of usual care in this organization prior to the study. For the few physician leaders who reported any policies, the recommended practice was to use questions embedded in the EHR system for which there is no evidence, and which are not included in guidelines [7]. These findings underline the need for formalized SBIRT implementation programs, incorporating the use of evidence-based instruments, to ensure that

Table 2 "Unhealthy drinkers" who received brief interventions or referral to treatment (BI/RT) by treatment arm

	PCP			NPP & MA			Control			p values[2]
	N screened positive	N received BI/RT	%	N screened positive	N received BI/RT	%	N screened positive	N received BI/RT	%	
Medical center										
1	90	51	56.67	1916	47	2.45	185	1	0.54	b, c
2	129	16	12.40	1849	24	1.30	41	1	2.44	b''', c
3	51	8	15.69	123	5	4.07	216	3	1.39	b', c''
4	241	141	58.51	1829	96	5.25	6	0	0.00	b'', c
5	145	17	11.72	229	23	10.04	142	3	2.11	a', b''
6	246	120	48.78	2114	69	3.26	19	1	5.26	b', c
7	394	200	50.76	172	9	5.23	26	0	0.00	b, c
8	503	153	30.42	1776	47	2.65	137	9	6.57	a'', b, c
9	306	15	4.90	54	16	29.63	9	0	0.00	a''', c
10	697	545	78.19	4260	140	3.29	175	7	4.00	b, c
11	306	115	37.58	1259	55	4.37	176	5	2.84	b, c
All	3108	1381	44.43	15581	531	3.41	1132	30	2.65	b, c

[1] Chi-square tests were used to compare the proportions of patients screened between each of the two intervention arms vs. control as well as between the two intervention arms

[2] a: p<0.0001, NPP & MA vs. Control. a' p<0.01, NPP & MA vs. Control. a'': p<0.05, NPP & MA vs. Control. a''': p<0.10, NPP & MA vs. Control. b: p<0.0001, PCP vs. Control. b': p<0.001, PCP vs. Control. b'': p<0.01, PCP vs. Control. b''': p<0.10, PCP vs. Control. c: p<0.0001, NPP & MA vs. PCP. c': p<0.01, NPP & MA vs. PCP. c'': p<0.05, NPP & MA vs. PCP

Table 3 Patient-, physician- and system-level factors associated with delivery of screening by treatment arm

	PCP Arm					NPP & MA Arm				
	Coefficient value	Std. err.	OR	95% CI	p value	Coefficient value	Std. err.	OR	95% CI	p value
Patient level										
Age										
18–24 vs. ≥60	−0.1018	0.0430	*0.90*	*(0.83, 0.98)*	*0.018*	−0.1726	0.0656	*0.84*	*(0.74, 0.96)*	*0.009*
25–44 vs. ≥60	−0.1582	0.0303	*0.85*	*(0.80, 0.91)*	*0.000*	−0.1329	0.0426	*0.88*	*(0.81, 0.95)*	*0.002*
45–59 vs. ≥60	−0.1074	0.0280	*0.90*	*(0.85, 0.95)*	*0.000*	−0.1319	0.0408	*0.88*	*(0.81, 0.95)*	*0.001*
Gender										
Female vs. Male	−0.2447	0.0217	*0.78*	*(0.75, 0.82)*	*0.000*	−0.2008	0.0305	*0.82*	*(0.77, 0.87)*	*0.000*
Comorbid psychiatric conditions										
Yes vs. no	0.1231	0.0269	*1.13*	*(1.07, 1.19)*	*0.000*	0.2436	0.0383	*1.28*	*(1.18, 1.38)*	*0.000*
Chronic diseases										
Yes vs. no	0.1934	0.0243	*1.21*	*(1.16, 1.27)*	*0.000*	0.3407	0.0345	*1.41*	*(1.31, 1.50)*	*0.000*
Physician level										
Age										
(per 1 year increase)	−0.2183	0.0034	*0.80*	*(0.80, 0.81)*	*0.000*					
Gender										
Female vs. male	1.1647	0.0247	*3.21*	*(3.05, 3.36)*	*0.000*					
Race/ethnicity										
Non-white vs. white	1.4355	0.0263	*4.20*	*(3.99, 4.42)*	*0.000*					
Years of services at the health plan										
(per 1 year increase)	0.2587	0.0032	*1.30*	*(1.29, 1.30)*	*0.000*					
Specialty										
Non-internal medicine vs. internal medicine	3.0877	0.0366	*21.93*	*(20.41, 23.56)*	*0.000*					
System level										
Colocation of AOD and primary care departments										
Yes vs. no	−2.3244	0.0689	*0.10*	*(0.09, 0.11)*	*0.000*	−0.4432	0.2274	*0.64*	*(0.41, 1.00)*	*0.051*
MA/PCP ratio at the clinic	−0.4393	0.0493	*0.64*	*(0.59, 0.71)*	*0.000*	3.0850	0.0748	*21.87*	*(18.89, 25.32)*	*0.000*
Ave. visit time	0.3606	0.0097	*1.43*	*(1.41, 1.46)*	*0.000*	0.1379	0.0104	*1.15*	*(1.12, 1.17)*	*0.000*
Number of PCPs trained at the clinic	−0.0387	0.0047	*0.96*	*(0.95, 0.97)*	*0.000*					

A three-level multivariate logistic model adjusting for clustering effects within physician and clinic was run for each of the two intervention arms

PCP primary care physicians, *NPP* non-physician providers, *MA* medical assistants, *AOD* alcohol and other drug

patients obtain optimal primary care treatment, including addressing alcohol as a potential complicating factor in many prevalent health conditions.

Implementation by physicians versus non-physicians

In this cluster randomized controlled trial in adult PC, we compared implementation of alcohol SBIRT in three arms: physician-delivered, non-physician-delivered and Control. Consistent with prior research [22], screening rates were much higher in the NPP and MA arm than PCP arm, and both had higher rates than the Control arm. Generally, this pattern was true across all sites, with some exceptions, particularly one medical center in which MAs (who were trained as part of the NPP and MA arm) "floated" between the NPP and MA and Control arm clinics, resulting in similar screening rates. Two of the medical centers had slightly higher rates in the Control than PCP arm due to some MAs "floating" into the Control arm.

MAs are well-placed to provide alcohol screening and it is consistent with their role to collect and record vital signs in the EHR, including weight, height, blood pressure and (in KPNC) smoking screening and exercise [67]. The NPP and MA arm's steadily improving screening rates from 38 % in month 1 to 60 % in month 12 suggests that barriers to screening that MAs may encounter are temporary and may be addressed through managers' use of ongoing monitoring and performance feedback reports and practice. Improvements may also have been affected by booster sessions and technical assistance visits, which

Table 4 Patient-, physician- and system-level factors associated with delivery of BI/RT by treatment arm

	PCP Arm					NPP & MA Arm				
	Coefficient value	Std. err.	OR	95% CI	p value	Coefficient value	Std. err.	OR	95% CI	p value
Patient level										
Age										
18–24 vs. ≥60	0.2127	0.2119	1.24	(0.82, 1.87)	0.315	0.3589	0.2019	1.43	(0.96, 2.13)	0.075
25–44 vs. ≥60	−0.1290	0.1755	0.88	(0.62, 1.24)	0.462	0.2557	0.1632	1.29	(0.94, 1.78)	0.117
45–59 vs. ≥60	−0.1571	0.1730	0.85	(0.61, 1.20)	0.364	0.5254	0.1615	*1.69*	*(1.23, 2.32)*	*0.001*
Gender										
Female vs. Male	−0.5081	0.1166	*0.60*	*(0.48, 0.76)*	*0.000*	−0.4701	0.1067	*0.62*	*(0.51, 0.77)*	*0.000*
Comorbid psychiatric conditions										
Yes vs. no	0.1489	0.1403	1.16	(0.88, 1.53)	0.289	0.2391	0.1121	*1.27*	*(1.02, 1.58)*	*0.033*
Chronic diseases										
Yes vs. no	−0.0359	0.1165	0.96	(0.77, 1.21)	0.758	0.2444	0.0995	*1.28*	*(1.05, 1.58)*	*0.014*
Physician level										
Age										
(per 1 year increase)	−0.0608	0.0161	*0.94*	*(0.91, 0.97)*	*0.000*					
Gender										
Female vs. male	0.2221	0.1932	1.25	(0.86, 1.82)	0.250					
Race/ethnicity										
Non-white vs. white	−0.5904	0.1599	*0.55*	*(0.41, 0.76)*	*0.000*					
Years of services at the health plan										
(per 1 year increase)	0.0614	0.0152	*1.06*	*(1.03, 1.10)*	*0.000*					
Specialty										
Non-internal medicine vs. internal medicine	−0.2045	0.1932	0.82	(0.56, 1.19)	0.290					
System level										
Colocation of AOD and primary care departments										
Yes vs. no	−0.1525	0.5258	0.86	(0.31, 2.41)	0.772	0.6106	0.4493	1.84	(0.76, 4.44)	0.174
MA/PCP ratio at the clinic	−3.1177	0.3265	*0.04*	*(0.02, 0.08)*	*0.000*	−0.4583	0.3325	0.63	(0.33, 1.21)	0.168
Ave. visit time	0.3111	0.0546	*1.36*	*(1.23, 1.52)*	*0.000*	0.0106	0.0529	1.01	(0.91, 1.12)	0.841
Number of PCPs trained at the clinic	−0.1695	0.0360	*0.84*	*(0.79, 0.91)*	*0.000*					

A three-level multivariate logistic model adjusting for clustering effects within physician and clinic was run for each of the two intervention arms

BI/RT brief intervention or referral to treatment, *PCP* primary care physicians, *NPP* non-physician providers, *MA* medical assistants, *AOD* alcohol and other drug

minimized discomfort with screening through reframing and normalizing it as a routine part of health care. Normalizing was accomplished by acknowledging that drinking is common in our culture and not problematic if within low-risk limits, and by comparing alcohol screening to asking about smoking and exercise—both are routinely addressed in KPNC's primary care clinics.

Different approaches to screening may also be more efficient and increase rates in the NPP and MA delivery model. The two NPP and MA clinics with the highest rates attributed success to the use of paper forms provided to patients by the receptionist and collected by MAs, who simply recorded responses in the EHR screening form; an approach they already used for other screening activities. This "paper and pencil" screening may increase workflow efficiency and increase quality and reliability of screening [68]. It may be that PCPs were less likely to consistently record screening when it was performed because of their many competing priorities, whereas MAs were more likely to record screening in the EHR tool because they were more closely supervised and monitored.

The BI/RT results were counter to prior research which found good implementation rates among non-physicians [22]. The PCP arm rates were 44.4 % versus the NPP and MA arm's 3.4 %. This was the pattern in most medical centers, with one exception where two physicians provided interventions themselves. When examining a population-based intervention rate (i.e., the proportion of all patients seen who received BI/RT), the PCP arm still had an advantage (0.63 versus 0.24 %).

The lower BI/RT rate in the NPP and MA arm was counter to our hypothesis that non-physician providers would have higher BI/RT rates. Several factors may have contributed to low BI/RT rates in the NPP and MA arm. First, because this was a naturalistic implementation study, we trained non-physician providers working in the health system rather than using research or externally or grant-funded clinicians, who may have different characteristics and motivations (because of being paid by a research study and invested in the success of the intervention) rather than having an existing operational role with competing duties. Non-physician providers were not always available immediately and thus the workflow often required an additional appointment either by phone or in person, or required phoning the provider when possible via a "consult phone", which meant a delay. Second, exam room availability was often an issue, which translated into concerns about backlogs if interventions were provided there. Third, providers reported that patients were resistant to seeing the non-physician providers, regardless of whether they were told that the discussion would be about their alcohol screening results or whether a more vague script about "healthy lifestyle" was used.

Overall, the findings from the current study suggest an efficient, but less complex workflow of MA screening followed by BI/RT by physicians, consistent with how other preventive services are delivered in this health system [69]. It also parallels recent findings that alcohol screening by staff and follow-up by clinicians is associated with more frequent use of screening and intervention [70]. These findings are also consistent with aspects of the Consolidated Framework on Implementation Research (CFIR) model [45]. The CFIR suggests that evidence-based interventions with greater complexity (such as the NPP and MA delivery model examined here) are less likely to be implemented. Also consistent with the CFIR framework, the lack of resources in the form of sufficient available time of non-physician providers and exam rooms were barriers to implementation of interventions and referrals in the NPP and MA arm. Further, the CFIR suggests that high compatibility of new evidence-based interventions with existing roles and duties can increase implementation as is the case for adding alcohol screening for MAs who already ask about other health behaviors (smoking and exercise).

One potential disadvantage with the physician-delivered intervention is that physicians reported shorter interventions (5 min average) versus non-physicians (23 min average). Yet longer interventions may not significantly increase effectiveness [71]. Physicians reported that the single item screening question required less than 1 min. We did not gather more specific information on how long providers spent on brief interventions versus referrals to specialty treatment.

These results may raise questions about the ability of currently predominant primary care models to use non-physician clinical team members to perform SBIRT and other new evidence-based practices. Team-based care has potential for addressing behavioral health problems including unhealthy alcohol and tobacco use and depression and for improving health conditions affected by these problems such as hypertension and obesity [72, 73]. Yet, a recent study documented staffing models in primary care practices which participated in a nationwide US team-based care initiative and found that even among those designated as patient-centered medical homes, fewer than 23 % employed health educators, pharmacists, social workers, nutritionists or community service coordinators and fewer than half employed care coordinators [74]. Ideally, medical home models and integrated care systems would include adequate levels of behavioral health care staff, on-call and readily available to deliver behavioral health interventions such as multiple-session brief interventions for unhealthy alcohol use [75]. Further, sufficient exam room space is needed to prevent backlogs, and the purpose of exam rooms may need to be expanded so that care coordination and behavioral services can be provided. Alternatively, primary care office design may need to be reconsidered so that sufficient non-physician provider consult room spaces are interspersed next to exam rooms.

In addition to increased team staffing, performance measures linked to incentives could aid implementation. The CFIR model and the experience at the US VA Health System, where alcohol SBIRT is mandated by an internal performance measure [41, 76], suggest that policies such as performance measures may increase implementation. Yet to date there are no external performance measures applicable to private, capitated systems or to US Federally Qualified Health Centers. Recently released findings that fewer than one in six Americans reported being asked about or discussing their alcohol consumption with a health professional are striking, given that the USPSTF has recommended it in general medical settings since 2004 [7]. In the system studied here, MA screening and physician intervention were found to be a feasible solution for implementation of SBIRT. Without structural changes in primary care practices that would improve their ability to provide consistent team-based care, MA to physician workflow may be one viable approach, and may also be considered for other underutilized USPSTF recommended services [46] such as depression screening. Full implementation of SBIRT likely also requires a time frame of more than 1 year for both individual providers and organizations to progress through stages of readiness for change in order to achieve optimal results.

Predictors of implementation within each model

In both PCP and NPP and MA arms, younger patients were less likely to be screened; this was counter-intuitive given their higher prevalence of unhealthy drinking [77, 78] and also counter to prior research [79]. Similarly, in general, younger patients were not more likely to receive BI/RT, though in the NPP & MA arm, patients aged 45–59 who screened positive were more likely to receive BI/RT than those aged 60 or older. Physicians may assume that unhealthy drinking is "to be expected" in younger patients, and thus not be as concerned about identifying it. Also, the training emphasized the link between alcohol and chronic conditions, which may have made it easier for physicians to screen and discuss drinking among older patients at risk for such conditions.

Consistent with results suggesting that men are more likely to binge drink, male patients were more likely to be screened and receive BI/RT in both arms. This is consistent with prior research indicating that men are more likely to be screened [79–81] and raises concerns given that women are less likely to seek alcohol intervention and treatment and may be more vulnerable to adverse health effects of unhealthy use [82]. That more individuals with psychiatric and chronic disease diagnoses were screened than those without (in both arms) is also consistent with prior research [79] and with the emphasis in the provider training on the relationship of unhealthy alcohol use to adverse health effects and reduced medication adherence [83]. However, psychiatric and chronic conditions only predicted receiving BI/RT in the NPP and MA arm. Such patients are generally more likely to see non-physician providers for chronic conditions, e.g., for behavioral interventions related to diabetes, so the intervention may have been paired with conversations about their chronic condition.

As found in prior research, female physicians were more likely than male to screen [44, 84], though there was no difference by physician gender in providing BI/RT. Physicians from non-White and Latino ethnic/racial groups were more likely to screen, although White physicians were more likely to record providing BI/RT. Few studies have examined these characteristics as predictors of SBIRT; the large sample size and racial/ethnic diversity of the provider sample allowed us to examine this. More research is needed to understand these differences in screening and BI/RT rates between gender and racial/ethnic groups. For example, some national studies have found higher rates of alcohol abuse in whites than some other ethnic groups and in men than women [85, 86]. Perhaps these differences in screening may reflect that physicians with healthier habits themselves (which was unmeasured in this study) are more likely to provide counseling [87]. Alternatively, the findings may reflect gender and ethnic differences in communication styles in which case additional or different approaches to training may particularly be needed for these subgroups.

Consistent with a greater focus on preventive care, a specialty of Family Medicine or training other than Internal Medicine was related to screening, but this characteristic did not affect BI/RT rates. Physicians newer to the system were less likely to both screen and intervene. Perhaps longer experience in the system may help physicians to practice more efficiently, leaving time for preventive screening and intervention.

Consistent with studies suggesting lack of screening is due to time constraints [28, 88], longer visits were related to higher odds of screening in both arms and intervention in the PCP arm. Provision of BI/RT was not related to appointment time in the NPP and MA arm likely because the intervention usually required a separate visit. However, having a higher ratio of MAs per physician increased the likelihood of screening in the NPP and MA arm. Having more MAs did not seem to off-load the work of physicians enough in the PCP arm to result in higher rates of screening or intervention as we had expected, and in fact was related to a lower odds of screening and BI/RT. This may be because a higher MA ratio is a reflection of a busier clinic.

Some findings on system-level predictors were counter-intuitive. Having more physicians trained in SBIRT in a medical center was related to lower odds of screening. The findings that co-location between primary care and specialty AOD treatment clinics was associated with a lower likelihood of receiving screening or intervention are also counter to the ideas that proximity of specialty treatment would increase awareness and that easier patient access to specialty treatment would increase physician confidence in discussing alcohol with patients. More research is needed to understand how co-location affects primary care clinician behavior, and whether there is a confounding factor related to both variables.

Study strengths and limitations

Conducting this study in real-world busy clinics, and using existing staff are important characteristics of an implementation study, and at the same time enhance both limitations and strengths. We could not control the schedules or priorities of clinic managers or providers or the movement of staff across clinics. However, using existing staff is important for understanding whether a model is feasible and sustainable regardless of externally funded interventionists.

Provider factors not examined include outcome expectancies, concerns about intrusiveness, beliefs that SBIRT is ineffective, negative attitudes about patients with alcohol problems, and self-efficacy; these have been previously well-documented [65, 79, 89–97].

Similar to studies for other health conditions, use of EHR data means that our data on screening and BI/RT are limited to that documented in the EHR. Yet this approach allowed for studying the natural process of care, studying a large number of patients, and having a population-based sample of patients and providers, rather than limiting our sample to those willing to be recruited into a study.

This study is the first to examine implementation of the NIAAA Guide for SBIRT [8] in adult primary care in a private, non-profit US health care system. It also uses an established EHR, a mechanism recommended by the field [15, 46], and known to be salient in predicting better implementation of primary care practices [98–101]. EHR use is also more generalizable to the future of private US health care settings because of Phase III Meaningful Use requirements [102].

Because of the large sample size, some statistically significant differences may not be clinically meaningful. Variations in the pattern of results across medical centers highlight the importance of including multiple medical centers or clinics when studying factors that influence implementation.

A further limitation is that data on alcohol use disorder screening were not recorded for a considerable proportion of those who screened positive for unhealthy alcohol use. We thus were unable to examine the proportion of those screening positive on the alcohol use disorders screen who received RT.

Finally, it is not known how the study's findings would generalize to systems with fewer exam room constraints or systems in which clinical health educators are dedicated to SBIRT (which would allow for same-time, warm hand-offs to exam room consultations). Moreover, currently predominant primary care models do not include health educators or behavioral specialists [74].

Conclusions

Our findings from this randomized trial of physician versus non-physician alcohol SBIRT implementation suggest that a model of MA screening and physician intervention may have the highest odds of implementation in currently predominant primary care models. Further, in large organizations such as this one, where policies and practices for systematic screening were not in place prior to training, implementation may take a longer time period than 1 year after an initial training and a higher "dosage" of quality improvement and feedback; longer time frames may be required for provider change [17] and full implementation, as has been found in the VA [68]. Many facilitators of implementation, such as organizational and provider stages of readiness for change [45] may increase over time after a new initiative begins. Informed by this study, a model using MA screening and physician intervention was adopted by Kaiser Permanente Northern California across all adult primary care clinics in June of 2013 for annual, evidence-based alcohol screening and intervention or referral to specialty treatment [103]. Future research is needed across systems that have implemented SBIRT to examine duration of time since initial implementation and duration and amount of related quality improvement activities as factors predicting SBIRT implementation outcomes. Research is also needed on whether implementation of BI and RT by non-physicians is more effectively implemented within fully realized and staffed medical home models.

Abbreviations

AOD: alcohol and other drug; BI: brief intervention; EHR: electronic health record; MA: medical assistant; NIAAA: US National Institute on Alcohol Abuse and Alcoholism; NPP: non-physician provider; PCP: primary care physician; RT: referral to treatment; SBIRT: screening, brief intervention and referral to treatment; USPSTF: United States Preventive Services Task Force.

Authors' contributions

JM, FC, CW and SS obtained funding and devised the concept for the clinical trial design, and analysis. JM, CW, DP, TR, SA, DS and SS developed the training curriculum. FC and WL conducted data acquisition and performed the statistical analyses. JM, FC, CW, DS, SA, TB, DD, CC and SS designed the concept for the paper, interpreted the results and drafted the manuscript. All authors read and approved the final manuscript.

Author details

[1] Kaiser Permanente Northern California, 1800 Harrison, Oakland, CA 94612, USA. [2] Division of Research, Kaiser Permanente Northern California, 2000 Broadway, Oakland, CA 94612, USA. [3] Department of Psychiatry, University of California, San Francisco, 401 Parnassus Ave, San Francisco, CA 94143, USA. [4] The Permanente Medical Group, Kaiser Northern California, 1201 Fillmore Street, San Francisco, CA 94115, USA.

Acknowledgements

We thank Agatha Hinman and Sabrina Wood for editorial assistance with the manuscript. We thank the KPNC Chemical Dependency Quality Improvement Committee and KPNC Chemical Dependency Program Directors and Addiction Medicine Physicians for their partnership, particularly Carol Havens, MD, Barrett Levine, MD, Michael Rubino, MD, Karen Spedowfski, PhD, and Matthew Tarran, PhD. We also thank the physicians, medical assistants, clinical health educators, behavioral medicine specialists, nurses, and managers of KPNC's adult and family medicine departments for their participation in the quality improvement activities related to this study. We especially thank Don Mordecai, M.D. and Sheryl Sun, M.D, for their strong leadership support of this project and of implementation of alcohol screening, brief intervention and referral to treatment within KPNC adult primary care. Thanks are also due to Richard Saitz, MD who led a "Train the Trainers" workshop for this project.

Funding/Support and role of the sponsor

This study was funded by the National Institute on Alcohol Abuse and Alcoholism (R01 AA018660). The sponsors had no role in the design and conduct of the study; collection, management, analysis, and interpretation of the data; preparation, review, and approval of the manuscript; and decision to submit the manuscript for publication.

Competing interests

The authors all declare that they have no conflicting interests.

References

1. US Department of Health and Human Services, National Institute on Alcohol Abuse and Alcoholism. 10th special report to the US Congress on alcohol and health : highlights from current research from the Secretary of Health and Human Services. Rockville, MD: US Department of Health and Human Services. June 2000. http://pubs.niaaa.nih.gov/publications/10Report/10thSpecialReport.pdf. Accessed 8 Oct 2015.
2. Rehm J, Room R, Monteiro M, Gmel G, Graham K, Rehn N, et al. Alcohol as a risk factor for global burden of disease. Eur Addict Res. 2003;9(4):157–64.
3. Stahre M, Roeber J, Kanny D, Brewer RD, Zhang X. Contribution of excessive alcohol consumption to deaths and years of potential life lost in the United States. Prev Chronic Dis. 2014;11:E109.
4. Kaner E, Bland M, Cassidy P, Coulton S, Deluca P, Drummond C, et al. Screening and brief interventions for hazardous and harmful alcohol use in primary care: a cluster randomised controlled trial protocol. BMC Public Health. 2009;9:287.
5. Bertholet N, Daeppen JB, Wietlisbach V, Fleming M, Burnand B. Reduction of alcohol consumption by brief alcohol intervention in primary care: systematic review and meta-analysis. Arch Intern Med. 2005;165(9):986–95.
6. O'Donnell A, Anderson P, Newbury-Birch D, Schulte B, Schmidt C, Reimer J, et al. The impact of brief alcohol interventions in primary healthcare: a systematic review of reviews. Alcohol Alcohol. 2014;49(1):66–78.
7. Moyer VA, Preventive Services Task Force. Screening and behavioral counseling interventions in primary care to reduce alcohol misuse: US preventive services task force recommendation statement. Ann Intern Med. 2013;159(3):210–8.
8. National Institute on Alcohol Abuse and Alcoholism. Helping patients who drink too much: a clinician's guide, updated 2005 edition. US Department of Health and Human Services [NIH Publication No. 07–3769], Rockville, MD. 2005. http://pubs.niaaa.nih.gov/publications/Practitioner/CliniciansGuide2005/clinicians_guide.htm. Accessed 8 Oct 2015.
9. Canadian Centre on Substance Abuse (CCSA) and College of Family Physicians of Canada (CFPC). Alcohol screening, brief intervention and referral: a clinical guide. In: Alcohol screening, brief intervention & referral helping patients reduce alcohol-related risks. College of Family Physicians of Canada and Canadian Centre on Substance Abuse. 2012. http://www.sbir-diba.ca/. Accessed 6 Jan 2015.
10. McKnight-Eily LR, Liu Y, Brewer RD, Kanny D, Lu H, Denny CH, et al. Vital signs: communication between health professionals and their patients about alcohol use–44 states and the District of Columbia, 2011. MMWR Morb Mortal Wkly Rep. 2014;63(1):16–22.
11. Garnick DW, Horgan CM, Merrick EL, Hoyt A. Identification and treatment of mental and substance use conditions: health plans strategies. Med Care. 2007;45(11):1060–7.
12. Bradley KA, Williams EC, Achtmeyer CE, Volpp B, Collins BJ, Kivlahan DR. Implementation of evidence-based alcohol screening in the Veterans Health Administration. Am J Manag Care. 2006;12(10):597–606.
13. Saitz R. Unhealthy alcohol use. N Engl J Med. 2005;352(6):596–607.
14. Kuehn BM. Despite benefit, physicians slow to offer brief advice on harmful alcohol use. JAMA. 2008;299(7):751–3.
15. Saitz R, Svikis D, D'Onofrio G, Kraemer KL, Perl H. Challenges applying alcohol brief intervention in diverse practice settings: Populations, outcomes, and costs. Alcohol Clin Exp Res. 2006;30(2):332–8.
16. Stewart SH, Miller PM. Alcohol screening and intervention in medical and surgical settings. In: Miller PM, Kavanagh DJ, editors. Translation of addictions science into practice. New York: Elsevier Science; 2007. p. 379–98.
17. Nilsen P. Brief alcohol intervention–where to from here? Challenges remain for research and practice. Addiction. 2010;105(6):954–9.
18. Centers for Medicaid and Medicare Services. Screening, Brief Intervention, and Referral to Treatment (SBIRT) services. Medicare Learning Services. 2014, June. http://www.cms.gov/Outreach-and-Education/Medicare-Learning-Network-MLN/MLNProducts/downloads/SBIRT_Factsheet_ICN904084.pdf. Accessed 7 July 2015.
19. Kaner E, Bland M, Cassidy P, Coulton S, Dale V, Deluca P, et al. Effectiveness of screening and brief alcohol intervention in primary care (SIPS trial): pragmatic cluster randomised controlled trial. BMJ. 2013;346:e8501.
20. van Beurden I, Anderson P, Akkermans RP, Grol RP, Wensing M, Laurant MG. Involvement of general practitioners in managing alcohol problems: a randomized controlled trial of a tailored improvement programme. Addiction. 2012;107(9):1601–11.
21. Williams EC, Johnson ML, Lapham GT, Caldeiro RM, Chew L, Fletcher GS, et al. Strategies to implement alcohol screening and brief intervention in primary care settings: a structured literature review. Psychol Addict Behav. 2011;25(2):206–14.
22. Babor TE, Higgins-Biddle J, Dauser D, Higgins P, Burleson JA. Alcohol screening and brief intervention in primary care settings: implementation models and predictors. J Stud Alcohol. 2005;66(3):361–8.
23. Babor TF, Higgins-Biddle JC, Dauser D, Burleson JA, Zarkin GA, Bray J. Brief interventions for at-risk drinking: patient outcomes and cost-effectiveness in managed care organizations. Alcohol Alcohol. 2006;41(6):624–31.
24. Cutrona SL, Choudhry NK, Stedman M, Servi A, Liberman JN, Brennan T, et al. Physician effectiveness in interventions to improve cardiovascular medication adherence: a systematic review. J Gen Intern Med. 2010;25(10):1090–6.
25. Georgeu D, Colvin CJ, Lewin S, Fairall L, Bachmann MO, Uebel K, et al. Implementing nurse-initiated and managed antiretroviral treatment (NIMART) in South Africa: a qualitative process evaluation of the STRETCH trial. Implement Sci. 2012;7:66.
26. Denberg TD, Ross SE, Steiner JF. Patient acceptance of a novel preventive care delivery system. Prev Med. 2007;44(6):543–6.
27. Tsai AG, Wadden TA. Treatment of obesity in primary care practice in the United States: a systematic review. J Gen Intern Med. 2009;24(9):1073–9.
28. Rahm AK, Boggs JM, Martin C, Price DW, Beck A, Backer TE, et al. Facilitators and barriers to implementing Screening, Brief Intervention, and Referral to Treatment (SBIRT) in primary care in integrated health care settings. Subst Abus. 2015;36(3):281–8.
29. Substance Abuse and Mental Health Services Administration. Systems-level Implementation of Screening, Brief Intervention, and Referral to Treatment. Rockville, MD: Substance Abuse and Mental Health Services Administration. 2013. Report No.: Technical Assistance Publication (TAP) Series 33. HHS Publication No. (SMA) 13-4741. http://store.samhsa.gov/shin/content//SMA13-4741/TAP33.pdf. Accessed 31 Aug 2015.
30. Hudson SV, Ohman-Strickland P, Cunningham R, Ferrante JM, Hahn K, Crabtree BF. The effects of teamwork and system support on colorectal cancer screening in primary care practices. Cancer Detect Prev. 2007;31(5):417–23.
31. Selby JV, Schmittdiel JA, Lee J, Fung V, Thomas S, Smider N, et al. Meaningful variation in performance: what does variation in quality tell us about improving quality? Med Care. 2010;48(2):133–9.
32. Aira M, Kauhanen J, Larivaara P, Rautio P. Factors influencing inquiry about patients' alcohol consumption by primary health care physicians: qualitative semi-structured interview study. Fam Pract. 2003;20(3):270–5.
33. Keurhorst MN, Anderson P, Spak F, Bendtsen P, Segura L, Colom J, et al. Implementing training and support, financial reimbursement, and referral to an internet-based brief advice program to improve the early identification of hazardous and harmful alcohol consumption in primary care (ODHIN): study protocol for a cluster randomized factorial trial. Implement Sci. 2013;8:11.
34. Miller NS, Sheppard LM, Colenda CC, Magen J. Why physicians are unprepared to treat patients who have alcohol- and drug-related disorders. Acad Med. 2001;76(5):410–8.
35. Yarnall KS, Pollak KI, Ostbye T, Krause KM, Michener JL. Primary care: is there enough time for prevention? Am J Public Health. 2003;93(4):635–41.
36. Johnson M, Jackson R, Guillaume L, Meier P, Goyder E. Barriers and facilitators to implementing screening and brief intervention for alcohol misuse: a systematic review of qualitative evidence. J Public Health (Oxf). 2011;33(3):412–21.

37. Thomas CP, McCarty D. Appendix D: adoption of drug abuse treatment technology in specialty and primary care settings. In: Harwood HJ, Myers TG, editors. New treatments for addiction: behavioral, ethical, legal, and social questions. Washington, DC: National Academies Press; 2004. p. 140–72.
38. Spandorfer JM, Israel Y, Turner BJ. Primary care physicians' views on screening and management of alcohol abuse: inconsistencies with national guidelines. J Fam Pract. 1999;48(11):899–902.
39. Miller PM, Stockdell R, Nemeth L, Feifer C, Jenkins RG, Nietert PJ, et al. Initial steps taken by nine primary care practices to implement alcohol screening guidelines with hypertensive patients: the AA-TRIP project. Subst Abus. 2006;27(1–2):61–70.
40. Rose HL, Miller PM, Nemeth LS, Jenkins RG, Nietert PJ, Wessell AM, et al. Alcohol screening and brief counseling in a primary care hypertensive population: a quality improvement intervention. Addiction. 2008;103(8):1271–80.
41. Lapham GT, Achtmeyer CE, Williams EC, Hawkins EJ, Kivlahan DR, Bradley KA. Increased documented brief alcohol interventions with a performance measure and electronic decision support. Med Care. 2012;50(2):179–87.
42. Satre DD, Leibowitz A, Mertens JR, Weisner C. Advising depression patients to reduce alcohol and drug use: factors associated with provider intervention in outpatient psychiatry. Am J Addict. 2014;23(6):570–5.
43. Ewing GB, Selassie AW, Lopez CH, McCutcheon EP. Self-report of delivery of clinical preventive services by US physicians. Comparing specialty, gender, age, setting of practice, and area of practice. Am J Prev Med. 1999;17(1):62–72.
44. Friedmann PD, McCullough D, Saitz R. Screening and intervention for illicit drug abuse: a national survey of primary care physicians and psychiatrists. Arch Intern Med. 2001;161(2):248–51.
45. Damschroder LJ, Aron DC, Keith RE, Kirsh SR, Alexander JA, Lowery JC. Fostering implementation of health services research findings into practice: a consolidated framework for advancing implementation science. Implement Sci. 2009;4:50.
46. Institute of Medicine. Improving the quality of health care for mental and substance-use conditions. Quality Chasm Series. Washington, DC: National Academies Press; 2006.
47. Anderson P, Wojnar M, Jakubczyk A, Gual A, Segura L, Sovinova H, et al. Managing alcohol problems in general practice in Europe: results from the European ODHIN Survey of General Practitioners. Alcohol Alcohol. 2014;49(5):531–9.
48. Bendtsen P, Anderson P, Wojnar M, Newbury-Birch D, Mussener U, Colom J, et al. Professional's attitudes do not influence screening and brief interventions rates for hazardous and harmful drinkers: results from ODHIN study. Alcohol Alcohol. 2015;50(4):430–7.
49. Garg AX, Adhikari NK, McDonald H, Rosas-Arellano MP, Devereaux PJ, Beyene J, et al. Effects of computerized clinical decision support systems on practitioner performance and patient outcomes: a systematic review. JAMA. 2005;293(10):1223–38.
50. Ryan J, Doty MM, Abrams MK, Riley P. The adoption and use of health information technology by community health centers, 2009–2013. New York: The Commonwealth Fund. May 2014. http://www.commonwealthfund.org/publications/issue-briefs/2014/may/adoption-and-use-of-hit-by-chcs. Accessed 8 Oct 2015.
51. Abrams MK, Doty MM, Ryan J, Hall D, Riley P. Ready or not? How community health centers view their preparedness to care for newly insured patients. The Commonwealth Fund. May 2014. http://www.commonwealthfund.org/publications/issue-briefs/2014/may/ready-or-not-how-chcs-view-their-preparedness. Accessed 6 Oct 2015.
52. Schoen C, Osborn R, Squires DD, Doty MM, Rasmussen P, Pierson R, et al. A survey of primary care doctors in ten countries shows progress in use of health information technology, less in other areas. Health Aff (Millwood). 2012;31(2):2805–16.
53. Hall SD. AHRQ: Open source EHR improves care in developing nations. *Fierce EMR*. March 19, 2013. http://www.fierceemr.com/story/ahrq-open-source-ehr-improves-care-developing-nations/2013-03-19. Accessed 8 Oct 2015.
54. World Health Organization, World Intellectual Property Organization, World Trade Organization. Promoting Access to Medical Technologies and Innovation: Intersections Between Public Health, Intellectual Property and Trade. Geneva, Switzerland: World Health Organization; 2013.
55. Kaiser Permanente. Fast facts about Kaiser Permanente. Kaiser Permanente Share. 2011. http://xnet.kp.org/newscenter/aboutkp/fastfacts.html. Accessed 8 Oct 2015.
56. Terhune C. Report: Kaiser tops state health insurance market with 40 % share. Los Angeles Times. 2013. http://articles.latimes.com/2013/jan/29/business/la-fi-mo-health-insure-market-20130129. Accessed 8 Oct 2015.
57. Ray GT, Collin F, Lieu T, Fireman B, Colby CJ, Quesenberry CP, Van den Eeden SK, Selby JV. The cost of health conditions in a health maintenance organization. Med Care Res Rev. 2000;57(1):92–109.
58. Gordon NP. Similarity of the adult Kaiser Permanente membership in Northern California to the insured and general population in Northern California: statistics from the 2009 California Health Interview Survey. Kaiser Permanente Northern California Division of Research. 2012. http://www.dor.kaiser.org/external/chis_non_kp_2009/. Accessed 2015 Jul 29.
59. Harris AH, Bowe T, Finney JW, Humphreys K. HEDIS initiation and engagement quality measures of substance use disorder care: impact of setting and health care specialty. Popul Health Manag. 2009;12(4):191–6.
60. Selby JV, Schmittdiel JA, Fireman B, Jaffe M, Ransom LJ, Dyer W, et al. Improving treatment intensification to reduce cardiovascular disease risk: a cluster randomized trial. BMC Health Serv Res. 2012;12:183.
61. Smith PC, Schmidt SM, Allensworth-Davies D, Saitz R. Primary care validation of a single-question alcohol screening test. J Gen Intern Med. 2009;24(7):783–8.
62. Vinson DC, Kruse RL, Seale JP. Simplifying alcohol assessment: two questions to identify alcohol use disorders. Alcohol Clin Exp Res. 2007;31(8):1392–8.
63. National Institute on Alcohol Abuse and Alcoholism. Tips for cutting down on drinking. 2008. http://pubs.niaaa.nih.gov/publications/Tips/tips.pdf. Accessed 15 Oct 2014.
64. Boston University School of Medicine/Boston Medical Center. Alcohol screening and brief intervention curriculum. http://www.bu.edu/act/mdalcoholtraining/index.html. Accessed 7 July 2015.
65. Bradley KA, Chavez LJ, Lapham GT, Williams EC, Achtmeyer CE, Rubinsky AD, Hawkins EJ, Saitz R, Kivlahan DR. When quality indicators undermine quality: bias in a quality indicator of follow-up for alcohol misuse. Psychiatr Serv. 2013;64(10):1018–25.
66. Rothman KJ. No adjustments are needed for multiple comparisons. Epidemiology. 1990;1(1):43–6.
67. Coleman KJ, Ngor E, Reynolds K, Quinn VP, Koebnick C, Young DR, et al. Initial validation of an exercise "vital sign" in electronic medical records. Med Sci Sports Exerc. 2012;44(11):2071–6.
68. Williams EC, Achtmeyer CE, Thomas RM, Grossbard JR, Lapham GT, Chavez LJ, et al. Factors underlying quality problems with alcohol screening prompted by a clinical reminder in primary care: a multi-site qualitative study. J Gen Intern Med. 2015;30(8):1125–32.
69. Grant RW, Schmittdiel JA, Neugebauer RS, Uratsu CS, Sternfeld B. Exercise as a vital sign: a quasi-experimental analysis of a health system intervention to collect patient-reported exercise levels. J Gen Intern Med. 2014;29(2):341–8.
70. Nemeth LS, Miller PM, Nietert PJ, Ornstein SM, Wessell AM, Jenkins RG. Organizational attributes and screening and brief intervention in primary care. Addict Behav. 2013;38(11):2639–42.
71. Kaner EFS, Brown N, Jackson K. A systematic review of the impact of brief interventions on substance use and co-morbid physical and mental health conditions. Ment Health Subst Use. 2011;4(1):38–61.
72. Klatsky AL. Alcohol-associated hypertension: when one drinks makes a difference. Hypertension. 2004;44(6):805–6.
73. Luppino FS, de Wit LM, Bouvy PF, Stijnen T, Cuijpers P, Penninx BW, et al. Overweight, obesity, and depression: a systematic review and meta-analysis of longitudinal studies. Arch Gen Psychiatry. 2010;67(3):220–9.
74. Peikes DN, Reid RJ, Day TJ, Cornwell DD, Dale SB, Baron RJ, et al. Staffing patterns of primary care practices in the comprehensive primary care initiative. Ann Fam Med. 2014;12(2):142–9.
75. Fleming MF, Barry KL, Manwell LB, Johnson K, London R. Brief physician advice for problem alcohol drinkers: a randomized controlled trial in community-based primary care practices. JAMA. 1997;277(13):1030–45.

76. Williams EC, Rubinsky AD, Chavez LJ, Lapham GT, Rittmueller SE, Achtmeyer CE, et al. An early evaluation of implementation of brief intervention for unhealthy alcohol use in the US Veterans Health Administration. Addiction. 2014;109(9):1472–81.
77. Dawson DA, Grant BF, Chou SP, Pickering RP. Subgroup variation in US drinking patterns: results of the 1992 national longitudinal alcohol epidemiologic study. J Subst Abuse. 1995;7(3):331–44.
78. Mertens JR, Weisner C, Ray GT, Fireman B, Walsh K. Hazardous drinkers and drug users in HMO primary care: prevalence, medical conditions, and costs. Alcohol Clin Exp Res. 2005;29(6):989–98.
79. D'Amico EJ, Paddock SM, Burnam A, Kung FY. Identification of and guidance for problem drinking by general medical providers: results from a national survey. Med Care. 2005;43(3):229–36.
80. Weisner C, Matzger H. Missed opportunities in screening for alcohol problems in medical and mental health services. Alcohol Clin Exp Res. 2003;27(7):1132–41.
81. Volk RJ, Steinbauer JR, Cantor SB. Patient factors influencing variation in the use of preventive interventions for alcohol abuse by primary care physicians. J Stud Alcohol. 1996;57(2):203–9.
82. Greenfield SF, Back SE, Lawson K, Brady KT. Substance abuse in women. Psychiatr Clin North Am. 2010;33(2):339–55.
83. Bryson CL, Au DH, Sun H, Williams EC, Kivlahan DR, Bradley KA. Alcohol screening scores and medication nonadherence. Ann Intern Med. 2008;149(11):795–804.
84. National Center on Addiction and Substance Abuse at Columbia University. Missed opportunity: National Survey of Primary Care Physicians and Patients on Substance Abuse. Survey Research Laboratory, University of Illinois at Chicago, Chicago. 2000. http://www.casacolumbia.org/articlefiles/380-Missed%20Opportunity%20Physicians%20and%20Patients.pdf. Accessed 8 Oct 2015.
85. Caetano R, Baruah J, Chartier KG. Ten-year trends (1992 to 2002) in sociodemographic predictors and indicators of alcohol abuse and dependence among whites, blacks, and Hispanics in the United States. Alcohol Clin Exp Res. 2011;35(8):1458–66.
86. Grant BF, Dawson DA, Stinson FS, Chou SP, Dufour MC, Pickering RP. The 12-month prevalence and trends in DSM-IV alcohol abuse and dependence: United States, 1991–1992 and 2001–2002. Drug Alcohol Depend. 2004;74(3):223–34.
87. Frank E, Carrera JS, Elon L, Hertzberg VS. Predictors of US medical students' prevention counseling practices. Prev Med. 2007;44(1):76–81.
88. Satre DD, McCance-Katz EF, Moreno-John G, Julian KA, O'Sullivan PS, Satterfield JM. Using needs assessment to develop curricula for Screening, Brief Intervention and Referral to Treatment (SBIRT) in academic and community health settings. Subst Abus. 2012;33(3):298–302.
89. Anderson P, Laurant M, Kaner E, Wensing M, Grol R. Engaging general practitioners in the management of hazardous and harmful alcohol consumption: results of a meta-analysis. J Stud Alcohol. 2004;65(2):191–9.
90. Barnett NP, Monti PM, Cherpitel C, Bendtsen P, Borges G, Colby SM, et al. Identification and brief treatment of alcohol problems with medical patients: an international perspective. Alcohol Clin Exp Res. 2003;27(2):262–70.
91. Funk M, Wutzke S, Kaner E, Anderson P, Pas L, McCormick R, et al. A multicountry controlled trial of strategies to promote dissemination and implementation of brief alcohol intervention in primary health care: findings of a World Health Organization collaborative study. J Stud Alcohol. 2005;66(3):379–88.
92. Institute of Medicine. Crossing the quality chasm: a new health system for the 21st Century. Quality Chasm Series. Washington, DC: National Academy Press; 2001.
93. Kaner EF, Heather N, Brodie J, Lock CA, McAvoy BR. Patient and practitioner characteristics predict brief alcohol intervention in primary care. Br J Gen Pract. 2001;51(471):822–7.
94. Lock CA, Kaner EF. Implementation of brief alcohol interventions by nurses in primary care: do non-clinical factors influence practice? Fam Pract. 2004;21(3):270–5.
95. Nilsen P, Aalto M, Bendtsen P, Seppa K. Effectiveness of strategies to implement brief alcohol intervention in primary healthcare. A systematic review. Scand J Prim Health Care. 2006;24(1):5–15.
96. Ockene JK, Adams A, Hurley TG, Wheeler EV, Hebert JR. Brief physician- and nurse practitioner-delivered counseling for high-risk drinkers: does it work? Arch Intern Med. 1999;159(18):2198–205.
97. Ohman-Strickland PA, John Orzano A, Nutting PA, Perry Dickinson W, Scott-Cawiezell J, Hahn K, et al. Measuring organizational attributes of primary care practices: development of a new instrument. Health Serv Res. 2007;42(3 Pt 1):1257–73.
98. Chaudhry B, Wang J, Wu S, Maglione M, Mojica W, Roth E, et al. Systematic review: impact of health information technology on quality, efficiency, and costs of medical care. Ann Intern Med. 2006;144(10):742–52.
99. Zhou YY, Kanter MH, Wang JJ, Garrido T. Improved quality at Kaiser Permanente through e-mail between physicians and patients. Health Aff (Millwood). 2010;29(7):1370–5.
100. Hillestad R, Bigelow J, Bower A, Girosi F, Meili R, Scoville R, et al. Can electronic medical record systems transform health care? Potential health benefits, savings, and costs. Health Aff (Millwood). 2005;24(5):1103–17.
101. Holroyd-Leduc JM, Lorenzetti D, Straus SE, Sykes L, Quan H. The impact of the electronic medical record on structure, process, and outcomes within primary care: a systematic review of the evidence. J Am Med Inform Assoc. 2011;18(6):732–7.
102. HealthIT.gov. How to attain meaningful use. EHR Incentives and Certification. http://www.healthit.gov/providers-professionals/how-attain-meaningful-use. Accessed 8 Oct 2015.
103. McKnight-Eily L. Communication between health professionals and their patients about alcohol use. Vital Signs Town Hall Teleconference sponsored by Centers for Disease Control and Prevention Office for State, Tribal, Local and Territorial Support. 2014. http://www.cdc.gov/stltpublichealth/townhall/presentations/2014/vs-january.pdf. Accessed 8 Oct 2015.

Prevalence and factors associated with use of khat: a survey of patients entering HIV treatment programs in Ethiopia

Alan R. Lifson[1*], Sale Workneh[2], Tibebe Shenie[2], Desalegn Admassu Ayana[3], Zenebe Melaku[4], Lemlem Bezabih[2], Hiwot Tekle Waktola[2], Behailu Dagne[2], Rose Hilk[1], Ken C. Winters[5] and Lucy Slater[6]

Abstract

Background: Khat, a plant native to East Africa, has psychoactive constituents similar to amphetamine. Chronic khat use can lead to psychological dependence with multiple physical and mental health harms, complicating clinical management of people living with HIV. In two Ethiopian cities where khat is common, we evaluated prevalence and correlates of khat use among patients new to HIV care.

Methods: During 2013–2014, we surveyed 322 patients recently enrolled in HIV clinics in Dire Dawa and Harar about khat use, demographics, smoking and alcohol use, clinical illness, food insecurity, and social support. We analyzed factors associated with khat use in the past year, as well as heaviest use of khat (based on greatest number of hours used in a typical month).

Results: 242 (75%) respondents reported lifetime khat use; 209 (65%) reported khat use during the previous year. 54% of khat users started before age 19 years. Although 84% believed that using khat every day is dangerous for health if you have HIV, khat was used in the previous year a median of 5 h/days and 30 days/month; 21% said they felt a need to cut down or control their khat use but had difficulty doing so. Those using khat were more likely to report smoking (46%) and alcohol use (49%) compared to non-khat users (1 and 31% respectively). Those reporting heaviest khat use ($\geq$180 h/typical month) were more likely to rate their health status as poor, have an underweight BMI ($\leq$18.5 kg/m^2), report more symptoms of chronic illness, and agree with more statements indicating a negative physical quality of life. In multivariate analysis, heavy users were more likely to be male, Muslim, and non-married.

Conclusions: Khat use was common among HIV patients entering care, and associated with symptoms of poorer physical health. Over half started khat use when they were young. Although most believed khat is harmful for HIV patients, a number of respondents reported some difficulty controlling their drug use. In settings where khat is legal and widely utilized, developing interventions for responsible use represent an important health priority as part of comprehensive care for people living with HIV.

Keywords: HIV, Khat, Amphetamine, Sub-Saharan Africa, Ethiopia

Background

Khat, or *Catha edulis*, is a flowering plant native to East Africa which is legal to grow, sell and consume in Ethiopia and used for its stimulant effects [1–3]. Most often the fresh leaves and shoots are chewed, although it can also be made into a tea or paste. The psychoactive constituents of khat, cathinone and cathine, are structurally similar to amphetamine. Immediate effects of khat may include euphoria, feelings of increased alertness and energy, hyperactivity, appetite suppression, and lack of fatigue. Acute psychological effects of khat use may include paranoia, hyperactivity, mania, withdrawal or isolation, and aggressive behavior [1–3]. Chronic khat

*Correspondence: lifso001@umn.edu
[1] Division of Epidemiology and Community Health, University of Minnesota, 1300 S. Second Street, Suite 300, Minneapolis, MN 55454-1015, USA
Full list of author information is available at the end of the article

use can lead to psychological dependence, manic behavior, violence, psychosis and other mental disorders [1, 3, 4]. Physical consequences of khat use can include hypertension and cardiovascular disease [2, 3, 5].

Khat use has been described as common in many Ethiopian populations [6–12]. A household survey of 1200 adults from one rural Ethiopian community found that 32% were khat users [6]. One survey of youth 15–24 years found 38% used khat in the previous year [12], while another study of high school students found 24% were khat chewers [9]. A survey of a representative sample of adults from throughout Ethiopia found wide geographic disparities in prevalence of khat use; in one high-prevalence community (Dire Dawa), 52% reported a lifetime history of khat use, of whom 58% reported use every day during the previous year [7].

Ethiopian studies show a relationship between khat use and unsafe sex, which may predispose to human immunodeficiency virus (HIV) infection [7, 12, 13]. Ethiopian khat users were more likely to have multiple sexual partners, to have sex with a non-regular partner, to exchange sex for money and to report a history of a genital ulcer [7, 12]. In one case-control Ethiopian study, khat use was associated with a twofold increased risk of HIV infection [13].

Despite the suggestion of significant overlap between the khat and HIV epidemics in Ethiopia, there are very limited data on prevalence and patterns of khat use in people living with HIV. This is particularly important since studies suggest that khat users may have poorer adherence to HIV therapy [7, 11], complicating their medical management. In addition to the physical and mental health harms that may be associated with khat, khat use has also been associated with an increased prevalence of smoking and alcohol use [10, 11], each of which can have their own adverse health effects for people with HIV [14, 15].

During 2013–2014, we enrolled patients in a 12 month prospective study from HIV clinics in two Ethiopian cities where khat use is especially common. Because we were interested in evaluating the impact of khat use on retention in clinical care, we chose those patients who had recently (within the last 3 months) enrolled in HIV care. Studies from Ethiopia and elsewhere show that loss to follow-up may be greatest within the first 6 months after entering care [16, 17], and it is patients new to care who are often most clinically and psychologically vulnerable.

We report results from our baseline survey evaluating prevalence and correlates of khat use in the previous year among patients newly enrolled in HIV clinics. Because khat use was relatively common in this population, we also analyzed factors associated with the heaviest use of khat, based on those with the greatest number of hours khat was used in a typical month during the preceding year.

Methods

Study setting

Adult patients (≥18 years) newly enrolled in HIV care (within previous 3 months) were identified and sequentially offered enrollment at two HIV clinics: Dil Chora regional hospital in Dire Dawa, and Hiwot Fana hospital (operated by Haramaya University) in Harar. Dire Dawa is a city located in eastern Ethiopia, with an estimated 2012 population of 262,884 [18], and is a major commercial and industrial hub. Harar is an ancient city and cultural heritage site in the highlands of eastern Ethiopia, with an estimated 2012 population of 110,457 [18]. Dire Dawa and Harar were selected as two cities with large HIV clinics, and where khat is commonly grown and used. Data from the Ethiopian Demographic and Health Survey reported an HIV seroprevalence of 4.0% in the Dire Dawa region and 2.8% in the Harari region [19]. In the same survey, although 11% of all Ethiopian women reported ever chewing khat, rates were 27% and 39% in the Dire Dawa and Harari regions, respectively [19]. Similarly, 28% of Ethiopia men reported ever chewing khat, but in the Dire Dawa and Harari regions, these rates were 79 and 82% respectively [19].

Data collection

A survey verbally administered in Amharic to participants included assessment of: (a) demographic characteristics, (b) khat use and attitudes, (c) smoking and alcohol use, (d) clinical illness, (e) food insecurity, and (f) social support. Survey items were adapted from other surveys plus our previous questionnaires with Ethiopian HIV patients [20–22]. Questions were translated into Amharic, and then pilot tested to ensure adequacy of translation, clarity, and cultural appropriateness.

Khat use questions included lifetime use and use within the previous year; for those reporting use in the prior year, we asked about days used in a typical month, and hours used in a typical day. To quantify khat use in the past year, we created summary scores of typical hours used per month, defined as the product of typical hours used per day and typical days used per month. We defined heavy khat use as the top quartile (greatest use) of typical hours used per month. We asked whether participants felt the need to cut down or control their khat use but had difficulty doing so; we also asked whether they used khat within a half hour after waking, used it in places one shouldn't (e.g., church, work), and used it even if they were sick in bed.

We inquired about and quantified use of alcohol and tobacco. Those who reported drinking in the past year were asked how many days they drank alcohol during a typical month, and how many drinks they took in a typical day when they did drink; the number of drinks during a typical month was then calculated as the product of drinks/day and days/month.

Severity of clinical illness was assessed by asking about specific symptoms of chronic illness (e.g., fever or diarrhea lasting ≥1 month), as well as by asking nine quality of life (QOL) questions related to perceived physical health; for example, if someone said they were bothered "some" or "very much" by physical problems related to their HIV, this was considered to represent a negative physical QOL response. Summary scores were created based on the number of negative QOL responses that were provided. Selected data were also abstracted from the participant's HIV clinic record, including most recent CD4+ count, World Health Organization (WHO) clinical stage [23], and height and weight to calculate body mass index (BMI).

Participants were asked three questions about food insecurity in the past 3 months, such as whether they "sometimes" or "often" went to bed hungry, ate smaller or fewer meals, or went a whole day without eating because there was not enough food.

Participants were also asked whether they agreed or not with eight statements indicating social connectedness and social support from others, such as whether they had someone to talk to in times of stress. Summary scores were created based on the numbers of positive social support statements that were agreed to.

Analysis

Confidence intervals (CI) are reported for selected proportions, standard deviation (SD) for mean values, and interquartile range (IQR) for median values. Predictors of both any khat use in the past year and heavy khat use were evaluated using Chi square for categorical variables, and *t* tests for continuous variables. Multivariate analysis was conducted using logistic regression. All data were double-entered; any discrepancies between entries were reconciled by checking the original data collection forms. All analyses were conducted using SAS version 9.3 (SAS Institute Inc., Cary, NC).

Human subjects

Institutional Review Board approval was obtained from the University of Minnesota, and Federal Democratic Republic of Ethiopia's Ministry of Science and Technology. Informed consent was obtained from all participants. For their time and effort, participants were reimbursed 70 Ethiopian birr (about $3.50 US) at the time of the survey.

Results

Study participants

Of 322 participants, 60% were from Dil Chora Hospital and 40% from Hiwot Fana. Characteristics of study participants are summarized in Table 1. Mean age was 33.8 years (range 18–70). Many participants had advanced clinical disease; 35% were WHO stage 3 or 4, and the median CD4+ count was 179 cells/mm^3 (IQR = 90,346). The median BMI was 19.6 kg/m^2 (IQR = 17.2, 22.0); 37% were ≤18.5 kg/m^2, considered underweight.

When asked to rate their overall health, 48% said very poor or poor. When asked 7 specific questions about symptoms over the past month, responses included chronic fatigue (71%), weight loss (58%), chronic pain (51%), chronic fever (40%), chronic cough (39%), chronic diarrhea (15%) and oral pain/sores (20%); 56% of patients had three or more of these symptoms. In response to nine questions about physical QOL, 86% gave a negative response to at least one QOL statement. For example

Table 1 Characteristics of patients from Dil Chora (Dire Dawa) and Hiwot Fana (Harar) Hospital HIV clinics (N-322)

	Number and % of total[a]
Gender	
Male	145 (45%)
Female	177 (55%)
Age (years)	
≤25	52 (16%)
26–35	166 (52%)
>35	104 (32%)
Marital	
Single	79 (25%)
Married	114 (35%)
Widow	45 (14%)
Other (divorced, separated)	84 (26%)
Education	
No school	81 (25%)
Some primary school	108 (34%)
Above primary school	133 (41%)
Religion	
Orthodox Christian	195 (61%)
Muslim	101 (31%)
Protestant/other	26 (8%)
Occupation	
Day labor	113 (36%)
Housewife	42 (13%)
Business (e.g., merchant)	34 (11%)
Civil servant	28 (9%)
Other	50 (16%)
Unemployed	48 (15%)

[a] Missing data excluded from analysis

66% said they were bothered "some" or "very much" by physical problems related to their HIV, 64% said physical pain limited their activities, and 47% said they did not have enough energy for everyday life. The mean number of negative QOL statements agreed to was 4.8 (SD = 3.3).

Twenty-seven percent gave positive responses ("sometimes"/"often") to one or more questions about food insecurity in the past 3 months; for example 19% reported sometimes or often going to bed hungry because there was not enough food. When asked 8 questions about social support or connectedness, 26% agreed with fewer than three positive statements. For example, 48% said they did not know of anyone who would help them if they needed it, and 38% said they did not have a feeling of closeness with anyone. The mean number of responses indicating positive social support was 4.9 (SD = 3.0).

Khat use

Two hundred forty-two (75%) respondents (84% of men and 68% of women) reported ever using khat during their lifetime. Among lifetime users, age at first use was ≤12 years for 6%, 13–15 years for 16%, 16–18 years for 31%, and ≥19 years for 46%. Two hundred nine (65%, 95% CI 59–70%) respondents reported using khat within the previous year. Among those using khat in the previous year, the median number of days used in a typical month was 30 (daily use) (IQR = 10,30); during a typical day, khat was chewed a median of 5 h (IQR = 4,8). The median number of hours used in a typical month was calculated as 120 (IQR = 45,180 h). Sixty-nine respondents, or 21% (95% CI 17–26%) of all persons interviewed, reported using khat ≥180 h during a typical month.

Participants who used khat in the previous year were asked several questions concerning perceptions of khat's health risks and their own drug use (Table 2). Three quarters believed khat use was dangerous for one's health if one was HIV-positive, and 21% felt the need to cut down or control use but had difficulty doing so (Table 2).

Correlates of khat use in past year

By demographic characteristics, those who used in khat in the previous year were more likely to be male, Muslim and (of borderline significance) day laborers, and less likely to be married and Protestant (Table 3). Those using khat were also more likely to rate their health status as poor, and (of borderline significance) to have an underweight BMI. Khat users reported a mean of 3.1 chronic symptoms compared to 2.5 among non-users ($p = 0.009$), a mean of 4.9 negative QOL statements versus 4.5 among non-users ($p > 0.10$), and a mean of 4.8 positive social support statements vs. 5.0 among non-users ($p > 0.10$).

Correlates of heavy khat use

Because khat use was relatively common in this population, we analyzed factors associated with the heaviest use of khat, defined as a calculated total of ≥180 h during a typical month, or the top quartile among current khat users. The comparison group was those with a calculated total of <180 h use in a typical month, including those who reported no use within the previous year.

By demographic characteristics, those who used khat >180 h in the past year were more likely than other participants to be male and Muslim, and less likely to be married and Protestant (Table 3). Heavy users were also more likely to rate their health status as poor and to have an underweight BMI. Heavy khat users reported a mean of 3.9 chronic symptoms compared to 2.7 among others ($p < 0.001$), a mean of 6.1 negative QOL statements vs. 4.4 among others ($p < 0.001$), and a mean of 4.4 positive social support statements versus 5.0 among others ($p > 0.10$).

Multivariate analysis was conducted to identify demographic predictors of heavy khat use, entering all variables shown in Table 4 into the model. Factors independently associated with heavy khat use included male gender [odds ratio (OR) 2.36, 95% CI 1.23, 4.52] and Muslim religion (OR 2.55, 95% CI 1.34, 4.87); those who were married were less likely to report heavy use (OR 0.38, 95% CI 0.19, 0.77) (Table 4).

Table 2 Attitudes about khat use among those Reporting use within the previous year, Dil Chora (Dire Dawa) and Hiwot Fana (Harar) Hospital HIV Clinics (N = 209)

	% responding affirmatively
Using khat is dangerous for your health if you have HIV	75
Using khat every day is dangerous for your health if you have HIV	84
Have you ever felt a need to cut down or control your khat use but had difficulty doing so?	21
Do you use khat within half an hour of waking up?	20
Do you find it difficult to not use khat in places where you shouldn't, such as work, church, school, or a hospital?	9
If you are so sick that you are in bed most of the day, or if you are so sick that you have to cut back on your normal activities or routines, do you still use khat?	8

Table 3 Characteristics of patients from Dil Chora (Dire Dawa) and Hiwot Fana (Harar) Hospital HIV clinics, comparing those who did and did not use khat in the previous year, and comparing heavy khat users (≥180 h in a typical month) to all other participants: univariate analysis

	% Who used khat		% who used khat	
	In past year (%)	p value	≥ 180 h/ month (%)	p value
Gender				
Male	75	<0.001	28	0.015
Female	56		16	
Age (years)				
≤25	62	0.519	19	0.556
26–35	63		20	
>35	69		25	
Marital				
Single	70	0.051	27	0.005
Married	56		11	
Other	70		27	
Occupation				
Day labor	73	0.054	25	0.491
Unemployed	60		23	
Other	60		19	
Education				
No school	59	0.197	27	0.281
Some primary school	71		18	
Above primary school	63		21	
Religion				
Orthodox Christian	63	<0.001	17	0.010
Muslim	76		31	
Protestant/Other	26		9	
BMI (kg/m²)				
≤18.5	71	0.066	29	0.011
>18.5	61		17	
WHO stage				
1–2	67	0.226	19	0.142
3–4	60		26	
Health (self-rated)				
Poor/very poor	71	0.039	26	0.030
Good/fair	60		16	
Food insecurity (last 3 months)				
Yes	72	0.123	23	0.728
No	62		21	

Other substance use

During the previous year, 30% of respondents reported smoking cigarettes or shisha (tobacco smoked with a hookah), and 43% reported drinking alcohol. Tobacco use in the past year was reported by 46% of those who also used khat in the previous year, compared to only 1% of those who did not use khat ($p < 0.001$). Those who used khat in the previous year reported smoking a mean of 5 cigarettes/day. Heavy khat users reported a mean of smoking 8 cigarettes/day.

Alcohol use in the previous year was reported by 49% of those reporting khat use in the previous year, compared to 31% of those who did not use khat ($p = 0.002$). Those who used khat in the previous year reported a mean of 36 drinks/month, compared to 11 drinks/month among those who did not use khat ($p < 0.001$). Heavy khat users reported a mean of 51 drinks/month.

Table 4 Demographic characteristics of patients from Dil Chora (Dire Dawa) and Hiwot Fana (Harar) Hospital HIV Clinics, comparing heavy khat users (≥180 h in a typical month) to all other participants: multivariate analysis

Demographic characteristic	Odds ratio (95% CI)	p value[a]
Gender		
Male (vs. female)	2.36 (1.23, 4.52)	0.010
Age		
≤25 years (vs. >35)	1.03 (0.42, 2.54)	0.978
26–35 years (vs. >35)	1.07 (0.55, 2.08)	
Marital		
Married (vs. other)	0.38 (0.19, 0.77)	0.007
Religion		
Muslim (vs. Orthodox Christian)	2.55 (1.34, 4.87)	0.009
Protestant (vs. Orthodox Christian)	0.55 (0.12, 2.57)	
Employment		
Day laborer (vs. other occupation)	1.33 (0.68, 2.60)	0.704
Unemployed (vs. other occupation)	1.20 (0.51, 2.84)	
Education		
No school (vs. above primary)	1.22 (0.56, 2.66)	0.413
Some primary school (vs. above primary)	0.73 (0.35, 1.51)	

[a] For overall demographic characteristic

Discussion

Among HIV patients newly enrolled in care at two large Ethiopian hospitals, we found a high prevalence of khat use, with 75% reporting lifetime use and 65% reporting use within the previous year. Among those using khat, over half reported chewing khat every day, and almost two-thirds used khat ≥5 h/day. Use of khat in the past year was also associated with poorer self-reported health status, a lower BMI, and a greater number of chronic symptoms. Heavy users (≥180 h in a typical month) reported all of these undesirable clinical outcomes, as well as a greater number of negative physical QOL statements.

Our study found that most persons who ever used khat had used it during the year prior to enrollment in care;

future analyses in this prospective study will compare khat use in the year before and after enrollment. Studies of khat have used different time frames to estimate recent use, such as past month [11] or past year [12]. Although we used past year, data from the 2011 Ethiopian Demographic and Health Survey using a 30 day time frame are consistent with our conclusions that most persons ever using khat have used it recently. Among men and women from the Harari region who ever used khat, 91 and 88% respectively had used one or more times it in the last 30 days; among men and women from Dire Dawa, corresponding rates were 85 and 96% [19].

HIV patients who reported khat use in the past year, especially heavy use, reported a greater number of chronic symptoms and a more negative physical QOL. Whether khat users who have such symptoms are more likely to use khat to help alleviate them, or whether chronic and habitual use causes increased symptomatology is unclear. However, other studies also report greater physical illness in khat users [6] and habitual khat use has been shown to be associated with a wide variety of physical and mental health harms, including cognitive impairment that may affect daily life activities [1–5, 24].

Khat users in our study were also significantly more likely to both use tobacco and drink alcohol. The association of khat use with both smoking and alcohol use has been reported from other studies as well [10, 11, 25]. We cannot say whether khat consumption predisposes users to use of these other substances (for example, use of alcohol to counteract stimulant properties of khat), or whether this association reflects underlying stressors or psychological factors that cause people to use multiple substances. Since both alcohol abuse and smoking can have negative health outcomes for HIV patients [14, 15], use of multiple substances may add to the adverse health effects potentially associated with khat.

Although khat is legal in Ethiopia and may be considered part of the lifestyle in some countries, it also has a potential for development of dependence [1, 3, 26, 27]. Although most respondents believed khat use (especially every day) was dangerous for health of HIV-infected individuals, use on a daily basis was common; 21% of current users reported that they felt a need to cut down or control their khat use but had difficulty doing so.

Our results have several implications for strategies to prevent or reduce khat use. Over half (54%) of khat users reported first use at age 18 years or younger. Given the prevalence of khat use in some populations of young people [8, 9], this supports the importance of drug education programs in schools and other settings where youth congregate. In addition to being a major cash crop, in certain communities khat has a social and cultural significance and acceptance [26, 28]. Rather than advocating for abstinence in all populations, a more balanced harm reduction approach that discourages excessive khat use or onset early in life may be more reasonable and favorable received [28].

Our study has several limitations. First, we chose for this study two cities where khat use is especially common; persons in different geographic areas may have a different prevalence and correlates of use. Second, khat use was self-reported, and some persons may have underreported their frequency of use. Third, associations between khat use and other factors in this survey do not necessarily imply temporality or causality. Finally, during khat sessions, leaves are kept in the mouth and typically chewed over several hours to release active components, and different khat plants may contain different concentrations of active cathinone products; therefore, the number of hours chewed may not strictly correspond with number of leaves ingested. As a statistical threshold, we chose the top quartile of hours khat was used in a typical month as the cut-point for heavy use. However, future studies, ideally in correlation to cathinone blood levels, can help to clarify how frequency and amount of use is associated with drug absorption and specific biological harms.

Conclusion

Among HIV positive Ethiopians entering care in two large eastern HIV clinics, two-thirds reported khat use within the past year, with a majority of these using khat on a daily basis. Use of khat, especially among heavy users, was associated with a number of measures of poorer physical health, including a greater number of chronic symptoms and poorer self-reported health status. In a setting where khat use is legal and widely utilized, defining patterns of responsible use and developing community-based interventions represent an important health priority to be included as part of a comprehensive care package for people living with HIV.

Abbreviations

BMI: body mass index; CI: confidence intervals; HIV: human immunodeficiency virus; IQR: interquartile range; QOL: quality of life; SD: standard deviation; WHO: World Health Organization.

Authors' contributions

AL was lead on planning and overseeing this study, conducting analysis, and writing the manuscript. All co-authors were involved in helping to develop the study design, and interpret study results, including SW, TS, LB, HTW, and BD who were directly responsible for implementing this project in Ethiopia. RH was responsible for data management. All co-authors provided feedback on this manuscript, including conclusions. All authors read and approved the final manuscript.

Author details

[1] Division of Epidemiology and Community Health, University of Minnesota, 1300 S. Second Street, Suite 300, Minneapolis, MN 55454-1015, USA. [2] Ethiopian Office, National Alliance of State and Territorial AIDS Directors, Addis

Ababa, Ethiopia. [3] College of Health and Medical Sciences, Haramaya University, Dire Dawa, Ethiopia. [4] International Center for AIDS Care and Treatment Program, Addis Ababa, Ethiopia. [5] Oregon Research Institute, Eugene, OR, USA. [6] Global Program, National Alliance of State and Territorial AIDS Directors, Washington, DC, USA.

Acknowledgements
We wish to thank the following individuals and organizations: Dil Chora Hospital in Dire Dawa, Hiwot Fana Hospital in Harar, the Dire Dawa Regional Health Bureau, Haramaya University, the National Alliance for State and Territorial AIDS Directors, and all of the HIV patients who participated in this study.

Competing interests
The authors declare that they have no competing interests.

Funding
Funding for this project was provided by the National Institute of Drug Abuse, National Institutes of Health, Grant Number: 1R21DA033131-01A1.

References

1. Pantelis C, Hindler CG, Taylor JC. Use and abuse of khat (Catha edulis): a review of the distribution, pharmacology, side effects and a description of psychosis attributed to khat chewing. Psychol Med. 1989;19:657–68.
2. Valente MJ, Guedes de Pinho P, de Lourdes Bastos M, Carvalho F, Carvalho M. Khat and synthetic cathinones: a review. Arch Toxicol. 2014;88:15–45.
3. Cox G, Rampes H. Adverse effects of khat: a review. Adv Psychiatr Treat. 2003;9:456–63.
4. Odenwald M, Neuner F, Schauer M, et al. Khat use as risk factor for psychotic disorders: a cross-sectional and case-control study in Somalia. BMC Med. 2005;3:5.
5. Al-Motarreb A, Al-Habori M, Broadley KJ. Khat chewing, cardiovascular diseases and other internal medical problems: the current situation and directions for future research. J Ethnopharmacol. 2010;132:540–8.
6. Belew M, Kebede D, Kassaye M, Enquoselassie F. The magnitude of khat use and its association with health, nutrition and socio-economic status. Ethiop Med J. 2000;38:11–26.
7. Berhane Y, Worku A. Alcohol and khat consumption and the association with HIV/AIDS prevention, care and treatment in Ethiopia. Ethiopian Public Health Association: Final report to U.S. Centers for Disease Control, December 2007.
8. Kebede D, Alem A, Mitike G, et al. Khat and alcohol use and risky sex behaviour among in school and out-of-school youth in Ethiopia. BMC Public Health. 2005;5:109.
9. Reda AA, Moges A, Biadgilign S, Wondmagegn BY. Prevalence and determinants of khat (Catha edulis) chewing among high school students in eastern Ethiopia: a cross-sectional study. PLOS ONE. 2012;7:e33946.
10. Tilahun M, Ayele G. Factors associated with Khat use among youths visiting HIV testing and counseling centers in Gamo Gofa, Southern Ethiopia. BMC Pub Health. 2013;13:1199.
11. Soboka M, Tesfaye M, Feyissa GT, Hanlon C. Khat use in people living with HIV: a facility-based cross-sectional survey from South West Ethiopia. BMC Psychiatry. 2015;15:69.
12. Alemu H, Mariam DH, Belay KA, Davey G. Factors predisposing out-of-school youths to HIV/AIDS-related risky sexual behaviour in Northwest Ethiopia. J Health Popul Nutr. 2007;25:344–50.
13. Abebe D, Debella A, Dejene A, et al. Khat chewing habit as a possible risk behaviour for HIV infection: a case-control study. Ethiop J Health Dev. 2005;19:174–81.
14. Lifson AR, Neuhaus J, Arribas JR, van den Berg-Wolf M, Labriola AM, Read TR. Smoking-related health risks among persons with HIV in the strategies for management of antiretroviral therapy clinical trial. Am J Pub Health. 2010;100:1896–903.
15. Molina PE, Bagby GJ, Nelson S. Biomedical consequences of alcohol use disorders in the HIV-infected host. Curr HIV Res. 2014;12:265–75.
16. Fox MP, Rosen S. Patient retention in antiretroviral therapy programs up to three years on treatment in sub-Saharan Africa, 2007–2009: systematic review. Trop Med Int Health. 2010;15(suppl 1):1–15.
17. Seyoum E, Mekonen Y, Kassa A, et al. ART Scale-up in Ethiopia: successes and challenges, January 2009. Addis Ababa: Ethiopia HIV/AIDS Prevention and Control Office, 2009. www.etharc.org/resources/download/finish/33/48.
18. GEOHIVE, Global population statistics. Ethiopia, main cities. www.geohive.com/cntry/ethiopia.aspx.
19. Central Statistical Agency [Ethiopia], ICF International. Ethiopia demographic and health survey 2011. Addis Ababa: Central Statistical Agency and Calverton, MD: ICF International, 2012. https://dhsprogram.com/pubs/pdf/FR255/FR255.pdf.
20. Department of Mental Health and Substance Abuse, World Health Organization: WHOQOL-HIV BREF. Geneva: World Health Organization, 2002. www.who.int/mental_health/evidence/WHOQOL-HIV%20BREF.pdf.
21. Cutrona CE, Russell DW. The provisions of social relationships and adaptation to stress. In: Jones WH, Perlman D, editors. Advances in Personal Relationships, vol. 1. Greenwich: JAI Press; 1987. p. 37–67.
22. Lifson AR, Workneh S, Hailemichael A, Demisse W, Slater L, Shenie T. Implementation of a peer HIV community support worker program in rural Ethiopia to promote retention in care. J Int Assoc Providers AIDS Care. 2015. pp 1–6. doi:10.1177/2325957415614648.
23. World Health Organization. WHO case definitions of HIV for surveillance and revised clinical staging and immunological classification of HIV-related disease in adults and children. Geneva: World Health Organization. 2007. www.who.int/hiv/pub/vct/hivstaging/en.
24. Colzato LS, Ruiz MJ, van den Wildenberg WPM, Hommel B. Khat use is associated with impaired working memory and cognitive flexibility. PLOS ONE. 2011;6:e20602.
25. Kassim S, Jawad M, Croucher R, Akl EA. The epidemiology of tobacco use among khat users: a systematic review. Biomed Res Int. 2015;2015:313692.
26. Manghi RA, Broers B, Khan R, Benguettat D, Khazaal Y, Zullino DF. Khat use: Lifestyle or addiction? J Psychoactive Drugs. 2009;41:1–10.
27. Kassim S, Al'absi M. Khat use is a neglected addictive behaviour. Addiction. 2015;111:179–80.
28. Odenwald M, Warfa N, Bhui K, Elbert T. The stimulant khat–another door in the wall? A call for overcoming the barriers. J Ethnopharmacol. 2010;132:615–9.

14

Predictive validity of two process-of-care quality measures for residential substance use disorder treatment

Alex H. S. Harris*, Shalini Gupta, Thomas Bowe, Laura S. Ellerbe, Tyler E. Phelps, Anna D. Rubinsky, John W. Finney, Steven M. Asch, Keith Humphreys and Jodie Trafton

Abstract

Background: In order to monitor and ultimately improve the quality of addiction treatment, professional societies, health care systems, and addiction treatment programs must establish clinical practice standards and then operationalize these standards into reliable, valid, and feasible quality measures. Before being implemented, quality measures should undergo tests of validity, including predictive validity. Predictive validity refers to the association between process-of-care quality measures and subsequent patient outcomes. This study evaluated the predictive validity of two process quality measures of residential substance use disorder (SUD) treatment.

Methods: Washington Circle (WC) Continuity of Care quality measure is the proportion of patients having an outpatient SUD treatment encounter within 14 days after discharge from residential SUD treatment. The Early Discharge measure is the proportion of patients admitted to residential SUD treatment who discharged within 1 week of admission. The predictive validity of these process measures was evaluated in US Veterans Health Administration patients for whom utilization-based outcome and 2-year mortality data were available. Propensity score-weighted, mixed effects regression adjusted for pre-index imbalances between patients who did and did not meet the measures' criteria and clustering of patients within facilities.

Results: For the WC Continuity of Care measure, 76 % of 10,064 patients had a follow-up visit within 14 days of discharge. In propensity score-weighted models, patients who had a follow-up visit had a lower 2-year mortality rate [odds ratio (OR) = 0.77, p = 0.008], but no difference in subsequent detoxification episodes relative to patients without a follow-up visit. For the Early Discharge measure, 9.6 % of 10,176 discharged early and had significantly higher 2-year mortality (OR = 1.49, p < 0.001) and more subsequent detoxification episodes.

Conclusions: These two measures of residential SUD treatment quality have strong associations with 2-year mortality and the Early Discharge measure is also associated with more subsequent detoxification episodes. These results provide initial support for the predictive validity of residential SUD treatment quality measures and represent the first time that any SUD quality measure has been shown to predict subsequent mortality.

Keywords: Quality measurement, Residential treatment, Continuing care, Retension

Background

In order to monitor and ultimately improve the quality of addiction treatment, professional organizations, health care systems, and addiction treatment programs must establish clinical practice standards and then operationalize these standards into reliable, valid, and feasible quality measures. Quality measures can help define and motivate guideline-congruent care, reveal gaps in the continuum of care, identify poor performers to whom quality improvement efforts can be targeted, and may provide an empirically-justified basis for performance-based

*Correspondence: Alexander.Harris2@va.gov
Center for Innovation to Implementation, Health Services Research and Development Service, VA Palo Alto Health Care System, Menlo Park, CA, USA

incentive programs. However, these benefits can only be realized if quality measures are valid and avoid unintended consequences, neither of which is a given [1, 2].

Improvement in clinically important outcomes is the most prominent goal of health care and therefore may seem like the only legitimate "gold standard" for measuring treatment quality. But using outcomes alone as quality measures presents at least three difficulties. First, post-treatment outcome data are often expensive and logistically difficult to collect. Second, using outcomes directly as quality measures requires risk adjustments for casemix and making debatable assumptions regarding missing baseline and follow-up data [3]. Third, outcome data alone cannot indicate if treatment access is sufficient or what structural and process changes might be needed to improve outcomes. Therefore, identifying treatment structure, access, and process measures in administrative data that reliably predict long-term outcomes is often the best available quality assessment method.

Predictive validity refers to the association between antecedent quality indicators (e.g., structural, access, and process-of-care measures) and subsequent quality indicators, such as patient outcomes. Associations between process-of-care measures and outcomes can be driven by many factors, including the fidelity with which the process can be operationalized with available data [4], selection of an appropriate outcome, the temporal proximity of the outcome to the clinical process, limited power to detect small effects, and potential bias due to unmeasured confounding factors [5]. Therefore, care and humility are indicated when interpreting the results of predictive validity studies. Regardless, if the presumed association between a process-of-care quality measure and patient outcomes cannot be demonstrated, the measure's validity should be considered suspect.

Formulating and implementing quality measures without careful empirical validation exposes all stakeholders to many risks, including promoting poor or incomplete care, and diverting effort and attention from potentially more important activities. Measures are often specified and implemented before enough data and/or interest accumulates to conduct validation studies. In diverse areas of medicine, even when careful validation is undertaken, the expected associations between process-of-care measures and outcomes are often absent or weaker than expected. Furthermore, when previously validated measures are put into use, particularly with incentives, changes in care or coding practices can lead to changes in predictive validity or other unintended consequences [6–10]. Addiction treatment quality measures have not been immune from these challenges [2, 11–15].

Residential addiction treatment programs are important features of the continuum of care for patients with SUD. As an intensive, relatively costly setting for SUD treatment, these programs are usually reserved for patients who need high levels of support, supervision, and stabilization before transitioning to outpatient continuing care. Two process-of-care measures have been proposed to capture elements of residential addiction program quality, one proposed by the Washington Circle and one by Rand and the Altarum Institute. The Washington Circle (WC) was a group of national experts that sought to improve the accessibility and effectiveness of SUD treatment through the use of quality measurement systems. One of the WC's major activities was developing quality measures for SUD treatment for publicly-funded and commercially-insured systems of care. One WC measure focuses on outpatient continuing care after residential treatment [16]. WC Continuity of Care is a dichotomous measure indicating whether or not a patient had an outpatient SUD treatment encounter within 14 days after discharge from residential treatment. The measure is intended to assess the minimum necessary service to provide quality treatment, but not necessarily optimal or sufficient continuity of care after residential treatment.

Garner et al. [17] evaluated the predictive validity of the WC Continuity of Care measure in a sample of 342 adolescents in long-term residential addiction treatment who were randomly assigned at discharge to either standard continuing care or an assertive continuing care condition. Overall, adolescent patients whose treatment met the WC Continuity of Care criterion were significantly more likely to have achieved recovery status (no alcohol or other drug use, abuse, or dependence symptoms while living in the community during the previous 30 days) at 3 months ($OR = 1.92$, $p < 0.05$). However, the predictive validity of this measure has never been evaluated in adult patients or beyond 3 months.

The other quality measure pertaining to residential SUD treatment was developed by RAND and the Altarum Institute as part of a national evaluation of mental health services commissioned by the US Veterans Health Administration (VHA). The measure taps the proportion of patients with SUD diagnoses admitted to residential SUD treatment who are discharged or self-discharge within 1 week of admission ("Early Discharge"). Patients who discharge early from residential addiction treatment programs typically have poorer outcomes and are more likely to be readmitted [18]. However, the strength of evidence for these associations is modest and the predictive validity of the Early Discharge quality measure itself has never been evaluated.

Therefore, the purpose of this study was to examine the predictive validity of these two process-of-care quality measures in the VHA, a large integrated health care system with extensive SUD treatment services. Because we lack data on more clinically detailed outcomes, such as improvements in symptoms and functioning, the primary outcomes in this study are 2-year mortality and patterns of utilization that might signify either successful stabilization in an outpatient setting or an escalation of symptoms requiring subsequent readmission or detoxification. Specifically, we hypothesized that WC Continuity of Care would be positively associated with subsequent outpatient SUD and mental health treatment after the 14-day post-discharge observation period and negatively associated with subsequent SUD and psychiatric inpatient admissions, detoxification episodes, as well as 2-year mortality. We hypothesized that these relationships would be in the opposite direction for the Early Discharge measure. If evidence can be found for the predictive validity of these measures, they could be used for system monitoring and quality improvement purposes in VHA's Mental Health Information System [19], or by other integrated health care systems.

Methods

Calculating the Continuity of Care measure

Using VHA's National Patient Care Database, we identified all patients with an SUD diagnosis who discharged to the community from one of VHA's 54 Substance Abuse Residential Rehabilitation Programs (SARRTPs; bed section codes: 27, 37, 85, 86, 88, 111) in fiscal year 2009 (FY09). We then determined whether each patient had an outpatient SUD visit within 14 days of discharge. SUD outpatient visits were defined as a clinical encounter in an SUD or mental health clinic in which an SUD diagnosis was recorded. Patients who transferred from the SARRTP to another residential setting were excluded from the denominator.

Calculating the Early Discharge measure

Using VHA's National Patient Care Database, we identified all patients with an admission to one of VHA's SARRTPs in FY09 with a SUD diagnosis, and determined whether each patient was discharged from the program to the community within 7 days. Although the denominators for the two measures are different (patients with admissions vs. patients with discharges), the samples largely overlap.

Outcomes

We examined if each measure was associated with the following utilization-based outcomes in the 6 months after each patient either met or did not meet the measures' criteria: Number of subsequent admissions to a SARRTP, number of admissions to other mental health residential or inpatient programs, number of outpatient encounters in SUD clinics, number of outpatient encounters in mental health clinics, and number of detoxification episodes. We also examined the association of each measure with 2-year mortality as determined by the VHA Vital Status file.

Propensity score modeling

Estimation of process-outcome associations from observational data is difficult because exposure to the process of care is non-random and often confounded with patient or program characteristics. Propensity score methods are often used to adjust for confounding. Here, a propensity score is defined as the probability of meeting a performance measure conditional on pre-treatment covariates. Several methods have been developed to calculate propensity scores. We used boosted regression to estimate each patient's propensity score for meeting each process-of-care measure. Boosted regression has been shown to produce models with less prediction error than other common methods [20]. One-year pre-index variables used in the propensity score models were age, gender, marital status (Y/N), race/ethnicity, co-morbid psychiatric diagnoses, traumatic brain injury, co-morbid medical diagnoses (e.g., diabetes, hepatitis C), homelessness, outpatient and residential SUD and mental health service utilization, and number of prior detoxification episodes.

Modeling associations between process measures and outcomes

For each process-of-care quality measure, using a propensity-score weighted [20], mixed-effects regression model, we evaluated if getting the measure-specified care (yes/no) was associated with patient-level outcomes beyond the possible effect of facility-level performance on the measure [21]. These models included VHA facility as a random effect and an exchangeable covariance structure. Utilization-based outcomes were modeled by mixed-effects, zero-inflated, negative binomial regression models. Two-year mortality was modeled in mixed-effects logistic regression models.

Facility-level variability

In order to assess the extent to which performance on these measures varied between facilities, we calculated descriptive statistics and histograms of the distributions of facility-level performance of the VHA facilities with residential SUD programs.

Results

For the WC Continuity of Care measure, 10,064 patients met the denominator criterion (i.e., discharged from a residential SUD treatment program in FY09) and 7648 (76 %) met the numerator criterion by having a follow-up visit within 14 days of discharge. The characteristics of patients who met versus did not meet the measure's numerator criterion are presented in Table 1, along with the characteristics of the "failed to meet" sample after weighting with propensity scores. Even, before propensity score weighting, the two groups were very similar on most characteristics. The most pronounced differences between patients meeting and not meeting the numerator criterion were the number of SUD outpatient visits in the previous 6 months (15.4 vs. 9.8), homelessness in the previous year (30.1 vs. 26.7 %), and HIV positive status (1.8 vs. 2.6 %). All of these differences were reduced or eliminated by the weighting procedure.

In propensity score-weighted models, patients whose care met the WC Continuity of Care measure had significantly more subsequent mental health admissions ($b = 0.15$, $p = 0.015$), significantly more mental health outpatient visits ($b = 0.42$, $p < 0.001$), and significantly more SUD outpatient visits ($b = 0.65$, $p < 0.001$). The measure was not significantly associated with number of subsequent admissions to residential SUD treatment programs or number of detoxification episodes. Notably, the odds of death in the two post-discharge years was significantly lower for patients who received the measure-specified continuity of care (4.35 vs. 5.57 %; OR = 0.77, $p = 0.008$). The unadjusted and propensity score-adjusted group differences in 2-year mortality and mean number of detoxifications in 6 months are presented in Table 2. Also, Fig. 1 shows substantial facility-level variation (41–99 %) in the WC Continuity of Care measure.

For the Early Discharge measure, 10,176 patients met the denominator criterion (i.e., admitted to a residential SUD treatment program in FY09) and 974 (9.6 %) met the numerator criterion by experiencing discharge within 7 days. The characteristics of patients who met versus did not meet the measure's numerator criterion are presented in Table 3, along with the characteristics of the "did not meet" sample after weighting with propensity scores. Unlike the WC Continuity of Care measure, it is considered undesirable to meet the numerator criterion for the Early Discharge measure. Again, even before propensity score weighting, the two groups were very similar on most characteristics. The most pronounced differences between patients meeting and not meeting the numerator criterion were in the number of mental health outpatient visits in the previous 6 months (15.8 vs. 13.8), Caucasian race (66.8 vs. 59.3 %), traumatic brain injury (4.3 vs. 2.7 %), and HIV positive status (2.7 vs. 1.8 %). All of these differences were reduced or eliminated by the weighting procedure.

In propensity score-weighted models, patients who met the numerator criterion for early discharge had significantly fewer mental health admissions ($b = -0.65$, $p < 0.001$), mental health outpatient visits ($b = -0.50$, $p < 0.001$), SUD outpatient visits ($b = -0.88$, $p < 0.001$), and admissions to residential SUD treatment programs ($b = -1.05$, $p < 0.001$) in the following 6 months. Patients discharging early also had significantly more subsequent detoxification episodes ($b = 0.11$, $p = 0.037$). Finally, the odds of death in the two post-discharge years was significantly higher in patients who discharged early and thereby met the numerator criterion (7.30 vs. 4.72 %; OR = 1.49, $p < 0.001$). The unadjusted and propensity score-adjusted group differences in 2-year mortality and mean number of detoxifications in 6 months are presented in Table 2. Also, Fig. 2 shows substantial facility-level variation in this measure from 0 to 46 %.

Table 1 Demographic and pre-index characteristics of patients meeting and not meeting the WC Continuity of Care numerator criterion

Characteristic	Met (N = 7648)	Did not meet (N = 2416)	Did not meet, weighted
Mean age (years)	49.1	49.8	49.1
Female	4.9 %	4.1 %	4.6 %
Caucasian	56.8 %	58.1 %	57.1 %
Married	21.8 %	22.2 %	22.0 %
Homeless in previous year	30.1 %	26.7 %	30.0 %
SUD outpatient visits	15.4	9.8	13.7
MH outpatient visits	14.5	12.0	13.0
Residential SUD admissions	0.07	0.08	0.07
Detoxification episodes	0.55	0.55	0.57
Co-morbid psychiatric diagnoses	80.1 %	80.0 %	80.7 %
Traumatic brain injury	2.9 %	2.6 %	2.6 %
HIV positive status	1.8 %	2.6 %	1.8 %

Separate co-morbid medical diagnoses were included in the model but not presented in this table. No notable differences existed in these variables

Table 2 Unadjusted and adjusted outcomes in patients meeting and not meeting measure criteria

Measure	Outcome	Patients meeting criteria	Patients not meeting criteria
WC Continuity of Care	Unadjusted 2-year mortality	4.50 %	5.92 %
	Adjusted 2-year mortality	4.35 %	5.57 %
	Unadjusted mean detoxes in 6 months	0.171	0.177
	Adjusted mean detoxes in 6 months	0.175	0.185
Early Discharge	Unadjusted 2-year mortality	7.30 %	4.72 %
	Adjusted 2-year mortality	6.29 %	4.29 %
	Unadjusted mean detoxes in 6 months	0.350	0.225
	Adjusted mean detoxes in 6 months	0.240	0.215

Adjustments refer to propensity score weighting in mixed effects regression models

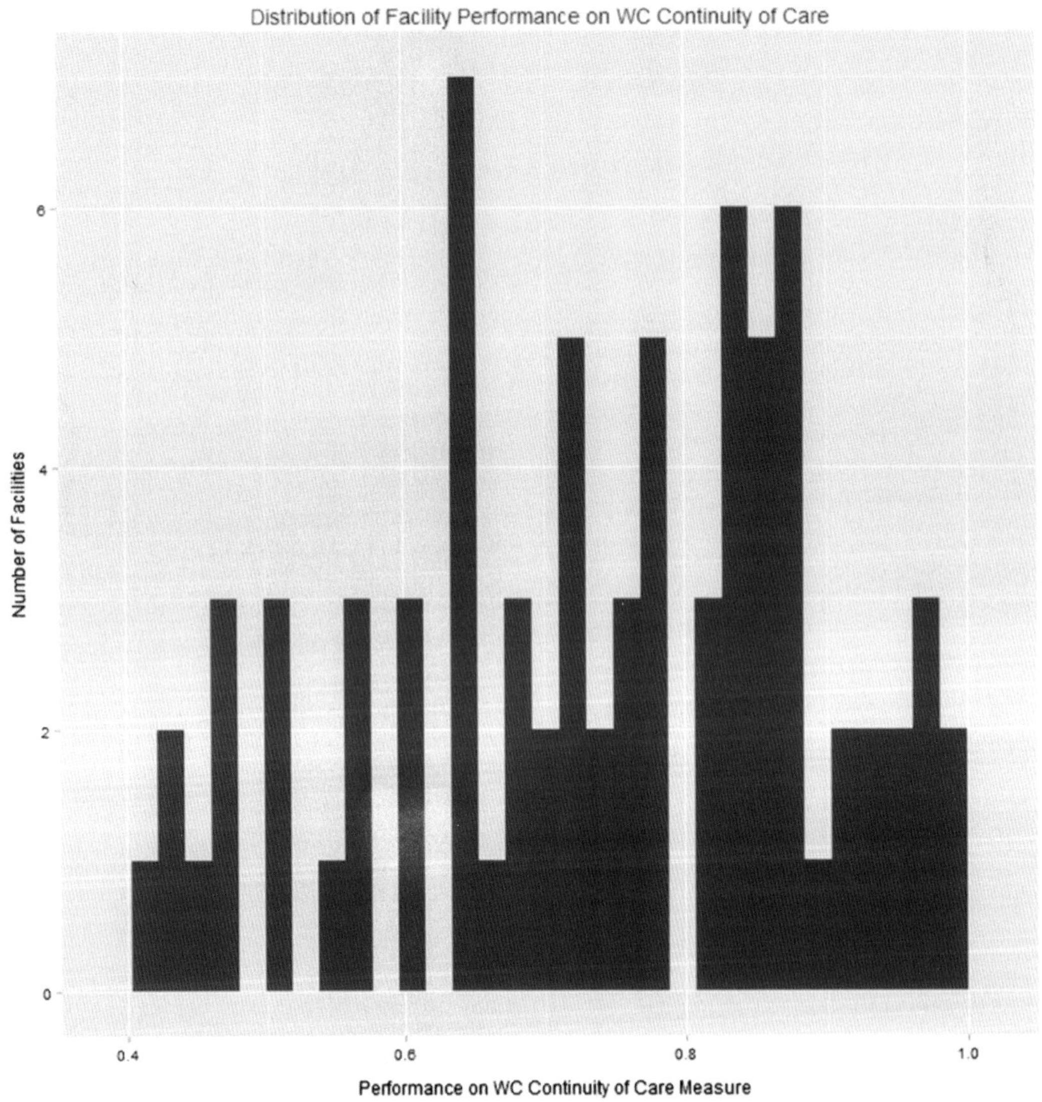

Fig. 1 Distribution of facility performance on WC Continuity of Care

Table 3 Demographic and pre-index characteristics of patients meeting and not meeting the Early Discharge numerator criterion

Characteristic	Met (N = 974)	Did not meet (N = 9202)	Did not meet, weighted
Mean age (years)	49.2	49.4	49.1
Female	5.7 %	4.5 %	5.3 %
Caucasian	66.8 %	59.3 %	65.6 %
Married	24.3 %	22.1 %	23.8 %
Homeless in previous year	29.2 %	29.4 %	29.6 %
SUD outpatient visits	15.8	14.1	15.4
MH outpatient visits	15.8	13.8	15.5
Residential SUD admissions	0.09	0.07	0.08
Detoxification episodes	0.72	0.54	0.70
Co-morbid psychiatric diagnoses	85.0 %	80.7 %	84.5 %
Traumatic brain injury	4.3 %	2.7 %	4.0 %
HIV positive status	2.7 %	1.8 %	2.2 %

Separate co-morbid medical diagnoses were included in the model but not presented in this table. No notable differences existed in these variables

Discussion

In this study, we examined the predictive validity of two process-of-care quality measures for residential SUD treatment in a large sample of patients in a very large integrated health care system. Ideally, data would have been available to examine the associations of these measures with near- and long-term changes in symptoms and functioning, instead of only administrative and utilization data. We originally had hypotheses about the relationships between these measures and patterns of utilization, such as outpatient SUD treatment engagement, that might signify successful stabilization, and patterns of utilization, such as subsequent readmission or detoxification, that might signify an escalation. However, the results indicated that more utilization specified in the measures was generally associated with more subsequent utilization of both types. In other words, markers of engagement in the health care system are associated with other markers of later engagement in the health care system. In retrospect, this is unsurprising and consistent with research in other clinical areas. The one type of utilization that ran counter to this general trend, however, was subsequent detoxification episodes. Although the WC Continuity of Care measure was unrelated to subsequent detoxification episodes, the Early Discharge measure (i.e., less initial utilization) was associated with significantly more subsequent detoxification episodes.

Even more impressive, both measures were associated with risk of death in the two post-discharge years in the expected directions: Continuity of Care with lower risk of death and Early Discharge with higher risk of death. These results are noteworthy given that mortality is a conceptually distal outcome of SUD treatment relative to, say, substance use. Previous efforts in the area of addiction and more broadly to examine associations between continuity of care and retention quality measures and outcomes have largely found none (e.g., [22–24]) with some exceptions (e.g., [17, 25, 26]). However, this is the first study of addiction treatment process measures to find associations with risk of death. It is possible but unlikely that the associations between these measures and risk of death are directly causal. Perhaps more likely is that these processes facilitate or are proxies for different levels of engagement with the health care system, which in turn affect mortality risk. Alternatively, these processes may be associated with unmeasured factors that are linked to mortality. In an event, finding SUD treatment process-of-care quality measures that are so strongly linked with subsequent risk of death is remarkable.

This study has several limitations. First, the VHA is a large integrated health care system serving US military Veterans. It is unknown to what extent these findings generalize to different health care systems or settings. Second, although patients who met the measures and patients who did not meet the measures were very similar on measured characteristics, and differences that did exist were trivial after propensity score weighting, these patients may have also differed on unmeasured characteristics, such as SUD severity or travel time to care, that could affect outcomes.

With these caveats in mind, it is still noteworthy that these two process-of-care quality measures for residential SUD treatment are linked to 2-year mortality risk, and the Early Discharge measure was associated with subsequent detoxification episodes. These results provide important new evidence supporting the predictive validity of the WC Continuity of Care measure and the Early Discharge measure, and thereby, affirming their value as tools to monitor the quality of residential SUD care for

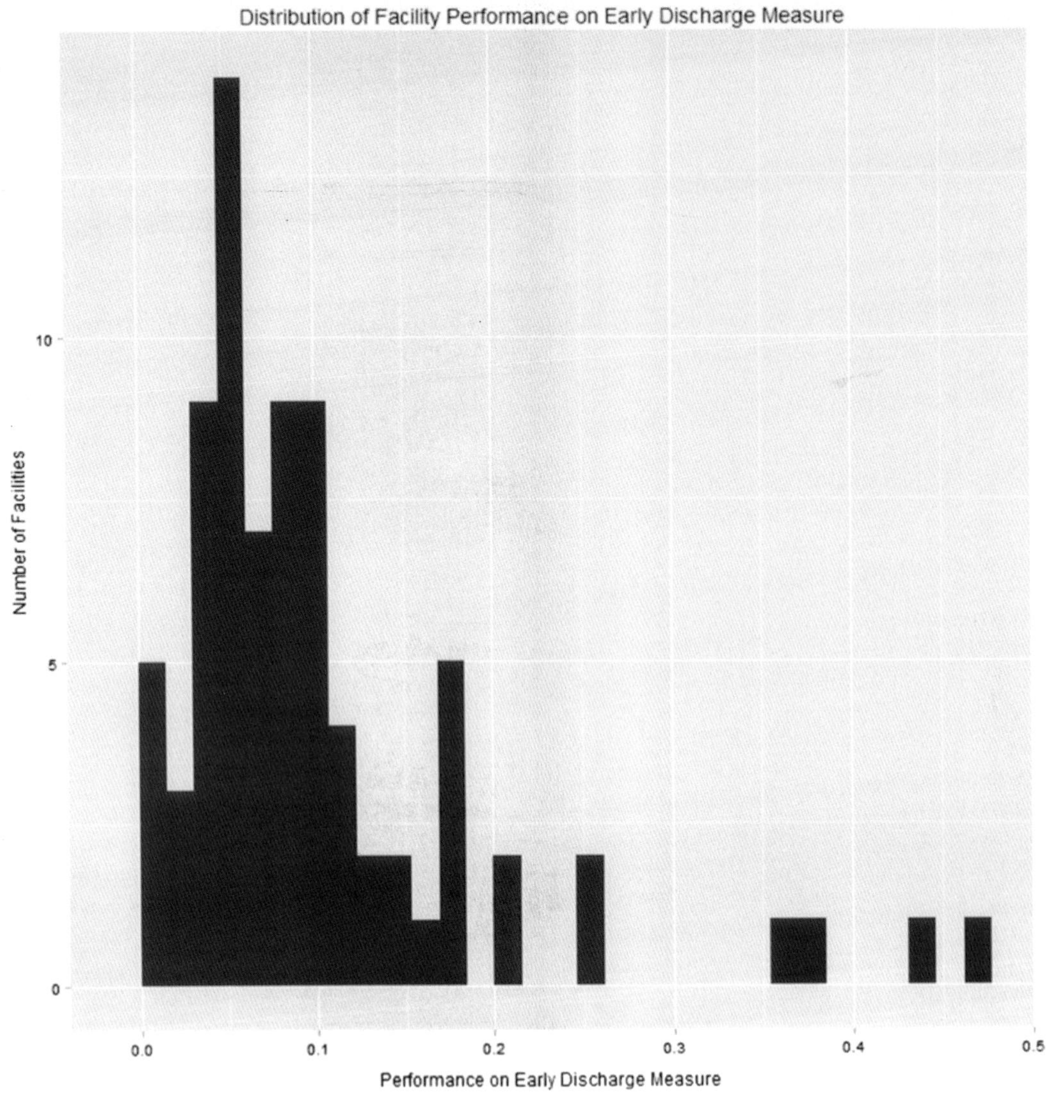

Fig. 2 Distribution of facility performance on Early Discharge measure

adults. Because these results were not guaranteed, we believe our study shows the importance of subjecting quality measures to validity checks before implementing them in clinical practice. Where these measures are implemented, especially if attached to incentives or consequences for providers or systems of care, it is critical to make sure that they do not drive unintended changes in practice (e.g., instituting a cursory follow-up program to meet the measure) that will dilute or destroy the process-outcome associations found in this study.

Abbreviations

SUD: substance use disorder; WC: Washington Circle; VHA: US Veterans Health Administration; SARRTP: Substance Abuse Residential Rehabilitation Programs; FY: fiscal year; OR: odds ratio.

Authors' contributions

AHSH, JWF, SMA, KH and JT conceived of the study and ASHH supervised the analysis and modeling. TB, LSE, TEP, and ADR participated in modeling decisions and conducted and interpreted analyses. All authors read and approved the final manuscript.

Acknowledgements

This study was funded by the VA Health Services Research and Development Service (Grants nos. SUS 99-015; IIR 10-370-2; RCS-14-232; RCS-04-141). The views expressed herein are not necessarily those of the Department of Veterans Affairs.

Competing interests

The authors declare that they have no competing interests.

References

1. Bradley KA, et al. When quality indicators undermine quality: bias in a quality indicator of follow-up for alcohol misuse. Psychiatr Serv. 2013;64(10):1018–25.
2. Harris AH, et al. Measuring the quality of substance use disorder treatment: evaluating the validity of the Department of Veterans Affairs continuity of care performance measure. J Subst Abuse Treat. 2009;36(3):294–305.
3. Iezzoni LI. The risks of risk adjustment. JAMA. 1997;278(19):1600–7.
4. Harris AHS, et al. Validation of the treatment identification strategy of the HEDIS addiction quality measures: concordance with medical record review. BMC Health Serv Res. 2011;11:73.
5. Parast L, et al. Challenges in assessing the process-outcome link in practice. J Gen Intern Med. 2015;30(3):359–64.
6. Werner RM, Bradlow ET. Relationship between Medicare's hospital compare performance measures and mortality rates. JAMA. 2006;296(22):2694–702.
7. Horn SD. Performance measures and clinical outcomes. JAMA. 2006;296(22):2731–2.
8. Wachter RM, et al. Public reporting of antibiotic timing in patients with pneumonia: lessons from a flawed performance measure. Ann Intern Med. 2008;149(1):29–32.
9. Walter LC, et al. Pitfalls of converting practice guidelines into quality measures: lessons learned from a VA performance measure. JAMA. 2004;291(20):2466–70.
10. Roth S, et al. Unintended consequences of a quality measure for acute bronchitis. Am J Manag Care. 2012;18(6):e217–24.
11. Harris AH, et al. HEDIS initiation and engagement quality measures of substance use disorder care: impact of setting and health care specialty. Popul Health Manag. 2009;12(4):191–6.
12. Harris AH, et al. Does meeting the HEDIS substance abuse treatment engagement criterion predict patient outcomes? J Behav Health Serv Res. 2010;37(1):25–39.
13. Dunigan R, et al. Engagement in outpatient substance abuse treatment and employment outcomes. J Behav Health Serv Res. 2014;41(1):20–36.
14. Garnick DW, et al. The Washington Circle engagement performance measures' association with adolescent treatment outcomes. Drug Alcohol Depend. 2012;124(3):250–8.
15. Harris AH, Humphreys K, Finney JW. Veterans affairs facility performance on Washington Circle indicators and casemix-adjusted effectiveness. J Subst Abuse Treat. 2007;33(4):333–9.
16. Garnick DW, et al. Adapting Washington Circle performance measures for public sector substance abuse treatment systems. J Subst Abuse Treat. 2009;36(3):265–77.
17. Garner BR, et al. The Washington Circle Continuity of Care performance measure: predictive validity with adolescents discharged from residential treatment. J Subst Abuse Treat. 2010;38(1):3–11.
18. Peterson KA, et al. Determinants of readmission following inpatient substance abuse treatment: a national study of VA programs. Med Care. 1994;32(6):535–50.
19. Trafton JA, et al. VHA mental health information system: applying health information technology to monitor and facilitate implementation of VHA Uniform Mental Health Services Handbook requirements. Med Care. 2013;51(3 Suppl 1):S29–36.
20. McCaffrey DF, Ridgeway G, Morral AR. Propensity score estimation with boosted regression for evaluating causal effects in observational studies. Psychol Methods. 2004;9(4):403–25.
21. Desai M, Begg MD. A comparison of regression approaches for analyzing clustered data. Am J Public Health. 2008;98(8):1425–9.
22. Harris AHS, et al. Measuring the quality of substance use disorder treatment: evaluating the validity of the Department of Veterans Affairs continuity of care performance measure. J Subst Abuse Treat. 2009;36(3):294–305.
23. Greenberg G, Rosenheck R, Fontana A. Continuity of Care and clinical effectiveness: treatment of posttraumatic stress disorder in the Department of Veterans Affairs. J Behav Health Ser Res. 2003;30:202–14.
24. Greenberg A, Rosenheck R, Seibyl C. Continuity of care and clinical effectiveness: outcomes following residential treatment for severe substance abuse. Med Care. 2002;40(3):246–59.
25. Adair CE, et al. Continuity of care and health outcomes among persons with severe mental illness. Psychiatr Serv. 2005;56(9):1061–9.
26. Greenberg GA, Rosenheck RA. Continuity of care and clinical outcomes in a national health system. Psychiatr Serv. 2005;56(4):427–33.

15

HIV treatment cascade among female entertainment and sex workers in Cambodia: impact of amphetamine use and an HIV prevention program

Sokunny Muth[1], Aynar Len[1], Jennifer L. Evans[2], Maly Phou[1], Sophal Chhit[3], Yuthea Neak[4], Song Ngak[1], Ellen S. Stein[2], Adam W. Carrico[5], Lisa Maher[6] and Kimberly Page[7*]

Abstract

Background: HIV prevalence remains high in Cambodia among female entertainment and sex workers (FESW), and amphetamine-type stimulant (ATS) use significantly increases risk of infection. A successful continuum of care (CoC) is key to effective clinical care and prevention. This study aimed to describe the HIV CoC in HIV-positive FESW. We examined CoC outcomes among HIV-positive FESW participating in the Cambodia Integrated HIV and Drug Prevention Implementation (CIPI) study, being implemented in ten provinces. CIPI is a trial aimed at reducing ATS use concomitant with the SMARTgirl HIV prevention program.

Methods: From 2013 to 2016, 1198 FESW $\geq$ 18 years old who reported multiple sex partners and/or transactional sex were recruited. We identified 88 HIV-positive women at baseline. We described linkage to care as 12-month retention and viral suppression (<1000 copies/mL). Logistic regression analyses were conducted to examine correlates of retention in care at 12 months, and viral suppression.

Results: Median age of the 88 HIV-positive women was 32 years [interquartile range (IQR) 28, 35]; 50% were working in entertainment venues and 50% as freelance sex workers; 70% reported SMARTgirl membership. In the past 3 months, women reported a median of 15 sex partners, 38% reported unprotected sex, and 55% reported using ATS. Overall, 88% were receiving HIV care, 83% were on antiretroviral therapy, 39% were retained in care at 12 months, and 23% were virally suppressed. SMARTgirl membership was independently associated with fourfold greater odds of 12-month retention in care (AOR = 4.16, 95% CI 1.38, 12.56). Those at high risk for an ATS use disorder had 91% lower odds of 12-month retention in care (AOR = 0.09, 95% CI 0.01, 0.72). Viral suppression was independently associated with SMARTgirl membership, older age, reporting of STI symptoms, worse symptoms of psychological distress, and greater numbers of sex partners.

Conclusions: This is the first study to characterize the HIV CoC in Cambodian FESW. While most women were successfully linked to HIV care, retention and viral suppression were low. Tailored programs like SMARTgirl, targeting the broader population of HIV-positive FESW as well as interventions to reduce ATS use could optimize the clinical and population health benefits of HIV treatment.

Trial registration This work reports data collected as part of a trial: NCT01835574. This work does not present trial results

*Correspondence: Pagek@salud.unm.edu
[7] Division of Epidemiology, Biostatistics and Preventive Medicine, Department of Internal Medicine, University of New Mexico, Albuquerque, NM, USA
Full list of author information is available at the end of the article

Keywords: HIV, Cambodia, Entertainment workers, Female sex workers, Amphetamines, HIV continuum of care, Treatment cascade

Background

HIV risk remains high in Cambodia among FESW. High numbers of sexual partners and non-injection ATS use are associated with elevated HIV risk and infection rates in this population [1–3]. Cambodia has achieved substantive progress in reducing the spread of HIV at a population level; the estimated number of new infections has fallen 95% from a peak of 24,348 in 1995 to 651 in 2015 [4]. Comprehensive deployment of basic HIV prevention programs including condom promotion, HIV voluntary counseling and testing, and high coverage of HIV antiretroviral treatment (ART), have contributed to these declines [5]. However, women engaged in entertainment and sex work remain disproportionately impacted [3]. In addition to individual risks, structural factors present challenges for HIV prevention among FESW. Anti-trafficking legislation aimed at suppressing human trafficking and sexual exploitation amplified HIV risks: brothel closures and migration of working women to entertainment venues and street-based sex work had negative impacts on access to HIV and STI prevention and health services [6]. Stigma, discrimination and violence further contribute to risk and negative health outcomes [7–9].

Cambodia has a national strategic goal of achieving elimination of new HIV infections by 2020. The National Center for HIV/AIDS, Dermatology and STI (NCHADS) Strategic Plan for HIV/AIDS and STI Prevention and Control in the Health Sector 2015–2020 outlines core phased strategies based on enhancing the HIV CoC including prevention, linkage and retention in care, enhanced quality of care and elimination of perinatal transmission [4]. The HIV CoC has been widely used to document engagement in care among people living with HIV [10]. The CoC includes measurable indicators from HIV detection through linkage and engagement in care and treatment. While measurement can vary, the framework can be applied widely or to key populations to inform HIV responses and document health disparities as it identifies losses at each step along the continuum [11–15]. CoC data on key populations, especially in FESW, are limited [16, 17].

The multiple circumstances and exposures that contribute to high risk for HIV infection in Cambodian FESW may also impact success along the HIV CoC. In particular, the high prevalence of problematic ATS use represents a major barrier to HIV treatment as prevention in this population. This is supported in part by prior research conducted predominantly in the United States (U.S.) where persons with HIV who use stimulants such as methamphetamine experience profound difficulties along the HIV CoC. People with HIV infection who use stimulants initiate ART at lower CD4 counts [18], are less likely to remain engaged in HIV care [19], and report difficulties with ART adherence that contribute to substantially elevated HIV viral load [18]. They may also experience faster disease progression [20, 21]. A threefold greater rate of AIDS-related mortality has been observed in crack-cocaine using women [22]. Women with HIV infection who use stimulants in the U.S. are also more likely to report engaging in HIV transmission risk behavior [23, 24], resulting in increased odds of onward HIV transmission where viral load is greater than 200 copies/mL [25]. We examine CoC outcomes among a sample of HIV-positive FESW participating in the Cambodia Integrated HIV and Drug Prevention Implementation (CIPI) Study being implemented in ten provinces in Cambodia [26, 27].

Study design and methods

Study sample and setting

In this paper, we restrict analyses to HIV-positive women who were enrolled in the CIPI Study. The CIPI Study targeted women at high risk of HIV infection in 10 provinces of Cambodia: female entertainment and sex workers (FESW). Specifics on the population and methods have been described in detail in a previous publication defining the protocol for the CIPI Study [26]. In brief, the study recruited and enrolled FESW who: (1) were biologically female; (2) aged ≥18 years; (3) reported ≥2 different sexual partners and/or transactional sex within the last month, (4) understood spoken Khmer language; and (5) were able to provide voluntary informed consent. Transactional sex was defined as exchanging sex for money, goods, or social favors. FESW work in a variety of venues including beer gardens, bars, massage, karaoke and other 'entertainment' establishments, as well as in other "freelance" venues including parks and guesthouses. In all provinces, CIPI outreach workers recruited women from multiple locations and locales where FESW were known to congregate or work. Outreach workers conducted a preliminary verbal screening for eligibility, described the study, answered questions, and invited women to attend the local study site (SMARTgirl Club) for eligibility evaluation and, if interested, study participation. HIV infection status and testing was not a criterion for participation in the CIPI study.

The CIPI Study was implemented within the SMARTgirl HIV prevention platform [26, 27], a widely disseminated 'standard of care' program launched nationally in 2008 to reduce HIV risk in women working in the high-risk entertainment sector [28]. SMARTgirl clubs exist in most provinces, and local community-based organizations maintain them and provide outreach to local women. The SMARTgirl program uses targeted communication tools and club events to disseminate health information, conduct and promote HIV testing, and referrals to health services including HIV care, sexually transmitted infection and reproductive health services. The CIPI Study integrated an ATS intervention and microenterprise opportunity within the existing SMARTgirl platform (described in [26, 27]).

Measures

At CIPI study visits, women were asked to complete an interviewer-administered survey regarding: sociodemographic information; work history including sex and entertainment work settings; sexual risk exposures, including number and types of partners, and condom use, and ATS exposures, both lifetime (at baseline) and in the past 3 months (at baseline and follow-up interviews); alcohol use, history of HIV testing and knowledge of antibody status; age and circumstances of first sex; experience of violence; health service utilization for HIV, STI and reproductive health; economic well-being; empowerment; and self-efficacy. ATS and alcohol use were assessed using the Alcohol Smoking and Substance Involvement Test (ASSIST), a validated screening measure for assessing alcohol and other substance use disorders [29]. Using validated cut off points for each substance use involvement score, the ASSIST indexes low, moderate, or high risk for the presence of disordered patterns of use. Psychological distress was assessed using the Kessler-10 (K-10), a validated, 10-item screening measure for mild, moderate, or severe distress that has shown superior validity in identifying depressive and anxiety disorders [30]. Each participant was instructed and asked to provide a urine specimen to be tested for ATS metabolites (i.e., methamphetamine and amphetamine). Urine is tested for adulteration using Specimen Validity Testing (SVT) (Innovation, Inc., San Diego, CA), and for ATS metabolites using the Innovacon Multi-Drug Screen Test Panel Dip Kit (Redwood Toxicology Laboratory, Inc., Santa Rosa, CA). Women were tested for prostate-specific antigen test (PSA), a biomarker of recent unprotected sex [31]. HIV testing was conducted at study entry (and subsequent visits) using a rapid antibody test in accordance with Cambodian National Guidelines, on women who consented to testing. Self-reported HIV testing history and results were obtained in interviews. We also linked all participants' names (with consent) to national records at the National Center for HIV, STD and Dermatology (NCHADS) to validate self-reported results, obtain results on participants who declined testing, and obtain date of first HIV detection for all women in the CIPI study, Participants who elected to receive HIV testing received concomitant HIV risk reduction counseling, and participants testing positive results were referred to HIV care services. Since HIV testing was voluntary within the CIPI study, review with NCHADS allowed us to examine and confirm HIV testing history on all women in the study. Time since HIV diagnosis was determined from this record review or for women who received a new HIV-positive results in the CIPI study, we used the date of that test to calculate the time since HIV diagnosis.

Detailed information on HIV CoC outcomes, including date of ART uptake and viral load was obtained through linking CIPI participant identifiers with SMARTgirl records and national surveillance data from NCHADS. We constructed a 5-stage HIV CoC with the following events: (1) diagnosed with HIV; (2) enrolled in HIV care; (3) initiation of ART; (4) retention in care for 12 months after initiating ART; and (5) viral suppression (i.e., HIV viral load less than 1000 copies/mL) [10, 12, 13]. Enrolled in HIV care was defined as having ever seen a medical practitioner (Nurse/Medical Assistant/MD) for HIV. ART initiation was defined as having started ART under the care of a medical practitioner. Retention was defined as having attended an appointment with an HIV medical practitioner within 12 months of ART initiation. NCHADS defines viral suppression as having at least one viral load test result less than 1000 copies/mL consistent with WHO guidelines [10].

Analyses

Cascade staging was assessed using both a "single" denominator (the number of HIV-positive women in the cohort) estimating loss as a proportion of those diagnosed, and with a "running" denominator wherein each indicator is assessed as a percent loss from the previous stage. The cascade figure was prepared using an "HIV States and Transitions" framework to summarize 'states' of participants within each state [13]. For bivariate analyses, we used Chi square and the Wilcoxon rank-sum tests, to test associations between categorical and continuous variables of interest, respectively, and CoC outcomes. Multivariable logistic regression analyses were performed to assess independent associations with 12-month retention in care following ART initiation as a primary outcome. Bivariate and multivariable analyses used robust standard errors. We also examined correlates of viral suppression as an exploratory outcome. Adjusting for time since HIV diagnosis, recent STI symptoms, and age at first sexual intercourse, factors were entered into a multivariable regression models if significantly associated ($p \leq 0.10$) in bivariate analyses, and retained if adjusted p values were ≤ 0.05. All statistical analyses were performed using Stata software, version 13.0 (StataCorp, College Station, TX).

Ethics

This study population experiences marginalization and is engaged in illegal behaviors. Sensitive behavioral and biological data were collected of this population. The study was conducted in compliance with ethical principles for human subjects research promoted by the Declaration of Helsinki developed by the World Medical Association [32]. Various procedures were adopted to ensure additional protection of all the women screened and enrolled in the trial including waiver of signed written informed consent. The consent process was conducted carefully to ensure potential participants understood the research objectives, procedures, risks and benefits, reimbursement, costs, and alternatives, and a short verbal assessment was conducted to ensure understanding. All women consented to have study information linked to NCHADS HIV records. The study protocol was reviewed and approved by the Cambodian National Ethics Committee, and the Institutional Review Boards (IRBs) of the University of California San Francisco and FHI360. The University New Mexico Health Sciences Center, University of Miami and University of New South Wales IRBs approved reliance agreements based on the UCSF IRB approval.

Results

Between June 2013 and May 2016, 88 (7.3%) women were identified with HIV infection among the 1198 who completed a baseline CIPI study visit. Their median age was 32 years (IQR 28, 35); 70.45% (n = 62) women reported being HIV infected at study entry, and 49 of these did not elect to be re-tested for HIV by the study. Twenty-six women who were identified as HIV positive on record linkage had self-reported either being HIV negative (N = 23) or never tested (N = 3), most (n = 18) also did not wish to be tested by the study. All women were aware that the study was working with NCHADS to obtain HIV results from testing conducted external to the CIPI Study. HIV-positive women were identified in all ten provinces participating in the CIPI study, but almost half (n = 41) were from two provinces: Phnom Penh (25%; n = 22) and Battambang (21.6%; n = 19). Over one-third (35%) reported never having attended school. Table 1 shows participant characteristics and risk exposures. Women were equally divided (50%) in reporting their primary work setting as either an entertainment venue or as free-lance/brothel based FESW. A majority (70%) were members of SMARTgirl, and 15% of members had attended a SMARTgirl club in the past month. All women (99%) reported multiple sex partners in the past 3 months. Unprotected sex in the past 3 months was reported by 38% of women. Twenty-eight women (32%) tested positive for PSA, indicating unprotected sex in the past 48 h. ATS use was prevalent by both self-report (55%) and urine screening (42%; indicating use in the past 48–72 h). We found 81% agreement between self-reported ATS use and ATS urine screening results. On the ASSIST, 51% scored moderate to high-risk for an ATS use disorder, and 51% were classified as being at similarly elevated risk for an alcohol use disorder. There were 27 (31%) participants that scored moderate or high-risk for clinically significant psychological distress on the K-10.

Figure 1 shows the HIV CoC. Of the 88 HIV-positive women, 88% (n = 77) were enrolled in care, 83% (n = 73) had initiated ART, 39% (n = 34) were retained in ART care at 12 months, and 23% (n = 20) were virally suppressed. The figure shows the proportions that advanced at each stage, and describes the "states" at each stage of the continuum. Using WHO guidelines [10], with a running denominator, we show that 59% of women who had been in care for 12 months were virally suppressed. Records from NCHADS showed that all women classified as virally suppressed (<1000 copies/mL), had undetectable viremia (<50 copies/mL).

Table 2 shows factors associated with 12-month retention in care after initiating ART. In multivariable analyses (Table 2), SMARTgirl membership was independently associated with fourfold greater odds of retention in care (Adjusted Odds Ratio (AOR) = 4.16, 95% CI 1.38, 12.56) compared to women who did not report membership. Women at high risk for an ATS use disorder based on ASSIST scores had 91% lower odds of 12-month retention (AOR = 0.09, 95% CI 0.01, 0.72). Women who reported any STI symptoms in the past 3 months had an elevated but not statistically significant adjusted odds of being retained in care, compared to those who did not report symptoms. Factors independently associated with viral suppression included age [per year increase; AOR 1.17 (95% CI 1.02, 1.34)]; number of sex partners in the past 3 months [per partner increase; AOR 1.01 (95% CI 1.00, 1.02)]; SMARTgirl membership [AOR 8.43; (95% CI 2.44, 29.09)]; self-reporting a sexually transmitted infection in the past 3 months [AOD 16.86 (95% CI 3.02, 94.09)], and scores indicating higher psychological distress on the Kessler (K10) scale (compared to low risk): AOR for Moderate Risk: 14.41 (95% CI 1.81–114.72); AOR for Severe Risk: 7.63 (95% CI 1.13, 51.45).

Table 1 Characteristics of HIV-positive FESW enrolled in the CIPI Study (N = 88)

Characteristic or exposure	N/median	(%)/IQR
Age (years)		
<20	1	(1)
20–29	27	(31)
30–39	55	(63)
≥40	5	(6)
SMARTgirl member (yes)	62	(70)
Length of time participant has been SMARTgirl member (months) (N = 62)		
<6	25	(40)
6–24	14	(23)
>24	23	(37)
SMARTgirl Club visit frequency in the past year (N = 58[a])		
≥1 time/month	9	(15)
<1 time/month	35	(60)
Never	14	(24)
Education (total years of school)		
None	31	(35)
Primary (1–6)	44	(50)
Secondary (7+)	13	(15)
Age of first sexual intercourse [median (IQR)]	18	(16–19)
Time since HIV diagnosis at baseline		
0, new infection[b]	29	(33)
1–12 month	18	(20)
>1–5 year	19	(22)
>5 year	22	(25)
Work setting (location worked most days in past month)		
Entertainment venue	44	(50)
Brothel/Freelance	44	(50)
Currently work for manager or boss (yes)	42	(48)
Income last month ($US)[c]		
<100	32	(36)
100–250	36	(41)
>250	20	(23)
Experienced food insecurity (last 3 months)		
Never	54	(61)
Rarely	16	(18)
Sometimes	8	(9)
Often	9	(10)
Experienced any physical or emotional violence (past 3 months)	47	(53)
Number of sexual of partners (last 3 months)		
<5	20	(23)
6–15	27	(31)
16–40	19	(22)
41–150	14	(16)
>150	8	(9)
Number of sexual partners [last 3 months; median (IQR)]	15	(6, 42.5)

Table 1 continued

Characteristic or exposure	N/median	(%)/IQR
Self-reported any unprotected sex (last 3 months)	33	(38)
PSA positive test	28	(32)
Self-reported use of ATS (past 3 months)	48	(55)
Tested for positive for ATS use at study visit	37	(42)
ATS ASSIST score		
<4	37	(42)
4–26	42	(48)
27+	9	(10)
Alcohol ASSIST score		
<11	37	(42)
11–26	33	(38)
27+	18	(20)
K10 Psychological distress (depression and anxiety)		
Low or No risk	37	(43)
Mild risk	23	(26)
Moderate risk	13	(15)
Severe risk	14	(16)
Self-reported symptoms of sexually transmitted infection (last 3 months)	19	(22)

[a] Restricted to the n = 58 SG members with non-missing data

[b] Time since diagnosis was determined by NCHADs records or as the date of testing from CIPI baseline for newly identified infections

[c] Average monthly household income in Cambodia in 2012 was US$56.53; in 2013, US$71.5; in 2014, US$89.98, and in 2015, US$91.14 (https://www.ceicdata.com/en/indicator/cambodia/annual-household-income-per-capita)

Discussion

This is the first study to characterize the HIV CoC in a group of Cambodian FESW. Although a high proportion of women were successfully linked and enrolled into HIV care, there were precipitous declines in the proportion who remained in care after initiating ART and achieving viral suppression: 43% of women who initiated ART were lost to follow up. These results are in stark contrast to estimates for the general Cambodian population, where 95% of those diagnosed and on ART are retained in care at 12 months [4]. Only one in four (23%) of the HIV-positive women in this study were virally suppressed. The proportion of women on ART who were virally suppressed (59%), however is not dissimilar to estimates in the general Cambodian population (64%) [4]. In contrast to other studies which include female sex workers, our results show that a high proportion were engaged in care and initiated treatment: 94% of those who enrolled in care initiated ART, compared to 28% in a recently published study of CoC outcomes in a South African FSW cohort [33]. Mountain et al. [17] show similar low rates of ART initiation in a meta-analysis of studies of FSW, with a pooled estimate of 39% ART initiation among ART eligible FSW in low and middle income countries. The proportion of virally suppressed

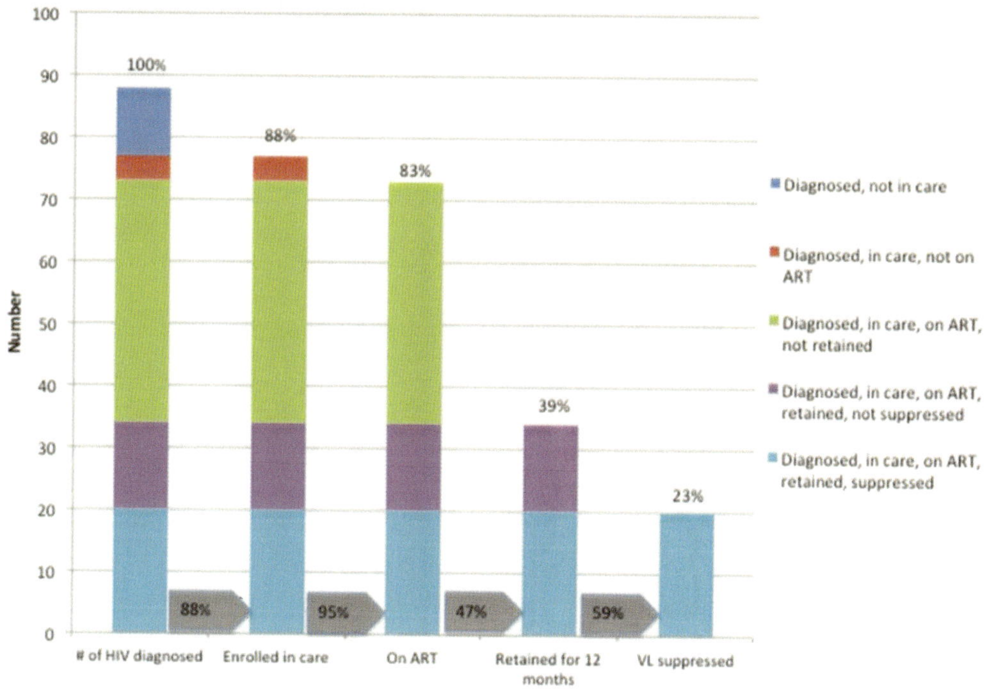

The figure illustrates five states in the Cascade of care. The proportions above the bars represent the % of all HIV infected women (fixed denominator) and the proportions between the bars (in the grey arrows) represent the % of women advancing by stage (running denominator).

Fig. 1 HIV cascade of care among FESW enrolled in the CIPI Study

participants in our study (59% of women retained) was similar (57%) to the pooled estimate in that study [17]. There are several potential reasons that FESW in Cambodia have poorer retention in care compared to the general population in Cambodia. Women working in the entertainment industry are very mobile, often moving between provinces, which likely impacts retention. Sex work is highly stigmatized in addition to being illegal in Cambodia, and some women may not feel that they can access care that is non-judgmental or responsive to their needs. That viral suppression in women in our sample who are engaged in care is comparable to that seen general population is encouraging. Expanded efforts targeting Cambodian FESW are clearly needed to optimize CoC indicators, especially the goal of successful engagement in care, which would contribute to reductions in HIV morbidity and mortality as well as decreased risk of onward HIV transmission in this high priority population. In Phnom Penh, there are currently two HIV clinics that serve key high-risk groups including FESW, and provide tailored services to women like space for their children during clinic visits. Expanding services that facilitate treatment engagement by FESW could will result in a higher proportion of women who achieve successful viral suppression.

Results also underscore the potential benefits of the SMARTgirl program for facilitating retention in care. SMARTgirl membership was associated with more than fourfold greater odds of 12-month retention after initiating ART, which highlights the potential benefits of continued implementation of SMARTgirl to optimize HIV treatment as prevention in this population. It was also associated with over eightfold higher odds of viral suppression. The SMARTgirl program, aimed at FESW, is designed to engage women in community HIV prevention efforts, principally by encouraging HIV testing and providing referrals to care for STIs and HIV infections. The SMARTgirl club and membership therein may be providing a larger platform for engagement and social mobilization [34] and which could be operationalizing broadly as a empowerment opportunity [35]. The broad reach of SMARTgirl could potentially be further leveraged as a platform to reach higher risk women, as has been done with the CIPI project [26], to implement multicomponent HIV prevention and care interventions.

Approximately half of participants screened positive for an ATS use disorder and/or an alcohol use disorder, and one-third screened with clinically significant psychological distress. Consistent with findings from the U.S. [19], those at highest risk for an ATS use disorder had 91% lower odds of 12-month retention after initiating ART. Expanded intervention approaches targeting ATS use, including conditional cash transfer with a

Table 2 Bivariate and multivariable results showing correlates of 12-month retention in HIV care among HIV-positive FESW enrolled in the CIPI study

Characteristic or risk exposure	12 Month retention in HIV Care (n = 34)					
	Bivariate			Multivariable		
	OR	95% CI	*p* value	AOR	95% CI	*p* value
Age (years)						
<20						
20–29	0.88	0.12, 6.29	0.90			
30–39	1.00	0.15, 6.55	1.00			
≥40	1.00	(ref[a])				
SMARTgirl member (yes)						
Yes	*2.75*	*0.96, 7.82*	*0.06*	*4.16*	*1.38, 12.56*	*0.01*
Length of time participant has been SMARTgirl member (months)						
<6	1.00	(ref)				
6–24	3.83	0.95, 15.36	0.06			
>24	1.95	0.60, 6.35	0.27			
SMARTgirl Club visit frequency in the past year						
≥ 1/month	1.00	(ref)				
<1/month	0.49	0.12, 2.00	0.32			
Never	0.28	0.06, 1.28	0.10			
Age of first sexual intercourse (years)	0.89	0.76, 1.03	0.13	0.84	0.70, 1.02	0.08
Time since HIV diagnosis (months)	1.00	0.99, 1.01	0.67	1.00	0.99, 1.01	0.52
Work setting: Brothel/Freelance based (vs. Entertainment venue)	1.21	0.51, 2.88	0.66			
Currently work for manager or boss	1.71	0.71, 4.08	0.23			
Income last month ($US)						
<100	1.00	(ref)				
100–250	0.64	0.24, 1.73	0.38			
>250	0.86	0.27, 2.68	0.79			
Food insecurity (last 3 months)						
Never	1.00	(ref)				
Rarely	1.32	0.42, 4.13	0.63			
Sometimes	1.02	0.22, 4.77	0.98			
Often	1.36	0.33, 5.71	0.67			
Experienced emotional or physical violence in the last 3 months	1.18	0.49, 2.80	0.71			
Number of sexual partners (self-reported, last 3 months)	1.00	1.00, 1.01	0.37			
Any unprotected sex (self-reported, last 3 months)	0.70	0.28, 1.72	0.43			
PSA positive test	0.66	0.26, 1.71	0.40			
Use of ATS (self-reported, past 3 months) (yes vs. no)	0.50	0.21, 1.21	0.12			
Tested for positive for ATS use at study visit (vs. negative)	0.52	0.21, 1.27	0.15			
ATS assist score						
<4	1.00	(ref)		1	(ref)	
4–26	0.89	0.36, 2.20	0.81	1.20	0.42, 3.38	0.72
27+	0.16	0.02, 1.45	0.11	*0.09*	*0.01, 0.72*	*0.02*
Alcohol assist score						
<11	1.00	(ref)				

Table 2 continued

Characteristic or risk exposure	12 Month retention in HIV Care (n = 34)					
	Bivariate			Multivariable		
	OR	95% CI	*p* value	AOR	95% CI	*p* value
11–26	0.51	0.19, 1.38	0.18			
27+	0.75	0.24, 2.37	0.62			
K10 Psychological distress						
Low or no risk	1.00	(ref)				
Mild risk	0.58	0.18, 1.83	0.35			
Moderate risk	2.63	0.71, 9.72	0.15			
Severe risk	0.91	0.25, 3.30	0.89			
STI symptoms (self-reported, last 3 mo)	2.08	0.74, 5.86	0.16	3.00	0.83, 10.81	0.09

Italic values indicate exposures found to be independently and significantly associated with 12-month retention in care

[a] ref = Referent group

cognitive-behavioral aftercare group are being tested as part of the CIPI trial [26, 27]. If this intervention proves effective in reducing ATS use, it could be more widely implemented using the SMARTgirl platform to address gaps in the HIV CoC among FESW. The high prevalence of psychiatric distress is noteworthy. Our findings are consistent with another recent study in a sample of FESW from Phnom Penh and Siem Reap, wherein almost half (43.2%) screened positive for psychological distress [36]. In our analyses of correlates of viral suppression, women with increased risk of psychiatric distress had higher odds of viral suppression. Further research should be done to examine this association, including the directionality and temporality of ART uptake and psychological well-being in FESW.

Multiple overlapping circumstances contribute to high HIV risk among Cambodian FESW, including individual sexual and drug risk exposures, low education and high poverty levels, and the negative impacts of public policy and policing [3]. In particular, violence serves as an important trigger for ATS use, and it is independently associated with unprotected sex among Cambodian FESW [6, 8, 9]. Central to many women's employment in entertainment venues is the requirement for highly sociable interactions with male customers and, for some women, this extends to transactional sex as an opportunity for income generation. ATS are used by many women to stay awake and work longer and see more clients, which also contributes to HIV risk [2, 37]. Expanded access to ART now joins the backbone HIV prevention platform of HIV testing, condom promotion and diagnosis, and treatment of STI as Cambodia aims for HIV elimination.

Our study has several limitations. First, the sample size is small, and results may not reflect the HIV CoC among all Cambodian FESW living with HIV. For some women we relied on self-report HIV status; however only women who reported a previous positive test were not tested by the study. Some (n = 26) women were diagnosed with HIV by the study, and although we obtained data after a year of diagnosis, including this recently diagnosed group could have led to conservative estimates of 12-month retention following ART initiation and viral suppression during this period. Viral suppression is defined in Cambodia as viral loads <1000 copies/mL, and this definition could potentially include women who had previously been virally suppressed, but who subsequently experienced breakthrough viremia and were no longer suppressed. The low numbers of viral suppression outcomes also impact risk estimates, and measures of excess risk found in multivariable analyses predicting this outcome should be interpreted with caution due to wide confidence intervals. This is an observational study, and the association seen with SMARTGirl membership should be interpreted with caution as this could reflect population characteristics rather than the effects of the program.

Despite these limitations, this study is the first to characterize the HIV CoC in Cambodian FESW, articulate the benefits of targeting this population for optimizing retention in HIV care, and identify ATS use as a risk factor for sub-optimal retention following ART initiation. These findings provide important information for sustaining and strengthening combination HIV prevention with this high priority population in order to eliminate HIV transmission in Cambodia by 2020.

There is increasing awareness that to meet the ambitious UNAIDS 90-90-90 HIV treatment targets and to get to zero new infections, efforts must be made to extend services and retain in care those who are most disenfranchised and at the highest risk for HIV disease progression and onward HIV transmission [38]. Improvements in the CoC states will optimize health outcomes and reduce

HIV transmission risk [39]. Targeting FESW who use ATS will optimize the benefits of ART treatment. Leveraging existing programmatic platforms such as SMART-girl, will enhance coverage to HIV-positive FESW, and potentially reduce attrition at all stages of the CoC.

Authors' contributions

The CIPI trial is part of a five-year research program led by KP and ESS. KP, AWC, JLE, LM, and CS conceived the research questions and designed the CIPI intervention with contributions from MS and SN. All authors were part of a trial design group led by KP. KP drafted the manuscript with contributions from MS, AWC, ESS, JLE, PM, LA, and LM. All authors commented on and approved the final version of the manuscript. All authors read and approved the final manuscript.

Author details

[1] FHI360, Phnom Penh, Cambodia. [2] Department of Epidemiology and Biostatistics, and Global Health, University of California, San Francisco, San Francisco, CA, USA. [3] Department of Mental Health and Substance Abuse, Ministry of Health, Phnom Penh, Cambodia. [4] National Authority for Combating Drugs, Phnom Penh, Cambodia. [5] Public Health Sciences and Psychology, University of Miami, Coral Gables, FL, USA. [6] The Kirby Institute for Infection and Immunity, UNSW Australia, Sydney, Australia. [7] Division of Epidemiology, Biostatistics and Preventive Medicine, Department of Internal Medicine, University of New Mexico, Albuquerque, NM, USA.

Acknowledgements

We are grateful to Amy Weissman for supporting the implementation of this project, Chhim Srean for coordinating data management in the field in its early phases and Hong Naysim for her invaluable work in the field as a supervisor and facilitator for the aftercare groups. We acknowledge the gracious and considerate involvement of the following organizations involved in data collection: Provincial Health Departments, Provincial AIDS and STI programs, Pre-ART/ART clinics in 10 provinces, Chouk Sar Association and the AIDS Health Foundation. We are indebted and grateful for the ongoing support of numerous non-governmental organizations involved in the implementation of this project including the Cambodian Women for Peace and Development, Phnom Srey Organization for Development, Poor Family Development and KHEMERA. Finally, this research would not be possible without the support from the Cambodia National Ministry of Health, Department Mental Health and Substance Abuse and the National Authority for Combating Drugs.

Competing interests

The authors declare that they have no competing interests.

Funding

The study is funded by the US National Institutes of Health (NIH), National Institute on Drug Abuse (1R01 DA033672; Page & Stein, PIs). The funder is not involved in the study design; collection, management, analysis and interpretation of data; writing of the report; and the decision to submit the report for publication. The content is solely the responsibility of the authors and does not necessarily represent the official views of the NIH. LM is supported by an Australian National Health and Medical Research Council (NHMRC) Senior Research Fellowship.

References

1. Couture MC, Sansothy N, Sapphon V, Phal S, Sichan K, Stein E, Evans J, Maher L, Kaldor J, Vun MC, et al. Young women engaged in sex work in Phnom Penh, Cambodia, have high incidence of HIV and sexually transmitted infections, and amphetamine-type stimulant use: new challenges to HIV prevention and risk. Sex Transm Dis. 2011;38(1):33–9.
2. Couture MC, Evans JL, Sothy NS, Stein ES, Sichan K, Maher L, Page K. Correlates of amphetamine-type stimulant use and associations with HIV-related risks among young women engaged in sex work in Phnom Penh, Cambodia. Drug Alcohol Depend. 2012;120(1–3):119–26.
3. Page K, Stein E, Sansothy N, Evans J, Couture MC, Sichan K, Cockroft M, Mooney-Somers J, Phlong P, Kaldor J, et al. Sex work and HIV in Cambodia: trajectories of risk and disease in two cohorts of high-risk young women in Phnom Penh, Cambodia. BMJ Open. 2013;3(9):e003095.
4. USAID: 2016 strategic direction summary Cambodia country operational plan. http://www.pepfar.gov/documents/organization/257617.pdf (2016). Accessed 4 Nov 2016.
5. Vun MC, Fujita M, Rathavy T, Eang MT, Sopheap S, Sovannarith S, Chhorvann C, Vanthy L, Sopheap O, Welle E, et al. Achieving universal access and moving towards elimination of new HIV infections in Cambodia. J Int AIDS Soc. 2014;17:18905.
6. Maher L, Dixon T, Phlong P, Mooney-Somers J, Stein E, Page K. Conflicting rights: how the prohibition of human trafficking and sexual exploitation infringes the right to health of female sex workers in Phnom Penh, Cambodia. Health Hum Rights. 2015;17(1):E102–13.
7. Maher L, Mooney-Somers J, Phlong P, Couture MC, Stein E, Evans J, Cockroft M, Sansothy N, Nemoto T, Page K. Selling sex in unsafe spaces: sex work risk environments in Phnom Penh, Cambodia. Harm Reduct J. 2011;8(1):30.
8. Draughon Moret JE, Carrico AW, Evans JL, Stein ES, Couture MC, Maher L, Page K. Young Women's Health Study C: the impact of violence on sex risk and drug use behaviors among women engaged in sex work in Phnom Penh, Cambodia. Drug Alcohol Depend. 2016;161:171–7.
9. Decker MR, Crago AL, Chu SK, Sherman SG, Seshu MS, Buthelezi K, Dhaliwal M, Beyrer C. Human rights violations against sex workers: burden and effect on HIV. Lancet. 2015;385(9963):186–99.
10. WHO: metrics for monitoring the cascade of HIV testing, care and treatment services in Asia and the Pacific. http://www.searo.who.int/entity/hiv/documents/metrics/en/ (2014). Accessed 1 Nov 2016.
11. MacCarthy S, Hoffmann M, Ferguson L, Nunn A, Irvin R, Bangsberg D, Gruskin S, Dourado I. The HIV care cascade: models, measures and moving forward. J Int AIDS Soc. 2015;18:19395.
12. Medland NA, McMahon JH, Chow EP, Elliott JH, Hoy JF, Fairley CK. The HIV care cascade: a systematic review of data sources, methodology and comparability. J Int AIDS Soc. 2015;18:20634.
13. Powers KA, Miller WC. Critical review: building on the HIV cascade: a complementary, "HIV States and Transitions" Framework for describing HIV diagnosis, care, and treatment at the population level. J Acquir Immune Defic Syndr. 2015;69(3):341–7.
14. Haber N, Pillay D, Porter K, Barnighausen T. Constructing the cascade of HIV care: methods for measurement. Curr Opin HIV AIDS. 2016;11(1):102–8.
15. Lourenco L, Colley G, Nosyk B, Shopin D, Montaner JS, Lima VD, Group SHAS. High levels of heterogeneity in the HIV cascade of care across different population subgroups in British Columbia, Canada. PLoS ONE. 2014;9(12):e115277.
16. Risher K, Mayer KH, Beyrer C. HIV treatment cascade in MSM, people who inject drugs, and sex workers. Curr Opin HIV AIDS. 2015;10(6):420–9.
17. Mountain E, Mishra S, Vickerman P, Pickles M, Gilks C, Boily MC. Antiretroviral therapy uptake, attrition, adherence and outcomes among HIV-infected female sex workers: a systematic review and meta-analysis. PLoS ONE. 2014;9(9):e105645.
18. Carrico AW, Riley ED, Johnson MO, Charlebois ED, Neilands TB, Remien RH, Lightfoot MA, Steward WT, Weinhardt LS, Kelly JA, et al. Psychiatric risk factors for HIV disease progression: the role of inconsistent patterns of antiretroviral therapy utilization. J Acquir Immune Defic Syndr. 2011;56(2):146–50.
19. Horvath KJ, Carrico AW, Simoni J, Boyer EW, Amico KR, Petroll AE. Engagement in HIV medical care and technology use among stimulant-using and nonstimulant-using men who have sex with men. AIDS Res Treat. 2013;2013:121352.

20. Carrico AW. Substance use and HIV disease progression in the HAART era: implications for the primary prevention of HIV. Life Sci. 2011;88(21–22):940–7.
21. Carrico AW, Shoptaw S, Cox C, Stall R, Li X, Ostrow DG, Vlahov D, Plankey MW. Stimulant use and progression to AIDS or mortality after the initiation of highly active antiretroviral therapy. J Acquir Immune Defic Syndr. 2014;67(5):508–13.
22. Cook JA, Burke-Miller JK, Cohen MH, Cook RL, Vlahov D, Wilson TE, Golub ET, Schwartz RM, Howard AA, Ponath C, et al. Crack cocaine, disease progression, and mortality in a multicenter cohort of HIV-1 positive women. AIDS. 2008;22(11):1355–63.
23. Morin SF, Myers JJ, Shade SB, Koester K, Maiorana A, Rose CD. Predicting HIV transmission risk among HIV-infected patients seen in clinical settings. AIDS Behav. 2007;11(5 Suppl):S6–16.
24. Molitor F, Truax SR, Ruiz JD, Sun RK. Association of methamphetamine use during sex with risky sexual behaviors and HIV infection among non-injection drug users. West J Med. 1998;168(2):93–7.
25. Rodger AJ, Cambiano V, Bruun T, Vernazza P, Collins S, van Lunzen J, Corbelli GM, Estrada V, Geretti AM, Beloukas A, et al. Sexual activity without condoms and risk of HIV transmission in serodifferent couples when the HIV-positive partner is using suppressive antiretroviral therapy. JAMA. 2016;316(2):171–81.
26. Page K, Stein ES, Carrico AW, Evans JL, Sokunny M, Nil E, Ngak S, Sophal C, McCulloch C, Maher L. Protocol of a cluster randomised stepped-wedge trial of behavioural interventions targeting amphetamine-type stimulant use and sexual risk among female entertainment and sex workers in Cambodia. BMJ Open. 2016;6(5):e010854.
27. Carrico AW, Nil E, Sophal C, Stein E, Sokunny M, Yuthea N, Evans JL, Ngak S, Maher L, Page K. Behavioral interventions for Cambodian female entertainment and sex workers who use amphetamine-type stimulants. J Behav Med. 2016;39(3):502–10.
28. FHI: SMARTgirl Program Review: providing HIV/AIDSI prevention and care for entertainmentworkers. https://www.fhi360.org/sites/default/files/media/documents/Program%20Review%20-%20SMARTgirl%2C%20Providing%20HIVAIDS%20Prevention%20and%20Care%20for%20Entertainment%20Workers%2C%20Reporting%20Period%20October%202008-June%202010.pdf. 2011.
29. Humeniuk R, Ali R, Babor TF, Farrell M, Formigoni ML, Jittiwutikarn J, de Lacerda RB, Ling W, Marsden J, Monteiro M, et al. Validation of the alcohol, smoking and substance involvement screening test (ASSIST). Addiction. 2008;103(6):1039–47.
30. Furukawa TA, Kessler RC, Slade T, Andrews G. The performance of the K6 and K10 screening scales for psychological distress in the Australian National Survey of Mental Health and Well-Being. Psychol Med. 2003;33(2):357–62.
31. Evans JL, Couture MC, Stein ES, Sansothy N, Maher L, Page K. Biomarker validation of recent unprotected sexual intercourse in a prospective study of young women engaged in sex work in Phnom Penh, Cambodia. Sex Transm Dis. 2013;40(6):462–8.
32. World Medical Association. Declaration of Helsinki. http://www.wmanet/en/30publications/10policies/b3/indexhtml (2014). Accessed 17 June 2014.
33. Schwartz S, Lambert A, Phaswana-Mafuya N, Kose Z, McIngana M, Holland C, Ketende S, Yah C, Sweitzer S, Hausler H et al. Engagement in the HIV care cascade and barriers to antiretroviral therapy uptake among female sex workers in Port Elizabeth, South Africa: findings from a respondent-driven sampling study. Sex Transm Infect 2016;93(4):290–296.
34. Lippman SA, Chinaglia M, Donini AA, Diaz J, Reingold A, Kerrigan DL. Findings from Encontros: a multilevel STI/HIV intervention to increase condom use, reduce STI, and change the social environment among sex workers in Brazil. Sex Transm Dis. 2012;39(3):209–16.
35. Shannon K, Strathdee SA, Goldenberg SM, Duff P, Mwangi P, Rusakova M, Reza-Paul S, Lau J, Deering K, Pickles MR, et al. Global epidemiology of HIV among female sex workers: influence of structural determinants. Lancet. 2015;385(9962):55–71.
36. Brody C, Chhoun P, Tuot S, Pal K, Chhim K, Yi S. HIV risk and psychological distress among female entertainment workers in Cambodia: a cross-sectional study. BMC Public Health. 2016;16(1):133.
37. Maher L, Phlong P, Mooney-Somers J, Keo S, Stein E, Couture MC, Page K. Amphetamine-type stimulant use and HIV/STI risk behaviour among young female sex workers in Phnom Penh, Cambodia. Int J Drug Policy. 2011;22(3):203–9.
38. UNAIDS: UNAIDS. 90-90-90: an ambitious treatment target to help end the AIDS epidemic. Geneva, Switzerland: UNAIDS, 2014. http://www.unaids.org/sites/default/files/media_asset/90-90-90_en_0.pdf. 2014.
39. Skarbinski J, Rosenberg E, Paz-Bailey G, Hall HI, Rose CE, Viall AH, Fagan JL, Lansky A, Mermin JH. Human immunodeficiency virus transmission at each step of the care continuum in the United States. JAMA Intern Med. 2015;175(4):588–96.

Insights from individuals successfully recovered from cannabis use disorder: natural versus treatment-assisted recoveries and abstinent versus moderation outcomes

David C. Hodgins* and Jonathan N. Stea

Abstract

Background: Increasing understanding of the pathways and processes of recovery from cannabis use disorder may help in designing effective and attractive interventions to promote recovery. We report insights from individuals who had successfully recovered from cannabis use disorder with a variety of pathways. Recovered individuals describe their perceptions of why they developed the problem, why they were successful in recovering, and the advice they would offer to individuals with similar problems.

Methods: Media announcements were used to recruit 119 volunteers who met lifetime but not past year criteria for cannabis use disorder. Participants were asked open-ended questions which were content analyzed and compared between individuals who whose recoveries were treatment-assisted (45%) versus natural (55%) and between individuals who were abstinent (57%) versus those who continued non-problematic consumption (43%).

Results: Participants most frequently described their problems as having developed due to the use of cannabis to *cope*, because of *environmental and social influences*, and *enjoyment of the positive effects*. Success in recovery was attributed to *focusing on reasons for change*, *goal commitment to change*, and *conquering denial/self-deception*. Treatment-assisted participants were more likely to perceive that they overcame their cannabis problem due to *treatment/self-help* and *conquering underlying issues*, whereas naturally recovered participants were more likely to describe *focusing on reasons for change*, *will power*, and *lost enjoyment/lifestyle change*. Treatment-assisted participants were more likely to recommend *seeking help/social support* and naturally recovered participants were more likely to endorse reflecting *on reasons for change*, *engaging in hobbies/distracting activities*, and *stimulus control/avoidance/change social environment*. The majority recommended professional treatment (79.1%) and self-help materials (76.9%), and a little over half (53.2%) would also recommend natural recovery.

Conclusions: These insights from people with lived experience further support previous research that treatment-assisted and natural recoveries are for the most part similar with respect to the recovery process. However, participants, whether or not they had had treatment involvement, recommended the use of treatment and self-help materials to sharpen their focus on the reasons to change and to enhance their commitment to change. At the same time, they saw value in the efforts of individuals to recovery without help.

Keywords: Cannabis, Marijuana, Cannabis use disorder, Natural recovery, Treatment, Recovery pathways

*Correspondence: dhodgins@ucalgary.ca
Department of Psychology, University of Calgary, 2500 University Drive NW, Calgary, AB T2N 1N4, Canada

Background

Rates of cannabis use and cannabis use disorder (CUD) are rising in North America, and CUD is a common presenting issue in addiction treatment [20, 32]. However, treatment-seeking rates are low relative to the numbers of people with the disorder [17] and rates of natural recovery are significant [3, 8]. Increasing our understanding of the pathways and processes of recovery may help in designing effective and attractive interventions to promote recovery.

A growing body of literature supports the efficacy of a variety of interventions for CUD [14]. However, only a few empirical studies of the recovery process from CUDs have been reported. Cunningham et al. [9] interviewed former frequent cannabis users about their reasons for stopping. The most common explanations included emotional maturation and taking on new roles and responsibilities. Boyd et al. [4] interviewed cannabis users who had quit using at least once in the past about change strategies. Participants described changing their environment to be the most helpful strategy and help from professionals as the least helpful strategy. Ellingstad interviewed a more defined group of former daily cannabis users who had quit for at least 1 year without the assistance of treatment [11]. The major reasons described for resolving their problem were increasingly viewing cannabis as negative, experiencing more negative effects, and change being related to a broader lifestyle shift. Strategies cited as helpful in quitting included involvement in activities unrelated to cannabis use, avoidance of triggers to use, and lifestyle changes. Finally, in the only prospective study, Swift et al. [30] followed a group of 200 long-term cannabis users for a 1-year period during which time nearly two-thirds attempted to reduce or stop using. The top reasons for these change attempts were physical or psychological health effects, boredom with using, concerns they were using too much, lack of money, and lifestyle circumstances.

One limitation of the existing research is that samples generally include individuals with relatively brief periods of reduction or cessation of use, and therefore, the results may not be relevant for understanding the longer-term recovery process, which typically occurs after multiple change attempts. The only study that focused on stable recoveries, specifically, is the Ellingstad study [11] of abstinent individuals who had naturally recovered (i.e., did not attend treatment). We extended this research by comparing the experiences of individuals who had recovered with and without the assistance of treatment, either though abstinence from any use or moderation of use [29]. The treatment-assisted and abstinence groups exhibited higher levels of lifetime severity of cannabis problems than the natural and moderation groups. This association between severity of problem and recovery pathways has been found for other addictive behaviours including alcohol, heroin, and gambling [3]. Interestingly, however, despite the different pathways to recovery, the motivators and processes of recovery were mostly similar for the different groups. Regardless of whether they sought treatment or not, or whether they become abstinent or moderated their use, recovered individuals most frequently described their motivations for tackling recovery as a conscious choice that was related to their cannabis use becoming incompatible with their self-image and lifestyle, and related to their use causing negative psychological concerns. They described relying most frequently on cognitive strategies such as thinking about the negative consequences of their use or the benefits of less use as well as a variety of behavioural strategies (decreasing time spent with other users, avoidance of cues to use, involvement in incompatible activities).

These descriptions of pathways and processes of recovery are potentially helpful in the development of treatment approaches and treatment system policies. For example, the association between severity and treatment pathway is consistent with the tenets of stepped care models that offer increasingly intense treatment for increasingly severe problems. However, given that the treatment processes appear similar in the different pathways, it is important to delve deeper into individual experiences for a more complete understanding of the recovery process. In the present report we describe further insights from individuals who have successfully recovered from cannabis use disorder, contrasting treatment-assisted and natural pathways, and abstinent and moderation outcomes. Comparing these groups potentially provides the broad perspective necessary to conceptualize treatment systems. Specifically, we summarize individual perceptions of why they developed the problem, why they were successful in recovering, and the advice they would offer to individuals with similar problems. The perspective of people with lived experience is increasingly recognized as central to planning interventions that are both effective and attractive [24].

Methods

Participants

Media announcements were used to recruit 119 volunteers for an in-person interview who met lifetime but not past year criteria for cannabis use disorder [2], according to the Composite International Diagnostic Interview (CIDI) [21]. Recruitment ads asked for individuals who were willing to share information about their recovery, which might be helpful in designing future treatment programs for other people. Other inclusion criteria were age 18 years and older, ability to read and write English, and willingness to refrain from any alcohol or illicit drug use for at least 8 h prior to the interview. In addition, participants were asked to provide, if possible, the name of a family member or friend who would be able to corroborate their cannabis use history.

The sample was 30% female and 70% male with a mean age of 37.3 years. The mean age of first use of cannabis was 14.7 years (SD = 3.0) and the mean age of onset of CUD was 20.0 years (SD = 6.5). The median length of recovery was 5 years. A history of treatment was reported by 53 individuals (45%). Sixty-eight (57%) were categorized as abstinent (no cannabis use for at least 12 months) and 51 (43%) reported some non-problematic use. Individuals reporting use most frequently reported using once or twice in the past 12 months (59%) or monthly (20%), although 6% reported weekly use and 16% almost daily use. Other demographic details are provided in Stea et al. [29] and Additional file 1: Table S1.

Interview

As the final section of a longer in-person interview that queried in detail cannabis use history, mental health comorbidity, and recovery efforts, and strategies, participants were asked a series of open-ended questions about the recovery process. Responses were probed for clarity and were recorded in writing by the interviewer. A number of areas were queried. First participants were asked: "What advice would you give to help another person with a marijuana problem"? Next they were asked whether they would recommend another person to reduce use to non-problematic levels or to quit completely (and why), and whether they would recommend that another person seek professional help or self-help materials or overcome the problem on their own without professional assistance. Participants were asked to describe their understanding of why they personally developed a marijuana problem, and finally, they were asked to describe their understanding of why they were able to overcome their problem. Participants could provide multiple responses to each question.

Data analysis

Responses were content analysed [5] with the aid of NVivo software [25]. An inductive approach was used as no a priori hypotheses were proposed. One individual derived categories reflecting responses to each of the above questions (JS), and then an independent rater used the category labels and a brief one sentence category description to code each response. Inter-rater reliability was assessed using percentage agreement and Kappa coefficients. Kappa greater than .80 was set as the minimum level of agreement a priori. Disagreements were resolved through discussion to provide a final categorization of each response. Frequency counts were calculated for the total sample, and for abstinence versus moderation subgroups (recovery use status), and the treatment-assisted versus natural recovery subgroups (recovery pathway), which were compared using Chi squared tests, with Bonferroni correction to the alpha level according to the number of categories. In the case where a significant result was obtained on a particular dependent variable for both recovery use status and recovery pathway, follow-up tests were conducted that controlled for the effects of each respective factor in order to elucidate the relationship with the dependent variable.

Results

Perceived etiology

Ten categories of perceived personal etiology were uncovered and interrater reliability was excellent (percent agreement = 89.8, Kappa = .88). Participants identified a mean of 1.6 (SD = 0.7) categories and group comparisons revealed no differences between the abstinence- ($M = 1.7$, $SD = 0.7$) and moderation ($M = 1.6$, $SD = 0.8$) recovery use status groups, F (1, 115) = 0.1, *ns*, or between the treatment-assisted ($M = 1.7$, $SD = 0.8$) and natural recovery ($M = 1.6$, $SD = 0.7$) pathways groups, F (1, 115) = 0.4, *ns*. Table 1 displays the percentage of participants that endorsed each category (Additional file 1: Table S2 provides category descriptions). The top three categories reported were: *used cannabis to cope* (43.7%), *environment/social influence* (41.2%), and *enjoyment/boredom/positive perceptions of cannabis* (23.5%). The category of *used cannabis to cope* reflected participant responses wherein cannabis was used to escape, self-medicate, and avoid emotional problems. The category of *environment/social influence* reflected participant responses wherein peer pressure and being around cannabis users was thought to contribute to the development of the cannabis problem. The category of *enjoyment/boredom/positive perceptions of cannabis* included enjoyment of the high, boredom, and positive perceptions of cannabis being helpful or fun in some way (e.g., mind enhancing/expanding, creating a philosophical and/or silly environment) was thought to contribute to the development of the cannabis problem.

While no differences emerged between the recovery use status, three differences emerged between the recovery pathway. Specifically, the treatment-assisted group was more likely to endorse the categories of *used cannabis to cope* (54.7 vs. 34.8%) and *genetics/predisposition* (20.8 vs. 1.5%), whereas the natural recovery group was more likely to endorse the category of *enjoyment/boredom/positive perceptions of cannabis* (31.8 vs. 13.2%). With a Bonferroni correction for 10 comparisons ($\alpha = .005$), only

Table 1 Percentage of participants that endorsed perceived etiology categories for the total sample and group comparisons

Category (%)	Total sample ($N=119$)	Recovery use status			Recovery pathway		
		AB ($n=68$)	MOD ($n=51$)	χ^2	TAR ($n=53$)	NR ($n=66$)	χ^2
Used cannabis to cope	43.7	47.1	39.2	0.7	54.7	34.8	4.7*
Environment/social influence	41.2	38.2	45.1	0.6	39.6	42.4	0.1
Enjoyment/boredom/positive perceptions of cannabis	23.5	20.6	27.5	0.8	13.2	31.8	5.7*
Addictive personality	14.3	11.8	17.6	0.8	17.0	12.1	0.6
Genetics/predisposition	10.1	14.7	3.9	3.7	20.8	1.5	12.0***
Habit/dependence/addiction	9.2	11.8	5.9	*ns*[i]	7.5	10.6	*ns*[i]
Loss of control	7.6	8.8	5.9	*ns*[i]	9.4	6.1	*ns*[i]
Cannabis per se causes the addiction	6.7	5.9	7.8	*ns*[i]	1.9	10.6	*ns*[i]
No problem actually existed	4.2	5.9	2.0	*ns*[i]	0.0	7.6	*ns*[i]
Denial/self-deception/ignorance/choice	3.4	1.5	5.9	*ns*[i]	3.8	3.0	*ns*[i]

Chi square values represent Pearson Chi square values. Absolute Chi square values are reported. *AB* abstinence; *MOD* moderation; *NR* natural recovery; *TAR* treatment-assisted recovery

[i] Fisher's exact test was used instead of Pearson Chi square because expected cell counts were less than 5

*$p<.05$; **$p<.01$; ***$p<.001$

the difference between the treatment-assisted group and the natural recovery group on the *genetics/predisposition* category remained statistically significant.

Perceived causes of recovery success

Twelve categories of participants' perceived causes of their recovery success showed excellent inter-rater reliability (percentage agreement = 83.3%, Kappa = .81, see Additional file 1: Table S3 for category descriptions). Participants identified a mean of 1.5 ($SD=0.8$) categories. Group comparisons on the mean number of categories revealed no differences between the abstinence- ($M=1.5$, $SD=0.7$) and moderation ($M=1.6$, $SD=0.8$) recovery use status groups, F (1, 115) = 0.1, *ns*, or between the treatment-assisted ($M=1.5$, $SD=0.7$) and natural recovery ($M=1.6$, $SD=0.8$) pathways, F (1, 115) = 0.2, *ns*. As can be seen in Table 2, the top three major categories reported by the total sample were: *focused on reasons for change* (36.1%), *goal commitment to change* (31.9%), and *conquered denial/self-deception* (25.2%). The category of *focused on reasons for change* reflected participant responses wherein recovery success was attributed to thinking about reasons for change and goal pursuit. The category of *goal commitment to change* reflected participant responses wherein recovery success was attributed to having strong motivation and commitment to change. The category of *conquered denial/self-deception* reflected participant responses wherein recovery success was attributed to a found sense of self-awareness or realization that cannabis was a problem.

While no differences emerged between the recovery use status groups, five differences emerged between the recovery pathways groups. Specifically, the treatment-assisted group was more likely to endorse the categories of *treatment/self-help* (24.5 vs. 4.5%) and *conquered underlying issues* (11.3 vs. 0.0%), whereas the natural recovery group was more likely to endorse the categories of *focused on reasons for change* (47.0 vs. 22.6%), *will power* (15.2 vs. 3.8%), and *lost enjoyment/lifestyle change* (13.6 vs. 1.9%). With a Bonferroni correction for 12 comparisons ($\alpha=.004$), only the difference between the treatment-assisted group and the natural recovery group on the *treatment/self-help* category remained statistically significant.

Recovery advice

Strategies

Content analysis was used to derive thirteen categories of hypothetical advice provided by participants to help another person with a cannabis problem. Excellent inter-rater reliability was obtained (percentage agreement = 91.0%, Kappa = .90, see Additional file 1: Table S4 for category descriptions). Participants identified a mean of 1.8 ($SD=1.7$) pieces of advice, with no differences between the abstinence- ($M=1.9$, $SD=0.9$) and moderation ($M=1.7$, $SD=0.9$) use status groups, F (1, 115) = 2.3, *ns*, or between the treatment-assisted ($M=1.7$, $SD=0.9$) and natural recovery ($M=1.9$, $SD=0.9$) groups, F (1, 115) = 0.8, *ns*. As can be seen in Table 3, the top three major advice categories reported by the total sample were: *seek help/social*

Table 2 Percentage of participants that endorsed perceived causes of recovery success categories for the total sample and group comparisons

Category (%)	Total sample ($N=119$)	Recovery use status			Recovery pathway		
		AB ($n=68$)	MOD ($n=51$)	χ^2	TAR ($n=53$)	NR ($n=66$)	χ^2
Focused on reasons for change	36.1	35.3	37.3	0.0	22.6	47.0	7.5**
Goal commitment to change	31.9	30.9	33.3	0.1	35.8	28.8	0.7
Conquered denial/self-deception	18.5	14.7	23.5	1.5	18.9	18.2	0.0
Treatment/self-help	13.4	16.2	9.8	1.0	24.5	4.5	10.1***
Religious/spiritual guidance	12.6	14.7	9.8	0.6	13.2	12.1	0.0
Will power	10.1	13.2	5.9	1.7	3.8	15.2	4.2*
Lost enjoyment/lifestyle change	8.4	5.9	11.8	*ns*[i]	1.9	13.6	*s**[i]
Social support	8.4	7.4	9.8	*ns*[i]	11.3	6.1	*ns*[i]
Stimulus control/avoidance/changed social environment	5.9	4.4	7.8	*ns*[i]	5.7	6.1	*ns*[i]
Conquered underlying issues	5.0	7.4	2.0	*ns*[i]	11.3	0.0	*s***[i]
Luck/lack of cravings or withdrawal	3.4	1.5	5.9	*ns*[i]	3.8	3.0	*ns*[i]
Helping others	1.7	2.9	0.0	*ns*[i]	0.0	3.0	*ns*[i]

Chi square values represent Pearson Chi square values. Absolute Chi square values are reported. *AB* abstinence; *MOD* moderation; *NR* natural recovery; *TAR* treatment-assisted recovery

[i] Fisher's exact test was used instead of Pearson Chi square because expected cell counts were less than 5

*$p<.05$; **$p<.01$; ***$p<.001$

Table 3 Percentage of participants that endorsed advice for the total sample and group comparisons

Category (%)	Total sample ($N=119$)	Recovery use status			Recovery pathway		
		AB ($n=68$)	MOD ($n=51$)	χ^2	TAR ($n=53$)	NR ($n=66$)	χ^2
Seek help/social support	37.8	47.1	25.5	5.8*	64.2	16.7	28.2***
Reflect on reasons for change	26.1	22.1	31.4	1.3	17.0	33.3	4.1*
Engage in hobbies/distracting activities	25.2	23.5	27.5	0.2	15.1	33.3	5.2*
Stimulus control/avoidance/change social environment	21.8	19.1	25.5	0.7	13.2	28.8	4.2*
Think positively	14.3	14.7	13.7	0.0	9.4	18.2	1.8
Face denial/self-deception	13.4	16.2	9.8	1.0	13.2	13.6	0.0
Change is a personal decision	11.8	13.2	9.8	0.3	7.5	15.2	*ns*[i]
Find underlying issue/motive for use	9.2	8.8	9.8	*ns*[i]	13.2	6.1	*ns*[i]
Quit	7.6	10.3	3.9	*ns*[i]	5.7	9.1	*ns*[i]
Research cannabis/addiction	5.0	4.4	5.9	*ns*[i]	5.7	4.5	*ns*[i]
Seek spiritual/religious guidance	5.0	7.4	2.0	*ns*[i]	3.8	6.1	*ns*[i]
Moderate use	2.5	4.4	0.0	*ns*[i]	3.8	1.5	*ns*[i]
Not sure/no answer	2.5	1.5	3.9	*ns*[i]	5.7	0.0	*ns*[i]

Chi square values represent Pearson Chi square values. Absolute Chi square values are reported. *AB* abstinence; *MOD* moderation; *NR* natural recovery; *TAR* treatment-assisted recovery

[i] Fisher's exact test was used instead of Pearson Chi square because expected cell counts were less than 5

*$p<.05$; **$p<.01$; ***$p<.001$

support (37.8%), *reflect on reasons for change* (26.1%), and *engage in hobbies/distracting activities* (25.2%). The category of *seek help/social support* reflected advice to seek a variety of forms of help, including from friends, family, and/or formal or professional help. The category of *reflect on reasons for change* included advice to think about the negative consequences of cannabis use, the reasons to change, and how life can be better without cannabis. The category of *engage in hobbies/distracting activities* reflected advice to occupy oneself via the pursuit of goals, hobbies, and other activities.

Several differences emerged among the groups. With respect to recovery status type, there was only one difference; the abstinence-oriented group was more likely to endorse the category of *seek help/social support* compared to the moderation-oriented group (47.1 vs. 25.1%); however, when recovery pathway was controlled for, there was no longer a significant relationship [treatment-assisted participants, χ^2 (1) = 3.2, *ns*; naturally recovered participants, χ^2 (1) = 0.2, *ns*]. With respect to recovery pathway, the treatment-assisted group was more likely to endorse the category of *seek help/social support* (64.2 vs. 16.7%)—this relationship remained significant after controlling for recovery use status [treatment-assisted participants, 72.2 vs. 18.8%, χ^2 (1) = 19.4, $p < .001$; naturally recovered participants, 47.1 vs. 14.7%, Fisher's exact test, *sig.*]—whereas the natural recovery group was more likely to endorse the categories of *reflect on reasons for change* (33.3 vs. 17.0%), *engage in hobbies/distracting activities* (33.3 vs. 15.1%), and *stimulus control/avoidance/change social environment* (28.8 vs. 13.2%). With a Bonferroni correction for 13 comparisons ($\alpha = .004$), only the difference between the treatment-assisted group and the natural recovery group on the *seek help/social support* category remained statistically significant.

Pathways

Participants were also asked to provide a number of recommendations about different recovery pathways, the results of which are displayed in Table 4. The majority of the total sample reported that they would recommend professional treatment (79.1%) and self-help materials (76.9%), and a little over half (53.2%) would recommend natural recovery (i.e., that a hypothetical person with a cannabis problem try to overcome the problem on their own without professional assistance). Interestingly, the moderation status group was significantly more likely to recommend natural recovery than the abstinent group (67.4 vs. 42.9%); however, when recovery pathway was controlled for, this relationship only remained significant among treatment-assisted participants (53.3 vs. 20.0%, Fisher's exact test, *sig.*), not naturally recovered participants [χ^2 (1) = 0.0, *ns*]. With respect to the recovery pathway group, the treatment-assisted group was significantly more likely to recommend self-materials

Table 4 Participant recommendations for the total sample and group comparisons

Variable	Total sample (*N* = 119)	Recovery use status			Recovery pathway		
		AB (*n* = 68)	MOD (*n* = 51)	χ^2	TAR (*n* = 53)	NR (*n* = 66)	χ^2
Recommend professional treatment for cannabis problem (% yes)	79.1[a]	79.1[b]	79.2[c]	0.0	86.5[d]	73.0[e]	3.1
Recommend self-help materials for cannabis problem (% yes)	76.9[f]	79.4	73.5[g]	0.6	86.8	68.8[h]	5.3*
Recommend natural recovery for cannabis problem (% yes)	53.2[j]	42.9[e]	67.4[k]	6.4*	30.0[l]	72.9[m]	20.0***
Recommend AB versus MOD (%)							
Quit	48.7	58.8	35.3	6.5*	62.3	37.9	7.0**
Depends on the person	24.4	19.1	31.4	2.4	17.0	30.3	2.8
Reduce/cut-back	19.3	13.2	27.5	3.8*	15.1	22.7	1.1
Neither or both	7.6	8.8	5.9	*ns*[i]	5.7	9.1	*ns*[i]

Chi square values represent Pearson Chi square values. Absolute Chi square values are reported. *AB* abstinence; *MOD* moderation; *NR* natural recovery; *TAR* treatment-assisted recovery

[i] Fisher's exact test was used instead of Pearson Chi square because expected cell counts were less than 5

[a] *n* = 115

[b] *n* = 67

[c] *n* = 48

[d] *n* = 52

[e] *n* = 63

[f] *n* = 117

[g] *n* = 49

[h] *n* = 64

[j] *n* = 109

[k] *n* = 46

[l] *n* = 50

[m] *n* = 59

*$p < .05$; **$p < .01$; ***$p < .001$

(86.8 vs. 68.8%), whereas the natural recovery group was significantly more likely to recommend natural recovery (72.9 vs. 30.0%); however, when recovery use status was controlled for, this latter relationship only remained significant among abstinence-oriented participants [71.4 vs. 20.0%, χ^2 (1) = 16.8, $p < .001$], not moderation-oriented participants (Fisher's exact test, *ns*).

When asked whether a person should reduce/cut-back or quit their cannabis use completely, the most popular response was to *quit* (48.7%), followed by *depends on the person* (24.4%), *reduce/cut back* (19.3%), and *neither or both* (7.6%). The abstinence-oriented group was significantly more likely to recommend that people quit (58.8 vs. 35.3%); however, when recovery pathway was controlled for, this relationship no longer remained significant [treatment-assisted participants, χ^2 (1) = 2.5, *ns*; naturally recovered participants, χ^2 (1) = 2.1, *ns*]. Moreover, the moderation status group was significantly more likely to recommend that people reduce/cut-back (27.5 vs. 13.2%). With respect to recovery pathway, the treatment-assisted group was significantly more likely to recommend that people quit compared to the natural recovery group (62.3 vs. 37.9%); however, when recovery status was controlled for, this relationship no longer remained significant [abstinence-oriented participants, χ^2 (1) = 3.6, *ns*; moderation-oriented participants, χ^2 (1) = 1.5, *ns*].

Discussion

Understanding the perceptions of people with lived experience about the development and resolution of a CUD is instructive in conceptualizing and promoting the process of recovery. Individuals with stable recoveries are one important informant group, but it is important that different experiences be represented, including different pathways and both abstinent and moderation outcomes. In this study, recovered individuals described their problems as having developed for multiple reasons, but in particular due to the use of cannabis to cope, because of environmental and social influences, and enjoyment of the positive effects. These perceptions align with research into the etiology of CUD insofar as coping motives for cannabis use have been found to be associated with the development of cannabis use disorders [6, 13]; environmental and social influences such as low parental monitoring, high peer group deviance, and cannabis availability have been found to predict cannabis initiation [15]; and perceived risk of harm has been found to be inversely associated with frequency of cannabis use [10, 12, 19]. Interestingly, we previously reported the responses of this sample to the Marijuana Motives Measure (MMM, [27]), which indicated that participants most often used cannabis for enhancement motives during their lifetime, followed by social, coping, expansion, and conformity motives [29]. This suggests that while participants believed that coping motives were the strongest contributor to the development of their cannabis problem, they more often used cannabis for other purposes (i.e., enhancement and social reasons), which highlights the pervasiveness of cannabis use during their lifetime.

Treatment-assisted participants were more likely to endorse *genetics/predisposition* compared to naturally recovered participants, whereas the latter group was more likely to endorse the reason of *enjoyment/boredom/positive perceptions of cannabis*. The fact that treatment-assisted participants more readily identified *genetics/predisposition* as an etiological category might reflect that they were taught this addiction model in treatment, but it is also possible that their CUDs were relatively and genuinely more influenced by genetic factors in light of their more frequent reports of family addiction problems [28]. There is indeed solid evidence that cannabis use and cannabis use disorders have heritable components [1, 33].

Participants were also asked to explain their understanding of why they were able to overcome their cannabis problem. The content analysis revealed that the top cited reasons were *focusing on reasons for change*, *goal commitment to change*, and *conquering denial/self-deception*. While there were no differences with respect to the recovery use status, treatment-assisted participants were more likely to perceive that they overcame their cannabis problem due to reasons of *treatment/self-help* and *conquered underlying issues*, whereas naturally recovered participants were more likely to cite the categories of *focused on reasons for change*, *will power*, and *lost enjoyment/lifestyle change*. These results suggest that participants attributed their recovery success to cognitive and motivational factors, which is consistent with our previous analyses demonstrating that cognitive strategies were the most helpful actions taken and maintenance factors involved in recovery [29]. These results support CBT-MET approaches to the treatment of CUDs [7, 14], and might suggest that an increased cognitive and motivational focus might be one way to improve psychosocial treatments [29].

Finally, participants were asked to provide advice and recommendations to help another hypothetical person with a cannabis problem. The top cited advice categories were to *seek help/social support*, *reflect on reasons for change*, and *engage in hobbies/distracting activities*. Interestingly, no differences emerged between the abstinence- and moderation-oriented participants. Whereas treatment-assisted participants were more likely to endorse the category of *seek help/social support* naturally recovered participants were more likely to endorse the categories of *reflect on reasons for change*, *engage in hobbies/distracting activities*, and *stimulus control/avoidance/change social environment*. These results differ from the advice provided by a sample of recovered gamblers participating in a treatment outcome study [31], whereby it was mostly indicated that there was nothing that could be done to aid in the decision to cease or reduce gambling, with a smaller proportion suggesting awareness-raising strategies (e.g., pointing out the negative consequences of problem gambling and arousing cognitive dissonance).

The majority of participants reported that they would recommend treatment and self-help materials to a hypothetical person with a cannabis problem. However, treatment-assisted participants were more likely to recommend self-help materials compared to naturally recovered participants, whereas the latter group was more likely to recommend natural recovery (i.e., try to resolve the cannabis problem without professional assistance), albeit only among those who were abstinent. Interestingly, moderation status participants who were treatment-assisted were more likely to recommend natural recovery than other participants, which might reflect a perceived lack of fit between their goals and the goals of the treatment program they attended. It is unclear to what extent these recommendations might be influenced in the future if moderation-focused treatments for cannabis use disorders become widely available. Additionally, the majority of participants reported that they would recommend abstinence to a hypothetical person with a cannabis problem, and not surprisingly, moderation status participants were more likely to recommend moderation compared to abstinent status participants.

These findings are limited in that the results are based on self-reports of volunteer participants. Use of open-ended questions with probing by interviews, and qualitative analysis is helpful given how little is known about the recovery process. However, it is impossible to know how representative these individuals are of the general recovery population, and how able individuals are at identifying recovery influences. In addition, although the cannabis use histories were corroborated by family and friend interviews [18], the findings are based upon participant retrospective attributions of events occurring a number of years ago. Assessing similar issues earlier in recovery may elicit somewhat different information.

Conclusions

It is timely and important that we attend to how to best promote recovery from CUD. With the recent trend towards cannabis decriminalization and legalization, it remains unclear to what extent these legal changes might impact the incidence of cannabis use disorders. While the majority of individuals who use cannabis will not develop a problem, a substantial minority of individuals who will develop a problem deserve greater access to non-stigmatizing and improved treatment options. With a view towards informing evidence-based clinical practice, the present study explored the recovery process from cannabis use disorders in the context of multiple recovery pathways, the findings of which hold a number of implications for policy and practice. These insights from people with lived experience further support previous research that treatment-assisted and natural recoveries are for the most part similar with respect to the recovery process, which is consistent with Klingemann's contention that there exists a shrinking gap between the natural recovery and treatment outcome literature [23]. The frequent attribution of the use of cannabis for coping with negative emotions reinforces the inclusion of emotional regulation training in treatment protocols and prevention efforts. The results for cannabis are also consistent with those for other substances, which supports the growing attention to transdiagnostic etiological and treatment models focusing on common elements [16, 22, 26].

However, participants, whether or not they had had treatment involvement, recommended the use of treatment and self-help materials to sharpen their focus on the reasons to change and to enhance their commitment to change. At the same time, they saw value in the efforts of individuals to recovery without help. As we have previously argued, these findings support the development of stepped care models that offer varying levels of support according to client wishes and needs [29]. Such models can include the provision of quality self-help materials by primary care providers and public health initiatives that promote self-directed efforts that are similar to treatment processes. The acknowledgement of moderation recovery outcomes within these models and self-help materials provides a more accurate and nuanced depiction of the recovery process, which might serve to de-stigmatize the non-isomorphic link between cannabis use and cannabis use disorder.

Authors' contributions

This research was conducted as part of a dissertation conducted by JS, under the supervision of DH. Both authors read and approved the final manuscript.

Acknowledgements

We appreciate the time and commitment of the volunteer participants.

Competing interests

The authors declare that they have no competing interests.

References

1. Agrawal A, Lynskey MT, Hinrichs A, Grucza R, Saccone SF, Krueger R, et al. A genome-wide association study of DSM-IV cannabis dependence. Addict Biol. 2011;16(3):514–8. https://doi.org/10.1111/j.1369-1600.2010.00255.x.
2. American Psychiatric Association. Diagnostic and statistical manual of mental disorders. 5th ed. Washington, DC: Author; 2013.
3. Bischof G, Rumpf HJ, John U. Natural recovery from addiction. In: Shaffer HJ, LaPlante DA, Nelson SE, editors. APA addiction syndrome handbook, vol. 2. Washington, D.C.: American Psychologial Association; 2012. p. 133–55.
4. Boyd SJ, Tashkin DP, Huestis MA, Heishman SJ, Dermand JC, Simmons MS, Gorelick DA. Strategies for quitting among non-treatment-seeking marijuana smokers. Am J Addict. 2005;14(1):35–42. https://doi.org/10.1080/10550490590899835.
5. Braun V, Clarke V. Using thematic analysis in psychology. Qual Res Psychol. 2006;3:77–101.
6. Bujarski SJ, Norberg MM, Copeland J. The association between distress tolerance and cannabis use-related problems: the mediating and moderating roles of coping motives and gender. Addict Behav. 2012;37(10):1181–4. https://doi.org/10.1016/j.addbeh.2012.05.014.
7. Copeland J, Gates P, Pokorski I. A narrative review of psychological cannabis use treatments with and without pharmaceutical adjunct. Curr Pharm Des. 2016;22(42):6397–408. https://doi.org/10.2174/1381612822666160831094811.
8. Cunningham JA. Untreated remissions from drug use: the predominant pathway. Addict Behav. 1999;24(2):267–70.
9. Cunningham JA, Toneatto T, Koski-Jannes A. Why do people stop their drug use? Results from a general population survey. Contemp Drug Probl. 1999;26:695–710.
10. Dennis M, Babor TF, Roebuck MC, Donaldson J. Changing the focus: the case for recognizing and treating cannabis use disorders. Addiction. 2002;97:4–15.
11. Ellingstad TP, Sobell LC, Sobell MB, Eickleberry L, Golden CJ. Self-change: a pathway to cannabis abuse resolution. Addict Behav. 2006;31(3):519–30. https://doi.org/10.1016/j.addbeh.2005.05.033.
12. Foster KT, Arterberry BJ, Iacono WG, McGue M, Hicks BM. Psychosocial functioning among regular cannabis users with and without cannabis use disorder. Psychol Med. 2017. https://doi.org/10.1017/S0033291717003361.
13. Fox CL, Towe SL, Stephens RS, Walker DD, Roffman RA. Motives for cannabis use in high-risk adolescent users. Psychol Addict Behav. 2011;25(3):492–500. https://doi.org/10.1037/a0024331.
14. Gates PJ, Sabioni P, Copeland J, Le Foll B, Gowing L. Psychosocial interventions for cannabis use disorder. Cochrane Database Syst Rev. 2016;5:CD005336. https://doi.org/10.1002/14651858.cd005336.pub4.
15. Gillespie NA, Neale MC, Legrand LN, Iacono WG, McGue M. Are the symptoms of cannabis use disorder best accounted for by dimensional, categorical, or factor mixture models? A comparison of male and female young adults. Psychol Addict Behav. 2012;26(1):68–77. https://doi.org/10.1037/a0026230.
16. Griffiths MD. Components model of addiction within a biopsychosocial framework. J Subst Use. 2005;10:191–7. https://doi.org/10.1080/14659890500114359.
17. Hasin DS, Grant B. NESARC findings on increased prevalence of marijuana use disorders-Consistent with other sources of information. JAMA Psychiatry. 2016;73(5):532. https://doi.org/10.1001/jamapsychiatry.2015.3158.
18. Hodgins DC, Stea JN. Psychometric evaluation of a lifetime version of the Marijuana Problems Scale. Addict Behav Rep. 2018;8:21–4. https://doi.org/10.1016/j.abrep.2018.05.001.
19. Johnston LD, Miech RA, O'Malley PM, Bachman JG, Schulenberg JE, Patrick ME. Monitoring the future. National survey results on drug use 1975–2017: overview. Key findings on adolescent drug use. Ann Arbor: Institute for Social Research, Univeristy of Michigan; 2018.
20. Kerridge BT, Mauro PM, Chou SP, Saha TD, Pickering RP, Fan AZ, et al. Predictors of treatment utilization and barriers to treatment utilization among individuals with lifetime cannabis use disorder in the United States. Drug Alcohol Depend. 2017;181:223–8. https://doi.org/10.1016/j.drugalcdep.2017.09.032.
21. Kessler RC, Ustun TB. The world mental health (WMH) survey initiative version of the world health organization (WHO) composite international diagnostic interview (CIDI). Int J Methods Psychiatr Res. 2004;13(2):93–121.
22. Kim HS, Hodgins DC. Component model of addiction treatment: a pragmatic transdiagnostic treatment model of behavioral and substance addictions. Front Psychiatry. 2018 **(in press)**.
23. Klingemann H, Sobell MB, Sobell LC. Continuities and changes in self-change research. Addiction. 2010;105(9):1510–8. https://doi.org/10.1111/j.1360-0443.2009.02770.x.
24. Nelson G, Macnaughton E, Curwood SE, Egalite N, Voronka J, Fleury MJ, et al. Collaboration and involvement of persons with lived experience in planning Canada's At Home/Chez Soi project. Health Soc Care Community. 2016;24(2):184–93. https://doi.org/10.1111/hsc.12197.
25. NVivo. NVivo qualitative data anlysis software. Version 9.0: QSR International Pty, Ltd. 2010.
26. Shaffer HJ, LaPlante DA, Labrie JW, Kidman RC, Donato AN, Stanton MV. Toward a syndrome model of addiction: multiple expressions, common etiology. Harvard Rev Psychiatry. 2004;12:367–74.
27. Simons J, Correia CJ, Carey KB, Borsari BE. Validating a five-factor marijuana motives measure: relations with use, problems, and alcohol motives. J Couns Psychol. 1998;45(3):265–73. https://doi.org/10.1037/0022-0167.45.3.265.
28. Stea JN (2013). Recovery from cannabis use disorders: abstinence versus moderation and treatment-assisted recovery versus natural recovery. (PhD), University of Calgary, Calgary.
29. Stea JN, Yakovenko I, Hodgins DC. Recovery from cannabis use disorders: abstinence versus moderation and treatment-assisted recovery versus natural recovery. Psychol Addict Behav. 2015;29(3):522–31. https://doi.org/10.1037/adb0000097.
30. Swift W, Hall W, Copeland J. One year follow-up of cannabis dependence among long-term users in Sydney, Australia. Drug Alcohol Depend. 2000;59(3):309–18.
31. Toneatto T, Dragonetti R. Effectiveness of community-based treatment for problem gambling: a quasi-experimental evaluation of cognitive-behavioral vs. twelve-step therapy. Am J Addict. 2008;17(4):298–303. https://doi.org/10.1080/10550490802138830.
32. United Nations Office on Drugs and Crime. 2014 world drug report. Vienna: United Nations; 2014.
33. Verweij KJ, Zietsch BP, Liu JZ, Medland SE, Lynskey MT, Madden PA, et al. No association of candidate genes with cannabis use in a large sample of Australian twin families. Addict Biol. 2012;17(3):687–90. https://doi.org/10.1111/j.1369-1600.2011.00320.x.

Patterns of HIV testing, drug use, and sexual behaviors in people who use drugs: findings from a community-based outreach program in Phnom Penh, Cambodia

Gitau Mburu[1], Chanrith Ngin[2], Sovannary Tuot[2], Pheak Chhoun[2], Khuondyla Pal[2] and Siyan Yi[2,3*]

Abstract

Background: People who use drugs are an important priority for HIV programs. However, data related to their utilization of HIV services are limited. This paper reports patterns of HIV testing, drug use, and risk and service perception among people who use drugs. Study participants were receiving HIV and harm reduction services from a community-based program in Phnom Penh, comprised of itinerant peer-led outreach and static drop-in centers.

Methods: This was a mixed-methods study conducted in 2014, comprising of a quantitative survey using a structured questionnaire, followed by two focus group discussions among a sub-sample of survey participants. Participants were recruited from hotspots in five HIV high-burden communes using a two-stage cluster sampling method. Quantitative descriptive analyses and qualitative thematic analyses were performed.

Results: This study included 151 people who use drugs with a mean age of 31.2 (SD = 6.5) years; 77.5% were male and 39.1% were married. The most common drugs used were methamphetamines (72.8%) and heroin (39.7%), and 38.0% injected drugs in the past 3 months. Overall, 83.3% had been tested for HIV in the past 6 months, of whom 62.5% had been tested by peers through community-based outreach. However, there were ongoing HIV risks: 37.3% were engaging in sex on drugs, only 35.6% used a condom at last sexual intercourse, and 10.8% had had a sexually transmitted infection in the last 6 months. Among people who reported injecting drugs in the past 3 months, 27.5% reported re-using needles/syringes. Almost half (46.5%) perceived themselves as being at lower risk of HIV compared to the general population. Qualitative results contextualized the findings of low perception of HIV risks and suggested that although services were often unavailable on weekends, at night, or during national holidays, peer-led community-based outreach was highly accepted.

Conclusions: A peer-led community-based approach was effective in reaching people who use drugs with HIV and harm reduction interventions. To mitigate ongoing HIV risks, expanding access to combination prevention interventions and implementing strategies to enable people who use drugs to objectively assess their HIV risks are required. Additionally, community-based programs should collect data along the care continuum, to enable decentralized tracking of progress towards 90–90–90 goals at local levels.

Keywords: 90–90–90 targets, HIV testing, HIV risk, People who use drugs, People who inject drugs, Cambodia

*Correspondence: siyan@doctor.com
[2] KHANA Center for Population Health Research, No. 33, Street 71, Phnom Penh, Cambodia
Full list of author information is available at the end of the article

Background

Prompt HIV diagnosis, timely linkage to care, early treatment, retention in care, and sustained viral suppression are all essential for optimal impact of antiretroviral therapy (ART) in reducing morbidity and mortality from human immunodeficiency virus (HIV) [1–4]. The time-sensitive sequencing of clinical and operational events that commence with an HIV diagnosis and end with long term viral suppression epitomize the continuum of HIV care [5].

However, significant loss to follow-up of people living with HIV occurs in the various steps between HIV testing and viral suppression [6, 7], resulting in an undesirable cascade [5]. Hence, a paradigm shift focusing on proportions of people living with HIV that are tested, linked to care, retained in care, adherent to ART, and achieving sustained viral suppression is increasingly framing outcomes of HIV care. The UNAIDS 90–90–90 targets, which aim to ensure that 90% of all people living with HIV know their status, 90% of all diagnosed people living with HIV receive ART, and 90% of all persons receiving ART achieve viral suppression [8], capture this paradigm shift.

Achievement of these global goals will depend on their attainment among all people living with HIV and key populations including people who use drugs [9]. People who use drugs constitute one of the most vulnerable populations to HIV. Unsafe drug use accounts for a third of newly diagnosed HIV infections outside sub-Saharan Africa [10], and 10% of all HIV infections globally [11]. Drug use is particularly widespread in Asia [12], and its impact on HIV is increasing [13]. In Cambodia, where the national HIV prevalence is 0.3% among the general population, people who use drugs are disproportionately affected, with a prevalence of 4.0% among people who use non-injecting drugs and 24.8% among individuals who inject them [14].

Given the importance of people who use drugs in the global HIV epidemic, it is essential that early testing, linkage, retention, and viral suppression are achieved among these groups. Currently, however, very few countries are well poised to attain the 90–90–90 targets in people who use drugs by 2020. A recent review revealed a significant lack of data related to HIV care continuum among people who use drugs. In the few countries where data are available, care outcomes among people who use drugs are significantly below 90–90–90 targets [9]. Individual studies have reported that people who use drugs have low rates of ART coverage [15], HIV testing [9], adherence [16], retention [17], and viral suppression [9, 17]. Although contextual differences exist, these poor outcomes are generally caused by a range of individual, social, legal, health system, and other structural barriers [13, 18, 19]. In addition, effective models for promoting the widespread reach and entry of people who use drugs into HIV care are generally limited globally [20].

Cambodian national response has placed an emphasis on key populations, including people who use drugs, in order to achieve the 90–90–90 target and eliminate new HIV infections under Cambodia 3.0 [21]. A recent review reported that, of the estimated 72,607 people living with HIV, 60,336 (83%) are diagnosed, 54,769 (75%) are receiving ART, and 50,935 (70%) are virally suppressed. As such, Cambodia is one of the few countries on track to achieve 90–90–90 targets [22]. However, this review did not evaluate care continuums for specific populations (e.g., key populations), which—authors assert—would more directly inform programming strategies for these populations [22].

In Cambodia, there are still gaps in the data and strategic information on the HIV situation and response, in particular among key affected populations [23]. The national estimated number of people who use non-injecting drugs and people who inject drugs was 13,000 and 1300, respectively [14]. However, precise 90–90–90 estimates among these populations are unavailable. Like many other countries, strategic information in each step along the continuum for people who use drugs is limited [14]. One of the five key objectives of the National Strategic Plan on Harm Reduction is strengthening the strategic information base [23].

In this paper, we report patterns of HIV testing, drug use, and sexual behaviors among people who use drugs who were receiving HIV and harm reduction services from a community-based HIV program in Phnom Penh. We also report their self-perception of HIV risk and views regarding community-based services they were receiving, in order to provide information that could improve services for this population. We conclude this paper with a brief discussion of the potential implications of our findings in relation to 90–90–90 targets in Cambodia.

Methods

Study design

This was a mixed-methods study that was composed of a large quantitative cross sectional survey, with a smaller qualitative component comprising focus group discussions (FGDs).

Study settings

The research was conducted among people who use drugs in Phnom Penh, who were in contact with a community-based program known as Sustainable Action against HIV and AIDS in Communities (SAHACOM). SAHACOM was implemented over a 5-year period ending in December 2014, focusing on key populations [24, 25]. The project was implemented by KHANA, a leading HIV non-governmental organization working through numerous community-based organizations (CBOs).

The project utilized a community-based approach to empower and create ownership of the project among key populations, including people who use drugs. The model was composed of itinerant peer-based outreach, and static drop-in centers. Through this model, key population peers were hired by CBOs to provide HIV and harm reduction services to people who use drugs, including HIV education, condoms, clean needles, and syringes. Through peer involvement, the model transformed people who currently or formerly used drugs from passive service recipients to active providers of services [26].

Besides providing the above services in their own localities, peers referred people who use drugs to the static drop-in centers, which were part of community-level infrastructure, where methadone, harm reduction counselling, peer discussions, personal care, needles, syringes, and condoms, among other commodities, were provided. In addition, people who use drugs in contact with the outreach teams were encouraged to form and attend peer discussions at drop-in centers for education purposes.

At the end of the implementation period, data were collected to assist in evaluation of the project. The purpose of the evaluation was to understand the HIV testing and prevention needs of the participants, and their perception of the SAHACOM services. Mixed methods were used to allow contextualization of quantitative survey data. This is a widely used approach of linking quantitative and qualitative data within implementation research [27, 28].

Participant selection

By the time the SAHACOM was implemented, the estimated total number of people who use drugs in Phnom Penh was 4188; of these 1068 injected drugs. In Phnom Penh, SAHACOM was implemented in 33 communes with high concentration of people who use drugs out of 96 communes in the city. Although accurate general population size for these communes was not available, strategic information related to HIV suggested that these 33 communes covered approximately 1969 people who use drugs, of whom 353 injected drugs. A two-stage cluster sampling method was used to select participants for the quantitative component. At the first stage, the research team identified five communes with at least 20 people who use drugs to be included in the study. A list of 'hotspots' where people who use drugs and congregated was made based on geographical clustering of high risk behaviors as is practiced elsewhere [29]. At the second stage, all people who use drugs in the selected hotspots were approached and invited to participate in the study, and were screened for eligibility.

Potential participants were included in the study if they: (1) were at least 18 years of age, (2) had used any form of illicit drugs in the past 3 months, (3) were able to present themselves on the day of the interview, and (4) were able to provide informed consent to participate in the study. Of the 192 people screened, 22 were excluded, leaving 170 eligible participants. For the qualitative component, a convenience-based subsample was selected from the primary participants in the quantitative phase. At the end of quantitative data collection, participants were invited to take part in focus group discussions based on interest, convenience, availability, and willingness to consent. The participant selection process is illustrated in Fig. 1.

Study tools development

The quantitative questionnaire was developed in English, translated into Khmer, back-translated to English, and pretested to ensure that it was culturally suitable and clearly understandable. Standardized questions were adapted from previous studies and Demographic and Health Surveys [14, 30, 31] to document participants' socio-demographic characteristics (e.g. age, sex, marital status, education, occupation, income, residence, and mobility), drug use characteristics (e.g. age of initiation, frequency, method and types and circumstances of drug use, sharing of needles or syringes, as well as history of drug-related arrests and voluntary rehabilitation or incarceration/imprisonment), HIV-related characteristics (e.g. prior HIV testing, venue of HIV testing and counselling, and sources of HIV education), sexual behaviors (e.g. sexual activity, number of sex partners, consistency of condom use, history of STI symptoms, whether STI treatment was sought, and nature of facility from which treatment for STI was sought), and self-perceived risk of HIV. To get a sense of participants' self-perceived risk of HIV, participants were asked to indicate whether they thought they were at lower, same, or higher risk, relative the general population.

Similarly, a topic guide for qualitative focus groups was developed in English, translated into Khmer, back-translated to English, pretested, and adjusted accordingly following piloting. The objective of the qualitative component was to contextualize and provide insights to the quantitative findings. The focus group topic guide questions were open ended and explored participants' drug use behaviors, HIV testing experiences, sexual behaviors, perceived risk of HIV, and perception of services they were receiving through the SAHACOM.

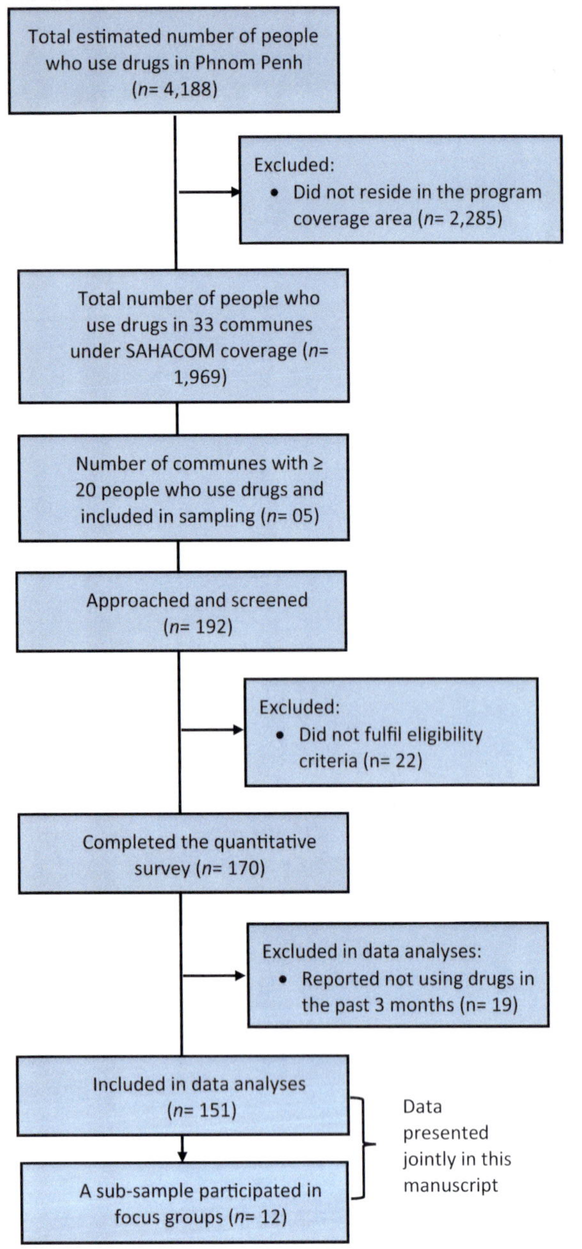

Fig. 1 Participant selection process

Data collection

Data were collected by researchers in private rooms in drop-in centers. Before data collection, researchers were provided with an overview of the study objectives and trained on the questionnaire filling techniques including error checking, focus group facilitation, privacy assurance, confidentiality, and data protection. Questionnaires were administered face-to-face to 170 participants, each lasting 30–45 min. At the end of survey questionnaires, participants were invited to participate in the focus groups.

Interested and consenting participants were provided with appointment schedules to attend the discussions. Invitation to take part in the focus groups was not based on types of drugs used, as long as participants had participated in the quantitative survey. In total, two focus group sessions, each with six participants, were conducted on the premises of CBOs. Recruitment for the focus groups was guided by saturation of themes, rather than by prespecified sample size as recommended in qualitative studies [32]. At the end of the second focus group session, it was clear that additional discussions would not yield further insights and recruitment was halted. The focus groups lasted 45–60 min, were tape-recorded, and were conducted in the local Khmer language.

Data analyses

Quantitative data were coded and entered into a computer using Epi Data version 3 (Odense, Denmark). Double data entry was performed to limit errors. Logic checks were performed, and 19 participants who reported that they had not used any illicit drugs in the past 3 months were excluded from the analyses. Summary of frequencies for nominal and ordinal variables was documented. Descriptive analyses were used to compute means for continuous variables. SPSS version 20.0 (IBM Corporation, New York, USA) was used for all data analyses.

Qualitative audio data were transcribed and transcripts translated to English from Khmer and imported into NVivo (QSR International). Thematic data analysis [33] was then conducted inductively within the original aims of the study, in order to provide context for the quantitative findings regarding sexual and injecting behaviors, nature of services received by participants, and participants' perception of those services. Nodes were created, and populated with appropriately labelled codes. Codes were populated with textual segments refined using constant comparison approach [34], and then categorized based on similarities to generate overarching themes [32, 33]. Verbatim quotes were extracted from participants' transcripts and displayed in the text to aid transparency of interpretation as recommended [35]. Qualitative text and quotes were presented alongside quantitative data in order to contextualize or explain survey findings in an integrated fashion [36].

Ethical considerations

This study was approved by the National Ethics Committee for Health Research (No. 082NECHR). Verbal consent was obtained from each participant. Before consenting, participants were informed of their right to discontinue their participation at any time, without any consequences. Names and contact information of the researchers were provided to participants for use in case they had any questions. Identifiable data were not collected on questionnaires; instead, unique codes were utilized in order to protect confidentiality of participants. Participant were compensated approximately US$5 for their time and transport to participate in the study.

Results

Socio-demographic characteristics

In total, 151 people who use drugs participated in the survey, whose mean age was 31.2 (SD = 6.5) years; a subsample of whom (n = 12) participated in the focus groups. Of the total participants, 77.5% were male; 39.1% were married, 40.4% were single, and 20.5% were either divorced or widowed. In addition, 14.6% were unemployed, and the sample was generally non-migratory, having lived in their current locations for a mean of 19 years (Table 1).

Drug use practices

As shown in Table 2, 38.0% of the total participants had injected drugs in the past 3 months. On average, participants started using drugs at the age of 21.3 (SD = 6.5) years, and had used drugs for the past 8.4 years. The most common drugs used were amphetamines (72.8%) and heroin (39.7%). Although most participants used drugs either with friends (54.4%) or alone (31.1%), a notable proportion (14.5%) used drugs with their sexual partners. More than half (55.3%) of the overall sample had been referred to a rehabilitation center in their lifetime, and 21.9% had been sent to the center in the past 12 months. A third (31.3%) had ever been incarcerated/imprisoned due to drug possession and other offences.

Table 1 Socio-demographic characteristics of participants

Variables	Number (%)
Mean age (years, ±SD)	31.2 ± 6.5
Gender	
Male	117 (77.5)
Female	34 (22.5)
Marital status	
Married	59 (39.1)
Divorced, widow	31 (20.5)
Single	61 (40.4)
Mean years of schooling completed (±SD)	5.2 ± 4.1
Main occupation	
Unemployed	22 (14.6)
Laborer	33 (21.9)
Self-employed business	45 (29.8)
Office worker	10 (6.6)
Other	41 (27.2)
Monthly income (US$, ±SD)	313.7 ± 601.0
Currently living with:	
Parents	41 (27.2)
Spouse/partner	60 (37.7)
Friend/colleagues	19 (12.6)
Siblings/relatives	14 (9.3)
Alone	17 (11.3)
Mean length of residency in Phnom Penh (in months, ±SD)	233.6 ± 149.3

SD standard deviation

Less than a third (27.5%) of participants who injected drugs in the past 3 months reported that they had used a needle that had been used by someone else the last time they injected. Contextualizing this finding a participant explained that, "we *stopped sharing syringe...we try to prevent it*" (respondent # 1, focus group 1), while another asserted that, "*we take a methadone regularly, stopped injecting and stopped sharing syringes*" (respondent # 4, focus group 1). Participants mentioned that peer educators were an important source of syringes for the participants. Besides commodity supplies, participants relied on peer educators for "*transportation service to get methadone*" (respondent # 4, focus group 1).

However, participants raised concerns regarding a lack of supplies on weekends or other days when national holidays and ceremonies were being held. One participant asserted that, "*on Saturday and Sunday, if we don't have, we need to buy*" (respondent # 6, focus group 1), because as explained by another participant, "*they just don't work at weekends but Monday to Friday they come to meet people at local*" (respondent # 5, focus group 1). Participants also explained that re-using or sharing needles was common at night when getting syringes or needles was limited:

> "*Sometimes, people inject around 12 or 1 at night, so during that time no one comes to provide you syringes or needles*" (respondent # 2, focus group 2).

Despite this gap in service provision, participants asserted the value of outreach suggesting that, "*they do not come and provide services all the time; however, their services reduce the cost of our expenses*" (respondent # 2, focus group 1).

HIV counselling and testing

As shown in Table 3, 96.0% had ever been tested for HIV in lifetime, and 83.3% had received an HIV test in the past 6 months. In addition, 97.2% had received counselling during their most recent HIV test. A majority (62.5%) of the HIV testing was delivered through community- or peer-initiated counseling and testing, with a minority (9.0%) having been provided through voluntary counseling and testing centers. In addition, 86.6% had received HIV education in the past 12 months, and although most participants received this information

Table 2 Drug use practices among the study participants

Variables	Number (%)
Type of drugs used in the past 3 months	
Methamphetamines	110 (72.8)
Heroin	60 (39.7)
Other (ecstasy, sniffed glue, marijuana, etc.)	5 (3.3)
Mean duration of drug use (months, ±SD)	103.8 ± 68.7
Mean age at first time of illicit drug use (years, ±SD)	21.3 ± 6.5
Frequency of illicit drug in the past 3 months	
Everyday	77 (51.3)
Almost everyday	21 (14.0)
A few times a month	24 (16.0)
A few times a week	27 (18.0)
People with whom you used drugs the last time	
Alone	47 (31.1)
Friend	82 (54.4)
Sexual partner/sweetheart	22 (14.5)
Reason to led you try illicit drugs for the first time	
I tried it by myself	45 (29.8)
Someone gave it to me or forced me to use it	6 (4.0)
Tried it with friends	81 (53.6)
Other	19 (12.6)
Injected drugs in the past 3 months	57 (38.0)
Used a used needle when injected drugs the last time ($n = 57$)	14 (27.5)
Shared needles at last drug injection ($n = 57$)	8 (15.7)
Perceived that needle/syringes are easy to find ($n = 57$)	50 (87.7)
Have been arrested for drug use or trafficking	70 (46.4)
Have ever been sent to a drug rehabilitation center	83 (55.3)
Have been sent to a rehabilitation center in the past 1 year	33 (21.9)
Had ever been incarcerated/imprisoned	50 (33.1)
Main cause of most recent incarceration/imprisonment	
Drug use or possession	11 (22.4)
Drug-related crimes (e.g. theft)	31 (63.3)
Other crimes (non-drug related)	7 (14.3)

from several different sources, the most common source of HIV education was peer educators or outreach workers (89.2%). These qualitative data suggested that community-based outreach program was an important source of HIV education, counselling and testing which was relatively acceptable to participants.

Contextualizing these findings, qualitative focus groups supported the view that HIV testing and education provided by peers and outreach workers were acceptable to participants. Referring to these peers and outreach workers, a focus group participant affirmed that, "*they help us to know that we are reactive HIV.... if we are HIV positive we go to get ART*" (respondent # 1, focus group 2). This participant further commented that, "*the organization always comes to educate us.*" (respondent # 1 focus group 2), while others contrasted access to testing in health facilities by asserting that they found outreach services easily accessible "*because they come two times per day*" (respondent # 6, focus group 2).

Table 3 Access to HIV counselling, testing, and education

Variables	Number (%)
Ever tested for HIV	144 (96.0)
Tested for HIV in the past 6 months ($n = 144$)	120 (83.3)
Place for last HIV testing ($n = 144$)	
Voluntary counseling and testing center	13 (9.0)
Community/peer-initiated testing	90 (62.5)
Public health center/clinic/hospital	31 (21.5)
Private clinic/hospital	10 (6.9)
Received result of the most recent HIV test ($n = 144$)	143 (99.3)
Received counseling for the last HIV test ($n = 144$)	139 (97.2)
Received HIV education in the past 12 months	129 (86.6)
Source of HIV education in the past 12 months ($n = 129$)	
Mass media (television/radio/newspaper)	60 (46.2)
Poster/billboard	34 (26.2)
Peer educator or outreach worker	116 (89.2)
Voluntary counseling and testing session	28 (21.5)
Health staff	43 (33.1)
Self-perceived level HIV risk compared to the general population	
Higher	52 (36.1)
Same	19 (13.2)
Lower	67 (46.5)
Don't know	6 (4.2)

HIV human immunodeficiency virus

Sexual behaviors

As shown in Table 4, 37.3% of the participants reported having sex while intoxicated with drugs. In addition, 10.8% had been diagnosed with an STI in the past 6 months. At the same time, 41.1% reported having been involved in sexual intercourse in the past 3 months, and only 35.6% reported using a condom in their last sexual intercourse act.

Table 4 Sexual behavior among the study participants

Sexual behaviors	Number (%)
Diagnosed with an STI in the past 6 months	16 (10.8)
Sought treatment for most recent STI symptom ($n = 16$)	2 (11.1)
Facility where the most recent STI was treated	
Public health center/hospital ($n = 2$)	1 (50.0)
Non-governmental clinic/hospital ($n = 2$)	1 (50.0)
Had sexual intercourse in the past 3 months	59 (41.3)
Used condom in last sexual intercourse ($n = 59$)	21 (35.6)
Had sexual intercourse when intoxicated ($n = 59$)	22 (37.3)

STI sexually transmitted infections

Qualitative data provided additional insights regarding the inconsistent condom use. In particular, narratives from the focus groups suggested that participants did not believe that they needed to use condoms with their spouses because they trusted them. Asked why they were not using condoms, participants responded by saying that, *"I trust my wife"* (respondent # 6, focus group 1), *"Yes, I believe my wife"* (respondent # 5, focus group 1), among other similar responses.

HIV risk perception

As shown in Table 3, a majority of participants (56.5%) viewed themselves to be at the same or lower risk of HIV infection compared to the general population. Although there were other reasons for not using condoms, such as a *"desire to have a child"* (respondent # 3, focus group 1), the finding of low condom use among the sample is relevant as it corroborates the low self-perception of HIV risk among the participants. While responding to a question regarding whether he thought he was at risk of HIV, a participant stated that, *"I have only my wife, I don't have any other partners"* (respondent # 4, focus group 1), showing that participants viewed HIV risk as external to themselves and their drug-using behaviors.

Further exploration of this issue in the focus groups suggested that participants believed that their increased knowledge was contributing to their protection from HIV, and they were no longer at high risk of HIV. When asked whether they thought their group was a high-risk group, participants contrasted the previous lack of knowledge with their current situation, stating that:

> *"Firstly, we didn't have a support from NGOs, secondly we don't have a counseling from NGOs and that made us lack knowledge about health care or prevention, so it made us a high risk group"* (respondent # 5, focus group 2).

This participant, who belonged to a specific peer discussion group of drug users in one of the drop-in centers went on to state that:

> *"Now, I think my group is a low-risk group, because we have a lot of knowledge from NGOs that come to educate us"* (respondent # 5, focus group 2).

These sentiments were supported by others who emphasized the changes in risks occurred due to the changes in sexual and injecting behaviors, primarily due to increased supply of harm reduction commodities. In a typical response regarding why they thought they were at low risk of HIV, a participant stated that, "previously, we didn't have condoms to use and didn't have any NGOs coming to provide them" (respondent # 2, focus group 2). Others also referred to condoms, stating that their HIV risk was reduced "because we have NGOs who taught about using condoms; now we know how to use it, especially to prevent STIs" (Respondent # 6, FGD 1).

Apart from availability of condoms, few participants also referred to availability of clean syringes as giving them a sense that they were at low risk. For instance, one participant mentioned that, "as for now, we do not have any disease because we use new syringes" (respondent # 1, focus group 1). As can be noted from the above excerpts, participants felt that, apart from knowledge per se, their use of preventive interventions was protecting them from HIV. Within these discussions, it emerged that the use of these comodities was enhanced by their free provision:

> *"Now we have NGOs to provide them, it isn't like before when we didn't have and we needed to buy"* (respondent # 4, focus group 1).

Discussion

This paper describes important information regarding access to HIV testing among people who use drugs. The study reports a high level of access to HIV testing in the context of ongoing injecting and sexual risks, and in a country where a quarter of people who inject drugs (24.8%) are HIV infected [14]. The high proportion of participants who had ever been tested (96.0%), or were tested in the last 6 months (83.3%) is notable given the generally low rates of testing among people who use drugs reported from other settings [9, 37, 38].

A number of factors may have contributed to this observation, the most likely being the model of community-based outreach, which embraced the deployment of community support volunteers, peer facilitators, and peer educators to provide services. The majority of those who were tested accessed testing from these peer providers rather than voluntary counseling and testing centers. The proportion of participants tested for HIV was high despite the perceived low risk of HIV. This approach may also have mitigated transport, administrative, attitudinal, and trust-related barriers which deter testing of people who use drugs in conventional health facilities [39, 40].

The utilization of drop-in centers and community-level infrastructure to provide methadone, personal care, counselling and education, needles, syringes, condoms, and other commodities may have synergistic effects on the uptake of these HIV and harm reduction interventions. Qualitative findings suggested that methadone was perceived as providing opportunities to reduce drug injecting, while increasing uptake of clean needles and syringes.

These findings endorse the use of methadone to mitigate risks [41, 42], and the use of community-based outreach model for providing integrated HIV and harm-reduction services [43]. Other studies have shown that the use of socially familiar infrastructure, such as community-based drop-in centers can act in synergy with the use of peer counsellors or educators or outreach workers to enhance HIV testing, entry into HIV care, and uptake of harm-reduction interventions [20, 39, 44, 45].

In spite of the close contact with peer-based outreach services, our findings highlighted ongoing risks of HIV infection among the study sample. Study participants believed that their knowledge of HIV and adoption of safer injecting practices reduced their risk of HIV. While this might be the case, participants were still exposed to significant risks. The low perceived level of risk, combined with a low rate of condom use among those who are sexually active, engagement in sex while intoxicated, and the occasional sharing of needles, operate together to escalate potential for HIV infection.

These enduring risks suggest a need for additional prevention interventions and delivery strategies tailored to participants' risk profile. For instance, despite the advantages of peer outreach model, a lack of outreach services over weekends, nights, and bank holidays increased risky injecting behaviors. While firm conclusions may not be made about the impact of these gaps, these findings suggest a need for innovative methods such as self-dispensing or vending machines for needles and syringes for participants who encounter these temporal shortages. On the other hand, PrEP might be useful in situations where condom use is intended but does not occur, which is relevant for couples, given that almost half of the participants were in stable relationships yet condom use with spouses was sub-optimal.

In addition, a sixth of participants used drugs with their sexual partners, further lending weight to other calls that testing and prevention services should be extended to sexual partners of people who use drugs [46]. Use of methamphetamine and other drugs during sex, colloquially termed 'chemsex,' is associated with higher sexual HIV transmission risks [47, 48], and requires to be addressed through specifically tailored information. Given the noted disconnect between perceived risks and actual HIV risk behaviors, further expansion of the scope of HIV education is required to enable participants objectively assess and understand their HIV risks. For instance, models of estimating actual risks [49] could be incorporated into educational efforts.

Limitations of the study

The study involved participants who were already in contact with peer outreach. It is therefore possible that this recruitment bias may have affected our results related to participants' uptake of HIV testing and perception towards peer-led community-based outreach. A reason for the finding that participants held the perception that they had lower HIV risk compared to the general population may have related to their recent HIV testing. Moreover, the proportion of participants who were already HIV positive was not known as participants were not required to divulge their HIV status. Consequently, the relationship between recent test results and risk perception could not be explored in this study. All participants were recruited in Phnom Penh, limiting generalizability to other people who use drugs nationally. Participants in the focus groups were selected based on convenience, which may exacerbate this selection bias. Despite application of eligibility criteria designed to retain participants that were currently using drugs, a small minority reported they had not used any form of illicit drugs in the past 3 months. More broadly, the methodology used in this study largely depended on participants self-reporting, and some participants skipped some questions, which may have introduced further limitations.

Implications for future research

Despite these limitations, our findings are consistent with research in Cambodia and elsewhere showing the effectiveness of community-based outreach in reaching people who use drugs [20, 50]. While this study reports on uptake of HIV testing, downstream data on linkage and retention on ART was unavailable, yet are central in the care continuum. Besides, the extent to which the program contributed to achievement of the first 90 in the 90–90–90 targets cannot be deduced because of lack of denominators and prior rates of testing. This is due to lack of local level strategic information regarding numbers of people at risk. Nationally, past efforts predominantly focused on increasing HIV testing, with significant limited focus on the continuum on local levels [23]. This was certainly the case in 2014 when this study was conducted [23].

However, the Health Sector Strategic Plan IV (2015–2020) includes strategies for improving the strategic information base as one of its cross-cutting strategy. Generation of localized data will enable programs monitor their contributions to 90–90–90 targets better, within their catchment areas. In addition, focus on the care continuum is central to the relatively recent approach—known as Boosted Continuum of Prevention to Care and Treatment—which aims to identify and reach new infections, ensure they are brought into care, and are retained in ART. This approach is targeted specifically to areas where new infections are occurring, among key populations, and should therefore be central to future community-based outreach programming and research.

Conclusions

The findings of this study demonstrate that utilization of peer outreach and community infrastructure familiar and close to people who use drugs such as drop-in centers could contribute to increasing uptake of HIV testing and other harm reduction interventions among these populations. Although the uptake of testing, needles, and syringes was high in this study, outstanding HIV risks were identified. Additional strategies are required to ensure that people at risk are enabled to have an objective understanding of their HIV risks and vulnerabilities of people who use drugs are mitigated in the study context.

Authors' contributions

SY and ST developed the study protocol and tools. GM, SY, and CN wrote the manuscript. ST, PC, and KP were responsible for data collection and data entry. ST, PC, KP, and CN supported study design, protocol development, and analyses of the study findings. All authors read and approved the final manuscript.

Authors' information

GM (MB.Ch.B, MPH) is a researcher at the Division of Health Research, Lancaster University, the United Kingdom. ST (MA) is Research Manager; PC (MPH) and KP (MHSc) are Research Fellow; and CN (Ph.D.) is Senior Research Advisor at KHANA Center for Population Health Research, Cambodia. SY (MD, MHSc, Ph.D.) is Director of KHANA Center for Population Health Research, Cambodia and Adjunct Professor at Touro University California, the United States.

Author details

[1] Division of Health Research, Lancaster University, Lancaster, UK. [2] KHANA Center for Population Health Research, No. 33, Street 71, Phnom Penh, Cambodia. [3] Center for Global Health Research, Touro University California, Vallejo, CA, USA.

Acknowledgements

Authors thank all participants, implementing partners and KHANA staff who made this study and the SAHACOM project possible. The SAHACOM project was funded by the United States Agency for International Development (USAID). Disclaimer: Content of this paper is the responsibility of the authors and does not reflect the view of USAID or our respective institutions.

Competing interests

The authors declare that they have no competing interests.

Funding

This study was financially supported by the United States Agency for International Development (USAID).

References

1. Ulett KB, Willig JH, Lin HY, Routman JS, Abroms S, Allison J, et al. The therapeutic implications of timely linkage and early retention in HIV care. AIDS Patient Care STDS. 2009;23(1):41–9.
2. Lundgren JD, Babiker AG, Gordin F, Emery F, Grund B, INSIGHT START Study Group, et al. Initiation of antiretroviral therapy in early asymptomatic HIV infection. N Engl J Med. 2015;373(9):795–807.
3. Mugavero MJ, Amico KR, Westfall AO, Crane HM, Zinski A, Willig JH, et al. Early retention in HIV care and viral load suppression: implications for a test and treat approach to HIV prevention. J Acquir Immune Defic Syndr. 2012;59(1):86–93.
4. Mellors JW, Munoz A, Giorgi JV, Margolick JB, Tassoni CJ, Gupta P, et al. Plasma viral load and CD4+ lymphocytes as prognostic markers of HIV-1 infection. Ann Intern Med. 1997;126(12):946–54.
5. Hill A, Pozniak A. HIV treatment cascades: how can all countries reach the UNAIDS 90–90–90 target? AIDS. 2015;29(18):2523–5.
6. Mugglin C, Estill J, Wandeler G, Bender N, Egger M, Gsponer T, et al. Loss to programme between HIV diagnosis and initiation of antiretroviral therapy in sub-Saharan Africa: systematic review and meta-analysis. Trop Med Int Health. 2012;17(12):1509–20.
7. Rosen S, Fox MP. Retention in HIV care between testing and treatment in sub-Saharan Africa: a systematic review. PLoS Med. 2011;8(7):e1001056.
8. Sidibe M, Loures L, Samb B. The UNAIDS 90–90–90 target: a clear choice for ending AIDS and for sustainable health and development. J Int AIDS Soc. 2016;19(1):21133.
9. Risher K, Mayer KH, Beyrer C. HIV treatment cascade in MSM, people who inject drugs, and sex workers. Curr Opin HIV AIDS. 2015;10(6):420–9.
10. Joint United Nations Programme on HIV/AIDS (UNAIDS). The gap report: people who inject drugs. Geneva: UNAIDS; 2014. p. 2015.
11. Mathers BM, Degenhardt L, Phillips B, Wiessing L, Hickman M, Strathdee SA, et al. Global epidemiology of injecting drug use and HIV among people who inject drugs: a systematic review. Lancet. 2008;372(9651):1733–45.
12. Aceijas C, Stimson GV, Hickman M, Rhodes T. Global overview of injecting drug use and HIV infection among injecting drug users. AIDS. 2004;18(17):2295–303.
13. UNAIDS. Global report. UNAIDS report on the global AIDS epidemic 2013. Geneva: UNAIDS; 2013.
14. Chhea C, Heng S, Tuot S. National population size estimation, HIV related risk behaviors, HIV prevalence among people who use drugs in Cambodia in 2012. Phnom Penh: National Authority for Combating Drugs and KHANA; 2014.
15. Mathers BM, Degenhardt L, Ali H, Wiessing L, Hickman M, Mattick RP, et al. HIV prevention, treatment, and care services for people who inject drugs: a systematic review of global, regional, and national coverage. Lancet. 2010;375(9719):1014–28.
16. Malta M, Magnanini MM, Strathdee SA, Bastos FI. Adherence to antiretroviral therapy among HIV-infected drug users: a meta-analysis. AIDS Behav. 2010,14(4):731–47.
17. Weber R, Huber M, Battegay M, Stahelin C, Castro Batanjer E, Calmy A, et al. Influence of noninjecting and injecting drug use on mortality, retention in the cohort, and antiretroviral therapy, in participants in the Swiss HIV Cohort Study. HIV Med. 2015;16(3):137–51.
18. Degenhardt L, Mathers BM, Wirtz AL, Wolfe D, Kamarulzaman A, Carrieri MP, et al. What has been achieved in HIV prevention, treatment and care for people who inject drugs, 2010–2012? A review of the six highest burden countries. Int J Drug Policy. 2014;25(1):53–60.
19. Tindal C, Cook K, Foster N. Theorising stigma and the experiences of injecting drug users in Australia. Aust J Prim Health. 2010;16(2):119–25.
20. Hayashi K, Wood E, Wiebe L, Qi J, Kerr T. An external evaluation of a peer-run outreach-based syringe exchange in Vancouver, Canada. Int J Drug Policy. 2010;21(5):418–21.
21. National Center for HIV/AIDS, Dermatology and STDs (NCHADS). Conceptual framework on virtual elimination of new HIV infections in Cambodia by 2020, Cambodia 3.0. Phnom Penh: NCHADS; 2012.
22. Granich R, Gupta S, Hall I, Aberle-Grasse J, Hader S, Mermin J. Status and methodology of publicly available national HIV care continua and 90–90–90 targets: a systematic review. PLoS Med. 2017;14(4):e1002253. https://doi.org/10.1371/journal.pmed.1002253.

23. National AIDS Authority. Cambodia Country Progress Report. Monitoring progress towards the UN political declaration on HIV and AIDS. Phnom Penh: National AIDS Authority; 2011. p. 2015.
24. Yi S, Tuot S, Chhoun P, Pal K, Ngin C, Choub SC, et al. Improving prevention and care for HIV and sexually transmitted infections among men who have sex with men in Cambodia: the sustainable action against HIV and AIDS in communities (SAHACOM). BMC Health Serv Res. 2016;16(1):599.
25. Yi S, Tuot S, Chhoun P, Brody C, Tith K, Oum S. The impact of a community-based HIV and sexual reproductive health program on sexual and healthcare-seeking behaviors of female entertainment workers in Cambodia. BMC infect Dis. 2015;15:221.
26. Sarkar S. Community engagement in HIV prevention in Asia: going from 'for the community' to 'by the community'–must we wait for more evidence? Sex Transm Infect. 2010;86(Suppl 1):i2–3.
27. Palinkas LA, Aarons GA, Horwitz S, Chamberlain P, Hurlburt M, Landsverk J. Mixed method designs in implementation research. Adm Policy Ment Health. 2011;38(1):44–53.
28. Creswell J. Research design: qualitative, quantitative and mixed methods approaches. Thousand Oaks, CA: Sage; 2003.
29. Wand H, Ramjee G. Targeting the hotspots: investigating spatial and demographic variations in HIV infection in small communities in South Africa. J Int AIDS Soc. 2010;13:41.
30. Heng S, Tuot S. Mid-term review of the sustainable action against HIV and AIDS in communities (SAHACOM). Phnom Penh: KHANA; 2013.
31. National Institute of Public Health National Institute of Statistics and ORC Macro. Cambodia Demographic and Health Survey 2010. Phnom Penh and Calverton, Maryland: National Institute of Public Health National Institute of Statistics, and ORC Macro; 2014.
32. Charmaz K. Grounded theory: objectivist and constructivist methods. In: Denzin NK, Lincoln YS, editors. Handbook of qualitative research. Thousand Oaks, CA: Sage; 2000. p. 509–35.
33. Bryman A. Social research methods. Oxford: Oxford University Press; 2012.
34. Silverman D. Interpreting qualitative data. Methods for analyzing talk text and inter-action. 2nd ed. London: Sage Publication; 2001.
35. Chiovitti RF, Piran N. Rigour and grounded theory research. J Adv Nurs. 2003;44(4):427–35.
36. Fetters MD, Curry LA, Creswell JW. Achieving integration in mixed methods designs—principles and practices. Health Serv Res. 2013;48(6 Pt 2):2134–56.
37. Niccolai LM, Toussova OV, Verevochkin SV, Barbour R, Heimer R, Kozlov AP. High HIV prevalence, suboptimal HIV testing, and low knowledge of HIV-positive serostatus among injection drug users in St. Petersburg, Russia. AIDS Behav. 2010;14(4):932–41.
38. Asher AK, Hahn JA, Couture MC, Maher K, Page K. People who inject drugs, HIV risk, and HIV testing uptake in sub-Saharan Africa. J Assoc Nurses AIDS Care. 2013;24(6):e35–44.
39. Sharma V, Sarna A, Luchters S, Sebastian M, Degomme O, Saraswati LR, et al. 'Women at risk': the health and social vulnerabilities of the regular female partners of men who inject drugs in Delhi, India. Cult Health Sex. 2015;17(5):623–37.
40. Bobrova N, Rhodes T, Power R, Alcorn R, Neifeld E, Krasiukov N, et al. Barriers to accessing drug treatment in Russia: a qualitative study among injecting drug users in two cities. Drug Alcohol Depend. 2006;82(Suppl 1):S57–63.
41. Low AJ, Mburu G, Welton NJ, May MT, Davies CF, French C, et al. Impact of opioid substitution therapy on antiretroviral therapy outcomes: a systematic review and meta-analysis. Clin Infect Dis. 2016;63(8):1094–104.
42. MacArthur GJ, van Velzen E, Palmateer N, Kimber J, Pharris A, Hope V, et al. Interventions to prevent HIV and Hepatitis C in people who inject drugs: a review of reviews to assess evidence of effectiveness. Int J Drug Policy. 2014;25(1):34–52.
43. Guise A, Seguin M, Mburu G, McLean S, Grenfell P, Islam Z et al. Integrated opioid substitution therapy and HIV care: a qualitative systematic review and synthesis of client and provider experiences. AIDS Care. 2017;29(9):1119–28.
44. Ti L, Hayashi K, Kaplan K, Suwannawong P, Wood E, Montaner J, et al. Willingness to access peer-delivered HIV testing and counseling among people who inject drugs in Bangkok, Thailand. J Commun Health. 2013;38(3):427–33.
45. Ti L, Hayashi K, Hattirat S, Suwannawong P, Kaplan K, Kerr T. 'Drug users stick together': HIV testing in peer-based drop-in centres among people who inject drugs in Thailand. Sex Health. 2015;12(3):263–8.
46. Kumar MS, Virk HK, Chaudhuri A, Mittal A, Lewis G. A rapid situation and response assessment of the female regular sex partners of male drug users in South Asia: factors associated with condom use during the last sexual intercourse. Int J Drug Policy. 2008;19(2):148–58.
47. Bourne A, Reid D, Hickson F, Torres-Rueda S, Weatherburn P. Illicit drug use in sexual settings ('chemsex') and HIV/STI transmission risk behaviour among gay men in South London: findings from a qualitative study. Sex Transm Infect. 2015;91(8):564–8.
48. Tavitian-Exley I, Vickerman P, Bastos FI, Boily MC. Influence of different drugs on HIV risk in people who inject: systematic review and meta-analysis. Addiction. 2015;110(4):572–84.
49. Martin NK, Vickerman P, Hickman M, Patterson TL, Rand E, Abramovitz D, et al. Overlapping substance using high-risk groups and infectious diseases: how dynamic modelling can evaluate risk and target HIV prevention. Addiction. 2016;111(9):1512–5.
50. Nazari SS, Noroozi M, Soori H, Noroozi A, Mehrabi Y, Hajebi A, et al. The effect of on-site and outreach-based needle and syringe programs in people who inject drugs in Kermanshah, Iran. Int J Drug Policy. 2016;27:127–31.

Development and differentiability of three brief interventions for risky alcohol use that include varying doses of motivational interviewing

Jennifer E. Hettema[1*], Stephanie A. Cockrell[1], Abigail Reeves[2], Karen S. Ingersoll[2], Paula J. Lum[3], Richard Saitz[4], Cristina M. Murray-Krezan[5] and Valerie A. Carrejo[1]

Abstract

Background: While brief intervention (BI) for risky alcohol use generally yields positive effects among those identified by screening, effect sizes are small and there is unexplained heterogeneity in outcome. The heterogeneity may be related to differences in intervention style and content, including elements of motivational interviewing (MI). To date, it has been difficult to interpret the role of MI in BI and these gaps in knowledge interfere with efforts to train, disseminate and implement BI that retains and maximizes efficacy. This study sought to develop BI protocols with varying doses of MI and test their differentiability. Differentiable BI protocols could allow for future studies that prospectively evaluate the role MI plays in affecting BI outcome.

Methods: We developed three intervention protocols: brief advice, standard BI (NIAAA Clinician's Guide), and MI-enhanced BI and administered them to 45 primary care patients who reported exceeding recommended drinking limits. We then rated the BI sessions for fidelity to the assigned protocol as well as MI consistency based on Motivational Interviewing Treatment Integrity (MITI) scale scores. The differentiability of BI protocols was determined by calculating fidelity to assigned protocols and comparing MITI scores using pairwise, Tukey-adjusted comparisons of least squares mean scores.

Results: High rates of fidelity to each protocol were achieved. The three BI protocols were also highly differentiable based on MITI scores.

Conclusions: The three interventions can be used in future trials to prospectively examine the role MI has in determining BI outcome.

Trial registration clinicaltrials.gov NCT02978027, retrospectively registered 11/28/16

Keywords: Motivational interviewing, Brief alcohol intervention in primary care, Treatment fidelity, Differentiable interventions, Risky alcohol use

Background

Screening and brief intervention (SBI) for risky alcohol use in primary care settings has demonstrated efficacy. In a meta-analysis of 23 controlled studies, patients identified by screening in primary care settings who received BI consumed less alcohol on average (3.6 fewer drinks per week) and were less likely to exceed limits (12% fewer) than control patients at one-year follow-up [1]. However, despite overall positive findings, there are high levels of variability in BI effects, with significant unexplained heterogeneity in outcomes [1–3]. In fact, the number of studies that do and do not find significant

*Correspondence: jhettema@salud.unm.edu
[1] Department of Family and Community Medicine, University of New Mexico, Albuquerque, NM, USA
Full list of author information is available at the end of the article

BI effects are nearly evenly split [4]. This variability may be attributable in part to differences in the intervention components and communication style that underlie tested BI protocols, including fidelity to motivational interviewing (MI).

MI is a patient-centered communication style that seeks to draw out and enhance patients' own motivation to change health behaviors [5]. Studies of SBI frequently report that the tested BI protocol was conducted in a manner that was consistent with an MI approach, but additional methodological details are often lacking. For example, Richmond et al. [6] briefly mention that "Patient counseling included techniques of motivational interviewing," Senft et al. [7]. mention that research staff "were trained in principles of motivational interviewing," Fleming et al. [8] included a workbook "based on the principles of motivational interviewing," and Reinhardt et al. [9] provided counseling sessions "based on motivational Interviewing," in which "the main content of each intervention was the enhancement of motivation." None of these examples provide a specific description of how MI was incorporated into the intervention.

There are several potential ways in which MI principles or skills could be integrated into BI. For example, interventionists could be trained to take a collaborative or empathic stance, to avoid potential roadblocks to communication such as labeling and unsolicited advice, to use specific frequencies of communication skills such as complex reflections, to conduct specific exercises, to adhere to different decision rules regarding patient readiness levels, or some combination of the above. Lack of methodological details regarding the content and structure of brief interventions makes it difficult to assess the moderating impact of MI dose on outcome across trials, and primary care-based meta-analyses to date have been unable to report on the impact of this construct [1–4].

Although MI has been found to be effective for addressing alcohol issues in medical care settings [10] and aligns with several principles of medical ethics [11], there are many barriers to implementing MI in brief medical interactions. Healthcare providers are faced with many competing priorities and limited time with patients, creating pressure to conduct preventive and behavioral health interventions as efficiently as possible [12]. Conducting MI, even its briefest applications, is more time consuming than simple advice giving. In addition, MI is a complex set of skills that requires flexible application and contingent responding to moment-to-moment changes in what patients say [5]. Proficiency in the approach requires extensive training time, ongoing supervision and resources that are often limited among medical trainees and clinicians. A recent review of MI training for healthcare professionals found that average training duration exceeded 1 day and in many cases such training failed to yield clinical improvements in MI proficiency [13]. Lastly, medical clinicians themselves often perceive barriers to implementing MI, including concerns about lack of time, low levels of perceived responsibility, low confidence, and lack of support [14].

To date, there is a dearth of empirical work examining mechanisms of behavior change in SBI for risky alcohol use [15]. Of the available research that has focused on the impact of MI within SBI, results have yielded mixed findings [16]. For example, Bertholet et al. [17] re-analyzed combined data from three controlled BI trials for proficiency in important MI behaviors and found no consistent predictors of outcome. In a similar secondary analysis designed to test the mediating link between MI-consistent behaviors such as open-questions, affirmations, and reflections, client change talk, and outcome proposed by the prevailing MI model [18], this hypothesized causal chain was only supported in specific conditions, such as with therapists who had more than 3 years experience [19].

There have been some attempts to compare different SBI approaches prospectively. For example, the Effectiveness of Screening and Brief Alcohol Intervention in Primary Care Trial (SIPS trial) compared three brief intervention conditions for hazardous drinkers in primary care settings: an informational leaflet, a brief advice session, and an MI-informed brief lifestyle counseling session [20]. Results of the SIPS showed no significant differences in drinking reduction between the three conditions at follow-up, although patients in the lifestyle counseling group had significantly increased readiness to change and satisfaction with the intervention. While this trial did compare different intensities of intervention, it was confounded by content and not specifically designed to allow for inferences regarding the role of MI strategies on outcome, as treatment modalities were additive, with all participants first receiving brief advice. Additionally, the content and structure of brief advice was not tightly controlled and study authors report that study interventionists, who were clinic-based providers, often extended into more therapeutic tasks.

More work has been done with regards to alcohol treatment, which may or may not be generalizeable to SBI in primary care. Here, findings are mixed, with some studies supporting the use of specific MI structure and content, and others not. For example, Morgenstern and colleagues attempted to dismantle the active components of MI treatment by prospectively comparing 4-sessions of MI, to non-directional MI, to a no treatment control condition and found similar outcomes across condition [21]. On the other hand, Field and colleagues compared brief advice, brief MI, and brief MI plus a feedback based telephone booster among trauma center patients who recently consumed alcohol and found that the BMI plus booster condition outperformed other treatments [22]. Apodaca conducted a recent secondary analysis of a brief intervention for college students with problems drinking and found that therapist use of Mi microskills such as reflections and open-questions produced both change and sustain talk [23]. This trend was also observed on a recent multivariate meta-analysis of MI process and outcome, which found that both therapist microskills and global ratings predicted change and sustain talk and that sustain talk was predictive of poor outcome, providing equivocal support for the proposed MI theory of change [24].

While we have evidence to suggest that primary care-based brief advice may be just as effective as MI with smoking cessation [25], the evidence is not clear for BI for risky alcohol use. One strategy for determining the impact of MI on BI efficacy is by prospectively comparing SBI protocols with varying doses of MI content. While mechanisms of action research have revealed variability in MI within clinical trials, to date, it has not been demonstrated that is possible to create interventions that are reliably differentiable while still maintaining consistency within a general BI structure. In the current study we sought to develop SBI protocols that were differentiable in terms of dose of MI, with the goal of prospectively comparing them in a future controlled trial.

Methods

Study procedures

Participants were recruited during regularly scheduled primary care visits at two university-operated community primary care clinics. While the university system electronic medical record prompts medical assistants to conduct alcohol screening annually during triage at primary care appointments, there is no standardized SBI protocol in place, compliance with screening is variable, and providers do not typically follow up regarding screening results. Patients attending the clinics were approached in the waiting room or the exam room prior to their scheduled visit to determine their interest in being screened for eligibility in the research study. Interested participants were asked to fill out a paper copy of the NIAAA screening questions ("Do you sometimes drink beer, wine, or other alcoholic beverages?, "How many times in the past year have you had 5 or more (4 for women) alcoholic drinks in one day?" [26], and the Alcohol Use Disorders Identification Test - Consumption (AUDIT-C) questionnaire [27], which includes three multiple choice questions measuring drinking frequency in the past year, number of drinks consumed on a typical drinking day, and frequency of risky drinking episodes in the past year. Inclusion criteria were endorsement of past year risky drinking, defined as any score other than zero in response to the NIAAA question about drinks in 1 day. Participants with an AUDIT-C score greater than 7, which indicates a likely alcohol use disorder were excluded, given that BI may not be sufficient for them. Eligible participants met with a researcher in a private exam room to provide informed consent. During their regularly scheduled primary care appointment, consenting patients were administered a baseline assessment and BI in their exam room prior to their provider visit or in a private adjacent office following their visit depending on the clinic flow and the availability of the clinician. Participants were randomly assigned to one of three distinct intervention conditions: BI based on the approach described in the NIAAA Clinician's Guide (NIAAA), Brief advice (BA), or an MI-enhanced NIAAA Clinician's Guide approach (MI). After the intervention, participants received a $25 gift card.

Baseline assessment

Following consent, participants completed a brief baseline assessment. The assessment was designed to be minimal to avoid potential assessment reactivity effects [28, 29]. Baseline assessment included a brief demographic form and a locator form to assist with later follow-up. Within the context of the SBI protocol, interventionists verbally re-administered the NIAAA heavy drinking episode screening question, determined drinking quantity and frequency, and assessed for AUDs using two questions related to drinking in harmful situations and drinking more than intended [26]. Participants who endorsed either of these criteria were further assessed for AUD by responding to questions that correspond to each DSM 5-criterion.

Intervention protocols

Interventions were adapted from the NIAAA protocol "Helping Patients Who Drink Too Much: A Clinician's Guide" [26]. All interventions were video recorded for later coding. Intervention protocols can be accessed in Additional files 1, 2 and 3.

NIAAA Clinician's Guide (NIAAA)

The NIAAA brief intervention was adapted directly from the NIAAA publication "Helping Patients Who Drink Too Much: A Clinician's Guide" [26]. This protocol includes both MI-consistent and MI-inconsistent elements. The protocol involves screening (see above) and then assessing for quantity and frequency using closed-ended questions. The guide has some ambiguity regarding strategies for assessing for alcohol use disorders. Although AUDIT-C inclusion criteria were designed to rule out patients with a likely alcohol use disorder, this screening tool does not have perfect sensitivity and it was still possible for patients to have an AUD upon further assessment. In this trial, assessment of alcohol use disorders was conducted using Vinson's [30] two questions described above, instead of the entire diagnostic checklist. Those exceeding recommended limits were told: "You're drinking more than is medically safe." They were shown a chart describing U.S. adult drinking patterns that included recommended drinking limits and the prevalence and consequences of exceeding them. The clinician then stated: "I strongly recommend that you cut down and I'm willing to help." The protocol called for assessment of readiness to change ("Are you willing to make changes in your drinking?"). For patients unwilling to make a change, the clinician was instructed to restate their concern, encourage self-reflection by asking the patient about reasons to cut down on drinking and barriers to change, and reaffirm willingness to help. For patients willing to make a change, the clinician was instructed to help the patient develop a plan to cut down within maximum limits, agree on specific steps and strategies, and provide a tip sheet on strategies for cutting down. The clinicians in the trial were specifically instructed to be warm and friendly. However, they were also instructed to avoid the use of MI micro-skills such as reflection, statements that infer the meaning underlying what patients have said, and not to differentially respond to change talk, by focusing on patients' motivations (versus barriers) to change.

Brief advice (BA)

The brief advice protocol was designed by removing MI-consistent elements from the NIAAA Clinician's Guide, while leaving other elements that were either not MI-consistent or neutral. The protocol involved screening and assessment using the same strategies described above. Patients exceeding recommended limits received the same feedback, information, and advice described above. All patients were then provided with a tip sheet on strategies for cutting down (e.g. pacing and spacing, keeping track, know your 'no') and encouraged to follow-up with a behavioral health provider with any questions or concerns. As above, the clinician in the trial was specifically instructed to be warm and friendly, but avoid the use of reflection and evocation of change talk.

MI-enhanced NIAAA Clinician's Guide (MI)

The MI intervention condition was also adapted from the NIAAA Clinician's Guide, with additional modification to include elements of MI. At the start of the protocol, clinicians were instructed to normalize SBI and ask the patient's permission before discussing alcohol use. The NIAAA screening questions were administered as designed, which is closed-ended. Otherwise, when possible, closed questions were reframed as open questions. Assessment of quantity, frequency, and AUD symptoms was done using open questions, followed by closed questions if additional clarification was needed. The ask-tell-ask technique was used to share feedback regarding the patient's risky drinking status and exchange information regarding U.S adult drinking patterns. Ask-tell-ask, involves asking patients what they know about a particular topic, providing information in a tailored way, and then asking the patient what they think of the information or how they might apply it. For patients low in readiness to make a change, clinicians built readiness using one of two structured MI tools: a scaling ruler or a road map. Scaling rulers involve asking patients to self-assess their perceived importance, confidence, or readiness to change and then strategically evoking change talk by inviting them to speak about why their assessment wasn't lower. The road map exercise involves evoking change talk by asking patients to imagine their life down two paths and to speak about the good things that might happen if they change and the bad things that might happen if they don't change. For patients high in readiness to change, the ask-tell-ask technique was used to explore the tip sheet on strategies for cutting down and develop an action plan. The MI intervention called for interventionists to use reflective listening statements and summaries throughout the protocol and differentially focus on the patient's reasons for change.

Fidelity and MI dose assessment

All intervention sessions were video recorded and objectively rated using two coding instruments. An independent fidelity coder rated all sessions and members of the research team co-rated a subset to establish estimates of interrater agreement. Research team members never coded their own sessions. Because of the different content and structure and each intervention, it was not possible to blind raters to condition. Fidelity checklists were developed specifically for each condition, and included yes, no, and not applicable check boxes for each step of the protocol. The total fidelity score was the proportion of protocol activities that were conducted that should have been conducted. The fidelity checklists are accessible in Additional files 1, 2, 3, 4, 5, and 6. Video recordings of interventions were also rated using the Motivational Interviewing Treatment Integrity Code 3.1.1 (MITI), a coding instrument designed to measure competence in MI that has demonstrated reliability and sensitivity [31, 32]. The MITI includes specific behavior counts thresholds, such as percent open questions, reflection to question ratio, and percent complex reflections, as well as assessment of global characteristics of the intervention, such as empathy and evocation. The MITI also has suggested benchmarks for beginning proficiency and competency.

Interventionists

The study interventionist was primarily the second author, a master's level social worker with extensive training in MI, however, the first author, a clinical psychologist, also conducted some sessions. Both are members of the Motivational Interviewing Network of Trainers (MINT) who completed a MINT "training for trainers (TNT)." Training for the study intervention involved extensive practice with mock patients until 95% fidelity measures were consistently met on all SBI protocols. The first author conducted bi-weekly feedback and supervision during the trial.

Statistical analysis

To determine the reliability of fidelity coding, intraclass correlation coefficients (ICCs) were calculated using a one-way random model for absolute agreement [33]. Cicchetti has recommended that ICCs be interpreted as follows: below 0.40 = poor; 0.40–0.59 = fair; 0.60–0.74 = good; and 0.75–1.0 = excellent [34]. To determine the differentiability of the three interventions, mean percent fidelity to each protocol was compared across the three conditions using one-way ANOVA. MITI scores were compared across the three conditions using pairwise, Tukey-adjusted comparisons of least squares mean scores. To reduce the possibility of spurious findings, a Bonferroni adjustment was made for 9 comparisons. Outcome measures met normality assumptions required for these analyses.

Results

Interrater agreement

Of the 45 sessions, 9 (20%) were co-rated to assess interrater agreement. Rates of interrater agreement were excellent for the fidelity checklist (ICC = 0.93, 95% CI = 0.72, 0.98). All MITI global scores (evocation, collaboration, autonomy support, direction, empathy) were also in the excellent range, with the exception of direction, which could not be calculated because there was no variability in rating. All behavior count threshold (% open questions, % complex reflections, reflection to question ratio, and % MI-adherent) interrater agreement estimates were also in the excellent range.

Participant flow

Of the 502 patients approached by researchers, 413 agreed to be screened for eligibility and 92 (22.3%) screened positive for risky drinking. Among ineligible screens, 291 did not report any past year risky drinking, and 5 exceeded the AUDIT-C upper cutoff. Other common reasons for ineligibility were lack of English fluency (n = 15) and pregnancy (n = 3). Of those who screened positive, 45 (48.9%) enrolled in the study: 15 were assigned to NIAAA, 14 were assigned to the BA, and 16 were assigned to MI. The primary reason for non-enrollment was lack of time.

Participant characteristics

Participants were predominantly female (60%) and 42% were Hispanic. On average, participants reported between 1 and 156 heavy drinking days in the past year (mean 26 (SD = 42)). AUDIT-C scores ranged from 3 to 7 (mean 4.6 (SD = 1.3)).

Timing

Mean time to complete SBI varied across conditions, with BA taking, on average, 7 min (SD = 6, Range 4–14), NIAAA 9 min (SD = 3, Range 6–18), and MI 17 min (SD = 6, Range 5–32).

SBI fidelity

Fidelity to intervention components, as measured by the fidelity checklists was high across all conditions. Overall, the clinician completed between 92 and 96% of protocol elements, with little variability within or across conditions. The mean percent fidelity did not differ across BA, NIAAA, and MI, which had respective scores of 96% (SD = 7%), 94% (SD = 6%), and 92% (SD = 6%) (p = 0.32).

MI differentiability

Significant differences between conditions were found for nearly all MITI constructs (Table 1). All differences were in the expected direction with MI showing the highest doses of MI, then NIAAA, and then BA. The MI condition met or exceeded MI competency standards on all measured domains with the exception of reflection to question ratio. BA and NIAAA did not contain levels of MI that are normally defined as meeting MI competency standards on any of the assessed domains, with the exception of percent complex reflections for the NIAAA condition.

Discussion

In this study, we found that it is possible to conduct high fidelity SBI with differing doses of MI. When implemented with risky drinking primary care patients our three SBI protocols yielded high, moderate, and low doses of MI based on MITI score assessments. This study lays for the groundwork for future research to prospectively compare the efficacy of SBI protocols with varying

Table 1 MITI scores among conditions

Skill	MITI 3.1.1 competency	BA (N = 13)		NIAAA (N = 15)		MI (N = 16)		Pairwise comparisons, p < 0.006*		
		Mean (SD)	99.4% CI+	Mean (SD)	99.4% CI	Mean (SD)	99.4% CI	BA v. NIAAA	BA v. MI	NIAAA v. MI
Evocation	4	1.9 (1.0)	(1.2, 2.5)	3.1 (1.0)	(2.4, 3.7)	4.8 (0.4)	(4.2, 5.4)	Yes	Yes	Yes
Collaboration	4	1.7 (0.9)	(1.1, 2.3)	3.0 (0.9)	(2.5, 3.5)	5.0 (0.0)	(4.5, 5.5)	Yes	Yes	Yes
Autonomy support	4	2.9 (0.5)	(2.5, 3.3)	3.6 (0.7)	(3.2, 4.0)	5.0 (0.0)	(4.6, 5.4)	Yes	Yes	Yes
Direction	4	5.0 (0.0)	–	5.0 (0.0)	–	5.0 (0.0)	–	–	–	–
Empathy	4	1.8 (0.9)	(1.1, 2.4)	2.9 (1.1)	(2.3, 3.5)	5.0 (0.0)	(4.4, 5.6)	Yes	Yes	Yes
Percent open questions	70%	0.0 (0.1)	(− 0.1, 0.1)	0.2 (0.1)	(0.1, 0.3)	0.4 (0.1)	(0.3, 0.4)	Yes	Yes	Yes
Percent complex reflections	50%	0.4 (0.2)	(0.2, 0.5)	0.5 (0.2)	(0.4, 0.6)	0.7 (0.1)	(0.6, 0.8)	No	Yes	No
Reflection to question ratio	2	0.6 (0.2)	(− 0.1, 1.2)	1.0 (1.2)	(0.4, 1.5)	1.5 (0.6)	(0.9, 2.0)	No	No	No
Percent MI adherent	90%	0.1 (0.2)	(− 0.1, 0.3)	0.3 (0.4)	(0.1, 0.4)	1.0 (0.0)	(0.8, 1.2)	No	Yes	Yes

+99.4% confidence intervals with type I error rate Bonferroni-corrected for 9 comparisons ($\alpha = 0.006$)

*P-values from pairwise, Tukey-adjusted comparisons of least squares mean scores, with additional Bonferroni adjustment for 9 comparisons

doses of MI. The protocols can be used in their current form to conduct such work and the MI protocol can provide a standardized MI-based SBI protocol for other work. The availability of these protocols may help to shine light on the unclear picture regarding the role of MI in SBI for risky alcohol use in primary care. Similarly, in the area of treatment and in other settings where the impact of MI structure and content on outcome is somewhat equivocal, the development of highly differentiable interventions may allow for improve prospective and retrospective analysis of effects.

The study has several strengths and limitations. The study sample was all English speaking and result may not be generalizeable to other clinic populations. The methods were tightly controlled resulting in strong internal validity and could be easily translated to a future prospective comparison of the interventions using an efficacy trial design. However, the current study does not necessarily reflect rates of fidelity or MI differentiability that might be observed in an effectiveness trial that involves real-world clinicians. Additionally, training and oversight of the study interventionist was much more intensive than might be feasible with non-research staff.

The protocols in the current study were also primarily conducted by one study interventionist. While this factor eliminates the risk of therapist effects confounding observed differences across SBI protocols, it may limit the generalizability of findings. Set the stage for other research that attempts to dismantle without clearly demonstrating idffereintiability.

Overall, this study represents an important contribution to the research base focused on mechanism of action of SBI for risky alcohol use in primary care. Conducting SBI with high doses of MI takes more time and requires more training and oversight, resulting in many feasibility barriers in the current medical training and practice environment. The current study provides researchers with a tool to address this important question. Future research should seek to compare the efficacy of the three SBI protocols, as well as determine the feasibility of training non-research clinicians to conduct the interventions with fidelity to both structure and MI dose, determine the intensity of training and support needed to yield such results and compare the protocols using a effectiveness trial design.

Conclusions

This study demonstrated that it is possible to create protocols for SBI for risky alcohol use that vary in MI dose, while maintaining fidelity to a structured SBI protocol. Fidelity ratings were consistently high and did not vary across the three SBI conditions, while nearly all measures of MI consistency varied across conditions in the expected direction. The only exception was reflection to question ratio, which may have been suppressed because of the screening and assessment questions at the beginning of the protocol. This study suggests that it is possible to unbundle SBI and MI to inform whether varying outcomes relate to the intensity of MI components in SBI protocols. Future studies should investigate potential differential outcomes of SBI protocols that contain no, little, or extensive MI skills and strategies.

Abbreviations

AUD: alcohol use disorders; AUDIT-C: Alcohol Use Disorders Identification Test - Consumption; BA: brief advice (intervention condition); BI: brief intervention; MI: motivational interviewing; MITI: motivational interviewing treatment integrity code; NIAAA: National Institute on Alcohol Abuse and Alcoholism; SBI: screening and brief intervention.

Authors' contributions

JEH, SAC, KSI, AR, PJL, RS, CMMK, VAC, JEH, SAC, KSI, and PJL conceptualized the work; JEH, SAC, AR collected the data; JEH and CMK analyzed the data; JEH, SAC and AR drafted the manuscript; JEH, SAC, KSI, AR, PJL, RS, CMMK, VAC provided critical revisions to the manuscript; JEH, SAC, KSI, AR, PJL, RS, CMMK, VAC approved the final manuscript and agree to be accountable for its content. All authors read and approved the final manuscript.

Author details

[1] Department of Family and Community Medicine, University of New Mexico, Albuquerque, NM, USA. [2] Department of Psychiatry and Neurobehavioral Sciences, University of Virginia, Charlottesville, VA, USA. [3] Department of Medicine, University of California San Francisco, San Francisco, CA, USA. [4] Department of Community Health Sciences, Boston University School of Public Health, Boston, MA, USA. [5] Department of Internal Medicine, University of New Mexico Health Sciences Center, Albuquerque, NM, USA.

Acknowledgements

Thank you to Krystal Bradford who assisted in data collection.

Competing interests

Jennifer Hettema is a consultant on a Substance Abuse and Mental Health Services Administration (SAMHSA) funded grant to the University of Nevada that focuses on developing and implementing training for health professional students in SBIRT (Screening, Brief Intervention, and Referral to Treatment). She serves as a nonpaid steering committee member for the Fetal Alcohol Syndrome Disorders Regional Training Center at the University of Nevada Reno. She is a a consultant for Train for Change, Inc. in which she provides motivational interviewing training and coaching and assists in developing curricula. She also owns two limited liability corporations, Transfer Innovations and Land of Enchantment Productions, which sell MI training videos and curricula that she developed.

Consent for publication

Not applicable.

Funding

This study was supported by a Grant (K23 AA020865) from the National Institutes on Alcoholism and Alcohol Abuse. The funding organization did not have any role in the design or conduct of the study; data collection management, analysis, or interpretation of the data; preparation, review or approval of the manuscripts; or the decision to submit the manuscript for publication.

References

1. Jonas DE, Garbutt JC, Amick HR, Brown JM, Brownley KA, Council CL, et al. Behavioral counseling after screening for alcohol misuse in primary care: a systematic review and meta-analysis for the U.S. Preventive Services Task Force. Ann Intern Med. 2012;157:645–54.
2. Kaner EF, Dickinson HO, Beyer F, Pienaar E, Schlesinger C, Campbell F, et al. The effectiveness of brief alcohol interventions in primary care settings: a systematic review. Drug Alcohol Rev. 2009;28(3):301–23.
3. Moyer A, Finney JW, Swearingen CE, Vergun P. Brief interventions for alcohol problems: a meta-analytic review of controlled investigations in treatment-seeking and non-treatment-seeking populations. Addiction. 2002;97(3):279–92.
4. Whitlock EP, Polen MR, Green CA, Orleans T, Klein J, U.S. Preventive Services Task Force. Behavioral counseling interventions in primary care to reduce risky/harmful alcohol use by adults: a summary of the evidence for the U.S. Preventive Services Task Force. Ann Intern Med. 2004;140(7):557–68.
5. Miller WR, Rollnick S. Motivational interviewing: helping people change. 3rd ed. New York: Guilford Press; 2013.
6. Richmond R, Heather N, Wodak A, Kehoe L, Webster I. Controlled evaluation of a general practice-based brief intervention for excessive drinking. Addiction. 1995;90:119–32.
7. Senft RA, Polen MR, Freeborn DK, Hollis JF. Brief intervention in a primary care setting for hazardous drinkers. Am J Prev Med. 1997;13(6):464–70.
8. Fleming MF, Lund MR, Wilton G, Landry M, Scheets D. The healthy moms study: the efficacy of brief alcohol intervention in postpartum women. Alcohol Clin Exp Res. 2008;32(9):1600–6.
9. Reinhardt S, Bischof G, Grothues J, John U, Meyer C, Rumpf H. Gender differences in the efficacy of brief interventions with a stepped care approach in general practice patients with alcohol-related disorders. Alcohol Alcohol. 2008;43(3):334–40.
10. Lundahl B, Moleni T, Burke BL, Butters R, Tollefson D, Butler C, et al. Motivational interviewing in medical care settings: a systematic review and meta-analysis of randomized controlled trials. Patient Educ Couns. 2013;93(2):157–68.
11. American Medical Association: Principles of medical ethics. http://www.ama-assn.org (2001). Accessed 22 Jul 2016.
12. Yarnall KSH, Pollak KI, Østbye T, Krause KM, Michener JL. Primary care: is there enough time for prevention? Am J Public Health. 2003;93(4):635–41.
13. Söderlund LL, Madson MB, Rubak S, Nilsen P. A systematic review of motivational interviewing training for general health care practitioners. Patient Educ Couns. 2011;84:16–26.
14. Hettema JE, Steele JM, Miller WR. Motivational Interviewing. Annu Rev Clin Psychol. 2015;1:91–111.
15. Heather N. Toward an understanding of the effective mechanisms of alcohol brief interventions. Alcohol Clin Exp Res. 2014;38:626–8.
16. Gaume J, McCambridge J, Bertholet N, Daeppen J-B. Mechanisms of action of brief alcohol interventions remain largely unknown—a narrative review. Front Psychiatry. 2014;5:108.
17. Bertholet N, Palfai T, Gaume J, Daeppen JB, Saitz R. Do brief alcohol motivational interventions work like we think they do? Alcohol Clin Exp Res. 2014;38:853–9.
18. Miller WR, Rose GS. Toward a Theory of Motivational Interviewing. Am Psychol. 2009;64(6):527–37.
19. Gaume J, Longabaugh R, Magill M, Bertholet N, Gmel G, Daeppen JB. Under what conditions? Therapist and client characteristics moderate the role of change talk in brief motivational intervention. J Consult Clin Psychol. 2016;84(3):211–20.
20. Kaner E, Bland M, Cassidy P, Coulton S, Dale V, Deluca P, et al. Effectiveness of screening and brief alcohol intervention in primary care (SIPS trial): pragmatic cluster randomized controlled trial. Br Med J. 2013;346:e8501.
21. Morgenstern JJ, Kuerbis A, Houser J, Amrhein P, Shao S, McKay JR. Dismantling motivational interviewing: Effects on initiation of behavior change among problem drinkers seeking treatment. Psychol Addict Behav. 2017;31:751.
22. Field C, Walters S, Marti CN, Jun J, Foreman M, Brown C. A multisite randomized controlled trial of brief intervention to reduce drinking in the trauma care setting: how brief is brief? Ann Surg. 2014;259:873–80.
23. Apodaca TR, Jackson KM, Borsari B, Magill M, Longabaugh R, Mastroleo NR, Barnett NP. Which individual therapist behaviors elicit client change talk and sustain talk in motivational interviewing? J Subst Abuse Treat. 2016;61:60–5.
24. Pace BT, Dembe A, Soma CS, Baldwin SA, Atkins DC, Imel ZE. A multivariate meta-analysis of motivational interviewing process and outcome. Psychol Addict Behav. 2017;31:524–33.

25. Hettema JE, Hendricks PA. Meta-analysis of motivational interviewing for smoking cessation. J Consult Clin Psychol. 2010;78:868–84.
26. National Institute on Alcohol Abuse and Alcoholism. Helping patients who drink too much: a clinician's guide. U.S. Department of Health and Human Services. 2005. http://pubs.niaaa.nih.gov/publications/Practitioner/CliniciansGuide2005/guide.pdf. Accessed 22 Jul 2016.
27. Bush K, Kivlahan DR, McDonell MB, Fihn SD, Bradley KA. The AUDIT alcohol consumption questions (AUDIT-C): an effective brief screening test for problem drinking. Arch Intern Med. 1998;158:1789–95.
28. Donovan DM, Bogenschutz MP, Perl H, Forcehimes A, Adinoff B, Mandler R, et al. Study design to examine the potential role of assessment reactivity in the Screening, Motivational Assessment, Referral, and Treatment in Emergency Departments (SMART-ED) protocol. Addict Sci Clin Pract. 2012;7:16.
29. McCambridge J, Kypri K. Can simply answering research questions change behavior? Systematic review and meta analyses of brief alcohol intervention trials. PLoS ONE. 2011;6(10):e23748.
30. Vinson DC, Kruse RL, Seal JP. Simplifying alcohol assessment: two questions to identify alcohol use disorders. Alcohol Clin Exp Res. 2007;31(8):1392–8.
31. Moyers TB, Martin T, Manuel JK, Hendrickson SM, Miller WR. Assessing competence in the use of motivational interviewing. J Subst Abuse Treat. 2005;28(1):19–26.
32. Moyers TB, Martin T, Manuel JK, Miller WR, Ernst D. Revised Global Scales: Motivational Interviewing Treatment Integrity 3.1.1 (MITI 3.1.1). University of New Mexico Center on Alcoholism, Substance Abuse and Addictions (CASAA). http://casaa.unm.edu/download/MITI3_1.pdf. Accessed 22 Jul 2016.
33. Shrout PE, Fleiss JL. Intraclass correlations: uses in assessing rater reliability. Psychol Bull. 1979;86:420–8.
34. Cicchetti DV. Guidelines, criteria, and rules of thumb for evaluating normed and standardized assessment instruments in psychology. Special section: normative assessment. Psychol Assess. 1994;6:284–90.

Barriers and facilitators affecting the implementation of substance use screening in primary care clinics: a qualitative study of patients, providers, and staff

Jennifer McNeely[1,2*], Pritika C. Kumar[1], Traci Rieckmann[3], Erica Sedlander[1], Sarah Farkas[4], Christine Chollak[1], Joseph L. Kannry[5], Aida Vega[5], Eva A. Waite[5], Lauren A. Peccoralo[5], Richard N. Rosenthal[6], Dennis McCarty[7] and John Rotrosen[4]

Abstract

Background: Alcohol and drug use are leading causes of morbidity and mortality that frequently go unidentified in medical settings. As part of a multi-phase study to implement electronic health record-integrated substance use screening in primary care clinics, we interviewed key clinical stakeholders to identify current substance use screening practices, barriers to screening, and recommendations for its implementation.

Methods: Focus groups and individual interviews were conducted with 67 stakeholders, including patients, primary care providers (faculty and resident physicians), nurses, and medical assistants, in two urban academic health systems. Themes were identified using an inductive approach, revised through an iterative process, and mapped to the Knowledge to Action (KTA) framework, which guides the implementation of new clinical practices (Graham et al. in J Contin Educ Health Prof 26(1):13–24, 2006).

Results: Factors affecting implementation based on KTA elements were identified from participant narratives. *Identifying the problem:* Participants consistently agreed that having knowledge of a patient's substance use is important because of its impacts on health and medical care, that substance use is not properly identified in medical settings currently, and that universal screening is the best approach. *Assessing barriers:* Patients expressed concerns about consequences of disclosing substance use, confidentiality, and the individual's own reluctance to acknowledge a substance use problem. Barriers identified by providers included individual-level factors such as lack of clinical knowledge and training, as well as systems-level factors including time pressure, resources, lack of space, and difficulty accessing addiction treatment. *Adapting to the local context:* Most patients and providers stated that the primary care provider should play a key role in substance use screening and interventions. Opinions diverged regarding the optimal approach to delivering screening, although most preferred a patient self-administered approach. Many providers reported that taking effective action once unhealthy substance use is identified is crucial.

Conclusions: Participants expressed support for substance use screening as a valuable part of medical care, and identified individual-level as well as systems-level barriers to its implementation. These findings suggest that screening programs should clearly communicate the goals of screening to patients and proactively counteract stigma, address staff concerns regarding time and workflow, and provide education as well as treatment resources to primary care providers.

*Correspondence: jennifer.mcneely@nyumc.org
[1] Department of Population Health, New York University School of Medicine, 550 First Avenue, VZ30 6th Floor, New York, NY 10016, USA
Full list of author information is available at the end of the article

Keywords: Substance use disorders, Drug abuse screening, Alcohol screening, Alcohol abuse, Drug abuse, Primary care, Qualitative research

Background

Alcohol and drug use are among the top ten causes of preventable death in the United States [1–4], but substance use disorders (SUDs) are greatly under-treated in the specialty addiction treatment system [5], and under-recognized in medical settings [6, 7]. Screening for alcohol use in adult primary care settings is recommended by the United States Preventive Services Task Force (USPSTF) and ranks as the third highest prevention priority for adults in the U.S [8–13]. The U.S. Surgeon General's report on addiction recommends screening for other drug use as well as alcohol, which is the current approach of federally-funded 'screening, brief intervention, and referral to treatment (SBIRT)' programs [14, 15]. Yet despite over a decade of concerted efforts to integrate substance use screening and interventions into mainstream medical care [16], primary care patients are rarely screened, assessed or treated for SUDs [6, 7, 17–22].

There is a rich literature on barriers to implementing screening for substance use in primary care [17–20]. In today's busy primary care practices, the time required for screening, challenges of integrating it into the clinical workflow, and poor quality of screening are the primary barriers. Most of the research documenting barriers to screening has been conducted with primary care physicians, but current primary care practice emphasizes a team-based approach and patient-centered care, and successful screening approaches typically involve other members of the care team performing the screening [23, 24]. The perspectives of non-physician clinical staff and patients are thus critical to developing effective implementation strategies, but have been underrepresented in the screening literature.

We sought to gain an understanding of substance use screening from a diversity of clinical stakeholders, as part of a multi-site study of the National Institute on Drug Abuse (NIDA) Clinical Trials Network (CTN). The overarching goal of this CTN study is to implement substance use screening using the NIDA CTN Common Data Elements (CDEs) in primary care clinics. The CDEs are validated substance use screening tools that have been selected for integration into electronic health records (EHRs) based on their accuracy and feasibility in medical settings [25, 26].

The conceptual model for the study is the Knowledge to Action (KTA) framework, which informs the selection and implementation of new clinical practices. Implementation models and frameworks can both guide the introduction of new practices, and inform our understanding of why the introduction of a given practice or intervention may succeed or fail [27]. While there is now a wealth of experience with implementing SBIRT through demonstration projects, it remains challenging to explain why certain approaches may have been successful in some settings but not in others, or to arrive at a set of key elements that are generally needed for the effective introduction of screening into health care settings [24]. The KTA framework was developed by implementation researchers based on a synthesis of 31 theories for planned action [28, 29]. It is considered a process model, meaning that it can be used to describe or guide the translation of research into practice [27]. Our study activities focus on the KTA 'action cycle,' and consist of adapting, implementing, and evaluating the use of substance use screening tools. This paper presents results of the initial phase of the larger CTN study, and used qualitative methods to identify current substance use screening practices, barriers to screening, and recommendations for its implementation in primary care clinics.

Methods

Design

Focus groups and individual interviews with clinical stakeholders were conducted to inform the development of EHR-integrated substance use screening tools, and strategies for their implementation in primary care clinics participating in the CTN study. A qualitative approach was used because we sought to gain an understanding of the attitudes of medical providers, clinical staff, and patients toward screening, and to elicit recommendations for introducing screening into these clinical sites. Focus groups elicited group norms and attitudes from each category of stakeholders, while individual interviews gathered more detailed information about the logistics of introducing EHR-integrated screening, and gave an in-depth understanding of primary care provider attitudes and perceived barriers. The study was approved by the Institutional Review Boards of NYU School of Medicine, Icahn School of Medicine at Mt. Sinai, and Oregon Health and & Science University.

Setting

The majority of data collection was done in one New York City health system that serves as the lead site for this CTN study, and has two participating primary care clinics. To gain additional insight from practitioners with greater SBIRT experience, we also conducted interviews at a second study site located in Portland, Oregon. Oregon introduced screening and brief intervention for alcohol and drug use in 2013 as an incentive measure for Coordinated Care Organizations (CCOs), under the state's health care transformation [30, 31]. Additionally, some of the Oregon participants for this study had interacted with a federally-funded SBIRT training program based at Oregon Health & Science University.

These urban, academic medical centers were chosen as sites for the CTN study because they have large networks of primary care practices, serve as training sites for multidisciplinary healthcare providers, are geographically diverse, and use Epic EHR software (Epic Systems Corporation). Epic is one of the most widely-utilized EHRs in the U.S. [32], and we chose Epic-using health systems in order to facilitate knowledge transfer between the study sites and enable future broad dissemination of the clinical tools that we plan to develop. Participating clinics within each health system were selected with a goal of providing a diversity of primary care practice settings. The two New York City sites were internal medicine clinics; one teaching practice that serves primarily a safety net patient population (NY-1), and one faculty practice (NY-2). The Portland (OR) sites were a family medicine and an internal medicine practice. At the time of the study, none of the sites had initiated systematic screening for alcohol or drug use.

Participants

Focus groups and individual interviews were conducted between June 2015 and February 2016, with a total of 67 participants. *Medical providers* were primary care providers (PCPs); medical assistants (MAs); or registered nurses (RNs). Our medical provider sample included both faculty and residents; although non-MD primary care providers (including nurse practitioners and Doctors of Osteopathy) were eligible to participate, our sample was composed entirely of MDs. *Patients* were individuals currently receiving care in one of the participating adult primary care clinics. A total of 11 focus groups were conducted at the New York clinics with faculty PCPs (two groups), residents (one group), MAs (two groups), RNs (one group), and patients (five groups). Because medical residents provided care at only one of the clinics, only one session was held with residents. At the smaller of the two New York clinics, RNs and MAs were combined into a single group. At the Oregon site, scheduling difficulties made it unfeasible to schedule and recruit participants for focus groups, and so only individual interviews were conducted.

Eight individual interviews were conducted with PCPs in Oregon (n = 6) and New York (n = 2). Individuals were selected for interviews using a critical case sampling approach [33, 34]. In New York, the interviews occurred after the focus groups, and were used to provide more in-depth exploration of questions or themes that were raised during the focus group sessions. The two PCPs selected for individual interviews were full-time faculty providers who had participated in a focus group and articulated good understanding of the clinic's operations. In Oregon, PCPs were individuals who were selected because of their SBIRT or health informatics experience, and were current full-time clinical faculty (n = 4) or primary care clinician informaticists (n = 2) at the study clinics.

To encourage participation, focus groups were held during regular scheduled meeting times and interviews were conducted on-site and during regular clinic hours. For focus groups with medical staff, all eligible individuals were invited by email to attend. For focus groups with patients, clinical staff distributed fliers with information about the group to patients presenting for care, and directed individuals who were interested to speak with a research assistant. All adult patients who were fluent in English were eligible to participate. Patients' medical providers were not involved in recruitment, and were not informed regarding participation of their patients in the study. All participants received an IRB-approved written information sheet, and the interviewer verbally summarized its content and solicited questions prior to each session. All participants and gave verbal consent to the interview and audio recording. Participants were not asked to review transcripts or provide feedback on our findings.

Methodology

The semi-structured interviews sought to evaluate constructs from the Knowledge to Action (KTA) framework that guide selection and implementation of new clinical practices; in this case, the inclusion of substance use screening in primary care clinics. Interview guides were developed by the CTN study Lead Investigator and followed the themes from the action phase of the KTA framework: identifying the problem; assessing barriers; and adapting to the local context. Interview guides (included as Additional file 1) covered views on the purpose, value, and acceptability of screening for substance use, current screening practices, opinions regarding providers' knowledge about substance use, and recommendations about the frequency and content of screening as well as how to integrate it into the clinical workflow. Interview guides for medical providers, staff, and patients covered the same general topics, but were tailored to the participant group (for example, interviews with patients addressed answering screening questions, while interviews with providers addressed delivering screening, receiving results, and clinical workflow). For medical providers, focus group and individual interview guides were similar, but individual interviews gave emphasis to personal experiences and attitudes, while focus groups emphasized current practices in the clinic and group attitudes regarding screening.

Data collection

Focus groups and interviews were conducted between June and November, 2015. The New York focus groups and interviews were conducted on-site at the clinics by the Lead Investigator (JM), who is a practicing PCP at a different New York City medical center. The interviews in Oregon were conducted by a psychologist (TR) who was the local site lead. Both interviewers have experience conducting qualitative health services research. Interviews were conducted in English. The average length of the focus groups and interviews was 45–60 min and all sessions were audio recorded. For each focus group, at least one member of the research staff observed the group and took field notes, while for individual interviews field notes were written by the interviewer following the session. Participants were given a small monetary amount for participation (staff received $50, patients received $20). Payments were calibrated to the amounts that are typically used for research in these clinical sites, and were higher for staff because they may have needed to take time away from paid clinical work in order to participate. Following each interview or focus group, participants were asked to complete a form collecting demographic information.

Data analysis

Interviews were transcribed verbatim from the audio recording, leaving out any names. A research assistant who attended all of the focus groups verified the transcripts by comparing them to the audio recordings. Transcripts were entered into Atlas ti (7.0) software for data management and analysis. Field notes were reviewed when needed by the interviewers (JM and TR) to facilitate recall, but were not included in the analysis.

Two researchers (PC and ES) reviewed each focus group and interview transcript. The initial review was done independently, and then the codes that each researcher had developed were discussed and redundancies were eliminated to arrive at an initial codebook. Transcripts were analyzed using thematic analysis; an inductive approach designed to identify and examine emerging themes from conceptual data that involves coding qualitative data using a list of themes found in the transcripts [35]. Initial codes and categories were developed to identify theoretically important concepts of the KTA. Emerging themes were mapped to the domains and constructs of the KTA after multiple readings of the transcripts. Several discussions were conducted among researchers (PCK, ES and JM) involved in the coding and analysis about the appropriateness of each code. Disagreements around codes, themes and subthemes were resolved by discussion among the team members and going back to the original transcripts and field notes. The final coding scheme consisted of 6 primary themes and 46 subthemes for provider transcripts and 4 primary themes and 38 subthemes for patient transcripts. Three researchers (PCK, ES and JM) concluded that thematic saturation was reached when no additional themes related to the KTA domains were emerging from the data.

Using the jointly developed codebook, ES coded all transcripts. Blinded to the coding of ES, PK coded a randomly selected 13 transcripts (20%) to establish inter-rater reliability. The Kappa coefficient for inter-rater reliability was 0.75 which is interpreted as excellent in qualitative literature [36]. In a final step, the themes and subthemes were aggregated into matrices, organized by the KTA domains, containing the most representative quotes from each interview. Matrix analyses visually display the range of related responses for each theme, to ensure that both majority and outlier responses are considered [37]. For example, the matrix for the theme 'identifying the problem' had columns named for each subtheme, and rows named for each interview type; cells were filled with quotes from the interviews that captured the subtheme.

Results

Demographic characteristics of the 67 participants are included in Table 1. Among the PCP participants, 29 were faculty and 5 were internal medicine residents. Two PCPs participated in both a focus group and an individual interview. A total of 15 medical assistants and 3 registered nurses participated. Most of the patient participants were over 45 years of age and female, and were primarily recruited from the New York teaching practice (NY-1 clinic).

Our results are described in three broad categories, based on the KTA framework. The first category, 'identifying the problem,' contains themes related to the value of screening and current practices. The second, 'assessing barriers,' includes themes related to individual-level and systems-level barriers to screening. The third category, 'adapting to the local context,' consists of recommendations from participants about implementing screening.

Identifying the problem

All stakeholder groups felt that identifying substance use is important for providing appropriate medical care.

Table 1 Characteristics of the 67 participants

Characteristic	Total N = 67	MDs N = 34	MAs and RNs N = 18	Patients N = 15
Age—mean (SD)	46 (SD = 12)	39 (11)	40 (SD = 9)	52 (SD = 13)
Age range	27–72	27–68	27–56	28–72
Age group				
26–35	21	14	6	1
36–45	19	10	6	3
46 +	25	8	5	11
Missing	2	2	1	0
Sex				
Female	49	21	14	12
Male	18	13	4	3
Hispanic				
No	50	30	10	10
Yes	14	2	8	4
Missing	3	2	0	1
Race				
Caucasian	23	19	2	1
Asian	14	13	1	0
Black	15	0	6	9
Other	10	0	6	4
Missing	5	2	3	1
Medical specialty	N/A		N/A	N/A
Internal medicine		29		
Family medicine		2		
Missing		3		
Patients seen per week	N/A		N/A	N/A
0–50		18		
51–100		11		
> 100		1		
Missing		4		

At the time of the study, none of the participating clinics had implemented a systematic approach to alcohol or drug screening, though they did have systems in place for tobacco screening. In this setting, participants felt that unhealthy alcohol and drug use among patients may go unidentified.

Left to the discretion of the provider, screening is not regularly done

Providers said that they asked about substance use during some visits, particularly during a patient's initial visit to the clinic or when pursuing a specific health complaint that may be alcohol- or drug-related. Drawbacks to this approach noted by providers were that the information may not be accurate, because patterns of substance use can change over time, or that patients may not feel comfortable disclosing substance use in an initial meeting with the provider. Participants noted that some patients may never be asked about alcohol or drug use, because screening depends on the provider, the patient's other medical problems, and the amount of time available.

Screening has value for medical care

Overwhelmingly, patients and providers agreed that substance use screening has value in primary care. Providers stated that knowing about a patient's substance use is critical to understanding their overall state of health, and that it impacts their care for other conditions.

Some PCPs talked about substance use being similar to other social determinants of health that impact disease risk and response to treatment, 'like whether they have a job and a place to live' (NY-1 Faculty MD focus group). Many providers discussed specific ways in which knowledge of substance use could affect their diagnoses, prescribing decisions, and care plans. As summarized by one PCP:

> *I do think it is probably both important and necessary, because I guess for two reasons. One, we are a point of intervention for something that might not otherwise be identified or discussed in somebody's life. But I also think it can be destructive. And I think people often don't know where to talk about it. So I think it's important to ask to give people that opportunity, but also to better understand who you're working with and whether that's part of why it's difficult to care for other identified disease processes.*
> *NY-1 Faculty MD interview*

Similar views were held by MAs and patients, who agreed that substance use affects overall health, and that medical providers need to know about substance use in order to provide good care. As stated by one MA: "Well, that would give the doctor information on how to take care of the patient, direct them to where they have to go if they need help, and help them with their care" (NY-2 MA focus group). Patients discussed that it was important for their medical providers knowing about substance use, to allow them to make accurate diagnoses and provide appropriate treatment. As one patient said, "And, yes, I want them to know everything about me so I can get the best possible diagnosis I can possibly get" (NY-1 Patient focus group).

In addition to providing overall knowledge about the patient's health, providers and patients also talked about specific ways in which screening for substance use adds value to the clinical encounter. Screening was felt to be a way of signaling to patients that talking about substance use is permissible, thus opening the door to a conversation that would not have otherwise have happened. Participants also noted that identifying substance use is a necessary first step toward helping patients with substance problems. Providers stated that primary care visits present an opportunity to identify and intervene upon unhealthy use. One expression of these views is from a PCP focus group:

> *Some patients actually want to be helped. And they may not ask for help unless you bring it up. So sometimes that's why they're actually here. But they won't tell you that. [Another participant, agreeing] "Patients don't…I mean, most patients won't bring it up themselves."*
> *NY-1 Faculty MD focus group*

Another way in which screening was thought to add value was by providing a 'teachable moment' for educating patients about substance use and related harms. This potential benefit was raised by both patients and PCPs, who felt that patients may not understand that their substance use is a health risk until they are specifically asked about it. As stated by a patient:

> *Some people don't know how to ask for help. Or sometimes they don't even realize that they need help. So maybe just talking about it with their doctor, you might not even realize how much you really do drink or how much you really do smoke unless someone asks you, oh, so how many drinks, you know… Like, how many drinks would you say that you had in a week? And if you're somebody that's like, oh, I don't have a problem. But if you think about it and be like, well, I have about ten drinks a week, you may begin to think like maybe I do have a problem. So, you know, it keeps that… It makes doctors and patients actually talk about their issues….*
> *NY-1 Patient focus group*

Assessing barriers to screening for substance use

Participants identified both individual-level and systems-level barriers to implementing substance use screening in primary care settings. Individual-level factors for patients included feeling uncomfortable disclosing substance use because they fear a negative reaction from their provider, concerns about confidentiality, and not being ready to discuss their substance use. Individual-level factors for providers included their knowledge and capacity to respond effectively to substance use. Systems-level factors included limitations imposed by the clinic's physical environment and lack of time.

Individual level barriers

Patients worry about how medical providers will react Patients and providers stated that patients may be uncomfortable disclosing substance use out of fear of being judged by their provider. They noted that the quality of the patient-provider relationship is an important determinant of whether patients will feel comfortable disclosing substance use. This viewpoint is captured in the following patient's statement:

> *You know, people are so afraid, I think sometimes of being judged. That sometimes it just creates this impediment in regards to being as forthcoming as you possibly can. I think the relationship [with the physician] is really the foundation…*
> *NY-2 Patient focus group*

Some patients expressed concern about unforeseen consequences of screening, if providers were to react negatively to a patient's disclosure of substance use. One patient speculated that if they felt uncomfortable with their provider's reaction it could impact their engagement in care, although they did not see this as a barrier for all patients.

> *Even, like, your doctor, it's like, well, maybe they'll look at me differently now. And then I'm uncomfortable coming. And then, so it could create this kind of like spiral of paranoia, you know. And then being uncomfortable and then feeling like, oh, now I have to leave. And like it could not end so well. You know what I mean? But then there's people who I think would be totally honest.*
> *NY-2 Patient focus group*

Patients are concerned about having substance use information in the medical record Patients also expressed concerns about substance use information appearing in their medical record, and how that could affect the care they receive from other providers. Some patients felt that having substance use information in their medical record could potentially impact their job, insurance payments for medical care, and providers' willingness to prescribe some medications (such as controlled substances). This overall unease with documentation of substance use was captured in the words of one patient:

> *…with the substance use being judged or, you know, against I guess societal expectations or whatever, I just think that that could also pose…you know, have someone feeling like I'm not too comfortable, you know, with that being in the records.*
> *NY-2 Patient focus group*

Providers were sensitive to patients' concerns about substance use information appearing in the medical record. One of the Oregon physicians with health information technology expertise discussed interacting with other healthcare providers who feel that it may not be appropriate to fully integrate substance use information into the EHR. A number of providers expressed heightened concern about documenting substance use, especially now that patients are often able to view their own medical records. This view is summarized here by one MA, but was similarly expressed by PCPs who worry about how patients will react to seeing substance use documented in their chart.

> *And it doesn't say confidential or whatever. So people are very worried. And it actually puts us at major risk when we start documenting all this stuff, that the patients will come back and say.. 'you said that I drank, you know, five bottles a day and I'm an alcoholic.' They read these things.*
> *NY-2 MA focus group*

Substance use is viewed differently from other medical conditions Patients talked about the stigma of substance use, and some felt that the patient gets blamed for having a substance use disorder. While this was not a theme in the provider interviews, patients were sensitive to how a patient with a substance use disorder could feel accused of bringing the condition upon themselves, and worried about how this would impact their treatment. As expressed by one patient:

> *I would think it would be something about substance use, because there's a stigma attached to it. Like, the fact that you maybe had cancer or you had heart disease, like you could say, well, that's not my fault. Like that's something that happened to me. And I overcame this, right? As opposed to the way the world looks at substance abuse as 'this is your fault, you did this to yourself' type of mentality. So I think that it would definitely be a difference between your previous medical conditions and substance abuse.*
> *NY-2 Patient focus group*

Patients may not be ready to disclose substance use Patients and providers discussed that an individual's own reluctance to acknowledge having a substance use problem, even to themselves, can pose a barrier to screening. Many participants stated that patients need to be ready to be honest with themselves about their substance use before they can be expected to disclose it to their medical providers. A related theme was that patients who are not ready and willing to receive help will not disclose substance use, and for these patients screening may be ineffective. This perspective was summarized by a patient:

> *And so if a person's willing to get honest and truthful about where they're at in their station in life.... Then it's good. But if the person is still addicted and deny their drug use or alcoholism or whatever it is, you know, the screening, I don't know how effective that would be.*
> *NY-1 Patient focus group*

Provider knowledge and training Both faculty and resident PCPs identified knowledge deficits as a barrier to providing screening and interventions to address substance use. Several providers stated that although they received training in addressing other behavioral health conditions, such as smoking cessation and depression treatment, they had less knowledge about alcohol and drug use. As a result, they felt poorly prepared to address substance use when it was identified. Knowledge was discussed as both a lack of education about substance use and as a lack of familiarity with assessing patients and linking them to appropriate treatment. As stated by one faculty PCP:

> *So that's a barrier for me, is like my own lack of knowledge of what's out there or what's reliable and good, and what the culture of those places is [so] that I can even advise my patients, [for example] 'Hey, I think this would be a good fit for you because,' or 'You might want to try to this first instead because.' And I think that's important when somebody is making a choice to try to do something like that.*
> *NY-2 Faculty MD focus group*

Although a small number of PCPs in our sample noted that they had received specialized training in substance use and felt comfortable with substance use interventions, they still felt that they would benefit from additional hands-on teaching, such as having a coach to observe their clinical interactions and offer feedback.

Residents in particular expressed discomfort with not knowing how to address a positive screening result, because they do not know how to treat it themselves and are unfamiliar with the treatment resources available in their clinic or in the community. As one resident noted, they may be knowledgeable about treating tobacco use, and feel confident with smoking cessation counseling, but they feel poorly prepared to intervene if a patient has alcohol or drug use.

> *I think for smoking I have a pretty good idea of like options for my patients. And I counsel them fairly often about it. And, you know, there's like medica-*

tion options and like all that sort of stuff. But for alcohol and drugs, like I have no idea like where to send them if they screen positive.
NY-1 Resident MD focus group

Patients themselves also expressed concern that providers may not have the proper training or knowledge to work with patients who report substance use. Some discussed substance use as a condition that requires specialized care, and one patient equated expecting physicians to address substance use with asking a cardiologist 'about what's going on with your foot.' While they were skeptical about doctors being able to intervene, patients did express more confidence in their ability to make referrals for treatment. As one patient stated,

But I don't believe that they know how to handle that. They would refer you to someone. But I don't think they would know what to do.
NY-2 Patient focus group

PCPs may fail to address a positive screening result Medical assistants expressed concern that primary care providers would not respond appropriately to patients with substance use problems. This would make them feel less comfortable screening, because they were not confident that it would ultimately help the patient.

Because I feel like if he'll tell me, a patient, oh yeah, I'm an alcoholic, I need help. Like she said with the depression, here's a box of tissues, sit outside. And then the doctor doesn't address it. And he says, 'I told you I had this problem and nothing was done.' And I'm sorry, but then we have care coordinators, navigators, like all these resources but they feel nobody's there to help them. So like we're in the middle. Then you feel bad. Here they come again. This is the second time you ask me this question, and they didn't help me the first time so I'm not going to answer. We've had that.
NY-2 MA focus group

System-level barriers

A number of systems-level barriers were identified by providers. The main barriers identified were lack of space and privacy in the clinic, poor access to treatment for patients with substance use disorders, and the time pressures of primary care visits.

Lack of privacy Medical assistants felt strongly that screening for substance use should be done individually and in a private room. Many reported that they did not have enough privacy in their workspace, and that screening under these conditions would be disrespectful to patients. One MA expressed that screening in their current space would make patients angry.

The space is so tight. And the space is so limited... She used to have...I don't know if you still do, two chairs in the same room, two patients at the same time, two MAs working. How are you going to ask that kind of question to a patient? They're going to fly, right, they're going to be very angry. I mean, that's something very private.
NY-1 MA focus group

Lack of treatment resources for patients with substance use problems Medical providers stated that better systems are necessary for delivering effective treatment to patients with SUDs, and that this needs to be in place before initiating a screening program. Several providers mentioned that they do not know where to refer patients, and that they lack resources in the clinic to help patients with substance use problems. As one resident expressed, it is discouraging for providers to feel that they cannot connect patients to appropriate care.

And I feel like the limitations on where we can refer people afterwards. Like, well, you don't quality for inpatient rehab. So I guess, what are we going to do? Try to go to AA? It didn't really feel like we were providing that much of a service...
NY-1 Resident MD focus group

Most providers and patients discussed substance use treatment as something that happens outside the primary care clinic, and requires referral to a community-based program. However, some providers expressed hope that there would be more primary care-integrated treatment in the future, particularly with the increased use of medication for addiction treatment. This perspective was summarized by one of the Oregon PCPs:

It doesn't do any good to screen for anything that you don't have a treatment for or can't access a treatment for, and I think there is hope as medicated medication assisted treatments expand into primary care. You know, the providers will have more tools available to them. Hopefully, we'll have more counseling resources as a result of the Affordable Care Act and mental health parity in primary care, but right now most primary care clinics don't.
OR Faculty MD interview

Providers who worked in clinics that had a social worker or behavioral health specialist saw them as a valuable member of the care team, but stated that insufficient resources are devoted to integrated care for substance use in the primary care setting. Specifically, one provider noted that their clinic has one substance use counselor for 'several thousand patients in internal medicine,' and that despite the high level of need, the funding for this position is constantly in jeopardy because the counselor is unable to bill for services.

Time Overwhelmingly, medical providers and staff identified lack of time as a barrier to addressing substance use in primary care. They noted that visits are brief, and that there are usually multiple competing priorities, such as the patient's chief complaint and other medical conditions. An example was given by one physician:

> *And I'm thinking of one person in particular who comes in, and by the time we talked about his chronic pain and primary hyper- pulmonary hypertension, neuropathy and fall risk and depression, I rarely have time to get to his substance use screening issues. Even though I've been taking care of him for thirteen years now and I know that he has a remote history of alcohol use disorder, I rarely, in a single visit, will get to that.*
> *OR Faculty MD interview*

Relatedly, some providers felt that discussing substance use felt like 'opening a can of worms' that would be difficult to address. Some suggested that being able to bring patients back for a visit that focused just on substance use would help, but also noted that their schedules were usually so full that this may not be possible. These concerns were expressed by faculty and resident PCPs, and captured here in the words of a resident:

> *I think one of the other things is we're a little afraid of substance abuse in the sense of that, if it comes up I feel like in order to really deal with it there are a lot of psychosocial issues that are behind it. Like people have a lot of co-morbid mental illness. And those are just difficult and very time consuming issues for us. So you really need like a dedicated visit when that comes up.*
> *NY-1 Resident MD focus group*

Adapting knowledge to the local context

Participants made a number of recommendations for how to implement screening in their practices. There was broad agreement across stakeholder groups on some aspects of the screening approach, but differences of opinion regarding other aspects, such as who among the clinical staff should deliver screening.

What substances should screening address?

Screening should encompass tobacco, alcohol and other drugs There was broad consensus across stakeholder groups that screening should address all classes of substance use, rather than being confined to tobacco or alcohol alone. There were no participants who voiced a different opinion on this question. Some MDs additionally noted that screening should capture the full spectrum of severity, to identify patients with unhealthy use as well as more severe substance use disorders.

Should screening be universal or targeted?

Universal screening Most participants were in favor of universal screening, and stated that targeted screening is likely to miss patients who have unhealthy substance use, and would be less acceptable to patients. Some patients and MAs voiced strong opinions that targeted screening could be discriminatory. One patient equated it with a 'stop and frisk' approach to policing, which has been criticized for targeting minority populations in NYC. These views that targeted screening may be less accurate, and that it could be less comfortable for patients who feel singled out for screening, were summarized by one patient in a focus group:

> *Let's suppose they ask you if you're on drugs, if you're doing this, what are you doing, but they don't ask the other one then what would...I will be thinking why he would only ask me and not him? You understand what I'm trying to say? I mean, you can't just, you know, sit there and say, okay, you look like a drinker, you look like a smoker, you know whatever.*
> *NY-1 Patient focus group*

Targeted screening While universal screening was favored by most providers, some noted that screening all patients is inefficient, and could crowd out higher value care. They noted that universal screening may not be feasible given the time limitations in primary care. In one of the MA focus groups, it was mentioned that screening older patients (over the age of 70 years) may not be necessary, since they are less likely to have substance use problems. As one provider stated,

> *Inherently I would think, yeah, generalized screening. But then if we are thinking within the context of primary care visit, now am I doing that at the loss of something else, other problems? And, yes, everything is important. And if I do preventative services it will be five hours a visit. So here's where I pick and choose. I wanted the universal screening. But what gives more bang for my buck?*
> *NY-1 Faculty MD focus group*

How frequently should screening occur?

Annual screening PCPs and MAs commented on the frequency of screening. The majority felt that screening once per year is most appropriate, and stated that annual screening is typical for other conditions. Some recommended that screening be done as part of an annual visit, though they also acknowledged that not all patients will have a dedicated annual visit for preventive care.

> *I think it would be great if it was a routine part of general health screening. So every time you get your annual exam, you know, we ask about exercise. We ask about nutrition. We ask about psychosocial factors. And we include alcohol, substance abuse, depression screening in all of that.*
> *OR Faculty MD interview*

More than once a year A minority of participants felt that screening should occur more frequently, and possibly at every visit, because substance use behaviors can change over time. They expressed concern that substance use can escalate quickly, and that limiting screening to once per year could result in missed opportunities for early intervention with respect to new or resurgent substance use. This view was expressed by a MA, who stated:

> *I do think it should be more than once a year. Because you could go do through something midyear and then go see the doctor and that question doesn't pop up. And then you're depressed, and then it's not being taken care of and something serious later could happen.*
> *NY-2 Medical Assistant*

How should screening be administered?

Patient self-administered screening There was some discrepancy of opinion regarding how screening should be administered, but the majority of participants preferred a self-administered approach. Self-administered screening was favored by providers and staff because it could save time. There was also a perception that patients would be more comfortable disclosing substance use if they did not have to report it face-to-face. This view is illustrated in the following comment from a Registered Nurse:

> *If I'm the patient, I think I'll be more truthful just checking it on the form rather than a medical assistant asking me. It's kind of like if I'm taking drugs then I'll be embarrassed telling her.*
> *NY-1 RN focus group*

Face-to-face screening A minority of participants preferred that screening be done in person, while also noting that the patient's trust in the person asking the questions is important. Some participants, including patients and providers, expressed concern over recording substance use related information in writing, and felt it would be more comfortable to talk about it than putting it down on a form. As expressed by one patient:

> *Because sometimes you don't know where that form is going. You want it to be real personal. I want to talk to my doctor... I think that when people put it down on paper it becomes real.*
> *NY-1 Patient focus group*

There was also a broader discussion in some groups that medical providers spend too much time looking at the EHR, and that this makes care less personal and can be a barrier to developing patient-provider relationships. As expressed by a MA, this was a reason for preferring face-to-face screening:

> *Sometimes even these patients complain that the doctors are so busy with the computer, you know writing things while they're being seen...you know seeing the patient. So I think it's more personal when you have that contact face to face to discuss what your issues are.*
> *NY-2 MA focus group*

Who should administer screening, if it is done face-to-face?

There were differences of opinion regarding who in the clinic should administer screening. Among MDs, most preferred that screening be done by ancillary staff in the clinic, and usually identified screening as a MA role. In the participating clinical sites, it was common practice for the MAs to deliver depression screening, and substance use screening was perceived as being similar. For the minority of PCPs who believed that screening should be administered by physicians, reasons included that the MAs are already quite burdened, variation in the quality of screening delivered by MAs, and beliefs that patients have greater trust in their physicians than in other members of the care team. They also noted that because it is ultimately the provider who needs to address a positive screen, they may want to ask the questions themselves. Concerns about the quality of MA-delivered screening were expressed by one NY physician:

> *That's how...is the MA doing it? Is the MA looking at the screen and just asking the questions and not making eye contact and just checking off the boxes? ..Unless, again, it's like you know which MA has done it. And you know what they're like and what that rapport is...*
> *NY-2 Faculty MD focus group*

In contradistinction to the opinion of most PCPs, the majority of MAs and patients stated a preference for PCPs to deliver screening, if it is to be administered face-to-face. They felt that PCP screening was more likely to be accurate, and would give patients an opportunity to discuss or clarify their responses with the provider. Some patients felt that their physician was better able to interpret their body language and engage them in conversation about their responses. MAs felt that patients would be more comfortable giving sensitive information only to their PCP. Some patients also worried that information could be lost or distorted if it was collected by the MA and then passed along to the PCP. This viewpoint is captured in a statement from one patient:

> *And then sometimes it can also be a communication breakdown between the medical assistant and getting it to the doctor. I would be worried that my doctor wouldn't get it the way I would deliver it.*
> *NY-1 Patient focus group*

When should screening occur?

Prior to the medical encounter Most participants felt that screening should be done prior to the medical encounter, either in the waiting room or before the patient arrives in clinic. A number of providers noted that the most preferred option would be for screening to be completed electronically, ideally through the patient portal while the patient is at home, and then integrated into the EHR prior to the visit.

> *What I would want to do is all the questionnaires would be done online. As much as can be done before the appointment would be put on the tablet. So they would update their medication list online. They would do all their questionnaires. So they would upgrade all their information. And it would all be done and ready to go for the MA and the provider. So that would be my ideal world.*
> *OR Faculty MD interview*

During the clinic visit, in the exam room Patients and MAs discussed the timing and location of screening during course of the medical visit, and did not bring up the possibility of pre-visit screening. Some expressed concerns about privacy, and felt screening was best performed in the exam room, and not in the waiting area. Patients and MAs were less likely than MDs to discuss electronic approaches to screening. Some expressed pessimism about the feasibility or acceptability of electronic screening for patients, particularly those who are older or less familiar with computers. As one patient stated:

> *I'd rather do it on paper. Or if I'm not capable, have someone verbally ask me. I don't like computers. I'm not going to get into that. I wouldn't answer the questions if it was through the computer. That's me. And I find that a lot of my friends, the seniors, prefer the paperwork or someone to ask them, like a receptionist or something, you know.*
> *NY-1 Patient focus group*

Discussion

Through interviews with key clinical stakeholders, this study characterized current substance use screening practices, barriers to screening, and recommendations for its implementation in primary care clinics. Our approach is unique in capturing the views of patients, as well as those of primary care providers, residents, MAs, and RNs. To be successful in practice, screening must be acceptable to all of these groups. By including participants from two health systems that differ markedly both in their geography, their health care environment, and their experience with SBIRT, we captured diverse views.

In the KTA framework, essential early steps in implementation are to identify, address barriers, and adapt knowledge to the local context. This process is important for guiding implementation strategies. Over the past decade, many attempts to introduce screening and brief intervention (SBI) have faced challenges in their implementation, or have not been sustained in the absence of grant funding [24, 38–41]. We considered these interviews, which were conducted as the initial phase of a larger implementation study, to be essential for designing a screening strategy that would address as many stakeholder concerns as possible, and thus be more likely to be adopted and sustained.

Participants from all stakeholder groups felt strongly that screening for substance use is important for the quality and safety of medical care, and is an essential part of the patient's medical history. In order to make accurate diagnoses, manage other medical conditions, and provide appropriate preventive care, it is important for medical providers to know about a patient's substance use [42]. This is a benefit of screening that is frequently overlooked in current discussions about the efficacy of SBIRT programs for reducing drug use. Current USPSTF guidelines recommend alcohol SBI for adults in primary care settings (Grade B recommendation) [13], but the evidence is considered insufficient to support a similar recommendation for drugs [43]. Recent clinical trials of SBI have had mixed results, with two studies demonstrating no impact on drug consumption [44, 45], and one study showing short-term reductions [46]. Notably, the study by Gelberg et al. that did show reductions in drug use [46] employed patient self-administered screening and provided PCPs with a prompt and decision support encouraging them to offer very brief advice. This approach could address some of the important barriers identified by participants in our study, including patient fears about how providers will react, and provider lack of time and knowledge to intervene on unhealthy substance use. While more research is needed on primary care-based approaches to identifying and effectively addressing drug use [47], this does not diminish the importance of screening's role in informing clinical care for other health problems.

Importantly, we captured the views of patients on primary care-integrated screening and interventions. While there is a rich literature on medical provider attitudes in this area [48–56], much less is known about patient attitudes [57, 58]. One study in a Colorado health system, conducted by Rahm et al., interviewed primary care stakeholders, including patients as well as PCPs and clinical staff, about SBIRT implementation [58]. Similar to the views of patients captured in our interviews, patients in the Colorado study endorsed universal screening as part of routine care, felt that it could help open up patient-provider discussions about substance use, and expressed concerns about the confidentiality of this information when documented in the EHR. Our patient interviews also identified a number of additional individual-level barriers to screening, including fear of the medical provider's reaction, and the stigma associated with SUDs, which patients felt were not treated like other medical conditions. These concerns were similarly expressed by primary care patients in one prior study, also conducted in New York City [57], which found that patients considered substance use to be highly stigmatized, and felt that patients would only share this information with trusted primary care providers.

Providers have stated concerns about patients being uncomfortable with screening in previous studies evaluating screening implementation efforts [41, 59], but patient voices on this subject have not previously been well articulated. While some patients may feel comfortable raising the subject of substance use [51], our interviews indicate that many will not disclose this information unless they are reassured that they will not feel 'judged' by their providers or experience negative consequences from doing so. Our findings are consistent with previous literature showing that substance use disorders are among the most severely stigmatized health conditions [60]. This is particularly concerning in light of evidence that patients who feel stigmatized by providers have poor treatment outcomes [61, 62].

An additional theme from our patient interviews, which has not been highlighted in the screening implementation literature, is that patients lack confidence in their medical providers' ability to effectively address substance use. In the face of stigma and expectations of negative repercussions from disclosing substance use, patients need to feel that there is benefit to doing so. This benefit can only be realized if medical providers are prepared to deliver appropriate medical care and treatment interventions to patients with unhealthy substance use. While more research on patient attitudes toward screening is needed, our findings point to the importance of articulating the value and purpose of screening to patients, informing patients about exactly how their substance use information will be used, and addressing perceived negative attitudes and lack of knowledge among medical providers and staff as being highly important to the success of any screening program.

Our interviews with providers reiterated many of the individual- and systems-level barriers that have been found in prior research [48–56, 63]. Medical providers, including PCPs and MAs, repeatedly raised lack of time and competing demands during the primary care visit, and expressed concerns that physicians lack knowledge about substance use and addiction. Perhaps related to lack of knowledge about the spectrum of substance use that is typically identified via primary care screening, providers in our study seemed to conflate a positive screen with a need for addiction treatment, which would be accomplished by making a referral for specialty care. Providers voiced frustration about lack of access to treatment resources, and not knowing how to refer patients to treatment programs, but there was almost no mention of the potential role of PCPs themselves in providing treatment for substance use disorders. This finding echoes another recent primary care study, which found that PCPs frequently believed that treatment for alcohol use disorder requires intensive counseling resources and that specialty care is most effective [56]. More focused efforts are needed to engage patients in treatment, including primary care-based SUD treatment (e.g., office-based opioid and alcohol pharmacotherapy) or the use of on-site behavioral health providers who can assess and engage patients, and make warm hand-offs to specialty care. Our study indicates that having effective approaches to delivering treatment is important for cultivating PCP support for a substance use screening program.

Limitations

Our study has some limitations. While we included sites from very different parts of the U.S., both were academic medical centers located in urban areas. Individuals from rural areas, or in smaller community primary care practices, may have different views on substance use screening. Most interviews were done at the New York site, and we were not able to conduct any patient interviews or focus groups in Oregon, which gave us a more limited picture of stakeholder attitudes from this health system. PCPs in our sample included both residents and faculty, but all were physicians. This reflects the characteristics of our sites, in which the majority of primary care providers, and all individuals identified as having SBIRT or HIT expertise, were MDs. Licensed providers with different training, such as nurse practitioners or Doctors of Osteopathy, may have different views about screening. While we consider the inclusion of patients to be an important strength of the study, it proved difficult to recruit younger patients, and so their views may be underrepresented. This could be important, because younger patients may have higher rates of substance use, and greater concerns about issues such as the impact of screening on their employment or health insurance. Interviews were conducted only in English, which also excluded some patients. Because our objective was to capture the views of a general primary care patient population, we have little representation of patients with current alcohol and drug use disorders. Our interviews were conducted by the study PI (in New York) or the site Lead Investigator (in Oregon), which has the potential to introduce social desirability bias. However, we did not see direct evidence of this in the interviews, in which many participants spoke critically about the current system of care and about substance use screening and interventions.

Finally, we found that stigma and negative attitudes toward substance use were common themes in our interviews, particularly in the patient focus groups. While the KTA framework includes individual attitudes as 'barriers to knowledge use,' being a process model it focuses less on the factors that underlie negative attitudes, or on how attitudes may change through the process of implementing a new practice. Employing an additional theoretical model that more explicitly explores individual attitudes and behavior change may have been useful for fully exploring these themes.

Conclusion

This qualitative study can inform the design of substance use screening programs in primary care practices. Based on our findings, we have designed and are now testing a strategy that seeks to optimally utilize existing staff and resources to deliver screening in the participating clinics. We are implementing validated brief screening questionnaires, administered annually to all patients, using a patient self-administered approach when possible. Screening results will be paired with EHR-integrated clinical decision support to assist primary care providers in conducting a brief counseling intervention. We have improved the system for linking patients with high-risk substance use to care by identifying a clear process for referring patients to the clinic's existing social workers, training the social workers in brief intervention, and improving their knowledge of referral sources for addiction treatment. We are hopeful that educating medical providers about substance use and interventions will begin to address providers' negative attitudes toward patients with unhealthy alcohol and drug use, but more work is likely needed to address stigmatizing beliefs among providers and clinical staff. To directly address patient concerns about stigma, we plan to use signage and consistent language to communicate to patients that screening is universal, and is part of routine medical care.

Our findings provide general guidance regarding key elements of a screening implementation approach for primary care settings. Screening programs should clearly communicate the goals of screening to patients and seek to proactively counteract stigma, address staff concerns regarding time and workflow, and provide education as well as treatment resources to primary care providers. Without a significant infusion of resources (to support, for example, longer primary care visits, or more behavioral health staff), no screening strategy will be able to address all of the barriers that were identified. Patient concerns about the confidentiality of their screening results, and about how their providers will react, remain as important challenges to screening in medical settings. However, our understanding of stakeholder views can inform substance use screening implementation efforts by identifying important barriers that need to be acknowledged, and addressed to the extent possible, when initiating a screening program.

Abbreviations

CCO: Coordinated Care Organization; CTN: Clinical Trials Network; EHR: electronic health record; KTA: Knowledge to Action (implementation framework); MA: medical assistant; MD: medical doctor; NIDA: National Institute on Drug Abuse; PCP: primary care provider; PI: principal investigator; RN: registered nurse; SBI: screening and brief intervention; SBIRT: screening, brief intervention, and referral to treatment; USPSTF: United States Preventive Services Task Force.

Authors' contributions

JM, TR, JK, RNR, DM, JR: Conception and design. JM, TR, ES, PCK: Analysis and interpretation of the data. All authors: Drafting and revision of the manuscript. SF, CC, AV, EAW, LP: Administrative, technical, or logistic support. JM, PCK, SF, CC, AV, EAW, LP: Collection of data. All authors read and approved the final manuscript.

Author details

[1] Department of Population Health, New York University School of Medicine, 550 First Avenue, VZ30 6th Floor, New York, NY 10016, USA. [2] Division of General Internal Medicine, Department of Medicine, New York University School of Medicine, 550 First Avenue, New York, NY 10016, USA. [3] Greenfield Health and Department of Psychiatry, Oregon Health and Science University, 9450 SW

Barnes Suite 100, Portland, OR 97225, USA. [4] Department of Psychiatry, New York University School of Medicine, One Park Avenue, 8th Floor, New York, NY 10016, USA. [5] Division of General Internal Medicine, Department of Medicine, Icahn School of Medicine at Mt. Sinai, One Gustave L. Levy Place, New York, NY 10029, USA. [6] Department of Psychiatry, Icahn School of Medicine at Mt. Sinai, 1090 Amsterdam Avenue, New York, NY 10025, USA. [7] OHSU-PSU School of Public Health, Oregon Health and Science University, 3181 SW Sam Jackson Park Road, Portland, OR 97239, USA.

Acknowledgements
The authors wish to acknowledge Melanie Harris, Marie Payment, Patricia Novo, Carol Cushing, and Carmen Rosa, and for their assistance with the study.

Competing interests
The authors declare that they have no competing interests

Funding
Supported by National Institute on Drug Abuse cooperative awards: U10DA013035, UG1DA013035, and UG1DA015815.

References

1. Dowell D, et al. Contribution of opioid-involved poisoning to the change in life expectancy in the United States, 2000–2015. JAMA 2017;318(11):1065–7.
2. Horgan, CM, Skwara KC, Strickler G. Substance abuse: the nation's number one health problem. Robert Wood Johnson Foundation and Schneider Institute for Health Policy, 2001.
3. Mokdad AH, Marks JS, Stroup DF, Gerberding JL. Actual causes of death in the United States, 2000. JAMA. 2004;291(10):1238–45.
4. McGinnis JM, Foege WH. Actual causes of death in the United States. JAMA. 1993;270(18):2207–12.
5. Substance Abuse and Mental Health Services Administration. NSDUH data review: receipt of services for substance use and mental health issues among adults: results from the 2016 national survey on drug use and health. Rockville: Substance Abuse and Mental Health Services Administration; 2017. https://www.samhsa.gov/data/sites/default/files/NSDUH-DR-FFR2-2016/NSDUH-DR-FFR2-2016.pdf. Accessed 6 Feb 2018.
6. Edlund MJ, Unutzer J, Wells KB. Clinician screening and treatment of alcohol, drug, and mental problems in primary care: results from healthcare for communities. Med Care. 2004;42(12):1158–66.
7. Rehm J, Anderson P, Manthey J, Shield KD, Struzzo P, Wojnar M, et al. Alcohol use disorders in primary health care: what do we know and where do we go? Alcohol Alcohol. 2016;51(4):422–7.
8. O'Donnell A, Anderson P, Newbury-Birch D, Schulte B, Schmidt C, Reimer J, et al. The impact of brief alcohol interventions in primary healthcare: a systematic review of reviews. Alcohol Alcohol. 2014;49(1):66–78.
9. Solberg LI, Maciosek MV, Edwards NM. Primary care intervention to reduce alcohol misuse ranking its health impact and cost effectiveness. Am J Prev Med. 2008;34(2):143–52.
10. Whitlock EP, Polen MR, Green CA, Orleans T, Klein J. Behavioral counseling interventions in primary care to reduce risky/harmful alcohol use by adults: a summary of the evidence for the U.S. Preventive Services Task Force. Ann Intern Med. 2004;140(7):557–68.
11. Maciosek MV, Coffield AB, Edwards NM, Flottemesch TJ, Goodman MJ, Solberg LI. Priorities among effective clinical preventive services: results of a systematic review and analysis. Am J Prev Med. 2006;31(1):52–61.
12. Kaner EF, Dickinson HO, Beyer F, Pienaar E, Schlesinger C, Campbell F, et al. The effectiveness of brief alcohol interventions in primary care settings: a systematic review. Drug and Alcohol Review. 2009;28(3):301–23.
13. Moyer VA. Screening and behavioral counseling interventions in primary care to reduce alcohol misuse: U.S. preventive services task force recommendation statement. Ann Intern Med. 2013;159(3):210–8.
14. SBIRT: Screening, Brief Intervention, and Referral to Treatment 2014 [cited 13 Oct 2014]. http://www.integration.samhsa.gov/clinical-practice/SBIRT. Accessed 14 July 2017.
15. U.S. Department of Health and Human Services (HHS), Office of the Surgeon General, Facing Addiction in America: The Surgeon General's Report on Alcohol, Drugs, and Health. Washington; 2016.
16. Babor TF, McRee BG, Kassebaum PA, Grimaldi PL, Ahmed K, Bray J. Screening, Brief Intervention, and Referral to Treatment (SBIRT): toward a public health approach to the management of substance abuse. Subst Abuse. 2007;28(3):7–30.
17. Nilsen P. Brief alcohol intervention—where to from here? Challenges remain for research and practice. Addiction (Abingdon, England). 2010;105(6):954–9.
18. Nilsen P, Aalto M, Bendtsen P, Seppa K. Effectiveness of strategies to implement brief alcohol intervention in primary healthcare. A systematic review. Scand J Prim Health Care. 2006;24(1):5–15.
19. Kaner E. Brief alcohol intervention: time for translational research. Addiction (Abingdon, England). 2010;105(6):960–1.
20. Babor TF, Higgins-Biddle JC. Alcohol screening and brief intervention: dissemination strategies for medical practice and public health. Addiction. 2000;95(5):677–86.
21. Rieckmann T, Abraham A, Zwick J, Rasplica C, McCarty D. A longitudinal study of state strategies and policies to accelerate evidence-based practices in the context of systems transformation. Health Serv Res. 2015;50(4):1125–45.
22. Garnick DW, Horgan CM, Merrick EL, Hoyt A. Identification and treatment of mental and substance use conditions: health plans strategies. Med Care. 2007;45(11):1060–7.
23. Mertens JR, Chi FW, Weisner CM, Satre DD, Ross TB, Allen S, et al. Physician versus non-physician delivery of alcohol screening, brief intervention and referral to treatment in adult primary care: the ADVISe cluster randomized controlled implementation trial. Addict Sci Clin Pract. 2015;10(1):26.
24. Williams EC, Johnson ML, Lapham GT, Caldeiro RM, Chew L, Fletcher GS, et al. Strategies to implement alcohol screening and brief intervention in primary care settings: a structured literature review. Psychol Addict Behav. 2011;25(2):206–14.
25. NIDA CTN Common Data Elements. https://cde.drugabuse.gov/. Accessed 14 July 2017.
26. Ghitza UE, Gore-Langton RE, Lindblad R, Shide D, Subramaniam G, Tai B. Common data elements for substance use disorders in electronic health records: the NIDA Clinical Trials Network experience. Addiction. 2013;108(1):3–8.
27. Nilsen P. Making sense of implementation theories, models and frameworks. Implement Sci. 2015;10:53.
28. Graham ID, Logan J, Harrison MB, Straus SE, Tetroe J, Caswell W, et al. Lost in knowledge translation: time for a map? J Contin Educ Health Prof. 2006;26(1):13–24.
29. Kastner M, Straus SE. Application of the Knowledge-to-Action and Medical Research Council frameworks in the development of an osteoporosis clinical decision support tool. J Clin Epidemiol. 2012;65(11):1163–70. https://doi.org/10.1016/j.jclinepi.2012.04.011.
30. Oregon Health Authority. 2013 Quality Pool Reference Instructions. http://www.oregon.gov/oha/analytics/CCOData/Reference%20Instructions.pdf. Accessed 3 Mar 2017.
31. Rieckmann T, Renfro S, McCarty D, Baker R, McConnell KJ. Quality metrics and systems transformation: are we advancing alcohol and drug screening in primary care? Health Serv Res. 2017;. https://doi.org/10.1111/1475-6773.12716.
32. Medscape. Medscape EHR report 2016. http://www.medscape.com.ezproxy.med.nyu.edu/features/slideshow/public/ehr2016. Accessed 7 July 2017.
33. Patton MQ. Qualitative research and evaluation methods. 3rd ed. Thousand Oaks: Sage; 2002.
34. Patton MQ. Enhancing the quality and credibility of qualitative analysis. Health Serv Res. 1999;5(34):1189–208.
35. Boyatzis RE. Thematic analysis and code development: transforming qualitative information. London: Sage; 1998.
36. Fleiss JL. Statistical methods for rates and proportions. 2nd ed. New York: Wiley; 1981.
37. Averill JB. Matrix analysis as a complementary analytic strategy in qualitative inquiry. Qual Health Res. 2002;12:855–66.

38. Kaner E, Bland M, Cassidy P, Coulton S, Deluca P, Drummond C, et al. Screening and brief interventions for hazardous and harmful alcohol use in primary care: a cluster randomised controlled trial protocol. BMC Public Health. 2009;9:287. https://doi.org/10.1186/471-2458-9-287.
39. Hilbink M, Voerman G, van Beurden I, Penninx B, Laurant M. A randomized controlled trial of a tailored primary care program to reverse excessive alcohol consumption. J Am Board Fam Med. 2012;25(5):712–22.
40. van Beurden I, Anderson P, Akkermans RP, Grol RP, Wensing M, Laurant MG. Involvement of general practitioners in managing alcohol problems: a randomized controlled trial of a tailored improvement programme. Addiction (Abingdon, England). 2012;107(9):1601–11.
41. Williams EC, Achtmeyer CE, Young JP, Rittmueller SE, Ludman EJ, Lapham GT, et al. Local implementation of alcohol screening and brief intervention at five Veterans Health Administration primary care clinics: perspectives of clinical and administrative staff. J Subst Abuse Treat. 2016;60:27–35.
42. Berger D, Bradley KA. Primary care management of alcohol misuse. Med Clin N Am. 2015;99(5):989–1016.
43. U.S. Preventive Services Task Force. Screening for Illicit Drug Use: U.S. Preventive Services Task Force Recommendation Statement. 2008. https://www.uspreventiveservicestaskforce.org/Page/Document/UpdateSummaryFinal/drug-use-illicit-screening. Accessed 14 July 2017.
44. Roy-Byrne P, Bumgardner K, Krupski A, Dunn C, Ries R, Donovan D, et al. Brief intervention for problem drug use in safety-net primary care settings a randomized clinical trial. J Am Med Assoc. 2014;312(5):492–501.
45. Saitz R, Palfai TPA, Cheng DM, Alford DP, Bernstein JA, Lloyd-Travaglini CA, et al. Screening and brief intervention for drug use in primary care the ASPIRE randomized clinical trial. J Am Med Assoc. 2014;312(5):502–13.
46. Gelberg L, Andersen RM, Afifi AA, Leake BD, Arangua L, Vahidi M, et al. Project QUIT (Quit Using Drugs Intervention Trial): a randomized controlled trial of a primary care-based multi-component brief intervention to reduce risky drug use. Addiction (Abingdon, England). 2015;110(11):1777–90.
47. Hingson R, Compton WM. Screening and brief intervention and referral to treatment for drug use in primary care: back to the drawing board. JAMA. 2014;312(5):488–9. https://doi.org/10.1001/jama.2014.7863.
48. Sterling S, Kline-Simon AH, Wibbelsman C, Wong A, Weisner C. Screening for adolescent alcohol and drug use in pediatric health-care settings: predictors and implications for practice and policy. Addict Sci Clin Pract. 2012;7(1):13.
49. Friedmann PD, McCullough D, Saitz R. Screening and intervention for illicit drug abuse: a national survey of primary care physicians and psychiatrists. Arch Intern Med. 2001;161(2):248–51.
50. Friedmann PD, McCullough D, Chin MH, Saitz R. Screening and intervention for alcohol problems. A national survey of primary care physicians and psychiatrists. J Gen Intern Med. 2000;15(2):84–91.
51. McCormick KA, Cochran NE, Back AL, Merrill JO, Williams EC, Bradley KA. How primary care providers talk to patients about alcohol: a qualitative study. J Gen Intern Med. 2006;21(9):966–72.
52. Spandorfer JM, Israel Y, Turner BJ. Primary care physicians' views on screening and management of alcohol abuse: inconsistencies with national guidelines. J Fam Pract. 1999;48(11):899–902.
53. Johnson M, Jackson R, Guillaume L, Meier P, Goyder E. Barriers and facilitators to implementing screening and brief intervention for alcohol misuse: a systematic review of qualitative evidence. J Public Health (Oxf). 2011;33(3):412–21. https://doi.org/10.1093/pubmed/fdq095.
54. Aira M, Kauhanen J, Larivaara P, Rautio P. Factors influencing inquiry about patients' alcohol consumption by primary health care physicians: qualitative semi-structured interview study. Fam Pract. 2003;20(3):270–5.
55. Yoast RA, Wilford BB, Hayashi SW. Encouraging physicians to screen for and intervene in substance use disorders: obstacles and strategies for change. J Addict Dis. 2008;27(3):77–97. https://doi.org/10.1080/10550880802122687.
56. Williams EC, Achtmeyer CE, Young JP, Berger D, Curran G, Bradley KA, et al. Barriers to and facilitators of alcohol use disorder pharmacotherapy in primary care: a qualitative study in five VA clinics. J Gen Intern Med. 2017. https://doi.org/10.1007/s11606-017-4202-z.
57. Spear SE, Shedlin M, Gilberti B, Fiellin M, McNeely J. Feasibility and acceptability of an audio computer-assisted self-interview version of the Alcohol, Smoking and Substance Involvement Screening Test (ASSIST) in primary care patients. Subst Abuse. 2016;37(2):299–305.
58. Rahm AK, Boggs JM, Martin C, Price DW, Beck A, Backer TE, et al. Facilitators and barriers to implementing Screening, Brief Intervention, and Referral to Treatment (SBIRT) in primary care in integrated health care settings. Subst Abuse. 2015;36(3):281–8.
59. Williams EC, Achtmeyer CE, Thomas RM, Grossbard JR, Lapham GT, Chavez LJ, et al. Factors underlying quality problems with alcohol screening prompted by a clinical reminder in primary care: a multi-site qualitative study. J Gen Intern Med. 2015.
60. Schomerus G, Lucht M, Holzinger A, Matschinger H, Carta MG, Angermeyer MC. The stigma of alcohol dependence compared with other mental disorders: a review of population studies. Alcohol Alcohol. 2011;46(2):105–12.
61. Brener L, von Hippel W, von Hippel C, Resnick I, Treloar C. Perceptions of discriminatory treatment by staff as predictors of drug treatment completion: utility of a mixed methods approach. Drug Alcohol Rev. 2010;29(5):491–7.
62. Luoma JB, Twohig MP, Waltz T, Hayes SC, Roget N, Padilla M, et al. An investigation of stigma in individuals receiving treatment for substance abuse. Addict Behav. 2007;32(7):1331–46.
63. Anderson P, Laurant M, Kaner E, Wensing M, Grol R. Engaging general practitioners in the management of hazardous and harmful alcohol consumption: results of a meta-analysis. J Stud Alcohol. 2004;65(2):191–9.

Alcohol consumption patterns and HIV viral suppression among persons receiving HIV care in Florida

R. L. Cook[1*], Z. Zhou[1], N. E. Kelso-Chichetto[1], J. Janelle[1,2], J. P. Morano[6], C. Somboonwit[7], W. Carter[8], G. E. Ibanez[9], N. Ennis[3], C. L. Cook[4], R. A. Cohen[3], B. Brumback[5] and K. Bryant[10]

Abstract

Background: Alcohol consumption has been associated with poor antiretroviral therapy (ART) adherence but less is known about its relationship to HIV viral suppression, or whether certain drinking patterns have a stronger association than others. The objectives of this study were to determine the association of different patterns of alcohol consumption to HIV viral suppression and ART adherence, and to determine whether any associations of alcohol with HIV viral suppression were mediated by poor ART adherence.

Methods: This observational study used baseline data from 619 HIV+ participants, recruited across 8 clinical and community settings across Florida as part of the Florida Cohort from 2014 to 2016. Alcohol consumption was measured by self-report, and grouped into four categories: heavy drinking (>7/week for women or >14 drinks/week for men); binge, but not heavy drinking (≥4 or >5 drinks/occasion for women and men, respectively), low level drinking (neither heavy nor binge), and abstinence. Serum HIV RNA measurements were obtained from statewide HIV surveillance data, and durable viral suppression was defined as achieving HIV viral suppression (<200 copies/ml) at every assessment in the past 12 months.

Results: The majority of the 619 participants were male (63%) and aged 45 or greater (65%). The proportion of participants with heavy, binge, low-level drinking and abstinence was 9, 25, 37 and 30%, respectively. Optimal ART adherence (≥95%) was reported by 68%, and 60% achieved durable viral suppression. In multivariable analysis controlling for demographic factors, drug use, and homelessness, heavy drinking (compared to abstinence) was associated with increased odds of failing to achieve durable viral suppression (OR 2.16, 95% CI 1.08–4.32) whereas binge drinking alone was not significantly associated with this outcome (OR 1.04, 95% CI 0.64–1.70). Both heavy drinking and binge drinking were significantly associated with suboptimal ART adherence. Mediation analyses suggested that only a small proportion of the relationship between heavy drinking and suboptimal viral suppression was due to poor ART adherence.

Conclusions: Exceeding weekly recommended levels of alcohol consumption (heavy drinking) was significantly associated with poor HIV viral suppression and ART non-adherence, while binge drinking was associated with suboptimal ART adherence in this sample. Clinicians should attempt to address heavy drinking in their patients with HIV.

Keywords: Alcohol consumption, Binge drinking, HIV, Viral suppression, ART adherence

*Correspondence: cookrl@ufl.edu
[1] Department of Epidemiology, College of Public Health and Health Professions and College of Medicine, University of Florida, PO Box 100231, Gainesville, FL 32610, USA
Full list of author information is available at the end of the article

Background

Despite widespread availability of antiretroviral therapy (ART) in the United States, viral suppression (<200 copies/ml) is achieved in only 25% of all persons living with HIV and 70% of those retained in care [1]. Lack of HIV viral suppression is associated with more rapid HIV disease progression, cardiovascular complications [2] and transmission of HIV within the community [1]. Therefore, strategies to improve HIV viral suppression are an important part of the current national HIV strategy [3].

Alcohol consumption is common in persons with HIV infection [4] and has been linked to several adverse health outcomes in this population [5]. Alcohol consumption could affect HIV viral suppression via both behavioral (e.g. ART adherence) and biological (e.g. immune dysfunction) mechanisms [5]. While researchers have consistently found an association between alcohol consumption and poor ART adherence [6, 7], relatively few studies have reported on the association of alcohol consumption to HIV viral suppression in the ART era [8]. These studies have produced mixed results, with some showing an association of alcohol use with HIV disease progression and poor viral suppression [9–11], while others find no significant association [12, 13].

Some of the differences in findings across different populations could be due to the way that alcohol exposure was defined, or whether or not the investigators controlled for potential confounding variables. In general, papers focusing on alcohol use feature a wide range of definitions to define alcohol consumption, ranging from "any" versus "none"; quantity/frequency of drinking (e.g. number of drinks per week), binge drinking (e.g. number of drinks consumed in one drinking session), to the presence of an alcohol use disorder. Differences in these definitions can lead to inconsistent results that are difficult to compare by study [14].

Alcohol consumption often overlaps with several other health conditions or behaviors that could be linked to poor HIV viral suppression, including social determinants of health (e.g. homelessness) [15, 16], comorbid behavioral health conditions (e.g. depression and anxiety) [17, 18], and other substance use [17–20]. These overlapping factors should be considered when making a conclusion about whether alcohol consumption does have an independent effect on HIV viral suppression.

Little is known about which specific patterns of drinking are most strongly associated with poor HIV viral suppression, and whether any associations can be explained by the impact of alcohol on ART adherence. Therefore, the objectives of this study were to determine the association of alcohol consumption to HIV viral suppression using two different definitions of alcohol consumption patterns (heavy use and binge-drinking), and to determine whether any associations could be explained by differences in ART adherence.

Methods

Participants

Between October 2014 and December 2016, we recruited 903 participants living with HIV/AIDS into the Florida Cohort. Initiated in 2014 and ongoing, the Florida Cohort collects self-reported information about demographic and behavioral factors that may affect health outcomes for persons with HIV/AIDS. Participants were recruited from a collaborative network of county health departments and community setting clinics throughout Florida (includes sites at Lake City, Gainesville, Tampa, Orlando, Sanford, Ft. Lauderdale, and Miami). Any person with HIV greater than 18 years of age was eligible to participate in the study. After providing written informed consent, participants completed an anonymous, self-administered questionnaire examining demographics, substance use, mental health symptoms, and HIV-related health behavior. In order to ensure that all interested and eligible persons could participate, study staff asked if assistance was needed to complete the questionnaire; in such cases the questionnaire was read to the participants. The survey took approximately 30–45 min to complete, and participants received a $25 incentive for their time.

With approval from the Florida Department of Health, survey responses were securely linked to medical records to obtain additional data on anti-retroviral medications, co-morbid health conditions, and laboratory test results, including HIV viral load and CD4+ T-cell count. Florida mandates that HIV viral load test results are reported to the statewide HIV surveillance system; for this reason, the surveillance information was able to be matched and linked for 97% of all study participants. The research procedures are approved by the institutional review boards (IRB) at the University of Florida, Florida International University, and the Florida Department of Health. In order to study the effect of alcohol on durable viral suppression, we limited this analysis to 619 participants who had been diagnosed with HIV for at least 1 year, who had at least 2 HIV viral load test results in the prior 12 months, and who did not have missing data for alcohol exposure. The 619 persons included in the analysis were not significantly different from those excluded for missing data about alcohol consumption in terms of age, race, or gender.

Measures

Alcohol consumption

Participants self-reported their alcohol consumption by answering the questions "In the past 12 months, how often did you have a drink containing alcohol" (options:

less than 1–3 times a month, 1–3 times a week, 4–6 times a week, every day), "How many standard drinks would you have on a typical day" (range 0 to 6+), and "How often did you have 4+ standard drinks for women or 5+ standard drinks for men on one occasion? (options: never, less than monthly, monthly, weekly, or daily/almost daily)". These three drinking items are based on the AUDIT-C, a 3-item scaled used to screen for drinking in primary care settings [21]. Using this information, plus the question "during the last 30 days, what is the largest number of drinks that you drank within a 24-h period", we defined two different patterns of alcohol consumption. Average weekly consumption was determined by multiplying the average quantity and frequency, and "heavy drinking" was defined as consuming more than 7 or 14 drinks/week for women or men [22]. Binge drinking focused on the amount consumed in one sitting, and was defined as consuming ≥4 or ≥5 drinks for women or men at least once a month in the past 12 months [22]. Because over 90% of heavy drinkers also reported binge drinking, we categorized each person into one of four categories: Heavy (regardless of binge status); binge (not including heavy drinking), low level drinking (any drinking that was not heavy or binge), or no current drinking (abstinence).

Covariates

The study questionnaire assessed socio-demographic variables, including age, gender, race and ethnicity, education and homelessness. The Personal Health Questionnaire Depression Scale (PHQ-8 score) and Generalized Anxiety Disorder 7-item scale (GAD-7) were used to assess current depressive symptoms (PHQ-8 score ≥10) and current anxiety symptoms (GAD-7 score ≥10), respectively [23, 24]. Current tobacco use was categorized as yes or no. We created a dichotomous summary variable that indicated any use of injected or non-injected illicit drugs in the past 12-months, including marijuana, cocaine/crack, heroin, pain medications (like oxycontin), sedatives, methamphetamine, ecstasy, and other stimulants.

Antiretroviral (ART) adherence

ART adherence was assessed by self-report, as this has been shown to correlate strongly with HIV outcomes and is simpler and less costly to obtain compared to other ART adherence assessment options [25, 26]. ART adherence was defined as the proportion of days in last 30 days they did not miss any medications, based on their response to the question, "In the last 30 days, how many days did you miss at least one dose of any of your HIV medication?", and was dichotomized as ≥95 versus <95% [27]. Adherence of 95% or greater is considered optimal adherence and has been associated with improved outcomes in terms of CD4 count and viral suppression [28, 29].

Viral suppression

HIV viral load values were obtained from HIV surveillance data. We considered the lab value closest to the time of baseline survey completion, and also all HIV viral load measures obtained up to 12 months prior to survey completion. We defined HIV viral suppression as an HIV-1 RNA test value ≤200 copies/ml. Durable viral suppression was achieved if all HIV viral load tests were suppressed viral load (≤200 copies/ml) in the past 12 months.

Data analysis

We first conducted a descriptive analysis comparing potential risk factors with the four patterns of drinking (heavy, binge, low, and none), using the Chi square test to assess for statistical significance across the 4 drinking categories. We compared the proportions of participants achieving durable HIV viral suppression and ≥95% ART adherence in each of the 3 drinking patterns compared to non-drinkers. We then conducted multivariable logistic regression analyses to identify the relationship of the different drinking patterns with durable viral load suppression, after controlling for demographic and behavioral characteristics that were significantly associated with durable viral suppression in bivariate analysis ($p < .10$). Crude and adjusted odds ratios with 95% confidence limits were reported. To assess whether the relationship of alcohol consumption to viral suppression was mediated by ART adherence, we conducted a mediation analysis [30]. The mediation analysis sought to differentiate the direct effects of heavy drinking on HIV viral suppression from indirect effects mediated by ART adherence. Because the dependent variable was not rare, we used a generalized linear model regression with a log link function for viral suppression, which produces estimates of risk ratios. No covariates were included due to convergence issues when fitting a log-linear model for the outcome. The mediation macro developed by Valeri and VanderWeele was used to calculate the bootstrap confidence intervals with 1000 bootstrap samples [30].

Overall, missing data on most covariates of interests were minimal (<3%). However, approximately 9% of participants did not report or partially reported the use of illegal drugs in the past year. In order to address the potential for biased estimates, multiple imputation was performed using fully conditional specification (FSC) method to generate 20 complete datasets. All variables in the multivariable model were used in the imputation.

All data analyses were performed in SAS version 9.4 (SAS Institute, Carry, NC, USA).

Results

Characteristics of the 619 study participants are presented in Table 1. The majority of the sample was male (63%), aged 45 years or greater (65%), and diverse in terms of race/ethnicity and education status (Table 1). Homelessness in the past year was reported among 16%. Current smoking and illicit drug use was reported by 53 and 58%, respectively. Symptoms of depression (31%) and anxiety (29%) were relatively common. Durable viral load suppression was achieved among only 60% of the sample. Among those currently using ART (94%), 68% reported optimal ART adherence. Thirty percent of the sample reported no use of alcohol in the past year, 9% met criteria for heavy drinking (exceeds weekly limits), 25% met criteria for binge drinking (but not heavy drinking), and 37% reported low level, non-binge drinking.

Descriptive analyses showing the distribution of potential covariates to the four drinking categories are shown in Table 2. Heavy and/or binge drinking were more common among those with less than a high-school education, those who smoked or used illicit drugs, persons who had been homeless in the past year, and persons with symptoms of depression or anxiety.

The proportion of persons with optimal ART adherence (≥95%) was significantly lower with each increasing category of alcohol consumption, compared to those who were abstinent (Fig. 1). Specifically, optimal ART adherence was reported by 80% of non-drinkers, 68% of low level drinkers, 58% of binge drinkers, and 51% of heavy drinkers. In contrast, durable viral suppression was significantly lower only in persons with heavy drinking (41%) compared to those who were abstinent (66%), but there was no significant difference in durable viral suppression in persons with low-level drinking (60%) or binge drinking alone (59%) compared to those who were abstinent (Fig. 2). In multivariable analyses, heavy drinking, compared to abstinence, was associated with suboptimal HIV viral load suppression in both crude analyses (OR 2.79; 95% CI 1.50–5.21) and adjusted analyses (OR 2.16; 95% CI 1.08–4.32) (Table 3). In contrast, binge drinking alone (without heavy drinking) was not associated with a significant change in overall rates of optimal viral suppression (unadjusted OR 1.35, 95% CI 0.87–2.10; adjusted OR 1.04, 95% CI 0.64–1.70) (Table 3).

In the mediation analysis, the majority of the relationship between heavy drinking and suboptimal HIV viral suppression was via a direct effect (RR 1.61, 95% CI 1.16,

Table 1 Baseline characteristics of persons living with HIV in the Florida Cohort (N = 619), 2014–2016

Baseline characteristics	No. (column %)
Gender	
Male	393 (63)
Female	226 (37)
Race	
Non-Hispanic White	137 (22)
Non-Hispanic Black	346 (56)
Hispanic	112 (18)
Other	24 (4)
Age group	
18–34	92 (15)
35–44	125 (20)
45–54	246 (40)
≥55	156 (25)
Education	
<High school	205 (33)
High school or equivalent	189 (31)
>High school	222 (36)
Homelessness	
No	513 (84)
Yes	96 (16)
Current smoking	
No	280 (47)
Yes	313 (53)
Any illicit drug use	
No	236 (42)
Yes	328 (58)
Current depressive symptoms	
No	416 (69)
Yes	188 (31)
Current anxiety symptoms	
No	428 (71)
Yes	174 (29)
Current ART use	
No	35 (6)
Yes	579 (94)
Current ART adherence	
<95%	177 (32)
≥95%	371 (68)
Durable viral load suppression	
≤200 copies/ml	369 (60)
>200 copies/ml	250 (40)
Drinking status	
Abstinence	184 (30)
Low, non-binge drinking	226 (37)
Binge drinking only	155 (25)
Heavy drinking	54 (9)

ART antiretroviral therapy

Table 2 Bivariate associations between covariates and alcohol consumption among the Florida Cohort (N = 619), 2014–2016

Characteristic	Drinking status (past year)					
	Total	N (Row %)				p value
		Abstinence	Low	Binge only	Heavy	
Gender						
Male	393 (63)	95 (24)	163 (41)	103 (26)	32 (8)	<.001
Female	226 (37)	89 (39)	63 (28)	52 (23)	22 (10)	
Race						
Non-Hispanic White	137 (22)	40 (29)	48 (35)	34 (25)	15 (11)	.95
Non-Hispanic Black	346 (56)	106 (31)	122 (35)	88 (25)	30 (9)	
Hispanic	112 (18)	30 (27)	47 (42)	27 (24)	8 (7)	
Other	24 (4)	8 (33)	9 (38)	6 (25)	1 (4)	
Age group						
18–34	92 (15)	17 (18)	41 (45)	26 (28)	8 (9)	.45
35–44	125 (20)	39 (31)	43 (34)	33 (26)	10 (8)	
45–54	246 (40)	79 (32)	83 (34)	59 (24)	25 (10)	
≥55	156 (25)	49 (31)	59 (38)	37 (24)	11 (7)	
Education						
<High school	205 (33)	69 (34)	50 (24)	57 (28)	29 (14)	<.001
High school or equivalent	189 (31)	52 (28)	77 (41)	48 (25)	12 (6)	
>High school	222 (36)	60 (27)	99 (45)	50 (33)	13 (6)	
Homelessness						
No	513 (84)	154 (30)	194 (38)	122 (24)	43 (8)	.08
Yes	96 (16)	23 (24)	29 (30)	33 (34)	11 (11)	
Current smoking						
No	280 (47)	97 (35)	112 (40)	58 (21)	13 (5)	<.001
Yes	313 (53)	77 (25)	105 (34)	92 (29)	39 (12)	
Any illicit drug use						
No	236 (42)	99 (42)	80 (34)	46 (19)	11 (5)	<.001
Yes	328 (58)	54 (16)	132 (40)	101 (31)	41 (13)	
Current depressive symptoms						
No	416 (69)	127 (31)	156 (38)	106 (25)	27 (6)	.08
Yes	188 (31)	53 (28)	63 (34)	48 (26)	24 (13)	
Current anxiety symptoms						
No	428 (71)	123 (29)	170 (40)	104 (24)	31 (7)	.04
Yes	174 (29)	54 (31)	50 (29)	49 (28)	21 (12)	
Current ART Adherence[a]						
<95%	177 (32)	32 (18)	64 (36)	59 (33)	22 (12)	<.001
≥95%	371 (68)	130 (35)	136 (37)	82 (22)	23 (6)	
Durable ART suppression						
≤200 copies/ml	369 (60)	121 (33)	135 (37)	91 (25)	22 (6)	.01
>200 copies/ml	250 (40)	63 (25)	91 (36)	64 (26)	32 (13)	

[a] Among participants who were currently taking ART. p values represent Chi square tests that the distribution of the variable varies by alcohol pattern

2.05), with a smaller yet significant indirect effect mediated via poor ART adherence (RR 1.05, 95% CI 1.00, 1.13) (Table 4). Although the overall effect of binge drinking on suboptimal HIV viral suppression was not significant (Table 4), the data suggest that indirect effects (mediated by poor ART adherence) could be more important when considering the relationship of binge drinking to suboptimal HIV viral suppression.

Table 3 Crude and adjusted associations between alcohol consumption and lack of durable viral load suppression among PLWH in the Florida Cohort (N = 619), 2014–2016

Characteristic	Crude estimates			Adjusted estimates		
	OR	95% CI	p value	AOR	95% CI	p value
Gender (ref = male)						
Female	0.83	0.60–1.17	.29	0.72	0.49–1.06	.09
Race (ref = Non-Hispanic White)						
Non-Hispanic Black	2.04	1.34–3.10	.69	1.85	1.17–2.94	.009
Hispanic	1.12	0.65	<.001	1.08	0.60	.80
Other	0.93	0.36	.88	0.71	0.26	.51
Age group (ref ≥ 55)						
18–34	3.77	2.18–6.51	<.001	3.99	2.21–7.20	<.001
35–44	2.95	1.78–4.87	<.001	2.80	1.64–4.76	<.001
45–54	1.82	1.17–2.84	.007	1.69	1.06–2.69	.03
Education (ref > high school)						
<High school	2.11	1.42–3.14	<.001	1.79	1.13–2.84	.01
High school or equivalent	1.74	1.16–2.60	.007	1.48	0.95–2.31	.09
Homelessness (ref = no)						
Yes	2.38	1.53–3.71	<.001	1.87	1.14–3.07	.01
Current smoking (ref = no)						
Yes	2.00	1.43–2.80	<.001	1.46	0.99–2.16	.06
Illicit drug use (ref = no)						
Yes	1.46	1.04–2.06	.03	1.17	0.78–1.75	.44
Depressive symptoms (ref = no)						
Yes	1.02	0.72–1.45	.92	–	–	–
Anxiety symptoms (ref = no)						
Yes	1.27	0.89–1.81	.19	–	–	–
Drinking status (ref = abstinence)						
Low drinking	1.29	0.86–1.94	.21	1.19	0.76–1.88	.45
Binge drinking only	1.35	0.87–2.10	.18	1.04	0.64–1.70	.87
Heavy drinking	2.79	1.50–5.21	.001	2.16	1.08–4.32	.03

PLWH persons living with HIV, *OR* odds ratio, *AOR* adjusted odds ratio, *CI* confidence limits

Discussion

In this sample of persons living with HIV infection in Florida, heavy alcohol consumption was associated with approximately twice the odds of having suboptimal HIV viral suppression compared to non-drinkers, even when accounting for several potential confounding variables. In contrast, adults who reported occasional binge drinking but did not meet criteria for heavy drinking were not as a group significantly different from non-drinkers in terms of overall durable HIV viral suppression. The findings demonstrate that differences in the way that alcohol consumption is measured and defined can result in different conclusions about the relationship of alcohol consumption with HIV-related health outcomes or behaviors.

Heavy drinking was also significantly associated with suboptimal ART adherence, so we assessed whether the association of heavy drinking to suboptimal HIV viral suppression was mediated by poor ART adherence. We found that only a small, albeit significant, proportion of the association was via an indirect (mediation) pathway. These findings suggest that much of the relationship between heavy drinking and suboptimal HIV viral suppression maybe due to other mechanisms such as direct biological effects of alcohol on the immune system or to the effects of alcohol on behavior, including engagement in care and persistence on ART therapy [31].

Approximately a quarter of the population met criteria for binge drinking but not for heavy drinking, and given that binge drinking was associated with suboptimal ART adherence, it was somewhat surprising that binge drinking was not also associated with poor HIV viral suppression. It could be that current ART medications are more forgiving in terms of ART adherence [32], or there could be other unmeasured differences between the heavy drinkers and binge drinkers in this sample. Our findings are also consistent with other research that has generally

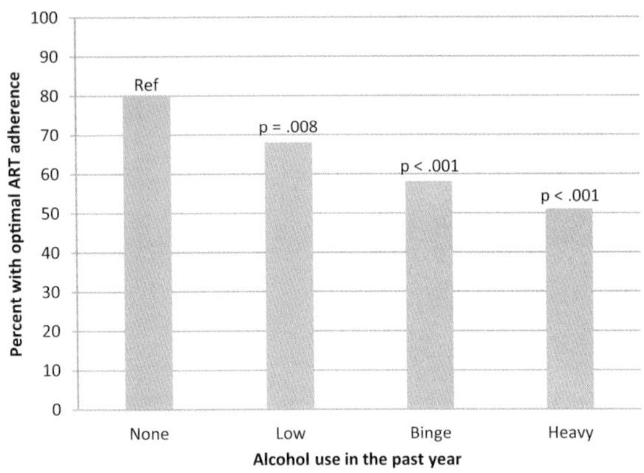

Fig. 1 Proportion of 579 persons with HIV who are receiving ART that report optimal (≥95%) adherence to antiretroviral treatment in the previous month, according to alcohol consumption classification. Binge drinking defined as exceeding daily (but not weekly) drinking recommendations, and heavy drinking defined as exceeding weekly drinking recommendations. Florida Cohort, 2014–2016

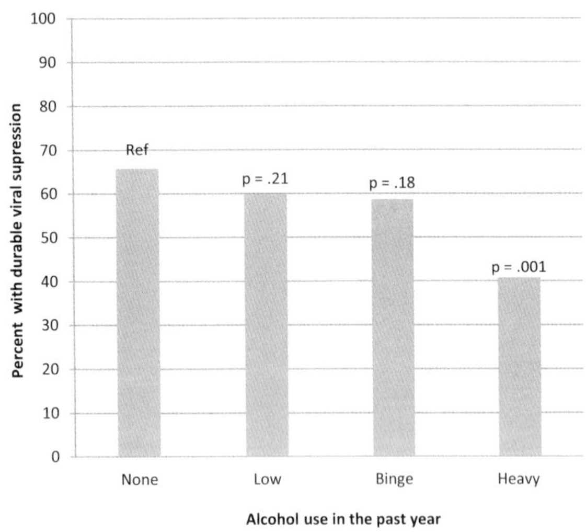

Fig. 2 Proportion of 619 persons with HIV with durable HIV viral suppression (HIV viral load undetectable or <200 copies/ml at each test in the past year). Binge drinking defined as exceeding daily (but not weekly) drinking recommendations, and heavy drinking defined as exceeding weekly drinking recommendations. Florida Cohort, 2014–2016

found the highest levels of alcohol consumption, but not all alcohol use patterns, to be associated with poor HIV viral suppression [9–11].

The evidence for a causal relationship between alcohol consumption and poor HIV viral suppression is supported by longitudinal data showing that increases in drinking correlate with worse viral suppression [9], and some evidence that a reduction in alcohol consumption

Table 4 Direct and indirect risk ratios for suboptimal HIV viral suppression for various alcohol consumption patterns

	Low drinking	Binge only	Heavy drinking
Direct effect	0.97 (0.76, 1.20)	1.02 (0.79, 1.26)	1.61 (1.16, 2.05)*
Indirect effect	1.00 (0.97, 1.03)	1.04 (1.01, 1.10)*	1.05 (1.00, 1.13)*
Total effect	0.97 (0.75, 1.20)	1.07 (0.82, 1.32)	1.70 (1.24, 2.18)*

Florida Cohort (N = 619), 2014–2016

* $p < .05$. The indirect effect represents the effect mediated by ART adherence

is associated with improved HIV viral suppression [33]. However, several limitations of the current study warrant mention. Although we used an item from a validated scale [26], self-reported ART adherence tends to over-estimate adherence. We chose to use a traditional cut-point of 95% adherent to distinguish adequate from inadequate adherence, although viral suppression can be now achieved with lower adherence (e.g. 80%) with more recent ART regimens [32]. Our sample was a convenience sample of persons who had been in care during the previous year, thus may not represent the entire population of persons living with HIV. The proportion of persons who met criteria for heavy drinking (exceeding weekly drinking limits) was also somewhat lower than the proportion found in other samples of PLWH. We likely under-estimated actual consumption, in part, due to limited response options on our alcohol assessment instrument. Although we adjusted for several factors that could have represented confounding variables that were the true cause of poor outcomes, it is possible that some unmeasured variables were the true cause of poor viral suppression in the heavy drinkers. These limitations are balanced somewhat by our ability to obtain HIV viral suppression information from statewide HIV surveillance, and by the diversity of our sample across gender, race, and location.

Detectable HIV viremia is associated with HIV disease progression and transmission of HIV virus to others, providing both individual and public health reasons to try to improve this outcome. If alcohol consumption contributes to HIV treatment failure, then interventions to address heavy alcohol consumption should become more routine in HIV clinical and public health settings. Our findings help reinforce the potential benefits of screening and brief intervention for alcohol problems in HIV care settings [22], especially when persons are having difficulties maintaining consistent HIV viral suppression. Future research should also seek to identify and address other mechanisms, such as retention in care, that could be affected by heavy alcohol consumption. We also need better strategies to identify which specific drinkers are in greatest need of intervention, and to identify and demonstrate the best strategies to help persons to reduce drinking.

Abbreviations

HIV: human immunodeficiency virus; ART: antiretroviral treatment; PLWH: persons living with HIV.

Authors' contributions

RC helped design the study, oversaw data analysis, wrote primary draft. ZZ and BB did data analysis, NKC helped design study and write paper. JJ, NW, CC, JM, RC helped to design the study questionnaire, JM, CS, WD, GI helped to collect data at different settings; KB helped design the overall study. All authors read and approved the final manuscript.

Author details

[1] Department of Epidemiology, College of Public Health and Health Professions and College of Medicine, University of Florida, PO Box 100231, Gainesville, FL 32610, USA. [2] Department of Medicine, University of Florida, Gainesville, FL, USA. [3] Department of Clinical and Health Psychology, University of Florida, Gainesville, FL, USA. [4] Department of Family, Community, and Health System Science, College of Nursing, University of Florida, Gainesville, FL, USA. [5] Department of Biostatistics, University of Florida, Gainesville, FL, USA. [6] Division of Infectious Diseases and International Medicine, University of South Florida Morsani College of Medicine, Tampa, FL, USA. [7] Department of Internal Medicine, University of South Florida Morsani College of Medicine, Tampa, FL, USA. [8] Florida Department of Health, Orange County Office of Clinical Services, Disease Investigation and Research, Orlando, FL, USA. [9] Department of Epidemiology, Florida International University, Miami, FL, USA. [10] National Institute on Alcohol Abuse and Alcoholism, Bethesda, MD, USA.

Competing interests

The authors declare that they have no competing interests.

Consent for publication

All authors declare that they consent to publication.

Funding

This work was supported by NIAAA Grant U24 AA022002, U24AA022003, and from the State of Florida via the University of Miami Miller School of Medicine Institute for AIDS and Emerging Infectious Diseases.

References

1. Skarbinski J, Rosenberg E, Paz-Bailey G, Hall HI, Rose CE, Viall AH, et al. Human immunodeficiency virus transmission at each step of the care continuum in the United States. JAMA Intern Med. 2015;175(4):588–96.
2. Langford SE, Ananworanich J, Cooper DA. Predictors of disease progression in HIV infection: a review. AIDS Res Ther. 2007;14(4):11.
3. FACT SHEET: The national HIV/AIDS strategy: updated to 2020. whitehouse.gov. 2015 (cited 2015 Sept 30). https://www.whitehouse.gov/the-press-office/2015/07/30/fact-sheet-national-hivaids-strategy-updated-2020. Accessed June 2017.
4. Monroe AK, Lau B, Mugavero MJ, Mathews WC, Mayer KH, Napravnik S, et al. Heavy alcohol use is associated with worse retention in HIV care. J Acquir Immune Defic Syndr. 2016;73(4):419–25.
5. Williams EC, Hahn JA, Saitz R, Bryant K, Lira MC, Samet JH. Alcohol use and human immunodeficiency virus (HIV) infection: current knowledge, implications, and future directions. Alcohol Clin Exp Res. 2016;40(10):2056–72.
6. Azar MM, Springer SA, Meyer JP, Altice FL. A systematic review of the impact of alcohol use disorders on HIV treatment outcomes, adherence to antiretroviral therapy and health care utilization. Drug Alcohol Depend. 2010;112(3):178–93.
7. Hendershot CS, Stoner SA, Pantalone DW, Simoni JM. Alcohol use and antiretroviral adherence: review and meta-analysis. J Acquir Immune Defic Syndr. 2009;52(2):180–202.
8. Vagenas P, Azar MM, Copenhaver MM, Springer SA, Molina PE, Altice FL. The impact of alcohol use and related disorders on the HIV continuum of care: a systematic review: alcohol and the HIV continuum of care. Curr HIV/AIDS Rep. 2015;12(4):421–36.
9. Barai N, Monroe A, Lesko C, Lau B, Hutton H, Yang C, et al. The association between changes in alcohol use and changes in antiretroviral therapy adherence and viral suppression among women living with HIV. AIDS Behav. 2017;21(7):1836–45.
10. Deiss RG, Mesner O, Agan BK, Ganesan A, Okulicz JF, Bavaro M, et al. Characterizing the association between alcohol and HIV virologic failure in a military cohort on antiretroviral therapy. Alcohol Clin Exp Res. 2016;40(3):529–35.
11. Sacamano PL, Farley JE. Behavioral and other characteristics associated with HIV viral load in an outpatient clinic. PLoS ONE. 2016;11(11):e0166016.
12. Conen A, Wang Q, Glass TR, Fux CA, Thurnheer MC, Orasch C, et al. Association of alcohol consumption and HIV surrogate markers in participants of the swiss HIV cohort study. J Acquir Immune Defic Syndr. 2013;64(5):472–8.
13. Sullivan KA, Messer LC, Quinlivan EB. Substance abuse, violence, and HIV/AIDS syndemic effects on viral suppression among HIV positive women of color. AIDS Patient Care STDS. 2015;29(Suppl 1):S42–8.
14. Cook RL, Clark DB. Is there an association between alcohol consumption and sexually transmitted diseases? A systematic review. Sex Transm Dis. 2005;32(3):156–64.
15. Kim TW, Kertesz SG, Horton NJ, Tibbetts N, Samet JH. Episodic homelessness and health care utilization in a prospective cohort of HIV-infected persons with alcohol problems. BMC Health Serv Res. 2006;27(6):19.
16. Gordon AJ, McGinnis KA, Conigliaro J, Rodriguez-Barradas MC, Rabeneck L, Justice AC, et al. Associations between alcohol use and homelessness with healthcare utilization among human immunodeficiency virus-infected veterans. Med Care. 2006;44(8 Suppl 2):S37–43.
17. Garey L, Bakhshaie J, Sharp C, Neighbors C, Zvolensky MJ, Gonzalez A. Anxiety, depression, and HIV symptoms among persons living with HIV/AIDS: the role of hazardous drinking. AIDS Care. 2015;27(1):80–5.
18. Paulus DJ, Jardin C, Bakhshaie J, Sharp C, Woods SP, Lemaire C, et al. Anxiety sensitivity and hazardous drinking among persons living with HIV/AIDS: an examination of the role of emotion dysregulation. Addict Behav. 2016;63:141–8.
19. Braithwaite RS, Fang Y, Tate J, Mentor SM, Bryant KJ, Fiellin DA, et al. Do alcohol misuse, smoking, and depression vary concordantly or sequentially? A longitudinal study of HIV-infected and matched uninfected veterans in care. AIDS Behav. 2016;20(3):566–72.
20. Green TC, Kershaw T, Lin H, Heimer R, Goulet JL, Kraemer KL, et al. Patterns of drug use and abuse among aging adults with and without HIV: a latent class analysis of a US Veteran cohort. Drug Alcohol Depend. 2010;110(3):208–20.
21. Bradley KA, DeBenedetti AF, Volk RJ, Williams EC, Frank D, Kivlahan DR. AUDIT-C as a brief screen for alcohol misuse in primary care. Alcohol Clin Exp Res. 2007;31(7):1208–17.
22. National Institute on Alcohol Abuse and Alcoholism. Helping patients who drink too much: a clinician's guide. National Institute on Alcohol Abuse and Alcoholism (NIAAA). 2008 (cited 2016 July 24). https://www.niaaa.nih.gov/guide.
23. Kroenke K, Spitzer RL, Williams JB. The PHQ-9: validity of a brief depression severity measure. J Gen Intern Med. 2001;16(9):606–13.
24. Spitzer RL, Kroenke K, Williams JBW, Löwe B. A brief measure for assessing generalized anxiety disorder: the GAD-7. Arch Intern Med. 2006;166(10):1092–7.
25. Mekuria LA, Prins JM, Yalew AW, Sprangers MAG, Nieuwkerk PT. Which adherence measure—self-report, clinician recorded or pharmacy refill—is best able to predict detectable viral load in a public ART programme without routine plasma viral load monitoring? Trop Med Int Health. 2016;21(7):856–69.

26. Wilson IB, Lee Y, Michaud J, Fowler FJ, Rogers WH. Validation of a new three-item self-report measure for medication adherence. AIDS Behav. 2016;20(11):2700–8.
27. Wilson IB, Fowler FJ, Cosenza CA, Michaud J, Bentkover J, Rana A, et al. Cognitive and field testing of a new set of medication adherence self-report items for HIV care. AIDS Behav. 2014;18(12):2349–58.
28. Mannheimer S, Friedland G, Matts J, Child C, Chesney M. The consistency of adherence to antiretroviral therapy predicts biologic outcomes for human immunodeficiency virus-infected persons in clinical trials. Clin Infect Dis. 2002;34(8):1115–21.
29. Paterson DL, Swindells S, Mohr J, Brester M, Vergis EN, Squier C, et al. Adherence to protease inhibitor therapy and outcomes in patients with HIV infection. Ann Intern Med. 2000;133(1):21–30.
30. Valeri L, Vanderweele TJ. Mediation analysis allowing for exposure-mediator interactions and causal interpretation: theoretical assumptions and implementation with SAS and SPSS macros. Psychol Methods. 2013;18(2):137–50.
31. Bae JW, Guyer W, Grimm K, Altice FL. Medication persistence in the treatment of HIV infection: a review of the literature and implications for future clinical care and research. AIDS. 2011;25(3):279–90.
32. Viswanathan S, Justice AC, Alexander GC, Brown TT, Gandhi NR, McNicholl IR, et al. Adherence and HIV RNA suppression in the current era of highly active antiretroviral therapy. J Acquir Immune Defic Syndr. 2015;69(4):493–8.
33. Cook RL, Zhou Z, Miguez MJ, Brumback B, Lewis J, Espinoza L, et al. Reducing alcohol consumption improved HIV viral suppression in women. Abstract presented at CROI, Seattle, WA; 2017.

21

Barriers to addiction treatment among formerly incarcerated adults with substance use disorders

Mandy D. Owens[1*], Jessica A. Chen[1], Tracy L. Simpson[2,3], Christine Timko[4,5] and Emily C. Williams[1]

Abstract

Background: Addiction treatment improves substance use and criminal recidivism outcomes among justice-involved individuals with substance use disorders, but is underutilized. Although information exists regarding barriers to addiction treatment among individuals with substance use disorders more generally, less is known about barriers among individuals with previous justice involvement. The purpose of this pilot study was to describe barriers to addiction treatment in a sample of adults with a substance use disorder who participated in a pilot trial of brief interventions and were recently released from jail.

Methods: Incarcerated individuals who were arrested for an alcohol- or drug-related crime and reported moderate or high alcohol use on the ASSIST ($n = 28$; 96.4% men) were recruited for a pilot trial of brief interventions to reduce substance use, which were delivered just prior to release from jail. After their release, participants completed the Barriers to Treatment Inventory (BTI), which included 25 numerical items and one open-ended question on additional barriers that provided qualitative data. We described frequency of quantitative responses and qualitatively coded open-ended data using seven previously identified domains of the BTI.

Results: The most commonly reported barriers assessed quantitatively were items related to Absence of Problem: "I do not think I have a problem with drugs" (42.8%), Privacy Concerns: "I do not like to talk about my personal life with other people" (35.8%), and Admission Difficulty: "I will have to be on a waiting list for treatment" (28.6%). Items related to Negative Social Support (e.g., "Friends tell me not to go to treatment") were rarely endorsed in this sample. Responses to the open-ended question also related to Absence of Problem, Privacy Concerns, and Admission Difficulty. Additional categories of barriers emerged from the qualitative data, including Ambivalence and Seeking Informal Assistance.

Conclusions: In this small sample of adults with a substance use disorder recently released from jail, barriers to treatment were frequently endorsed. Future research on larger samples is needed to understand barriers to treatment specific to justice-involved populations. Clinicians may consider using open-ended questions to explore and address barriers to addiction treatment among individuals with current or recent justice involvement.

Keywords: Barriers, Treatment, Substance use disorder, Jail, Inmates, Prisoners, Alcohol, Drugs

Background

Substance use disorders (SUD) are very common among those incarcerated by the criminal justice system: more than half of people in prison (58%) and nearly two-thirds of people in jail (63%) meet criteria for a SUD [1]. Individuals transitioning from jail or prison back into the community face many challenges, including being required to meet probation or parole conditions and expectations, reestablishing housing and employment that were lost while incarcerated, and stigma [2–5]. Those with a SUD also must contend with increased risk of mortality and returning to environments that increase the likelihood of substance

*Correspondence: mandy.owens@va.gov
[1] Health Services Research and Development, VA Puget Sound Health Care System, Department of Health Services, University of Washington, 1660 South Columbian Way, S-152, Seattle, WA 98108, USA
Full list of author information is available at the end of the article

use [2, 4, 6–8]. Additionally, 41% of all probationers are required to attend alcohol or drug treatment [9]. Although there is some evidence that legal pressure may improve retention in treatment, namely for those in short- or long-term residential treatment [10], many individuals may not seek treatment at all and still will drop out of outpatient treatment prematurely, despite severe consequences. For example, in a sample of 926 individuals who opted to attend addiction treatment in lieu of jail or prison, 59% dropped out of treatment, of whom 25% were reincarcerated [11]. Addiction care specifically geared towards the needs of justice-involved individuals may improve treatment engagement and mitigate retention challenges, reduce risk for returning to substance use, and help to prevent individuals' continued involvement with the justice system [2].

In the general population of U.S. residents 12 years and older, approximately 8.1% have a SUD, but only 11–14% of those with a SUD seek or get the treatment they need [12, 13]. Multiple barriers to treatment have been identified in general samples of persons with a SUD not specific to those who are justice-involved. For example, among two large, national samples of individuals with a SUD in the United States who were not seeking treatment [12, 14] and a sample of individuals with a SUD presenting to treatment, [15] barriers included not being ready to stop using alcohol or drugs, lacking resources (e.g., insurance), and not knowing where to seek treatment [12, 14, 15].

Individuals with a SUD who are justice involved face similar treatment barriers to individuals with a SUD more generally, including lack of health care and costs of treatment [5, 16] and not seeing their substance use as a problem [3, 5, 17]. These barriers were experienced across various groups of justice-involved individuals not in SUD treatment, including those who were incarcerated [7] or on probation or parole [5, 17] and those with both alcohol and other drug use disorders [3, 5]. Despite these similarities, justice-involved individuals with a SUD appear to face additional barriers, including stigma related to having a legal history [3, 7] or criminal justice agencies' preference to provide "drug-free treatment" that exclude pharmacotherapies for SUD [18].

However, there are limitations of prior studies of barriers to addiction treatment for justice-involved individuals. For example, some of these studies focused on specific subgroups, such as those with a drug use disorder [17] or women [7], when justice-involved individuals comprise a heterogeneous population. Other studies only examined barriers to medication-assisted treatments [18, 19]. Further, studies often queried participants on a finite selection of barriers rather than using open-ended questions (e.g., [5, 7]), which may not capture the full range of barriers experienced by this group. Given the low rates of treatment receipt among justice-involved individuals with a SUD and the subsequent consequences they may experience (e.g., re-arrest or reincarceration), there is a need for a more comprehensive understanding of barriers to addiction treatment among this group to inform more effective interventions that improve treatment retention and outcomes, and decrease recidivism. Thus, exploration of a broader range of barriers to treatment among justice-involved individuals with a SUD may be needed to help treatment programs and court systems reduce these barriers and/or directly address them with their clients.

To improve our understanding of barriers to addiction treatment experienced by justice-involved individuals with a SUD more generally, the purpose of the current pilot study was to describe barriers to addiction treatment reported among a small sample of recently incarcerated individuals with a SUD, including responses provided to an open-ended question of additional barriers. Given the small sample size and broad assessment of barriers to treatment that has not been done previously with justice-involved individuals with a SUD specifically, there were no a priori hypotheses and the study was exploratory.

Methods

Data source

The parent study took place between April 2014 and June 2015. The current study represents a secondary analysis of follow-up data collected from a pilot randomized clinical trial of a single, 1-h brief intervention to reduce substance use with participants who were recruited from a large detention center in the Southwestern United States. The pilot trial was advertised as a study on preparing for release from jail; thus, individuals were not necessarily treatment-seeking. Individuals were recruited while they were incarcerated via flyers and presentations, and all screening, informed consent, baseline assessments, and intervention procedures took place prior to their release from jail. Participants in the trial received either a motivational intervention to reduce substance use or an educational intervention on substance use and addiction within 14 days of their pending release from jail [20]. Participants were contacted to complete two follow-up interviews after their release from jail including a 1-month interview and a 3 to 6-month interview. All participants signed a consent form. All study procedures were approved by an institutional review board at the University of New Mexico.

The parent study enrolled 40 participants, of whom 25 completed at least one follow-up interview [20]. There were an additional 3 participants consented into the parent trial who completed a follow-up interview but were ultimately excluded from the parent trial analyses for various reasons (e.g., female participants were excluded from main analyses to reduce heterogeneity). The present study included these three additional participants for a total of 28 participants who completed at least one follow-up interview and, thus, responded to questions regarding barriers to treatment. Participants who completed a follow-up interview did not differ from those who did not on demographic characteristics, pre-incarceration substance use, or lifetime treatment or legal histories. For participants who completed both follow-up interviews, quantitative data from their 1-month interview only were used; qualitative responses were used from both interviews to maximize data.

Participants

Recruitment targeted individuals with an alcohol- or drug-related charge (e.g., driving under the influence, possession of a controlled substance), who were sentenced and had a release date, and agreed to participate in an in-person follow-up interview after their release. Of those who met these criteria, eligible individuals were further screened for: (a) having "moderate to high alcohol involvement" in the 3 months prior to their current incarceration as assessed by the Alcohol, Smoking, and Substance Involvement Screening Test (scores of 4 and above) [21], and (b) being released within 14 days. Exclusion criteria were: (a) scoring above 20 on the Mini Mental Status Exam [22], suggesting gross cognitive impairment; (b) reporting active psychotic symptoms as assessed by the Structural Clinical Interview for DSM-IV Diagnoses psychotic screening [23]; (c) lacking English proficiency; and (d) participating in the methadone maintenance program at the detention center, as they had more clinical contact throughout their incarceration than other individuals.

Data collection

At the baseline interview prior to their release, participants completed a battery of assessments (e.g., demographic information, treatment history) and provided post-release location information, including phone numbers, mailing addresses, and email addresses for themselves, friends and family members, and anyone else with whom they might have contact. Once released, participants were contacted to complete a 1-month interview (28–49 days post-release) and a 3 to 6-month interview (84–180 days post-release), both of which were conducted in-person. If participants were unable to complete the 1-month interview within the designated timeframe, they still were eligible to complete the 3 to 6-month interview.

Participants' blood alcohol contents were tested prior to beginning follow-up interviews to ensure they were less than 0.02 before proceeding. They then completed assessments that included substance use and treatment seeking behaviors since being released and barriers to treatment, and were compensated for their time ($25 for 1-month interview, $40 for 3 to 6-month interview).

Measures

Demographic information

Demographic information was assessed at the baseline interview. Participants' gender, age, race/ethnicity, and other demographic information were measured using the CASAA Demographics Interview form [24]. Diagnostic criteria for lifetime and current (12 months prior to baseline interview) alcohol use disorder and up to four non-alcohol SUDs were assessed using the Structural Clinical Interview for DSM-IV Diagnoses Substance Use Disorder module [23]. Participants also completed the Alcohol and Drug Use sections of the Addiction Severity Index [25], which provided information on lifetime alcohol and drug treatment episodes.

Substance use and treatment seeking

At the follow-up interviews, the Form-90 [26] was used to measure the percentage of days after release from jail without any use of alcohol or drugs. The parent study added an interview question to the Form-90 that queried any substance use treatment seeking behaviors (yes/no) since release from jail ("Any substance use treatment seeking behaviors?").

Barriers to treatment

Barriers were assessed at the follow-up interviews with the Barriers to Treatment Inventory (BTI) [15]. The BTI is a seven factor, 25-item self-report measure and individuals rated agreement with potential barriers (for list of items, see Table 1) on a 1–5 Likert-type scale (1 = Strongly Disagree, 5 = Strongly Agree). Rapp and colleagues [15] administered the full 59-item BTI to 312 individuals with a SUD presenting to an addiction treatment intake center and conducted the initial factor analysis. Of the original 59 items, a seven-factor model was found to have adequate fit and was comprised of 25 items [15]. The seven factors included: Absence of Problem (e.g., "I do not think I have a problem with drugs", "I do not think treatment will make my life better"), Negative Social Support ("I will lose my friends if I go to treatment", "My family will be embarrassed or ashamed if I go to treatment"), Fear of Treatment ("I have had a bad experience with treatment", "I am too embarrassed or ashamed to go to treatment"), Privacy Concerns ("I do not like to talk in groups", "I do not like to talk about my personal life with other people"), Time Conflict ("It will be hard for me to find a treatment program that fits my schedule"), Poor Treatment

Table 1 Sample characteristics among 28 adults with a SUD recently released from jail

	Mean (SD)	*n* (%)
Age (years)	35.1 (10.1)	
Male		27 (96.4%)
Race/ethnicity		
Hispanic		7 (25.0%)
Biracial/multiracial		7 (25.0%)
American Indian/Alaskan native		6 (21.4%)
Non-Hispanic White		5 (17.9%)
Other		3 (10.7%)
Days Incarcerated*	168.5 (106.9)	
Any current substance use disorder**		23 (85.2%)
Current alcohol use disorder**		19 (70.4%)
Current drug use disorder**		14 (51.9%)
Lifetime alcohol use disorder		28 (100.0%)
Lifetime drug use disorder		26 (92.9%)
Lifetime alcohol treatment episodes	3.9 (5.2)	
Lifetime drug treatment episodes	2.1 (3.1)	
Post-release percent days abstinent	67.9 (38.4)	
Post-release treatment seeking (formal or informal)		10 (35.7%)

*Data for $n=2$ participants were removed because they were incarcerated for more than 2 SD from the mean (range = 31–874 days)

**Data were available for $n=27$ participants only. Of the 27 participants with complete diagnostic data, the $n=4$ participants who did not meet criteria for any current substance use disorder all had been incarcerated in jail for more than 12 months

Availability ("I am moving too far away to get treatment", "I have difficulty getting to and from treatment"), and Admission Difficulty ("I have to go through too many steps to get into treatment") [15]. Cronbach's alphas for each factor domain ranged from 0.65 to 0.86 [15]. For the current study, responses to each item on the BTI were grouped into three types: Disagree (ratings of 1 or 2), Uncertain (rating of 3), and Agree (ratings of 4 or 5).

One open-ended question was added to the end of the BTI that asked, "Please describe any additional barriers to treatment in your own words." Participants provided written responses to this question.

Data analyses

Sample characteristics were described overall. The mean and standard deviation for each BTI item, as well as the *n* and percent that endorsed each response type (Disagree, Uncertain, Agree) were calculated. Each individual BTI item was described (rather than aggregated in previously identified BTI domains [15]) in order to describe the full range of barriers reported in this sample for this hypothesis-generating study. We then coded qualitative responses to the open-ended question of additional barriers using template analysis [27] (i.e., content analysis or thematic coding). In this approach, data are coded both inductively and deductively, thus allowing for coding of both a priori domains and emergent domains. The initial coding template was based on the seven factors (domains) of the BTI reported by Rapp et al. [15]. Two coders (M.D.O., J.A.C.) independently coded open-ended responses; discrepancies then were discussed by all authors until consensus was reached. Consistent with the recommendations by Sandelowski [28], we opted not to report frequencies of qualitative results, as the use of numbers may have detracted from making well-rounded interpretations of the data, particularly in the context of data generated from a single, open-ended survey question as opposed to an in-depth interview.

Results

Among the 28 participants who completed at least one follow-up interview, 11 completed only the 1-month interview, 6 completed only the 3 to 6-month interview, and 11 completed both. Responses to the open-ended question of additional barriers were examined for all completed interviews ($n=39$), of which four were left blank (10.3%). Just over half of participants included in the present study were randomized to the motivational intervention condition ($n=15$, 53.6%). Sample characteristics are provided in Table 1.

The means and standard deviations, as well as the number and percentage of participants endorsing items in each of the seven BTI domains are provided in Table 2. The most commonly endorsed barriers to addiction treatment were related to the domain Absence of Problem: "I do not think I have a problem with drugs" (42.8%) and "My drug use is not causing any problems" (32.2%), and Privacy Concerns: "I do not like to talk about my personal life with other people" (35.7%) and "I do not like to talk in groups" (32.2%). No participants endorsed four of the five barriers from the Negative Social Support domain: "I will lose my friends if I go to treatment", "People will think badly of me if I go to treatment," "Someone in my family does not want me to go to treatment," or "My family will be embarrassed or ashamed if I go to treatment."

Results of the qualitative data analysis are presented in Table 3. Coding identified responses consistent with a priori domains based on Rapp et al.'s factor analysis [15] as well as emergent domains. Within a priori domains, barriers related to Absence of Problem ("Don't need it"), Privacy Concerns ("I'm not completely comfortable with speaking in a group setting"), and Time Conflict ("Just pending court dates") were endorsed. Three emergent domains were identified in the data, including Ambivalence (e.g., "The fact that I enjoy the drug"), Seeking Informal Assistance (e.g., "I have yet to go to treatment

Table 2 Descriptive information from the Barriers to Treatment Inventory

	Mean	SD	Disagree *n* (%)	Uncertain *n* (%)	Agree *n* (%)
Absence of Problem	2.6	1.1			
I do not think I have a problem with drugs	3	1.5	12 (42.8)	4 (14.3)	12 (42.8)
No one has told me I have a problem with drugs	2.5	1.5	17 (60.7)	3 (10.7)	8 (28.6)
My drug use is not causing any problems	2.7	1.6	15 (53.5)	4 (14.3)	9 (32.2)
I do not think treatment will make my life better	2.3	1.2	18 (64.3)	6 (21.4)	4 (14.3)
I can handle my drug use on my own	2.9	1.4	12 (42.8)	8 (28.6)	8 (28.6)
I do not think I need treatment	2.5	1.3	17 (60.7)	4 (14.3)	7 (25.0)
Negative Social Support	1.8	0.5			
I will lose my friends if I go to treatment	1.8	0.7	23 (82.1)	5 (17.9)	0
Friends tell me not to go to treatment	2.0	1.0	23 (82.1)	2 (7.1)	3 (10.7)
People will think badly of me if I go to treatment	1.8	0.6	25 (89.3)	3 (10.7)	0
Someone in my family does not want me to go to treatment	1.6	0.6	26 (92.9)	2 (7.1)	0
My family will be embarrassed or ashamed if I go to treatment	1.5	0.6	26 (92.9)	2 (7.1)	0
Fear of Treatment	1.9	0.8			
I have had a bad experience with treatment	2.1	1.2	21 (75.0)	2 (7.1)	5 (17.8)
I am afraid what might happen in treatment	1.9	0.9	23 (82.1)	3 (10.7)	2 (7.1)
I am afraid of the people I might see in treatment	1.8	0.9	23 (82.1)	3 (10.7)	2 (7.1)
I am too embarrassed or ashamed to go to treatment	1.8	0.9	23 (82.1)	3 (10.7)	2 (7.1)
Privacy Concerns	2.7	1.2			
I do not like to talk in groups	2.6	1.4	18 (64.3)	1 (3.6)	9 (32.2)
I hate being asked personal questions	2.6	1.3	17 (60.7)	3 (10.7)	8 (28.6)
I do not like to talk about my personal life with other people	2.8	1.3	16 (57.2)	2 (7.1)	10 (35.7)
Time Conflict	2.2	0.9			
I have things to do at home that make it hard for me to get to treatment	2.1	1.0	21 (75.0)	3 (10.7)	4 (14.3)
It will be hard for me to find a treatment program that fits my schedule	2.3	1.0	17 (60.7)	8 (28.6)	3 (10.7)
Poor Treatment Availability	2.0	0.9			
I am moving too far away to get treatment	2.0	1.0	23 (82.1)	3 (10.7)	2 (7.1)
I do not know where to go for treatment	1.9	0.8	22 (78.6)	5 (17.9)	1 (3.6)
I have difficulty getting to and from treatment	2.1	1.2	20 (71.4)	2 (7.1)	6 (21.5)
Admission Difficulty	2.6	1.1			
I will have to be on a waiting list for treatment	2.7	1.2	12 (42.8)	8 (28.6)	8 (28.6)
I have to go through too many steps to get into treatment	2.5	1.1	16 (57.1)	6 (21.4)	6 (21.5)

1 Strongly disagree, *3* uncertain, *5* strongly agree. "Disagree" includes responses to both "Disagree" and "Strongly Disagree". "Agree" includes responses to both "Agree" and "Strongly Agree"

cause [sic] I want to try and see if the support im [sic] getting from my family will be enough..."), and Other, which included open-ended responses that were difficult to interpret or code (e.g., "AA meetings" and "The fact that alcohol is advertised all around").

Post-hoc analyses

To explore potential influences of reported barriers to treatment, independent samples t tests were conducted to examine between-group differences in endorsements of BTI items across study condition (from the parent trial, motivational intervention: $n=15$, educational intervention: $n=13$) and between those who did ($n=10$) and did not ($n=18$) report engaging in any treatment seeking behaviors after release from jail. Because we considered these between-group comparisons exploratory and not hypothesis-driven, there were no a priori power analyses conducted, and results are to be used for hypothesis generation.

Exploratory comparisons across study conditions suggested that, relative to those who received the educational intervention, participants randomized to receive the motivational intervention were more likely to agree with barriers related to Absence of Problem: "I do not have a problem with drugs" ($M=3.5$, $SD=1.3$ vs. $M=2.4$, $SD=1.5$; $t=2.169$, $p<.05$) and "I can handle my drug use on my own" ($M=3.4$, $SD=1.4$ vs. $M=2.2$, $SD=1.1$; $t=2.491$, $p<.05$; see Appendix A). There were no other between group differences by study condition identified in exploratory analyses.

Table 3 Examples of additional barriers identified in responses to open-ended question, organized by a priori and emergent domains

a Priori domains	Examples of responses from open-ended question
Absence of Problem	"Don't need it" "I just don't want to go to treatment. I'm fine on my own"
Negative Social Support	None listed
Fear of Treatment	"Don't want to, it hasn't helped in the past" "I just don't like the sound of it"
Privacy Concerns	"I'm not completley comfortable with speaking in a group setting" "Myself—hard to get myself open like that (hard to trust)"
Time Conflict	"Just pending court dates" "Not wanting to take the time to go"
Poor Treatment Availability	"Transportation and time avail. Ex: You have a 8 am drug treatment class in Bernalillo Cty-while I now live in Santa Fe city [sic]" "Transportation is an issue"
Admission Difficulty	"Just my misdemeanor situation prevents inpatients treatments to accept me. That's about it as far as I can see"
Emergent domains	
Ambivalence	"I don't have the motivation to go. I'm lazy" "The fact that I enjoy the drug"
Seeking Informal Assistance	"I have yet to go to treatment cause [sic] I want to try and see if the support im [sic] getting from my family will be enough"
Other	"AA meetings" "The fact that alcohol is advertised all around" "I have heard it all"
No barriers	"Currently attending treatment. I am ready to change my life for the better" "Currently I have no barriers"

Each response was coded using the barrier factor domains reported by Rapp et al. [15]. Responses that did not fit into an existing category were coded as emergent domains. Responses to open-ended questions came from all completed interviews ($n = 39$), of which four were left blank. One response included multiple barriers, so this was coded into two domains

Participants who reported seeking any post-release treatment appeared less likely than those who did not seek treatment to endorse one barrier from Absence of Problem: "I do not think treatment will make my life better" ($M = 1.6$, $SD = 0.7$ vs. $M = 2.7$, $SD = 1.2$; $t = 2.501$, $p < 0.05$), and two barriers related to Privacy Concerns: "I do not like to talk in groups" ($M = 1.9$, $SD = 0.9$ vs. $M = 3.0$, $SD = 1.5$; $t = 2.454$, $p < 0.05$) and "I hate being asked personal questions" ($M = 1.9$, $SD = 0.7$ vs. $M = 3.1$, $SD = 1.3$; $t = 2.993$, $p < 0.05$; see Appendix B). No other differences in reported barriers to treatment among those who sought versus did not seek treatment after release from jail were identified in post hoc analyses.

Discussion

This exploratory study used a survey with closed- and open-ended responses to describe barriers to addiction treatment in a small sample of recently-incarcerated adults with a SUD, a population among whom addiction treatment may be of paramount importance, is underutilized, and rarely tailored to their needs. Barriers to addiction treatment were frequently endorsed, but there were no barriers universally endorsed by this sample. Findings can be considered hypothesis-generating regarding barriers to treatment that might be specific to this population. These findings may be useful in informing future research and clinical efforts for individuals with a SUD with recent or current justice involvement.

Previous studies among justice-involved populations have identified lack of healthcare and related costs, limited availability of qualified healthcare providers, long wait times, stigma, and criminal justice agencies' procedures and preferences (e.g., exclusion of medication-assisted treatments due to preference to be "drug-free") as barriers to treatment [4, 5, 7, 18, 19, 29]. There were similarities in findings between studies on barriers to treatment with other justice-involved samples and the current study. Among justice-involved individuals choosing to attend treatment in lieu of incarceration, [17] 23.9% expressed no desire for treatment, which is similar to 25.0% of the current sample reporting "I do not think I need treatment". Rose et al. (2014) found that women incarcerated in jail also reported long wait lists as a barrier to treatment, although this was more common among this sample of women than the current sample (58.9% vs. 28.6%) [7]. Unfortunately, it often is difficult to make comparisons across studies due to variability in assessing barriers and differing samples. The present study is small, but potentially broader in inclusion criteria than previous studies, and adds to these previous studies by expanding the assessment of barriers. Indeed, we found that barriers not previously identified may be important to consider for this population, including perceiving Absence of Problem and Privacy Concerns. Knowledge of these potential barriers in combination with those previously identified in justice-involved individuals, such as Ambivalence, may provide counselors and criminal justice staff with more nuanced information to assist their clients in overcoming obstacles to seeking or staying in treatment.

A previous study also used the BTI, but with a sample of general treatment-seeking individuals with a SUD, [15] which presented the opportunity to compare rates of barriers to the current sample of justice-involved individuals with a SUD. Among this sample of treatment-seeking individuals, barriers to treatment included the Fear of Treatment, Time Conflict, and Poor Treatment

Availability, which also were endorsed by similar proportions of the current study sample. It is noteworthy, however, that participants in the present study sample endorsed Absence of Problem at a markedly higher rate than what was reported by Rapp et al., such as, "I do not think I have a problem with drugs" (42.8% vs. 12.5%) and "My drug use is not causing any problems" (32.2% vs. 8.0%). These discrepancies may be because the sample from Rapp et al. already had initiated the process of seeking addiction treatment, which often includes an acknowledgement of engaging in problematic substance use, compared to the current sample, who were not necessarily treatment-seeking. Alternatively, the present study selected for people reporting moderate to high alcohol use who may not have had much drug involvement. Because we did not alter the original scale to include both drugs and alcohol in these items, we may have inadvertently overestimated the degree to which our participants felt they had an "Absence of Problem." However, half of the sample met criteria for a current drug use disorder, suggesting that many individuals in this sample still were experiencing problems related to their drug use.

Though our sample was small, an interesting finding was the relatively few endorsements of barriers in the Negative Social Support domain. Specifically, participants in the present study did not endorse four of the five items, and only a small number endorsed "Friends tell me not to go to treatment" ($n=3$, 10.7%). In contrast, these barriers were more frequently endorsed by the treatment-seeking sample of individuals with a SUD reported by Rapp et al., although still in low proportions (proportions of agreement ranged from 7.4 to 16.0%) [15]. This finding suggests the possibility that justice-involved individuals with a SUD experience barriers related to Negative Social Support less frequently. While future research is needed to further explore this finding, these results suggest a possible intervention pathway—via the involvement of friends and family to encourage treatment engagement. Additionally, these findings may indicate that resources should be diverted to addressing other barriers, where they may have more impact.

In exploratory, post hoc analyses comparing barriers between participants randomly assigned to treatment conditions, barriers generally were endorsed by similar proportions. Groups did, however, differ on two items from the Absence of Problem domain ("I do not have a problem with drugs", "I can handle my drug use on my own"), with participants assigned to the motivational intervention reporting these barriers more frequently than those assigned to the education intervention. These findings are hypothesis-generating in suggesting that motivational interventions may not be helpful for increasing problem recognition among justice-involved individuals with a SUD, as they are designed to do, or may be unhelpful in this domain. Other studies with jail populations found null results of motivational interventions on other outcomes such as treatment engagement [30]. Of note, our results should be interpreted with caution, given the small sample, post hoc nature of these analyses, multiple comparisons, and that the parent study did not include a no-treatment control condition.

Similarly, in post hoc analyses comparing barriers reported between groups based on post-release treatment seeking, groups largely were similar. However, those who reported seeking treatment reported less apprehension about talking in groups or being asked personal or intrusive questions as a barrier. These findings highlight privacy as a potential concern among those who did not seek treatment, which may have clinical implications. This non-treatment-seeking group may prefer individual treatment or find pharmacotherapy less invasive and more beneficial than psychotherapy. However, research is needed in larger samples of justice-involved adults with a SUD who have and have not sought treatment to further explore this issue, and examine if pharmacotherapy could be a viable option for those with Privacy Concerns.

Findings from the present study suggest the possibility that barriers beyond those commonly identified may exist in this population. Two participants specifically referenced issues related to their justice involvement in the reporting of additional barriers that were coded under a priori domains ("Just pending court dates" coded as Time Conflict; and "Just my misdemeanor situation prevents inpatients treatments to accept me" coded as Admission Difficulty). Though justice-involvement was not, on its own, coded as an emergent barrier domain, it is possible that this population experiences specific enhanced barriers to treatment that were not cued by the generally phrased open-ended question we used regarding potential additional barriers to treatment. Additionally, it would be useful to better understand potential barriers identified with more in-depth qualitative work. For example, it would be informative to know if "pending court dates" refer to multiple demands on time or waiting to start treatment to know exact sentencing requirements, as well as to know how a "misdemeanor situation" may prevent someone from entering inpatient treatment (e.g., if someone is precluded from treatment while they wait for court dates). We had limited ability to assess these issues due to both small sample size and administration of one open-ended question without the opportunity to probe. Nonetheless, our study is hypothesis-generating regarding the need for broadening measures of barriers to treatment for persons involved with the criminal justice system, which can then inform future interventions for this population.

The present study is limited in several additional ways. First, this study had a small sample and thus the results presented here should be considered descriptive and hypothesis-generating. Given the small sample, we likely were underpowered to detect between-group differences across treatment condition assignment and report of post-release treatment receipt. The multiple exploratory comparisons we conducted between groups increase the risk of making a Type II error. Moreover, findings may not be representative of justice-involved individuals with a SUD more generally (e.g., those who are arrested without ever being incarcerated) because the sample only included individuals who were sentenced, had a substance use-related charge, were being released from a large Southwest detention center, and agreed to participate in a clinical trial, and recruitment targeted those with an alcohol use disorder (e.g., some may not have identified with needing "drug treatment"); this study also excluded those in the methadone maintenance program. The study recruited for individuals with an alcohol use disorder, but many questions of the BTI use language referring to drug use specifically (e.g., "I do not think I have a problem with drugs"), which may have influenced responses to these BTI items and resulted in overestimates of these barriers. Findings also may not be generalizable to women, and there may be additional barriers experienced by women not reflected in these results (e.g., competing basic needs related to childcare, added stigma [7]). Findings also may be biased by loss to follow-up. Though we compared participants across follow-up status and identified no differences, participants who did not complete either follow-up interview may experience more or different barriers to treatment (e.g., lacking reliable access to a phone, which may make it difficult to seek out treatment services). Further, many participants already had made changes to their alcohol and/or drug use by the time they completed the follow-up interview, which may have influenced their perceived need for treatment. Because this study was a secondary analysis of a pilot parent study that was not designed to investigate issues related to barriers to treatment, we may have missed some barriers to treatment (e.g., barriers to addiction treatment related to cost and lack of healthcare coverage did not emerge), which are commonly reported in the literature [5, 16]. We also did not assess some key issues that may influence barriers to treatment, such as conditions of release or probation or parole requirements (e.g., having more probation appointments interfering with ability to attend treatment) or provide external incentives to engage in treatment (e.g., SUD treatment is a condition of probation and compliance is associated with remaining out of jail or prison). Finally, participants were not given prompts or further opportunity to expand on potential barriers to treatment, as the BTI is a self-report measure rather than an interview.

Conclusions

Though this study is small, it contributes to the burgeoning literature on barriers to addiction treatment in a sample of individuals with a SUD with recent or current justice involvement. Results suggest that although barriers reported were variable across the sample and none were endorsed uniformly, recently incarcerated individuals with a SUD experience many barriers to treatment. While some barriers may be similar to those experienced by non-justice-specific populations with a SUD, findings from the present study indicate the possibility of unique barriers within this population of recently incarcerated adults. Specifically, it is possible that this population experiences greater barriers related to not seeing their substance use as a problem and fewer barriers related to Negative Social Support. There also may be barriers to treatment that are justice-specific, and these barriers may be missed by commonly-used instruments, such as the BTI. Results indicate a strong need for more research in larger samples to more comprehensively assess barriers in this population. Further, referring justice-involved individuals to the same addiction treatment designed for the general population (e.g., predominately group therapy) may result in barriers for them (e.g., not wanting to talk in groups) and be less effective. Clinicians working with justice-involved individuals with a SUD may want to use open-ended questions to explore potential barriers to addiction treatment, so that they may anticipate and plan for them. Better understanding barriers to treatment experienced by justice-involved individuals with a SUD is a promising area for research as it will ultimately help to inform new interventions aimed at increasing receipt of addiction treatment for this population.

Authors' contributions

MDO was the PI for the parent study and was involved in designing and conducting the pilot trial, and analyzing data for the current study and writing the manuscript. JAC assisted with qualitative analyses, interpreting results, and reviewing and writing the manuscript. TLS and CT assisted with interpreting results, and reviewing and writing the manuscript. ECW served as senior mentor for MDO and supervised qualitative analyses, as well as assisted with interpreting results, and reviewing and writing the manuscript. All authors read and approved the final manuscript.

Author details

[1] Health Services Research and Development, VA Puget Sound Health Care System, Department of Health Services, University of Washington, 1660 South Columbian Way, S-152, Seattle, WA 98108, USA. [2] Center for Substance Abuse Treatment and Education, VA Puget Sound Health Care System, Seattle, USA. [3] Department of Psychiatry and Behavioral Sciences, University of Washington, Seattle, WA, USA. [4] Center for Innovation to Implementation, VA Palo Alto Health Care System, Palo Alto, USA. [5] Department of Psychiatry and Behavioral Sciences, Stanford University, Palo Alto, CA, USA.

Acknowledgements
The authors would like to thank Barbara McCrady, Michael Bogenschutz, Theresa Moyers, J. Scott Tonigan, Katie Witkiewitz, Kylee Hagler, Lauren Rowell, the participants, and others for assisting with the design and conduct of the parent study.

Competing interests
The authors declare that they have no competing interests.

Ethics approval
All participants completed an informed consent process and signed a consent form. Procedures for this study were approved by an institutional review board the University of New Mexico.

Funding
The parent study was funded by the National Institute on Alcohol Abuse and Alcoholism (F31-AA023414) and by the Graduate Professional and Student Association at the University of New Mexico. Dr. Owens was supported by a VA Office of Academic Affiliations' Advanced Fellowship in Health Services Research and Development (TPH 61-000-20) as was Dr. Chen (TPH 61-000-14). Dr. Timko was funded by a Senior Research Career Scientist Award from VA HSR&D (RCS 00-001). Dr. Williams was funded by a Career Development Award from the Department of Veterans Affairs Health Services Research & Development (VA HSR&D) (CDA 12-276).

Appendix A: Post-hoc results of between-group differences by study condition

	Motivational		Educational		*t*-value
	Mean	SD	Mean	SD	
Absence of Problem	3.0	1.0	2.3	1.1	1.758
I do not think I have a problem with drugs	3.5	1.3	2.4	1.5	2.169*
No one has told me I have a problem with drugs	2.7	1.4	2.3	1.5	0.645
My drug use is not causing any problems	3.0	1.6	2.3	1.5	1.176
I do not think treatment will make my life better	2.5	1.1	2.0	1.2	1.201
I can handle my drug use on my own	3.4	1.4	2.2	1.1	2.491*
I do not think I need treatment	2.7	1.2	2.3	1.4	0.866
Negative Social Support	1.7	0.5	1.9	0.5	1.128
I will lose my friends if I go to treatment	1.7	0.6	2.0	0.8	1.228
Friends tell me not to go to treatment	1.7	0.8	2.2	1.2	1.282
People will think badly of me if I go to treatment	1.8	0.7	1.8	0.6	0.195
Someone in my family does not want me to go to treatment	1.5	0.5	1.8	0.7	1.663
My family will be embarrassed or ashamed if I go to treatment	1.6	0.6	1.5	0.7	0.566
Fear of Treatment	1.8	0.6	2.0	0.9	0.760
I have had a bad experience with treatment	2.0	1.0	2.3	1.5	0.648
I am afraid what might happen in treatment	1.7	0.6	2.2	1.1	1.503
I am afraid of the people I might see in treatment	1.8	0.8	1.8	1.1	0.087
I am too embarrassed or ashamed to go to treatment	1.7	0.8	1.8	1.1	0.319
Privacy Concerns	2.3	0.9	3.1	1.4	1.681
I do not like to talk in groups	2.3	1.0	3.0	1.7	1.364
I hate being asked personal questions	2.3	0.9	3.0	1.5	1.380
I do not like to talk about my personal life with other people	2.3	1.0	3.2	1.4	1.876
Time Conflict	2.1	0.9	2.2	0.9	0.173
I have things to do at home that make it hard for me to get to treatment	2.0	1.1	2.2	1.0	0.393
It will be hard for me to find a treatment program that fits my schedule	2.3	0.9	2.2	1.1	0.096
Poor Treatment Availability	1.9	1.0	2.1	0.7	0.500
I am moving too far away to get treatment	1.9	1.1	2.1	0.9	0.570
I do not know where to go for treatment	1.9	1.0	1.8	0.7	0.503
I have difficulty getting to and from treatment	1.9	1.2	2.4	1.3	0.960
Admission Difficulty	2.6	1.0	2.5	1.2	0.222
I will have to be on a waiting list for treatment	2.9	1.3	2.5	1.2	0.690
I have to go through too many steps to get into treatment	2.4	1.1	2.5	1.3	0.316

$n = 15$ received Motivational Intervention (treatment condition); $n = 13$ received Educational Intervention (control condition)
1 Strongly disagree, *3* Uncertain, *5* Strongly agree
*$p < 0.05$

Appendix B. Post-hoc results of between-group differences by post-release treatment seeking

	Sought treatment		Did not seek treatment		*t*-value
	Mean	SD	Mean	SD	
Absence of Problem	2.3	0.9	2.9	1.2	1.403
I do not think I have a problem with drugs	2.9	1.6	3.1	1.5	0.260
No one has told me I have a problem with drugs	2.1	1.3	2.7	1.5	1.090
My drug use is not causing any problems	2.7	1.6	2.7	1.6	0.053
I do not think treatment will make my life better	1.6	0.7	2.7	1.2	2.501*
I can handle my drug use on my own	2.3	1.3	3.2	1.3	1.678
I do not think I need treatment	1.9	1.0	2.9	1.3	2.056
Negative Social Support	1.7	0.6	1.8	0.5	0.571
I will lose my friends if I go to treatment	1.7	0.7	1.9	0.8	0.656
Friends tell me not to go to treatment	1.5	0.5	2.2	1.2	1.845
People will think badly of me if I go to treatment	1.9	0.7	1.8	0.5	0.499
Someone in my family does not want me to go to treatment	1.6	0.7	1.7	0.6	0.267
My family will be embarrassed or ashamed if I go to treatment	1.7	0.8	1.4	0.5	0.891
Fear of Treatment	2.0	0.9	1.9	0.7	0.247
I have had a bad experience with treatment	2.5	1.4	1.9	1.1	1.144
I am afraid what might happen in treatment	1.9	1.0	1.9	0.8	0.032
I am afraid of the people I might see in treatment	1.8	1.0	1.8	0.9	0.060
I am too embarrassed or ashamed to go to treatment	1.6	0.7	1.9	1.0	0.793
Privacy Concerns	2.1	0.8	3.0	1.3	2.251*
I do not like to talk in groups	1.9	0.9	3.0	1.5	2.454*
I hate being asked personal questions	1.9	0.7	3.1	1.3	2.993**
I do not like to talk about my personal life with other people	2.5	1.3	2.9	1.3	0.756
Time Conflict	1.9	0.9	2.3	0.9	1.173
I have things to do at home that make it hard for me to get to treatment	1.9	1.0	2.2	1.0	0.659
It will be hard for me to find a treatment program that fits my schedule	1.9	0.9	2.4	1.0	1.457
Poor Treatment Availability	1.7	0.7	2.1	0.9	1.336
I am moving too far away to get treatment	1.7	0.7	2.1	1.1	1.088
I do not know where to go for treatment	1.6	0.8	2.0	0.8	1.206
I have difficulty getting to and from treatment	1.8	1.0	2.3	1.3	1.096
Admission Difficulty	2.5	1.2	2.6	1.1	0.313
I will have to be on a waiting list for treatment	2.7	1.4	2.7	1.2	0.044
I have to go through too many steps to get into treatment	2.3	1.1	2.6	1.2	0.562

$n = 10$ reported seeking any type of treatment after release from jail; $n = 18$ reported that they did not seek any type of treatment after release
1 Strongly disagree, *3* Uncertain, *5* Strongly agree
$^*p < 0.05$; $^{**}p < 0.01$

References

1. Bronson J, Stroop J, Zimmer S, Berzofsky M. Drug use, dependence, and abuse among state prisoners and jail inmates, 2007–2009. Washington, DC: United States Department of Justice, Office of Juvenile Justice and Delinquency Prevention; 2017.
2. Chandler RK, Fletcher BW, Volkow ND. Treating drug abuse and addiction in the criminal justice system: improving public health and safety. JAMA. 2009;301(2):183–90.
3. Glynn LH, Kendra MS, Timko C, Finlay AK, Blodgett JC, Maisel NC, Midboe AM, McGuire JF, Blonigen DM. Facilitating treatment access and engagement for justice-involved veterans with substance use disorders. Crim Justice Policy Rev. 2016;27(2):138–63.
4. Binswanger IA, Nowels C, Corsi KF, Long J, Booth RE, Kutner J, Steiner JF. "From the prison door right to the sidewalk, everything went downhill," a qualitative study of the health experiences of recently released inmates. Int J Law Psychiatry. 2011;34(4):249–55.
5. Sung H-E, Mahoney AM, Mellow J. Substance abuse treatment gap among adult parolees: prevalence, correlates, and barriers. Crim Justice Rev. 2011;36(1):40–57.
6. Binswanger IA, Stern MF, Deyo RA, Heagerty PJ, Cheadle A, Elmore JG, Koepsell TD. Release from prison—a high risk of death for former inmates. N Engl J Med. 2007;356(2):157–65.
7. Rose SJ, LeBel TP, Begun AL, Fuhrmann D. Looking out from the inside: incarcerated women's perceived barriers to treatment of substance use. J Offender Rehabil. 2014;53(4):300–16.
8. Fox AD, Maradiaga J, Weiss L, Sanchez J, Starrels JL, Cunningham CO. Release from incarceration, relapse to opioid use and the potential for buprenorphine maintenance treatment: a qualitative study of the perceptions of former inmates with opioid use disorder. Addict Sci Clin Pract. 2015;10(1):2.

9. Bonczar TP. Characteristics of adults on probation, 1995. Traffic. 1997;4(9):10–2.
10. Perron BE, Bright CL. The influence of legal coercion on dropout from substance abuse treatment: results from a national survey. Drug Alcohol Depend. 2008;92(1):123–31.
11. Evans E, Li L, Hser Y-I. Client and program factors associated with dropout from court mandated drug treatment. Eval Program Plan. 2009;32(3):204–12.
12. Cohen E, Feinn R, Arias A, Kranzler HR. Alcohol treatment utilization: findings from the National Epidemiologic Survey on alcohol and related conditions. Drug Alcohol Depend. 2007;86(2–3):214–21.
13. Hedden SL. Behavioral health trends in the United States: results from the 2014 National Survey on Drug Use and Health: Substance Abuse and Mental Health Services Administration, Department of Heath & Human Services; 2015.
14. Substance Abuse and Mental Health Services Administration. Results from the 2012 National Survey on Drug Use and Health: Summary of national findings. In: NSDUH Series H-46, HHS Publication No(SMA) 13-4795. edn.: Substance Abuse and Mental Health Services Administration Rockville, MD; 2013.
15. Rapp RC, Xu J, Carr CA, Lane DT, Wang J, Carlson R. Treatment barriers identified by substance abusers assessed at a centralized intake unit. J Subst Abuse Treat. 2006;30(3):227–35.
16. Owens GP, Rogers SM, Whitesell AA. Use of mental health services and barriers to care for individuals on probation or parole. J Offender Rehabil. 2011;50(1):37–47.
17. Evans E, Li L, Hser Y-I. Treatment entry barriers among California's Proposition 36 offenders. J Subst Abuse Treat. 2008;35(4):410–8.
18. Friedmann PD, Hoskinson R Jr, Gordon M, Schwartz R, Kinlock T, Knight K, Flynn PM, Welsh WN, Stein LA, Sacks S. Medication-assisted treatment in criminal justice agencies affiliated with the criminal justice-drug abuse treatment studies (CJ-DATS): availability, barriers, and intentions. Subst Abuse Off Publ Assoc Med Educ Res Subst Abuse. 2012;33(1):9–18.
19. Matusow H, Dickman SL, Rich JD, Fong C, Dumont DM, Hardin C, Marlowe D, Rosenblum A. Medication assisted treatment in US drug courts: results from a nationwide survey of availability, barriers and attitudes. J Subst Abuse Treat. 2013;44(5):473–80.
20. Owens MD, McCrady BS. A pilot study of a brief motivational intervention for incarcerated drinkers. J Subst Abuse Treat. 2016;68:1–10.
21. Hides L, Cotton SM, Berger G, Gleeson J, O'Donnell C, Proffitt T, McGorry PD, Lubman DI. The reliability and validity of the alcohol, smoking and substance involvement screening test (ASSIST) in first-episode psychosis. Addict Behav. 2009;34(10):821–5.
22. Folstein MF, Folstein SE, McHugh PR. "Mini-mental state". A practical method for grading the cognitive state of patients for the clinician. J Psychiatr Res. 1975;12(3):189–98.
23. First M, Spitzer R, Gibbon M, Williams J. Biometrics research. New York State Psychiatric Institute; New York: 2002. Structured clinical interview for DSM-IV-TR axis I disorders, research version, patient edition. Clinical Trials Version (SCID-CT). 1995;9(2):92–104.
24. Demographics interview 2.2 (English version). https://casaa.unm.edu/inst/Demographic%20Interview%202_2.pdf. Accessed 1 Oct 2017.
25. McLellan AT, Kushner H, Metzger D, Peters R, Smith I, Grissom G, Pettinati H, Argeriou M. The fifth edition of the Addiction Severity Index. J Subst Abuse Treat. 1992;9(3):199–213.
26. Tonigan JS, Miller WR, Brown JM. The reliability of Form 90: an instrument for assessing alcohol treatment outcome. J Stud Alcohol. 1997;58(4):358–64.
27. King N. Template analysis. In: Cassell GSAC, editor. Qualitative methods and analysis in organizational research. London: Sage Publications; 1998. p. 118–34.
28. Sandelowski M. Real qualitative researchers do not count: the use of numbers in qualitative research. Res Nurs Health. 2001;24(3):230–40.
29. Marlow E, White MC, Chesla CA. Barriers and facilitators: parolees' perceptions of community health care. J Correct Health Care. 2010;16(1):17–26.
30. Prendergast ML, McCollister K, Warda U. A randomized study of the use of screening, brief intervention, and referral to treatment (SBIRT) for drug and alcohol use with jail inmates. J Subst Abuse Treat. 2017;74:54–64.

22

Racial/ethnic differences in the association between alcohol use and mortality among men living with HIV

Kara M. Bensley[1,2*], Kathleen A. McGinnis[3], David A. Fiellin[4], Adam J. Gordon[5,6], Kevin L. Kraemer[7,8], Kendall J. Bryant[9], E. Jennifer Edelman[4], Stephen Crystal[10], Julie R. Gaither[3,4], P. Todd Korthuis[11], Brandon D. L. Marshall[12], India J. Ornelas[1], K. C. Gary Chan[1], Julia C. Dombrowski[13], John C. Fortney[12], Amy C. Justice[3,4] and Emily C. Williams[1,2]

Abstract

Background: Increasing alcohol use is associated with increased risk of mortality among patients living with HIV (PLWH). This association varies by race/ethnicity among general outpatients, but racial/ethnic variation has not been investigated among PLWH, among whom racial/ethnic minorities are disproportionately represented.

Methods: VA electronic health record data from the Veterans Aging Cohort Study (2008–2012) were used to describe and compare mortality rates across race/ethnicity and levels of alcohol use defined by the Alcohol Use Disorders Identification Test-Consumption (AUDIT-C) questionnaire. Within each racial/ethnic group, Cox proportional hazards models, adjusted for age, disease severity, and comorbidities, compared mortality risk for moderate-risk (AUDIT-C = 4–7) and high-risk (AUDIT-C ≥ 8) relative to lower-risk (AUDIT-C = 1–3) alcohol use.

Results: Mean follow-up time among black (n = 8518), Hispanic (n = 1353), and white (n = 7368) male PLWH with documented AUDIT-C screening (n = 17,239) was 4.3 years. Black PLWH had the highest mortality rate among patients reporting lower-risk alcohol use (2.9/100 person-years) relative to Hispanic and white PLWH (1.8 and 2.3, respectively) (*p* value for overall comparison = 0.011). Mortality risk was increased for patients reporting high-risk relative to lower-risk alcohol use in all racial/ethnic groups [black adjusted hazard ratio (AHR) = 1.36, 95% confidence interval (CI) 1.12–1.66; Hispanic AHR = 2.18, 95% CI 1.30–3.64; and white AHR = 2.04, 95% CI 1.61–2.58]. For only white PLWH, mortality risk was increased for patients reporting moderate-relative to lower-risk alcohol use (black AHR = 1.09, 95% CI 0.93–1.27; Hispanic AHR = 1.36, 95% CI 0.89–2.09; white AHR = 1.51, 95% CI 1.28–1.77).

Conclusion: Among all PLWH, mortality risk was increased among patients reporting high-risk alcohol use across all racial/ethnic groups, but mortality risk was only increased among patients reporting moderate-risk relative to lower-risk alcohol use among white PLWH, and black patients appeared to have higher mortality risk relative to white patients at lower-risk levels of alcohol use. Findings of the present study further underscore the need to address unhealthy alcohol use among PLWH, and future research is needed to understand mechanisms underlying observed differences.

Keywords: HIV, Alcohol use, Mortality risk, Racial/ethnic disparities, Veterans

*Correspondence: kbensley@uw.edu
[1] Department of Health Services, Magnuson Health Sciences Center, University of Washington School of Public Health, 1959 NE Pacific St, Box 357660, Seattle, WA 98195-7660, USA
Full list of author information is available at the end of the article

Background

Alcohol use is common among people living with human immunodeficiency virus (HIV) and has known adverse effects on HIV-related outcomes. Alcohol use adversely influences health among patients living with HIV (PLWH) and is associated with lower receipt and poorer outcomes of HIV treatment, and ultimately with mortality among PLWH [1–5]. While no level of alcohol use appears to be "safe" for PLWH, risk of adverse outcomes is generally increased for those with higher severity of alcohol use relative to those who use alcohol at lower levels [1, 6].

HIV infection disproportionately impacts vulnerable populations [7] including racial/ethnic minorities. Mortality rates among PLWH also differ across racial/ethnic groups, with black PLWH having the highest mortality rates and Hispanic the lowest [8]. Racial/ethnic minority PLWH experience increased HIV stigma [9], socioeconomic disadvantage and increased persecution [10], and decreased access to care [3] that may make consequences of alcohol use worse for racial/ethnic minority [10] relative to white PLWH [11–15]. Due to these experiences, non-white PLWH may have increased risk of mortality associated with alcohol use relative to whites. Previous studies in non-HIV-specific populations demonstrate that racial/ethnic minorities have worse consequences at similar levels of alcohol use [16] and higher risk of mortality at lower levels of alcohol use than whites [17]. Thus, we hypothesize that racial/ethnic minority PLWH may also have worse consequences at similar levels of alcohol use and higher mortality risk at lower levels of alcohol use than white PLWH. Because risk factors and influences of health behaviors are likely to vary among racial/ethnic groups depending on their lived experiences, experts have called for studies to examine alcohol-related risk among vulnerable sub-populations of PLWH [5]. No prior study has examined whether the association between alcohol use and mortality varies across race/ethnicity among PLWH. Therefore, we evaluated whether the association between level of alcohol use and mortality differs across racial/ethnic groups in a national sample of PLWH.

Methods

Data source

The data source for this study is the Veterans Aging Cohort Study (VACS), an observational cohort of patients who receive care at the nationwide Veterans Health Administration (VA) starting October 1, 1997 [18]. VACS data were extracted from the VA Informatics and Computing Infrastructure data warehouse, a national VA repository that includes clinical and administrative data for all VA patients, as well as clinical alcohol screening data (collected using the Alcohol Use Disorders Identification Test Consumption (AUDIT-C) questionnaire among over 90% of VA outpatients) since 2008 [19].

Sample

We included all male PLWH with a documented AUDIT-C alcohol screening between October 1, 2008 and March 30, 2012 who reported any alcohol use in the past year (AUDIT-C scores > 0) and were documented to be one or more of the three major racial/ethnic groups in the United States: black, Hispanic, and/or white. Women, other minority groups, and patients with AUDIT-C scores indicating patients who reported no alcohol use in the past year (AUDIT-C = 0) were excluded. Though research of this type is needed among women and other minority groups, associations between alcohol use and outcomes vary based on gender [20–22], and the numbers of both women and other minorities with HIV who also report alcohol use at high levels are very small in VACS. Exclusion of patients reporting no alcohol use was done because the measure of alcohol used (AUDIT-C score) does not differentiate between lifetime abstainers and those who have become abstinent due to other reasons (e.g., declining health) among patients reporting no alcohol use [1, 6].

Predictor

Alcohol use was measured using the AUDIT-C, a validated screen for unhealthy alcohol use [23–25] and a measure of alcohol use severity [26, 27]. The AUDIT-C is also associated with phosphatidylethanol, a biomarker for alcohol use [28, 29]. AUDIT-C scores range from 0 to 12; scores of 0 represent patients reporting no alcohol use in the past year, and increasing scores are associated with increased risk of multiple medical outcomes [30, 31], alcohol use disorder symptoms [24–26, 32, 33], and mortality [4, 17, 28, 30, 34]. For this study, the first AUDIT-C documented during the study period for each patient was used to measure levels of alcohol use based on clinically meaningful AUDIT-C cut-off scores for male patients [25, 26]: lower-risk (AUDIT-C 1-3), moderate-risk (AUDIT-C 4-7), and high-risk (AUDIT-C 8-12). AUDIT-C screening is conducted as part of routine health screening at the VA, thus AUDIT-C scores are documented annually for over 90% of all established outpatients.

Outcome

Time to death by any cause was specified as the primary outcome. Survival time was measured from date of the first AUDIT-C screening during the study period until death or loss to follow-up/end of study censoring, July 23, 2014 [35]. Death was measured using a validated measure created by combining four databases tracking deaths among VA patients: the Patient Treatment File, tracking hospital deaths within the VA System; the Beneficiary Identification Records Locating System, tracking VA death benefits; the Medicare Vital Status File; and the

Social Security Death Master File, which has comparable completeness and accuracy to the National Death Index [36].

Effect modifier

Race/ethnicity was categorized as non-Hispanic black, Hispanic, and non-Hispanic white [37]. Because patients can identify with multiple racial/ethnic groups, race/ethnicity was hierarchically coded, first as Hispanic ethnicity, and then as black and then white, consistent with single-race/ethnicity classification by rarest to most common racial/ethnic groups [38].

Covariates

Age was categorized as < 50, 50–64, and 65 and older. Secondary measures of age were also derived: age as a continuous linear variable and age as a quadratic variable (age squared).

HIV disease severity Because HIV disease severity may confound the association between alcohol use and mortality [39], two measures of severity were described using the closest documented measure in the 6 months prior to and following AUDIT-C screening. These included: CD4 count (< 200, 200–500, > 500 cells/mm^3) and a binary measure of viral load suppression (HIV-1 RNA < 200 copies/mL). In adjusted models, CD4 count was used to account for HIV disease severity as these measures are highly correlated. A binary measure of receipt of antiretroviral therapy (ART) at baseline AUDIT-C measure (at least one pharmacy fill prior to or within 7 days after baseline AUDIT-C measure) was described across racial ethnic groups. *Other comorbid conditions* were measured based on International Classification of Diseases 9th Edition (ICD-9 CM) codes documented any time between the beginning of VACS (10/1/97) and the baseline AUDIT-C measure. These included: non-AIDS related cancers (bladder, breast, buccal cavity and pharynx, digestive system, Hodgkin's lymphoma, ill-defined cancer, kidney, leukemia, male genital system, melanomas, non-epithelial skin cancer, penile, prostate, stomach, testicular, ureter, urinary system), lung disease (chronic obstructive pulmonary disorder, asthma, or other lung disease), cardiovascular disease (congestive heart failure, myocardial infarction/coronary artery disease, peripheral vascular disease, ischemic stroke, stroke), hypertension, diabetes, hepatitis B, hepatitis C, anxiety, major depression, psychosis (e.g., schizophrenia), and post-traumatic stress disorder [40]. Body mass index (underweight < 18.5, normal/overweight = 18.6–29.9, obese > 30) was also included as HIV disease progression is associated with weight loss and wasting [41]; and higher BMI is associated with better HIV prognosis [42].

Other substance use measures included tobacco use (current, never, ever), determined based on documentation in an electronic clinical reminder [43], and current drug use (based on ICD-9 CM codes within 1 year prior to 6 months after AUDIT-C screening). These were also considered as covariates as both are associated with alcohol use and mortality.

Analyses

Population characteristics, as well as levels of alcohol use and mortality rates, were described and compared across racial/ethnic groups; comparisons were done using Chi square tests of independence. To test racial/ethnic differences in the association between alcohol use and mortality, we fit a Cox Proportional Hazards model with time to death as the outcome and level of alcohol use as the predictor and tested a multiplicative interaction between racial/ethnic group and level of alcohol use. A Wald test was used to evaluate the overall significance of the interaction at p value < 0.05, and adjusted hazard ratios were calculated to estimate associations between level of alcohol use and mortality within each racial/ethnic group. Models were first unadjusted (Model 1) and then adjusted additionally for: age (Model 2), age and HIV disease severity based on CD4 count (Model 3), and age, HIV severity, receipt of ART, and comorbidities (Model 4). The iterative modeling strategy allowed for hypothesis-generation regarding what factors may be driving associations observed. Multiple imputation models were used to account for missing data in Cox Proportional Hazards models, particularly missing values for CD4 count, BMI, and smoking. To assess whether including age as a continuous linear or quadratic variable would better fit the model (i.e., address any residual confounding by age), models using categorical, linear, quadratic variables for age were tested among complete cases, and model fit was compared using Akaike Information Criterion. Tests of model fit indicated similar fits and results across models, thus age was used as a categorical variable in the primary analyses. All analyses were conducted in Stata Version 13 [44].

Results

Eligible patients included 17,239 male PLWH; 49.4% were black, 7.9% were Hispanic, and 42.7% were white. The mean follow-up time was 4.3 years [Standard deviation (SD) = 1.3] for black, 4.3 (SD = 1.2) for Hispanic, and 4.4 (SD = 1.2) years for white PLWH.

Patient characteristics and levels of alcohol use differed across racial/ethnic groups (Table 1). Black patients had the highest prevalence of patients age 50–64, and were generally sicker than both white and Hispanic patients, having lower CD4 cell counts, higher viral loads, and

Table 1 Patient characteristics and AUDIT-C categories across racial/ethnic groups and overall

	Black n = 8518 (%)	Hispanic n = 1353 (%)	White n = 7368 (%)	p value	Overall n = 17, 239 (%)
Demographic characteristics					
Age					
< 50	38.2	39.5	37.7	< 0.001	38.1
50–64	55.9	52.3	49.1		52.7
65+	5.9	8.1	13.2		9.2
HIV disease severity					
CD4 count (< 200)[a]					
< 200	17.8	13.7	13.7	< 0.001	14.7
200–500	42.6	38.6	40.2		41.3
> 500	39.7	47.7	48.5		44.0
Viral load (≥ 500)[a]	32.1	22.6	19.4	< 0.001	26.0
HAART	73.4	76.1	76.7	< 0.001	75.0
Comorbid mental and physical health conditions					
Smoking status					
Never	24.5	30.9	29.5	< 0.001	27.1
Past	10.3	17.1	16.9		13.6
Current	65.3	51.9	53.6		59.3
Drug use	24.3	8.6	14.5	< 0.001	16.9
BMI[a]					
Underweight	3.7	1.5	2.5	< 0.001	3.0
Normal and overweight	76.7	79.7	79.5		78.2
Obese	19.6	18.8	18.0		18.8
Cancer (non-AIDS related)	6.4	7.0	12.6	< 0.001	9.1
Lung disease	17.5	17.6	19.9	< 0.001	18.5
Cardiovascular disease	12.2	11.8	15.1	< 0.001	13.4
Hypertension	49.2	38.4	40.3	< 0.001	44.5
Diabetes	14.3	15.8	12.2	< 0.001	13.5
Hepatitis B	10.2	13.2	8.1	< 0.001	9.5
Hepatitis C	28.4	14.7	26.0	< 0.001	22.3
Anxiety	11.6	18.9	18.8	< 0.001	15.3
Major depression	20.5	21.8	21.7	0.180	21.1
Psychosis (schizophrenia, schizoaffective, other)	13.2	11.8	13.6	0.014	12.6
PTSD	13.3	10.7	12.3	< 0.001	12.1
AUDIT-C categories					
AUDIT-C category					
Lower-risk (1–3)	74.2	76.9	78.2	< 0.001	76.1
Moderate-risk (4–7)	18.3	16.9	17.1		17.7
High-risk (8–12)	7.5	6.3	4.8		6.2

[a] Missing data about disease severity makes N = 14,880, N for BMI = 17,188, N for smoking = 16,958

higher proportions of current smoking, drug use, underweight or obese, hypertension, Hepatitis C, and PTSD. Black patients also included the highest proportion of patients reporting high and moderate risk alcohol use. Hispanic patients were generally younger, but had higher prevalence of hepatitis B than other racial/ethnic groups. White patients were generally older, and had better measures of HIV disease severity and receipt of ART than black patients (but similar to Hispanic patients). White PLWH also included the highest proportion with non-AIDS related cancer, lung disease, cardiovascular disease. White patients had the highest proportion of patients reporting lower-risk alcohol use.

Mortality rates varied across racial ethnic groups (Table 2). Among all PLWH reporting past-year alcohol use and those reporting lower-risk use, black patients had the highest mortality rates relative to Hispanic and white patients ($p = 0.01$ and < 0.01 respectively). There were no

Table 2 Mortality rates overall and by level of alcohol use and race for black, Hispanic, and white VA patients living with HIV (n = 17,239)

	Overall (n = 17, 239)		Black (n = 8518)		Hispanic (n = 1353)		White (n = 7368)		p value*
# of Deaths	2041		1042		128		871		*0.014*
	Mortality rate[a]	95% CI	Mortality rate[a]	95% CI	Mortality rate[a]	95% CI	Mortality rate[a]	95% CI	p value*
Overall (n = 17,239)	2.7	(2.6, 2.9)	2.9	(2.7, 3.1)	2.2	(1.8, 2.6)	2.7	(2.5, 2.9)	*0.0111*
Lower-risk (n = 13,119)	2.4	(2.3, 2.6)	2.7	(2.5, 2.9)	1.8	(1.4, 2.2)	2.3	(2.1, 2.5)	*0.0008*
Moderate-risk (n = 3044)	3.3	(3.0, 3.7)	3.1	(2.7, 3.5)	2.9	(2.0, 4.2)	3.7	(3.2, 4.3)	0.1507
High risk (n = 1076)	5.0	(4.4, 5.7)	4.5	(3.7, 5.3)	5.0	(3.2, 8.0)	5.9	(4.8, 7.3)	0.1419

[a] Mortality rate is calculated per 100 person-years

*p value determined by Chi square test for difference in number of deaths and log-rank test for difference in mortality rate, italicized if significant

significant differences in mortality rates across racial/ethnic groups among patients in the moderate or high-risk levels of alcohol use. As alcohol risk groups increased, mortality rates also increased overall and across all racial/ethnic groups.

In all Cox Proportional Hazards models, the association between levels of alcohol use and mortality varied significantly across racial/ethnic groups (p value of overall interactions for Models 1–4 < 0.001). Associations between level of alcohol use and mortality risk within racial/ethnic groups differed based on covariate adjustment (Table 3). In unadjusted models (Model 1), and models adjusted for age only (Model 2), moderate- relative to lower-risk alcohol use was associated with significantly increased mortality risk for all patients across racial/ethnic groups. In models additionally adjusted for disease severity (Model 3), moderate- relative to lower-risk alcohol use was significantly associated with increased mortality risk only for whites and Hispanics. In models adjusted additionally for comorbidities (Model 4), moderate- relative to lower-risk alcohol use was associated with significantly increased mortality risk only for white patients (Table 3). For all racial/ethnic groups, across all models (Models 1–4), high-risk alcohol use was significantly associated with greater mortality risk than lower-risk alcohol use. The magnitude of the association appeared to differ such

Table 3 Hazard ratios of mortality comparing moderate- and high-risk relative to lower-risk alcohol use among black, Hispanic, and white VA patients living with HIV: overall and by race/ethnicity

Alcohol use categories	Iterative modeling strategy	Overall		Black		Hispanic		White	
		(n = 17,239)		(n = 8518)		(n = 1354)		(n = 7376)	
		HR	95% CI	HR	95% CI	HR	95% CI	HR	95% CI
Lower-risk		Ref							
Moderate-risk	Model 1[a]	*1.37*	*(1.23, 1.53)*	*1.17*	*(1.00, 1.36)*	*1.63*	*(1.06, 2.49)*	*1.60*	*(1.37, 1.88)*
	Model 2[b]	*1.39*	*(1.25, 1.54)*	*1.20*	*(1.03, 1.40)*	*1.64*	*(1.07, 2.51)*	*1.59*	*(1.35, 1.86)*
	Model 3[c]	*1.34*	*(1.21, 1.50)*	1.15	(0.99, 1.34)	*1.56*	*(1.02, 2.39)*	*1.56*	*(1.33, 1.84)*
	Model 4[d]	*1.26*	*(1.13, 1.40)*	1.08	(0.92, 1.26)	1.36	(0.89, 2.08)	*1.50*	*(1.27, 1.76)*
High-risk	Model 1[a]	*2.04*	*(1.77, 2.35)*	*1.68*	*(1.39, 2.04)*	*2.80*	*(1.68, 4.66)*	*2.55*	*(2.03, 3.20)*
	Model 2[b]	*2.11*	*(1.83, 2.43)*	*1.66*	*(1.37, 2.02)*	*2.65*	*(1.59, 4.41)*	*2.85*	*(2.27, 3.58)*
	Model 3[c]	*1.92*	*(1.66, 2.21)*	*1.52*	*(1.25, 1.85)*	*2.49*	*(1.49, 4.15)*	*2.61*	*(2.08, 3.29)*
	Model 4[d]	*1.62*	*(1.40, 1.88)*	*1.35*	*(1.11, 1.64)*	*2.14*	*(1.28, 3.58)*	*2.01*	*(1.59, 2.55)*

Interactions between alcohol use categories and racial/ethnic groups were all significant (p < 0.001)

Italicsed results are significant at p value < 0.05

[a] Model 1 is unadjusted

[b] Model 2 is adjusted for age

[c] Model 3 is adjusted for age and CD4 count

[d] Model 4 is adjusted for age, disease severity (CD4 count), receipt of HAART, and comorbidities (non-AIDS related Cancers (bladder, breast, buccal cavity and pharynx, digestive system, Hodgkin's lymphoma, ill-defined cancer, kidney, leukemia, male genital system, melanomas, non-epithelial skin cancer, penile, prostate, stomach, testicular, ureter, urinary system), lung disease (COPD, asthma, or other lung disease), cardiovascular disease (congestive heart failure, MI/CAD, peripheral vascular disease, ischemic stroke, stroke), hypertension, diabetes, hepatitis B, hepatitis C, anxiety, psychosis (schizophrenia, schizoaffective disorder, other psychosis), PSTD, BMI, drug use, and lifetime tobacco use

that Hispanic and white PLWH had higher mortality risk than black PLWH at high-risk levels of alcohol use relative to lower-risk levels, although the confidence intervals overlapped in many cases.

To examine magnitude of associations across racial/ethnic differences, the effect of race/ethnicity on mortality risk within each AUDIT-C category was considered in secondary analysis (Table 4). Black patients had a significantly higher mortality risk compared to white and Hispanic patients at lower-risk levels of alcohol use in unadjusted models (Model 1), when adjusted for age only (Model 2), and when adjusted for age and HIV disease severity (Model 3). When comparing mortality risk across racial/ethnic groups at lower-risk levels of alcohol use in models adjusted for age, disease severity, and comorbidities (Model 4), black patients had significantly higher mortality risk than Hispanics, while Hispanics had lower mortality risk than white PLWH. Among PLWH reporting moderate-risk alcohol use, the only significant difference across racial ethnic groups was in fully adjusted models, such that both black and Hispanic patients had lower mortality risk than white patients. Among PLWH reporting high-risk alcohol use, there were no significant differences between Hispanic relative to white, nor among black relative to Hispanic patients (Models 1–4). However, in all models (Models 1–4) among patients reporting high-risk alcohol use, black patients had significantly lower mortality risk than white patients.

Discussion

In this national sample of male PLWH who receive VA care, associations between alcohol use and mortality varied across racial/ethnic groups. For all racial/ethnic groups, high-risk relative to lower-risk alcohol use was associated with increased risk of mortality. Moderate relative to lower-risk alcohol use was associated with statistically significant increased mortality risk for all racial ethnic groups in unadjusted models, but only among white patients in fully adjusted models. For black and Hispanic PLWH, point estimates suggested increased risk associated with moderate levels of alcohol use, but no statistically significant associations were observed in fully adjusted models.

These findings expand on current understanding of alcohol-related risk among PLWH. While previous studies among PLWH identified greater risk of mortality for patients with both moderate- and high-risk alcohol use

Table 4 Hazard ratios comparing mortality between racial/ethnic groups within each AUDIT-C category

Comparison by race/ethnicity	Lower-risk		Moderate-risk		High-risk	
	HR	95% CI	HR	95% CI	HR	95% CI
Black relative to white						
Model 1[a]	*1.15*	*(1.03, 1.28)*	0.84	(0.69, 1.01)	*0.76*	*(0.57, 1.00)*
Model 2[b]	*1.25*	*(1.12, 1.39)*	0.94	(0.77, 1.14)	*0.73*	*(0.55, 0.96)*
Model 3[c]	*1.17*	*(1.05, 1.31)*	0.86	(0.71, 1.05)	*0.68*	*(0.52, 0.90)*
Model 4[d]	0.99	(0.88, 1.11)	*0.71*	*(0.58, 0.87)*	*0.66*	*(0.50, 0.87)*
Hispanic relative to white						
Model 1[a]	*0.78*	*(0.61, 0.98)*	0.79	(0.53, 1.16)	0.85	(0.51, 1.41)
Model 2[b]	0.83	(0.66, 1.05)	0.86	(0.58, 1.27)	0.77	(0.46, 1.29)
Model 3[c]	0.81	(0.64, 1.02)	0.81	(0.55, 1.19)	0.77	(0.46, 1.28)
Model 4[d]	*0.75*	*(0.59, 0.94)*	0.68	(0.46, 1.00)	0.80	(0.48, 1.33)
Black relative to Hispanic						
Model 1[a]	*1.48*	*(1.17, 1.86)*	1.06	(0.72, 1.57)	0.89	(0.54, 1.46)
Model 2[b]	*1.50*	*(1.19, 1.89)*	1.09	(0.74, 1.61)	0.94	(0.57, 1.54)
Model 3[c]	*1.45*	*(1.15, 1.82)*	1.07	(0.73, 1.58)	0.89	(0.54, 1.46)
Model 4[d]	*1.32*	*(1.05, 1.66)*	1.05	(0.71, 1.55)	0.83	(0.50, 1.37)

[a] Model 1 is unadjusted

[b] Model 2 is adjusted for age

[c] Model 3 is adjusted for age and CD4 count

[d] Model 4 is adjusted for age, disease severity (CD4 count), receipt of HAART, and comorbidities (non-AIDS related Cancers (bladder, breast, buccal cavity and pharynx, digestive system, Hodgkin's lymphoma, ill-defined cancer, kidney, leukemia, male genital system, melanomas, non-epithelial skin cancer, penile, prostate, stomach, testicular, ureter, urinary system), lung disease (COPD, asthma, or other lung disease), cardiovascular disease (congestive heart failure, MI/CAD, peripheral vascular disease, ischemic stroke, stroke), hypertension, diabetes, hepatitis B, hepatitis C, anxiety, psychosis (schizophrenia, schizoaffective disorder, other psychosis), PSTD, BMI, drug use, and lifetime tobacco use

Italicsed results are significant at p value < 0.05

relative to those with lower-risk alcohol use [4, 28], findings from the present study suggest that these associations vary across racial/ethnic groups. Differences in the association between alcohol use and mortality may be driven by racial/ethnic differences in patients reporting high-risk or moderate-risk alcohol use, by differences in mortality risk among those reporting lower-risk alcohol use, which were used as a reference group in analyses comparing levels of alcohol use, or by residual confounding. While previous research suggested that racial/ethnic minorities may be at increased risk of mortality associated with alcohol use, our findings suggest a more complicated picture.

In this study, Hispanic PLWH had increased mortality among patients reporting high-risk, but not moderate-risk alcohol use, relative to those reporting lower-risk alcohol use, but decreased mortality relative to black patients reporting lower-risk levels of use in all models and marginally decreased mortality risk relative to white patients in unadjusted and fully adjusted models. There were fewer Hispanic patients than other racial/ethnic groups in this sample, and the model may have been insufficiently powered to detect differences among Hispanic patients. Further, previous research on alcohol use among Hispanics identified differences in alcohol-related outcomes based on acculturation to the United States, with higher levels of acculturation being associated with poorer alcohol-related outcomes [45, 46]. In this secondary data analysis, we did not have access to measures regarding contextual or cultural factors, thus, there may be unmeasured protective factors in this group that build resiliency against the ill effects of alcohol use.

Among black PLWH reporting any alcohol use, there was no significant difference in mortality risk among patients with moderate-risk relative to lower-risk alcohol use in fully adjusted models, although there was significant increased risk of mortality for high- relative to lower-risk alcohol use. These findings are consistent with previous research in general (non-HIV specific) outpatients [17]. Our comparisons of racial/ethnic groups within alcohol use levels may help explain these findings. Specifically, we found that black patients had increased mortality relative to white patients among PLWH reporting lower risk alcohol use, although this was attenuated by adjustment for comorbid conditions. Additionally, black patients had decreased mortality risk relative to white patients at higher-risk levels of alcohol use.

Reasons for the lack of increased risk of mortality among patients reporting moderate- and high-risk levels of alcohol use relative to those reporting lower-risk alcohol use among black PLWH are unknown, but may be due to contextual factors relating to alcohol use and competing health conditions. For example, previous studies have suggested that greater prevalence of adverse alcohol-related consequences among black relative to white persons [10, 16] relates to greater exposure to racism, and community-level contextual factors such as residence in low socioeconomic status areas leading to greater stress, with social norms promoting abstinence in black communities possibly leading to increased stigma for people who use alcohol, and surveillance by authorities leading to increased law enforcement involvement in black communities [10, 47–49]. However, there was no significant difference in alcohol-associated mortality risk comparing black to white patients at lower-levels of alcohol use when additionally adjusting for comorbidities (Model 4; Table 4), suggesting that competing health conditions may account for differences in mortality risk between black and white patients at lower-risk levels of alcohol use, and alcohol use may not be the strongest risk factor for death among black PLWH.

Competing health conditions may be more strongly associated with mortality, and may be bi-directionally associated with alcohol use. Thus, adjusting for health factors that may be exacerbated by alcohol use may have over-adjusted findings and attenuated the association between alcohol use and mortality. Black patients have increased risk of both prevalence of adverse health conditions and poor outcomes associated with these conditions relative to white patients, in part owing to substantial stigma and discrimination experienced by black persons due to racism [50]. For instance, in this sample, black patients had the highest proportion of hypertension, Hepatitis C, current tobacco use, and other drug use. These conditions may be more prevalent among black patients [51] or more strongly associated with poor outcomes among black patients [52, 53] due to contextual factors including racism [50, 54], and all are strongly predictive of mortality among PLWH [55–58]. Additionally, these conditions are bi-directionally associated with alcohol use [59, 60], and adjusting for these possible mediating factors may have over-adjusted the model. These measures, included only in Model 4 and disproportionately distributed among black patients, may have inadvertently adjusted away some pathways (e.g., racism) via which alcohol use would be associated with mortality for black PLWH.

Finally, it is possible that differential receipt of specialty addictions treatment across racial/ethnic groups could help explain findings of the present study. Specifically, black patients are more likely than white to receive specialty addictions treatment in the VA system [61, 62]. Therefore, it is possible that higher treatment receipt among black patients may account for lack of association between moderate-risk levels of alcohol use and mortality among black patients, and differences in mortality risk at high-risk levels of alcohol use between black and white patients. Future research is needed to investigate this issue.

The overall patterns observed in the data across racial/ethnic groups replicate findings from a similar study regarding associations between alcohol use and mortality among non-HIV-specific VA patients [17]. While previous studies show that non-white patients have worse consequences of alcohol use at similar levels to white patients [10, 16], there may be aspects of care at the VA that make this populations unique. Eligibility for VA services reduces disparities in access to care, which may reduce racial/ethnic disparities overall [63]. Additionally, there may be increased mortality risk for white PLWH at moderate risk levels of alcohol use, but not for racial/ethnic minorities, perhaps due to risk factors that make PLWH unique. Future research is needed to better understand and address contributing factors mediating the strength of associations between alcohol use and mortality risk.

Findings confirm risks of alcohol use at high-risk levels for all racial/ethnic groups and affirm recommendations for clinical interventions. Specifically, brief interventions are recommended for all primary care patients who drink above recommended limits, and specialty addictions treatment or alcohol use disorder medications are recommended for patients with more severe unhealthy alcohol use [64]. PLWH are at increased risk of under-receipt of alcohol related treatment, relative to patients without HIV [65, 66], and findings of the present study further underscore the need to address unhealthy alcohol use among PLWH. Increased access to alcohol-related care is needed, and should be offered across treatment settings, including both in primary care and HIV treatment settings [67–70].

There are several limitations to this study. This study used secondary clinical data and was observational. Thus, residual confounding (e.g., by socioeconomic status, sexual orientation, gender identity, or rural status, which were unmeasured or not included in this dataset) may be present. Socioeconomic status, in particular, is a known risk factor for poor outcomes among PLWH for which we did not have a measure [71], and adjustment for it decreased the association between alcohol use and mortality in a previous study [17]. Similarly, the study design did not allow identification of entry into VA care, which may be patterned by race and influence mortality and thus reflect an additional residual confounder. While the AUDIT-C has been validated across racial/ethnic groups [32], black patients may be more likely to under-report alcohol use due to stigma [72]. A previous study in VACS additionally showed that among patients reporting past-year abstinence from alcohol use, those with HCV had increased likelihood of biomarker-detected alcohol use [28], and black patients are overrepresented among VACS patients with HCV relative to those without HCV [73]. Black patients may also be more likely to overestimate the size of a standard drink [74], which may have misclassified alcohol use level among black patients in this study. Additionally, the AUDIT-C, while a validated screen for unhealthy alcohol use [23–25], is not an in-depth structured assessment of alcohol use. In this cohort, AUDIT-C is asked and documented by a clinician, and may be limited based on method of screening administration and results documentation [75], as well as by patient recall or social desirability bias [76]. Further, though alcohol use can vary over time within persons, alcohol use was also not considered to be a time-varying factor in this analysis. However, previous research assessing repeated alcohol screening scores [77] and research using AUDIT-C trajectory models indicates that the vast majority of patients remain in stable AUDIT-C categories over time [78]. Additionally, missing data, which was accounted for in this study using multiple imputation, may not be missing at random. There are also limitations to the external validity of this study. This study is only among men receiving care at the VA, and may not be generalizable to women veterans living with HIV and/or non-veterans. Additionally, PLWH in this study are already linked with care, and results will not be generalizable to PLWH not linked with care. Finally, alcohol use data is only available from 2008, when the AUDIT-C screening data became widely available in the VA. Future studies are needed examining these issues among women, non-veterans, and people living with HIV not linked to healthcare.

Future research is also needed to determine which factors mediate the association between alcohol use and mortality to understand variation in the association across racial/ethnic groups. Better understanding these mechanisms will be integral for designing policies and interventions to prevent mortality associated with alcohol use among all PLWH. Our findings are hypothesis-generating regarding potential mechanisms. For instance, our findings suggest the possibility that there were competing risks for mortality among more vulnerable racial/ethnic groups, as comorbid conditions and greater HIV disease severity were over-represented among black persons in this population. Similarly, white patients may have been more susceptible to the effects of alcohol use on ART. They were more likely to be on ART, which may have increased the influence of heavy alcohol use on risk of death (by affected adherence to ART) relative to black persons (who were less likely to receive ART). The influence of other potential moderating factors, such as receipt of alcohol-related care and rural status, should also be examined.

Despite limitations and need for further research, this study—conducted in a national sample of racially/ethnically diverse PLWH receiving care from the largest single provider of HIV care in the United States—is the first to our knowledge to evaluate the influence of alcohol use on mortality across racial/ethnic minority groups of PLWH. Findings from this study suggest that, similar to studies among general outpatients [17], associations between alcohol use and mortality vary across racial/ethnic groups. While associations vary in magnitude across racial/ethnic groups and may be dependent on other patient level factors within racial/ethnic groups, overall patterns were similar across groups. This highlights the need to increase access to alcohol-related care to address high-risk alcohol use across all racial/ethnic groups to decrease mortality risk among PLWH, while considering potential that competing health conditions may account for increased mortality risk among racial/ethnic minority PLWH at lower-risk levels of alcohol use.

Authors' contributions

Data for this study were obtained from the Veterans Aging Cohort Study (PI: Amy Justice, MD, MPH). All authors contributed to study design, protocol development, and data interpretation. KMB led literature review, study design, data analysis and interpretation, and manuscript writing; ECW served as senior mentor, guiding all stages of study design, analysis, interpretation, and presentation. KAM provided mentorship and guidance in study design, analysis, interpretation, and presentation. KCGC served as senior biostatistician, providing expertise on analysis. A version of this manuscript is included in the dissertation submitted in partial fulfillment of the requirements for the degree of Doctor of Philosophy from the University of Washington (completed by KMB in August 2017). All authors read and approved the final manuscript.

Author details

[1] Department of Health Services, Magnuson Health Sciences Center, University of Washington School of Public Health, 1959 NE Pacific St, Box 357660, Seattle, WA 98195-7660, USA. [2] VA Health Services Research and Development (HSRD) Denver Seattle Center of Innovation for Veteran-Centered and Value-Driven Care, VA Puget Sound Healthcare System, 1660 S. Columbian Way, Mailstop S-152, Seattle, WA 98108, USA. [3] VA Connecticut Healthcare System, West Haven Campus, 950 Campbell Avenue, West Haven, CT 06516, USA. [4] Yale School of Medicine, 333 Cedar St, New Haven, CT 06510, USA. [5] Salt Lake City VA, 500 Foothill Dr, Salt Lake City, UT 84148, USA. [6] University of Utah, 201 Presidents Cir, Salt Lake City, UT 84112, USA. [7] VA Pittsburgh Healthcare System, University Drive, Pittsburgh, PA 15240, USA. [8] University of Pittsburgh School of Medicine, 3550 Terrace St, Pittsburgh, PA 15213, USA. [9] National Institute on Alcohol Abuse and Alcoholism, 5635 Fishers Ln, Rockville, MD 20852, USA. [10] Rutgers University, 7 College Ave, New Brunswick, NJ 08901, USA. [11] Oregon Health & Science University, 3181 SW Sam Jackson Park Rd, Portland, OR 97239, USA. [12] Brown University School of Public Health, 121 S Main St, Providence, RI 02903, USA. [13] University of Washington School of Medicine, 1959 NE Pacific St, Seattle, WA 98195, USA.

Acknowledgements

Not applicable.

Competing interests

The authors declare that they have no competing interests.

data, due to patient confidentiality, and so are not publicly available. Data are however available from the authors upon reasonable request and with permission of VA, in compliance with current VA data management guidelines.

Consent for publication

Not applicable.

Funding

The funders of this study had no role in study design, data collection, analysis, interpretation and presentation, or in the decision to submit the manuscript for publication. Views presented in the manuscript are those of the authors and do not reflect those of the University of Washington, the National Institute on Alcohol Abuse and Alcoholism, the National Institutes of Health, the Department of Veterans Affairs, or the United States Government. This study was supported by the COMpAAAS/Veterans Aging Cohort Study, which is a CHAART Cooperative Agreement funded by the National Institutes of Health: National Institute on Alcohol Abuse and Alcoholism (U24-AA020794, U01-AA020790, U01-AA020795,U01-AA020799; U10 AA013566-completed) and in kind by the US Department of Veterans Affairs. This study was additionally funded by a 2017 Small Grant from the Alcohol and Drug Abuse Institute at the University of Washington (PI: Kara Bensley), and by a 2017 Pre-doctoral Fellowship from VA Puget Sound Research & Development awarded to Dr. Bensley. Dr. Bensley is also supported by Award Number T32AA007240, Graduate Research Training in Alcohol Problems: Alcohol-related Disparities, from the National Institute on Alcohol Abuse and Alcoholism. Dr. Williams is funded through a VA Health Services Research & Development Career Development Award (CDA 12-276).

References

1. Braithwaite RS, Conigliaro J, Roberts MS, Shechter S, Schaefer A, McGinnis K, et al. Estimating the impact of alcohol consumption on survival for HIV+ individuals. AIDS Care. 2007;19:459–66.
2. Braithwaite RS, Bryant KJ. Influence of alcohol consumption on adherence to and toxicity of antiretroviral therapy and survival. Alcohol Res Health J Natl Inst Alcohol Abuse Alcohol. 2010;33:280–7.
3. Hahn JA, Samet JH. Alcohol and HIV disease progression: weighing the evidence. Curr HIV/AIDS Rep. 2010;7:226–33.
4. Justice AC, McGinnis KA, Tate JP, Braithwaite RS, Bryant KJ, Cook RL, et al. Risk of mortality and physiologic injury evident with lower alcohol exposure among HIV infected compared with uninfected men. Drug Alcohol Depend. 2016;161:95–103.
5. Williams EC, Hahn JA, Saitz R, Bryant K, Lira MC, Samet JH. Alcohol use and human immunodeficiency virus (HIV) infection: current knowledge, implications, and future directions. Alcohol Clin Exp Res. 2016;40:2056.
6. Wandeler G, Kraus D, Fehr J, Conen A, Calmy A, Orasch C, et al. The J-curve in HIV: low and moderate alcohol intake predicts mortality but not the occurrence of major cardiovascular events. J Acquir Immune Defic Syndr 1999. 2015;71:302.
7. Frohlich KL, Potvin L. Transcending the known in public health practice: the inequality paradox—the population approach and vulnerable populations. Am J Public Health. 2008;98:216–21.
8. Centers for Disease Control and Prevention. HIV surveillance report, 2014 [Internet], 2015 Nov. Report No.: 26. http://www.cdc.gove/hiv/library/reports/surveillance.
9. Vanable PA, Carey MP, Blair DC, Littlewood RA. Impact of HIV-related stigma on health behaviors and psychological adjustment among HIV-positive men and women. AIDS Behav. 2006;10:473–82.
10. Zemore SE, Ye Y, Mulia N, Martinez P, Jones-Webb R, Karriker-Jaffe K. Poor, persecuted, young, and alone: toward explaining the elevated risk of alcohol problems among Black and Latino men who drink. Drug Alcohol Depend. 2016;163:31.
11. Martin JK, Tuch SA, Roman PM. Problem drinking patterns among African Americans: the impacts of reports of discrimination, perceptions of prejudice, and "risky" coping strategies. J Health Soc Behav. 2003;44:408–25.
12. Power R, Koopman C, Volk J, Israelski DM, Stone L, Chesney MA, et al. Social support, substance use, and denial in relationship to antiretroviral treatment adherence among HIV-infected persons. AIDS Patient Care STDs. 2003;17:245–52.

13. Elliott JC, Aharonovich E, O'Leary A, Wainberg M, Hasin DS. Drinking motives as prospective predictors of outcome in an intervention trial with heavily drinking HIV patients. Drug Alcohol Depend. 2014;134:290–5.
14. Murphy DA, Greenwell L, Hoffman D. Factors associated with antiretroviral adherence among HIV-infected women with children. Women Health. 2002;36:97–111.
15. Singh N, Berman SM, Swindells S, Justis JC, Mohr JA, Squier C, et al. Adherence of human immunodeficiency virus-infected patients to antiretroviral therapy. Clin Infect Dis. 1999;29:824–30.
16. Mulia N, Ye Y, Greenfield TK, Zemore SE. Disparities in alcohol-related problems among white, black, and Hispanic Americans. Alcohol Clin Exp Res. 2009;33:654–62.
17. Williams EC, Bradley KA, Gupta S, Harris AHS. Association between alcohol screening scores and mortality in black, Hispanic, and white male veterans. Alcohol Clin Exp Res. 2012;36:2132–40.
18. Fultz SL, Skanderson M, Mole LA, Gandhi N, Bryant K, Crystal S, et al. Development and verification of a "virtual" cohort using the National VA Health Information System. Med Care. 2006;44:S25–30.
19. Bradley KA, Williams EC, Achtmeyer CE, Volpp B, Collins BJ, Kivlahan DR. Implementation of evidence-based alcohol screening in the Veterans Health Administration. Am J Manag Care. 2006;12:597–606.
20. Chartier KG, Hesselbrock MN, Hesselbrock VM. Ethnicity and gender comparisons of health consequences in adults with alcohol dependence. Subst Use Misuse. 2013;48:200–10.
21. Witbrodt J, Mulia N, Zemore SE, Kerr WC. Racial/ethnic disparities in alcohol-related problems: differences by gender and level of heavy drinking. Alcohol Clin Exp Res. 2014;38:1662–70.
22. Zemore SE, Murphy RD, Mulia N, Gilbert PA, Martinez P, Bond J, et al. A moderating role for gender in racial/ethnic disparities in alcohol services utilization: results from the 2000 to 2010 National Alcohol Surveys. Alcohol Clin Exp Res. 2014;38:2286–96.
23. Bradley KA, Bush KR, Epler AJ, Dobie DJ, Davis TM, Sporleder JL, et al. Two brief alcohol-screening tests From the Alcohol Use Disorders Identification Test (AUDIT): validation in a female Veterans Affairs patient population. Arch Intern Med. 2003;163:821–9.
24. Bradley KA, DeBenedetti AF, Volk RJ, Williams EC, Frank D, Kivlahan DR. AUDIT-C as a brief screen for alcohol misuse in primary care. Alcohol Clin Exp Res. 2007;31:1208–17.
25. Bush K. The AUDIT alcohol consumption questions (AUDIT-C): an effective brief screening test for problem drinking. Arch Intern Med. 1998;158:1789.
26. Rubinsky AD, Dawson DA, Williams EC, Kivlahan DR, Bradley KA. AUDIT-C scores as a scaled marker of mean daily drinking, alcohol use disorder severity, and probability of alcohol dependence in a US general population sample of drinkers. Alcohol Clin Exp Res. 2013;37:1380–90.
27. Bradley KA, Kivlahan DR, Zhou X-H, Sporleder JL, Epler AJ, McCormick KA, et al. Using alcohol screening results and treatment history to assess the severity of at-risk drinking in Veterans Affairs Primary Care Patients. Alcohol Clin Exp Res. 2004;28:448–55.
28. Eyawo O, McGinnis KA, Justice AC, Fiellin DA, Hahn JA, Williams EC, et al. Alcohol and mortality: combining self-reported (AUDIT-C) and biomarker detected (PEth) alcohol measures among HIV infected and uninfected. J Acquir Immune Defic Syndr. 2017;1. https://doi.org/10.1097/QAI.0000000000001588
29. Justice AC, McGinnis KA, Tate JP, Xu K, Becker WC, Zhao H, et al. Validating harmful alcohol use as a phenotype for genetic discovery using phosphatidylethanol and a polymorphism in *ADH1B*. Alcohol Clin Exp Res. 2017;41:998–1003.
30. Kinder LS, Bryson CL, Sun H, Williams EC, Bradley KA. Alcohol screening scores and all-cause mortality in male Veterans Affairs patients. J Stud Alcohol Drugs. 2009;70:253–60.
31. Chavez LJ, Williams EC, Lapham G, Bradley KA. Association between alcohol screening scores and alcohol-related risks among female veterans affairs patients. J Stud Alcohol Drugs. 2012;73:391.
32. Frank D, DeBenedetti AF, Volk RJ, Williams EC, Kivlahan DR, Bradley KA. Effectiveness of the AUDIT-C as a screening test for alcohol misuse in three race/ethnic groups. J Gen Intern Med. 2008;23:781–7.
33. Dawson DA, Grant BF, Stinson FS, Zhou Y. Effectiveness of the derived alcohol use disorders identification test (AUDIT-C) in screening for alcohol use disorders and risk drinking in the US General Population. Alcohol Clin Exp Res. 2005;29:844–54.
34. Harris AHS, Bryson CL, Sun H, Blough D, Bradley KA. Alcohol screening scores predict risk of subsequent fractures. Subst Use Misuse. 2009;44:1055–69.
35. Breslow NE. Analysis of survival data under the proportional hazards model. Int Stat Rev Rev Int Stat. 1975;43:45.
36. Sohn M-W, Arnold N, Maynard C, Hynes DM. Accuracy and completeness of mortality data in the Department of Veterans Affairs. Popul Health Metr. 2006;4:2.
37. Office of Budget and Management. Revisions to the standards for the classification of federal data on race and ethnicity. Office of Budget and Management; 1997.
38. Mays VM, Ponce NA, Washington DL, Cochran SD. Classification of race and ethnicity: implications for public health. Annu Rev Public Health. 2003;24:83–110.
39. Giordano TP, Morgan RO, Kramer JR, Hartman C, Richardson P, White CA, et al. Is there a race-based disparity in the survival of veterans with HIV? J Gen Intern Med. 2006;21:613–7.
40. Goulet JL, Fultz SL, Rimland D, Butt A, Gibert C, Rodriguez-Barradas M, et al. Do patterns of comorbidity vary by HIV status, age, and HIV severity? Clin Infect Dis. 2007;45:1593–601.
41. Wheeler DA, Gibert CL, Launer CA, Muurahainen N, Elion RA, Abrams DI, et al. Weight loss as a predictor of survival and disease progression in HIV infection. Terry Beirn Community Programs for Clinical Research on AIDS. J Acquir Immune Defic Syndr Hum Retrovirol. 1998;18:80–5.
42. Jones CY, Hogan JW, Snyder B, Klein RS, Rompalo A, Schuman P, et al. Overweight and human immunodeficiency virus (HIV) progression in women: associations HIV disease progression and changes in body mass index in women in the HIV epidemiology research study cohort. Clin Infect Dis. 2003;37(Suppl 2):S69–80.
43. McGinnis KA, Brandt CA, Skanderson M, Justice AC, Shahrir S, Butt AA, et al. Validating smoking data from the Veteran's Affairs Health factors dataset, an electronic data source. Nicot Tob Res. 2011;13:1233–9.
44. StataCorp. Stata statistical software: release 13. College Station, TX: StataCorp LP; 2013.
45. Zemore SE. Acculturation and alcohol among Latino adults in the United States: a comprehensive review. Alcohol Clin Exp Res. 2007;31:1968–90.
46. Karriker-Jaffe KJ, Zemore SE. Associations between acculturation and alcohol consumption of Latino men in the United States. J Stud Alcohol Drugs. 2009;70:27–31.
47. Zapolski TCB, Pedersen SL, McCarthy DM, Smith GT. Less drinking, yet more problems: understanding African American drinking and related problems. Psychol Bull. 2014;140:188–223.
48. Jones-Webb R, Snowden L, Herd D, Short B, Hannan P. Alcohol-related problems among black, Hispanic and white men: the contribution of neighborhood poverty. J Stud Alcohol. 1997;58:539–45.
49. Karriker-Jaffe KJ, Zemore SE, Mulia N, Jones-Webb R, Bond J, Greenfield TK. Neighborhood disadvantage and adult alcohol outcomes: differential risk by race and gender. J Stud Alcohol Drugs. 2012;73:865–73.
50. Williams DR, Mohammed SA, Leavell J, Collins C. Race, socioeconomic status, and health: complexities, ongoing challenges, and research opportunities—race, SES, and health. Ann N Y Acad Sci. 2010;1186:69–101.
51. Hajjar I. Trends in prevalence, awareness, treatment, and control of hypertension in the United States, 1988–2000. JAMA. 2003;290:199.
52. Moolchan ET, Fagan P, Fernander AF, Velicer WF, Hayward MD, King G, et al. Addressing tobacco-related health disparities. Addiction. 2007;102:30–42.
53. Cooper H, Friedman SR, Tempalski B, Friedman R, Keem M. Racial/ethnic disparities in injection drug use in large US metropolitan areas. Ann Epidemiol. 2005;15:326–34.
54. Williams DR, Jackson PB. Social sources of racial disparities in health. Health Aff (Millwood). 2005;24:325–34.
55. Altice FL, Kamarulzaman A, Soriano VV, Schechter M, Friedland GH. Treatment of medical, psychiatric, and substance-use comorbidities in people infected with HIV who use drugs. Lancet. 2010;376:367–87.
56. Fischer MJ, Wyatt CM, Gordon K, Gibert CL, Brown ST, Rimland D, et al. Hepatitis C and the risk of kidney disease and mortality in veterans with HIV. J Acquir Immune Defic Syndr. 1999;2010(53):222–6.
57. Freiberg MS, Chang C-CH, Kuller LH, Skanderson M, Lowy E, Kraemer KL, et al. HIV infection and the risk of acute myocardial infarction. JAMA Intern Med. 2013;173:614.

58. Freiberg MS, McGinnis KA, Kraemer K, Samet JH, Conigliaro J, Curtis Ellison R, et al. The association between alcohol consumption and prevalent cardiovascular diseases among HIV-infected and HIV-uninfected men. JAIDS. 2010;53:247–53.
59. Lieber CS. Alcohol and hepatitis C. Alcohol Res Health. 2001;25:245–54.
60. Kahler CW, Strong DR, Papandonatos GD, Colby SM, Clark MA, Boergers J, et al. Cigarette smoking and the lifetime alcohol involvement continuum. Drug Alcohol Depend. 2008;93:111–20.
61. Bensley KM, Harris AHS, Gupta S, Rubinsky AD, Jones-Webb R, Glass JE, et al. Racial/ethnic differences in initiation of and engagement with addictions treatment among patients with alcohol use disorders in the Veterans Health Administration. J Subst Abuse Treat. 2017;73:34.
62. Glass JE, Perron BE, Ilgen MA, Chermack ST, Ratliff S, Zivin K. Prevalence and correlates of specialty substance use disorder treatment for Department of Veterans Affairs Healthcare System patients with high alcohol consumption. Drug Alcohol Depend. 2010;112:150–5.
63. Peterson K, McCleery E, Waldrip K. Evidence brief: update on prevalence of and interventions to reduce racial and ethnic disparities within the VA. VA Evid Based Synth Prog Evid Briefs [Internet]. Washington (DC): Department of Veterans Affairs (US); 2011. http://www.ncbi.nlm.nih.gov/books/NBK384611/. Cited 5 May 2017.
64. VA/DoD Clinical Guideline for the Management of Substance Use Disorders [Internet]. Washington, D.C.: The Management of Substance Use Disorders Work Group; 2015. https://www.healthquality.va.gov/guidelines/MH/sud/VADoDSUDCPGRevised22216.pdf.
65. Williams EC, Lapham GT, Shortreed SM, Rubinsky AD, Bobb JF, Bensley KM, et al. Among patients with unhealthy alcohol use, those with HIV are less likely than those without to receive evidence-based alcohol-related care: a national VA study. Drug Alcohol Depend. 2017;174:113–20.
66. Harris AHS, Kivlahan DR, Bowe T, Humphreys KN. Pharmacotherapy of alcohol use disorders in the Veterans Health Administration. Psychiatr Serv Wash DC. 2010;61:392–8.
67. Korthuis PT, Lum PJ, Vergara-Rodriguez P, Ahamad K, Wood E, Kunkel LE, et al. Feasibility and safety of extended-release naltrexone treatment of opioid and alcohol use disorder in HIV clinics: a pilot/feasibility randomized trial. Addict Abingdon Engl. 2017;112:1036–44.
68. Edelman EJ, Maisto SA, Hansen NB, Cutter CJ, Dziura J, Fiellin LE, et al. The starting treatment for ethanol in primary care trials (STEP trials): protocol for three parallel multi-site stepped care effectiveness studies for unhealthy alcohol use in HIV-positive patients. Contemp Clin Trials. 2017;52:80–90.
69. Edelman EJ, Hansen NB, Cutter CJ, Danton C, Fiellin LE, O'Connor PG, et al. Implementation of integrated stepped care for unhealthy alcohol use in HIV clinics. Addict Sci Clin Pract. 2016;11:1.
70. Sanchez M, Finnell D. Alcohol screening and brief intervention for persons living with HIV. J Assoc Nurses AIDS Care. 2017;28:266–78.
71. Pellowski JA, Kalichman SC, Matthews KA, Adler N. A pandemic of the poor: social disadvantage and the US HIV epidemic. Am Psychol. 2013;68:197–209.
72. Keyes KM, Hatzenbuehler ML, McLaughlin KA, Link B, Olfson M, Grant BF, et al. Stigma and treatment for alcohol disorders in the United States. Am J Epidemiol. 2010;172:1364–72.
73. Freiberg MS, Chang C-CH, Skanderson M, McGinnis K, Kuller LH, Kraemer KL, et al. The risk of incident coronary heart disease among veterans with and without HIV and hepatitis C. Circ Cardiovasc Qual Outcomes. 2011;4:425–32.
74. Kerr WC, Patterson D, Greenfield TK. Differences in the measured alcohol content of drinks between black, white and Hispanic men and women in a US national sample. Addiction. 2009;104:1503–11.
75. Williams EC, Achtmeyer CE, Thomas RM, Grossbard JR, Lapham GT, Chavez LJ, et al. Factors underlying quality problems with alcohol screening prompted by a clinical reminder in primary care: a multi-site qualitative study. J Gen Intern Med. 2015;30:1125–32.
76. Williams EC, Rubinsky AD, Chavez LJ, Lapham GT, Rittmueller SE, Achtmeyer CE, et al. An early evaluation of implementation of brief intervention for unhealthy alcohol use in the US Veterans Health Administration: early evaluation of VA's brief intervention. Addiction. 2014;109:1472–81.
77. Lapham GT, Rubinsky AD, Heagerty PJ, Achtmeyer C, Williams EC, Hawkins EJ, et al. Probability and predictors of patients converting from negative to positive screens for alcohol misuse. Alcohol Clin Exp Res. 2014;38:564–71.
78. Marshall BDL, Operario D, Bryant KJ, Cook RL, Edelman EJ, Gaither JR, et al. Drinking trajectories among HIV-infected men who have sex with men: a cohort study of United States veterans. Drug Alcohol Depend. 2015;148:69–76.

MySafeRx: a mobile technology platform integrating motivational coaching, adherence monitoring, and electronic pill dispensing for enhancing buprenorphine/naloxone adherence during opioid use disorder treatment

Zev Schuman-Olivier[1,2,3*], Jacob T. Borodovsky[1], Jackson Steinkamp[3,4], Qays Munir[1,3], Kyle Butler[1], Mary Ann Greene[1], Jonah Goldblatt[3,5], Hai Yi Xie[1] and Lisa A. Marsch[1]

Abstract

Background: While buprenorphine/naloxone (B/N) is approved for opioid use disorder treatment, effective delivery of B/N comes with significant challenges. Most notably, many patients do not take medication daily as prescribed; this non-adherence worsens treatment outcomes, increases healthcare costs, and leads to persistent worries of diversion among providers and policymakers. The present study examines the feasibility, usability, and acceptability of *MySafeRx*—a mobile technology platform integrating motivational coaching, adherence monitoring, and electronic pill dispensing designed to address the challenges of office-based opioid treatment (OBOT) with B/N.

Methods: The *MySafeRx* platform integrates electronic pill dispensers, text-messaging, and videoconferencing to provide supervised self-administration of medication and daily motivational coaching through an Android app interface. High-risk early adults (18–39 years old) who were enrolled in OBOT with B/N and had documented illicit opioid use in the past month during opioid agonist therapy ($n = 12$) participated in a 28-day single-arm observational study of the *MySafeRx* platform in addition to standard care.

Results: Two-thirds of participants who completed the study achieved an average of > 5 days per week of supervised B/N self administration. Visual confirmation of medication adherence was demonstrated for an average of 72% of study days among all participants. All participants achieved platform technical proficiency within 60 min, reporting good levels of usability and acceptability. Illicit opioid abstinence rates confirmed by urine toxicology increased by 53% during *MySafeRx* but fell 43% within 3 weeks post-intervention.

Conclusion: The *MySafeRx* medication adherence and remote coaching mobile platform is acceptable and can be feasibly implemented in real-world opioid use disorder treatment settings during high-risk periods (i.e., initial stabilization, after illicit opioid lapse), resulting in reduced illicit opioid use; however, the effect did not last after intervention completion, suggesting longer duration or extended taper of program may be needed.

ClinicalTrials.Gov NCT02942199 10/24/16 https://clinicaltrials.gov/ct2/show/NCT02942199

*Correspondence: zschuman@cha.harvard.edu
[3] Cambridge Health Alliance, Outpatient Addiction Services, Department of Psychiatry, Harvard Medical School, 26 Central Street, Somerville, MA 02143, USA
Full list of author information is available at the end of the article

Background

Opioid use disorder is a public health crisis. Opioid overdoses are the leading cause of death in the US for people under 50 [1], and more than 2.6 million Americans meet criteria for an opioid use disorder (OUD) [2]. Evidence-based opioid agonist treatments for OUD (i.e., buprenorphine, methadone) are currently utilized by healthcare practitioners to meet the growing treatment demand [3–5]. In particular, office-based buprenorphine treatment (OBOT) has been demonstrated to be an effective and safe means of treating OUD [6–8].

Despite the effectiveness of buprenorphine/naloxone (B/N) treatment [9–11], medication non-adherence still occurs. Masand, et al. define non-adherence as failing to take any prescribed doses (although patients who discontinue their medication after an initial period of adherence can also be correctly described as non-adherent), while full adherence is defined as taking all doses when and how they are prescribed. Partial adherence is defined as anything between full and non-adherence, including prolonged gaps in medication dosing, infrequent lapses, missed doses, incorrect dosing with less or more than prescribed, use of alternative route of administration, or change in dosing frequency [12]. Partial adherence and non-adherence are associated with reduced OBOT treatment retention [13], which in turn increases patients' risk of relapse and overdose death [14]. In a Clinical Trials Network study, youth with OUD who ingested B/N on less than 5 out of 7 days per week (~71% of study days) had significantly lower odds of remaining in treatment at 12 weeks (OR: 0.07 (0.01, 0.89), $p=0.04$). Similarly, OBOT patients who took B/N less than 80% of study days were 10 times more likely to relapse, and once patients left OUD treatment, the risk of opioid overdose increased rapidly [15, 16]. In addition, partial adherence to medication may be even more common than non-adherence with buprenorphine and leads to under-dosing [17]. Under-dosing not only increases rates of relapse and treatment dropout, but also increases opioid overdose susceptibility, as under-dosing medication may not achieve adequate mu-opioid receptor (MOR) blockade [18, 19]. Finally, adherence with B/N treatment reduces healthcare costs; one study showed a significant increase in total healthcare charges with < 80% adherence ($28,458 vs. $49,051; $p<0.01$) [20], suggesting that medication adherence is critical for cost as well as outcomes.

The reasons for non-adherence can be multifactorial including patient-, provider-, and systems-level causes. On the patient level, motivational (e.g., ambivalence about recovery, treatment and medication), psychological (e.g. shame and stigma about medication [21], untreated psychiatric co-morbidity [22]), developmental (e.g. young age [23, 24], difficulty accepting chronic illness and the concept of maintenance treatment [24, 25], focus on identity, relationships, children, and work instead of treatment [26, 27]) and logistical (e.g., living with others who are using such as siblings [23], far distance to clinic [28], lacking money for co-pay) causes are common. Provider-level causes include discord between patients and providers or counselors leading to withdrawal, as well as insufficient clinical and administrative support to monitor and address non-adherence through measures such as observed induction, supervised administration of medication, pill counts, and toxicology testing. On the systems level, inadequate insurance reimbursements, frequent prior authorization requests and maximum dose limits, lack of easily accessible psychosocial treatment, burdensome co-pays, and a black market for diverted buprenorphine impact adherence [29, 30].

The problem of non-adherence is a common concern with many medications [31], but it is a particularly crucial issue in B/N treatment, because B/N is a Schedule III opioid medication and non-adherence often results in diversion, defined as "the unauthorized rerouting or misappropriation of prescription medication to someone other than for whom it was intended" [29]. Numerous studies suggest that prescribed B/N is often diverted to people without access to legitimate prescriptions who generally use it for self-treatment or withdrawal prevention [32–35]. Clinicians prescribing B/N believe that medication non-adherence is associated with increased diversion, by sharing or selling to friends and family [24]. Prescribers, who often have limited tools for preventing medication misuse and diversion, fear attracting DEA involvement [36–38], which could plausibly cause them to avoid prescribing patients higher doses of medication even when it may be needed. Although the Drug Addiction Treatment Act of 2000 (DATA 2000) enables waivered physicians to prescribe B/N outside of federally-licensed Opioid Treatment Programs, less stable and more complex OUD patients are commonly required to show up for daily monitored B/N dosing or referred to daily methadone maintenance. Similarly, current clinical practice guidelines recommend more frequent visits during the early stage of B/N treatment [39]. These treatment models often require patients to travel significant distances every day or several times a week to receive medication [28], which can interfere with patients' abilities to maintain employment and provide childcare [2, 40] while they are already struggling with logistical and motivational barriers to participation in office-based treatment.

While mobile technology platforms have shown a moderate to high impact in enhancing chronic illness management and medication adherence in various primary care settings [41–44], limited experience with these platforms exists in OBOT settings. These multi-level gaps in treatment for unstable patients with OUD necessitate a low-cost intervention that can ensure daily B/N adherence, while also reducing medication diversion, enhancing treatment outcomes, and avoiding the increased time and travel burdens on patients caused by onsite supervised dosing programs [45, 46]. To provide a comprehensive solution to all of these issues, we developed the *MySafeRx* platform, a technology-based mobile intervention which integrates daily remote observation of medication self-administration, motivational recovery coaching, and secure electronic pill dispensers.

In this pilot study, we evaluated the feasibility, usability, and acceptability of the *MySafeRx* model for people with OUD in early adulthood (18–39 years old) who were prescribed B/N during periods of clinical instability. The primary aims of the present study were to demonstrate (1) feasibility of *MySafeRx,* by achieving supervised self-administration of B/N on > 5/7 days per week [13] for at least two-thirds of participants, with no reports of substantial B/N diversion; (2) usability, by having at least two-thirds of participants achieve at least 90% competency with the *MySafeRx* platform during 60 min of training and by having a mean usability of > 68, which is the cutoff of adequate usability on the well-validated system usability scale [47, 48]; and (3) acceptability, by achieving a mean overall participant satisfaction score of > 3 of 5 on a satisfaction scale at the end of the intervention period.

Methods

Study design

This was a single-arm, open-label clinical trial to receive 4 weeks of mobile recovery coaching and adherence monitoring via the *MySafeRx* program in conjunction with standard B/N OBOT. After signing informed consent, potential participants were asked to complete an initial survey battery to ensure eligibility. Eligible participants who were not excluded were invited to attend an in-office technology training session, which concluded with video-supervised self-administration of a B/N dose via the *MySafeRx* platform. We defined Day 1 of the study as the first day of video-supervised self-administration of a participant's B/N dose via the *MySafeRx* platform. Participants who chose to start the intervention by partaking in the Day 1 technology training AND in-office, video-supervised self-administration of B/N (N = 12) were asked to complete weekly feasibility, usability, and acceptability surveys via REDCap [49] for 4 weeks. Weekly urine toxicology screens were obtained through the clinical treatment protocol during the 4-week intervention and then for 4 additional weeks to monitor the effects of *MySafeRx* discontinuation on illicit opioid use.

Participants

Participants were recruited through referral from prescribers (n = 5) or OBOT nurse care managers (n = 2) in a regional OBOT network throughout the North Boston metropolitan region. Through regular email reminders and invitation of research coordinators to team meetings, OBOT providers were encouraged to refer unstable young adults who were struggling in OBOT while prescribed buprenorphine and at risk of termination from treatment OR who were recently inducted onto buprenorphine and felt to be at high risk of relapse in standard care. Those eligible were: (1) ages 18–39; (2) able to provide informed consent; (3) clinically diagnosed with opioid use disorder (DSM-5); (4) currently prescribed buprenorphine; (5) able to meet daily in a confidential place for scheduled videoconferencing; and (6) had an illicit positive opioid urine toxicology test in the past month or a missed urine toxicology with a self-report admission of past-month illicit opioid use while on opioid agonist treatment. Participants were excluded if they: (1) were unable to speak English or read the informed consent written at a 6th grade reading level; (2) were in their third trimester of pregnancy; (3) had cognitive deficits that may have limited their ability to complete study procedures; (4) had a medical requirement for twice-daily dosing of buprenorphine; (5) regularly used alcohol or benzodiazepines; or (6) exhibited signs of severe mental illness such as active suicidal ideation or psychosis. Participants were reimbursed with $60 for returning all the electronic devices, and up to $150 for study visit completion, including $30 for baseline visit, $30 for 2-week follow-up visit, $30 for 4-week follow-up visit, $2/day for completed check-in ($60 max).

MySafeRx platform overview

The *MySafeRx* platform provides motivational support and medication adherence monitoring for people with OUD and mental illness during periods of vulnerability or instability (e.g., early B/N OBOT stabilization, after illicit opioid use lapse during B/N OBOT). Furthermore, it creates an integrated remote adherence monitoring and recovery support network by facilitating real-time confidential information sharing and communication between the site clinicians taking care of the participant (e.g., OBOT nurses, substance abuse counselors, and the prescriber) and the trained Mobile Recovery Coaches (MRCs) who check-in with participants each day.

The platform integrates four key components: (1) secure electronic pill organizers with unique medication release codes that are transmitted via Android app; (2) mobile text messaging, primarily including (a) programmed alerts which maintain and communicate contingency expectations from the underlying treatment program (e.g., "You missed your urine toxicology test this week. You are at risk of a medication hold in 48 h. Please complete the required testing and contact your doctor about next steps as soon as possible to prevent a medication hold.") and (b) confidential communication with MRCs in order to initiate videoconferencing meetings (e.g., Are you available and in a private place for our video meeting within 5 min?") or other communication consistent with motivational interviewing principles (e.g., emphasizing autonomy when someone doesn't show up on video—"Taking your medication and what you want to talk about today is completely up to you, I will be available for the next 20 min if you want to meet."); (3) daily remote videoconferencing check-ins, which include brief motivational interventions delivered by trained MRCs; and (4) a standardized protocol for supervised self-administration of medication via videoconferencing. These components, described in detail below, are integrated through the *MySafeRx* smartphone application and web portal. Initial proof-of-concept usability testing and iterative refinement of the platform took place for 1.5 years prior to this study with participants (n=3) prescribed controlled substances for 3 months each during outpatient dual diagnosis treatment [50].

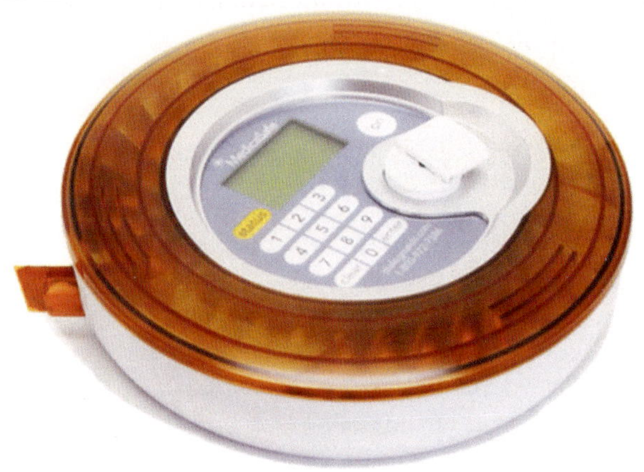

Fig. 1 MedicaSafe pill dispenser

Electronic medication dispenser and backup rescue lockbox

The MedicaSafe 3000 (www.medicasafe.com; Fig. 1) is a secure electronic medication dispensing device that uses unique random codes to unlock and dispense medication. MedicaSafe provided dispensers for the study free of charge. The *MySafeRx* system is designed so that the MRC can release this code to the participant during the adherence monitoring video encounter. The pill dispenser has the capacity to hold up to 30 days of medication (B/N tablets or films); however, for this study, the dispensers were refilled weekly onsite under the supervision of a registered nurse (RN) or medical doctor, and each MedicaSafe dispenser was filled with 6 days' worth of medication. To address concerns about patient safety, a Masterlock 5900D combination lockbox, which costs $20, was provided to each participant with a 1-day rescue dose in case of technology failure, which gave sufficient time to resolve any issues arising during the study. During the pilot we had to change the safety protocol from 2 days to 1-day rescue dosing because of insurance provider constraints. The participant's rescue lockbox code could be found by MRCs in the *MySafeRx* mobile application, allowing the MRC to release it in the case of dispenser failure or as the standard dose on the 7th day of each week. The rescue lockbox was refilled and the combination was reset and updated in the app at each weekly visit.

Mobile recovery coaching, training, and certification

Mobile recovery coaches (MRCs) were responsible for conducting daily mobile medication adherence and recovery coaching sessions through the *MySafeRx* mobile application, using secure Wi-Fi or broadband connections from their residences, which were located in multiple US states. A remote *MySafeRx* manager was available 24/7 to support MRCs in the event of emergency, technology issues, or to provide backup when participants missed sessions and needed to dose outside the scheduled session window. These MRCs used the mobile application to coordinate with the local site clinicians directly responsible for the patient's care.

Non-clinician mobile recovery coaches used a motivational interviewing (MI) framework for daily recovery coaching sessions. MI is an empathic, patient-centered conversational approach [51], which we selected as the theoretical background for the *MySafeRx* intervention because of its ability to focus on reducing ambivalence about taking medication and participating in treatment. All MRCs were required to pass a structured standardized patient interview designed by Dr. Theresa Moyers and Dr. Denise Ernst to assess MI competency using the Motivational Interviewing Treatment Integrity (MITI) Coding Manual 4.2 [52]. In order to be eligible for the 20-min standardized interview test, potential MRC candidates had to either already be Motivational Interviewing Network of Trainers (MINT) certified or had to participate in an introductory Motivational Interviewing (MI) training by *MySafeRx* staff and complete at least 6 weeks of supervised practice sessions with *MySafeRx* staff. After MRCs passed the MI competency interview test, participants were required to successfully complete a background check with references and a Criminal Offender Record Information (CORI) record check. Those who were successful then completed 2 h of interactive webinar training on how to use the *MySafeRx* platform and 90 min of safety and medication adherence training.

MRCs were scheduled to spend up to 840 min with each participant during the 4-week program. For this trial, we had 4 MRCs who worked on average 2–4 days per week. While the maximum daily capacity for a MRC was set at 10 participants, on the busiest day of the trial, the largest number of participants seen by a MRC during a single day was 4.

Smartphone application and web portal

The *MySafeRx* Android application provided an encrypted (AES 128-bit) HIPAA-compliant vehicle for text messaging and daily adherence monitoring via video-conferencing sessions. All videoconferencing was conducted using the Zoom Application Programmer Interface and was transmitted using the encrypted Secure Socket Layer protocol with resistance to video freezing [53]. Unique meeting room IDs were generated and transmitted securely over HTTPS to the coach and participant's Android devices.

The platform includes Android application user interfaces for both the MRC and the participant. The user interface for MRCs supports multiple functions: text messaging; session scheduling; initiating and conducting video sessions; recording medication adherence and substance use reports; releasing medication dose codes to open the dispenser; and securely communicating with clinicians and the *MySafeRx* manager. The participant user interface supports the following: text messaging; choosing a scheduled time to meet with a MRC; contacting the *MySafeRx* manager; and receipt of the dose code. The participant joins a video session with a MRC for motivational recovery coaching prior to receiving their medication each day, and the MRC uses the app to release the code needed to open the locked dispenser. Participants without an Android phone (n=5) were provided for 30 days duration a 4G LTE LG Android G pad 7-inch tablet valued at $120, which was connected through a program "family plan" costing $160 per month to maintain up to 4 devices.

Prescribers and assigned site clinician delegates (e.g., team nurse or counselor) used the *MySafeRx* web interface to access details of their patients' daily interactions with MRCs. The website provides clinicians with individual participant statistics, including medication adherence, drug/alcohol use, new physical or mental health symptoms, safety concerns, and triggers/high-risk events, reported daily by the MRCs in Daily Recovery Reports. We developed a software algorithm that produces a color-coded result for each day, representing various levels of concern about patient risk level: red (severe concern), yellow (moderate concern) and green (no concern). The color algorithm uses MRC-generated data to enable clinicians to rapidly digest information. Prescribers and delegates were responsible for responding in a clinically appropriate manner if notified of any non-adherence or clinically relevant symptoms. For non-urgent issues, prescribers can send messages through the website interface to MRCs as needed for addressing during the next morning's dosing period.

Daily workflow

Each participant scheduled daily session times through the Android application with a MRC based on availability. In order to avoid the common tendency of patients to withdrawal from a program if conflict, discord, regret about something they did, or other negative transference emerges with a certain counselor [54], participants were encouraged to work with a minimum of three MRCs on different days throughout the trial, fostering a positive transference with the overall program instead of any one individual coach. Daily sessions began with a text reminder from a MRC sent through the *MySafeRx* application at the scheduled time, followed by a text invitation to begin videoconferencing (Fig. 2). Session duration ranged from 10 to 45 min and included a brief motivational intervention. During the session, the MRC sent an access code to the participant through the application, which allowed the participant to dispense their daily medication dose from a secure electronic pill dispenser (MedicaSafe 3000). The MRC observed medication placement and checked for dissolution in the mouth.

After the session, the MRC completed a Daily Recovery Report through the Android application, documenting the participant's medication adherence, reported substance use, daily recovery goals, and other relevant notes. These reports were visible to other MRCs to allow collaborative team-based coaching and the clinicians who were clinically responsible for the participant's treatment. Further, in the event of a serious safety concern, homicidal or suicidal ideation, the use of illicit opioids, or consecutive days of medication non-adherence, all clinicians on the patient's care team were part of a rapid alert system that automatically notified them via email with a red-colored alert in the subject line. This email contained no protected health information (PHI); it merely advised all the participant's clinicians to log into the secure web portal to view the details of the event.

Safety and access to medication

In conjunction with the study Data Safety Monitoring Board, we developed management algorithms for MRCs and the *MySafeRx* manager to ensure that no patient who was motivated to take his/her medication was ever denied access to the medication. A backup MRC was

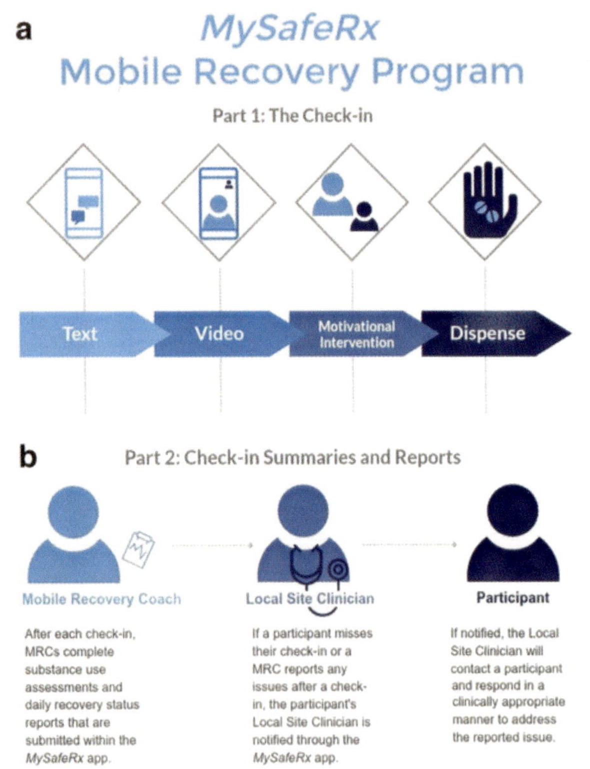

Fig. 2 MysafeRx mobile recovery program

always available if a participant missed their scheduled dosing time and the scheduled MRC was no longer available. We also opened an additional 4–5 PM scheduling window for participants who missed their morning scheduled time and who wanted to reschedule the dosing time. If someone was unable to join a videoconference (e.g., due to Internet connectivity issues), MRCs were instructed to provide the medication code by phone and to document this lapse in supervision of self-administration with a note to the participant's prescribing clinician. The prescribing clinician would then make the clinical decision about the relevance of this as a non-adherence event. After each perceived non-adherence event, the *MySafeRx* manager would reach out to the participant by phone. When the next contact with the participant was established, the manager would confirm the nature of the missed daily recovery check-in. Finally, for participants who missed scheduled appointments, the MRCs were encouraged to focus future motivational enhancement sessions on program-interfering behaviors in order to help participants understand and overcome their barriers to attending appointments on time. The intention of this process was to help shape long-term attendance behaviors, which would benefit treatment both during and after the study.

Measures

Baseline measures

Participants completed surveys about demographics, technology usage and attitudes [55], and substance use history. A doctoral-level provider conducted a psychiatric review of systems, using a DSM-IV SCID Screen [56], and the Montreal Cognitive Assessment [57] during the baseline screening visit. The Principal Investigator reviewed this information and the electronic health record for study participants, evaluating exclusion criteria, prior to scheduling the technology training and initial supervised dosing via the *MySafeRx* platform.

Primary outcomes measures

During the study, outcome measures were collected to assess acceptability, feasibility, and usability of the *MySafeRx* platform (NCT02942199).

1. Feasibility:

    (a) *Daily supervised adherence reporting* MRCs recorded through the application whether fully-supervised daily medication dosing and observed dissolution of medication in each participant's mouth occurred.
    Our primary aim was to demonstrate *feasibility* by achieving supervised self-administration of B/N for an average of at least 5 of 7 days per week during the study for at least two-thirds of participants. This cutoff was based on a study of youth with OUD showing a marked difference in attrition for youth above and below 5 days per week of medication adherence [13].

    (b) *Self-report monitoring survey of non-adherence and diversion* We also assessed the level of self-reported non-adherence and collected reports about diversion reported by MRCs, providers, or participants. Participants completed a weekly survey via REDCap reporting whether they took all of their medication in the past week. If the answer was no, then they were asked to enter the number of days during the past week when medication was missed (non-adherence). Participants were also asked whether they shared or sold any medication in the past week. If the answer was yes, then they were asked to enter the number of days during the past week when medication was shared or sold to others (diversion). These self-report data were only visible to research staff, and not a participant's referring prescriber and staff.

2. Usability:

    (a) *Technology training checklist (TTC)* After a maximum of 60 min of in-office training with the *MySafeRx* platform, study staff observed Day 1 in-office dosing session via the Android application and used the 10-item TTC to evaluate the participant's competency with *MySafeRx* and the MedicaSafe Dispenser. We aimed to demonstrate *usability* by having at least two-thirds of participants achieve 90% competency during 60 min of platform training on the TTC by the second day of platform use.

    (b) *System usability scale (SUS)* [58] This reliable and valid measure of a system's usability was completed by participants on Day 28. The scale is composed of 10 items on a 5-point Likert scale from "Strongly Disagree" to "Strongly Agree," with half of the items being reverse coded [r]. Sample items include "I think that I would like to use this system frequently"; "I found the system unnecessarily complex [r]"; "I thought the system was easy to use"; "I found the system very cumbersome to use [r]". The scale also included a section for open-ended comments. The scale is transformed following a standardized algorithm to provide a score ranging from 0 to 100, in which a 68 is the average score and is considered the cutoff for adequate usability (equivalent to a "C") while 79 is the cutoff for excellent usability (equivalent to an "A−"), with 75–80 being the equivalent of a "B+" [47, 48, 59]. We aimed to demonstrate *usability* by having a mean score greater than 68 on the SUS after 28 days using the integrated platform.

3. Acceptability:

    (a) *MySafeRx satisfaction scale* After completing the study, participants were asked to fill out a 13-item system satisfaction scale with four principal components: ease of use, NOT bothersome, helpful, and NOT hindering treatment goals [60]. The survey used a 5-point Likert scale ranging from "Strongly Disagree" to "Strongly Agree." We aimed to demonstrate *acceptability* with mean levels of overall satisfaction with the *MySafeRx* platform greater than 3 out of 5 after 28 days.

    (b) *Monitoring survey* This weekly questionnaire assessed overall acceptance of the integrated system by participant self-report. The survey used a 7-point Likert scale ranging from "Completely Disagree" to "Completely Agree." We aimed to demonstrate *acceptability* with mean levels of overall satisfaction with the *MySafeRx* platform greater than 4 out of 7 after 28 days.

4. Impact on abstinence from illicit opioids by week:

    (a) *Urine toxicology screens* Nurse care managers conducted urine toxicology screening at least weekly for all participants using a clinical program protocol that included regular and random urine screening. Participants consented to have the results of all toxicology screens conducted by clinical staff during the study window be collected and stored in a database by study staff. Urine collection was conducted in a bathroom without a sink following standard clinic protocol but was not observed. Sample temperature was checked immediately, while specific gravity, pH and creatinine were analyzed for each participant to evaluate for evidence of tampering. Participants agreed to toxicology testing for buprenorphine, illicit opioids, amphetamine, benzodiazepines, alcohol, cannabis, and cocaine. Urine toxicology used enzyme-mediated immunoassay techniques (Beckman Synchron, Beckman Coulter, Fullerton, CA), but rapid chromatographic immunoassays were used for oxycodone (Bio-Rad, Hercules, CA) and Liquid Chromatography/Tandem Mass Spectrometry were used for fentanyl testing (LabCorp). Urine toxicology results were recorded by the laboratory in the EMR and these results were extracted into REDCap by study staff. The study team identified the most recent pre-study urine screen prior to Day 1, and then from Day 1 the analysis algorithm captured the next 8 weeks of required weekly clinical toxicology testing. Weeks with negative urine screens were considered as opioid abstinent weeks for reporting outcomes.

Data analysis

The primary outcomes (feasibility, acceptability, and usability) warranted primarily descriptive data analysis due to small sample size ($n=12$), which was based on having a substantial cohort for usability testing determined by the 10 ± 2 rule [61]. We conducted secondary analyses on urine toxicology screening to understand the relationship between this medication adherence program and illicit opioid use. We evaluated whether the number of negative weeks of illicit opioid negative urine toxicology increased with time during the program, and if so, whether that increase would be maintained after completion of the 4-week *MySafeRx* program.

Results

Participants (N=12) were primarily Caucasian and English-speaking with a mean age of 31.33 (range 26–36) (Fig. 3). Use of cocaine (33.3%) and benzodiazepines (41.7%) were common in the 30 days prior to study participation. Mental health comorbidity was also common: 58.3% of participants had an anxiety disorder, 41.7% had a major depressive episode in the past, and 25% had a diagnosis of PTSD (Table 1). Two participants had mental health comorbidity which prevented them from completing all baseline study activities. Prior to starting the intervention phase, one participant was terminated from the study and another withdrew consent.

Feasibility

Two-thirds (8 of 12) of participants who completed the study achieved an average of > 5 days per week of supervised B/N self-administration. Mobile Recovery Coaches visually confirmed medication adherence for an average of 72% of study days for all participants. Ten of 12 participants reported perfect adherence via REDCAP self-report; however, dispenser data and coach reports demonstrated that only 1 of 12 had 100% adherence. No participant reported diverting medication by selling or sharing. Importantly, of the 12 study participants, only 10 returned their pill dispenser devices after 28 days (one reported it was stolen by her sister, while another was incarcerated, then moved out of town without returning it).

Usability

All participants achieved 90% competency after the first training session, which lasted on average ~ 42 min (range 15–60). The average System Usability Score was 78.8 (SD 14.8, range 60–100) at the end of participation. Individual question means, and standard deviations are provided in Additional file 1: Table S1. Only three of twelve participants left feedback in the open comment question, two indicating that the app was "good" and "works very well," and one indicating that the "app froze too often".

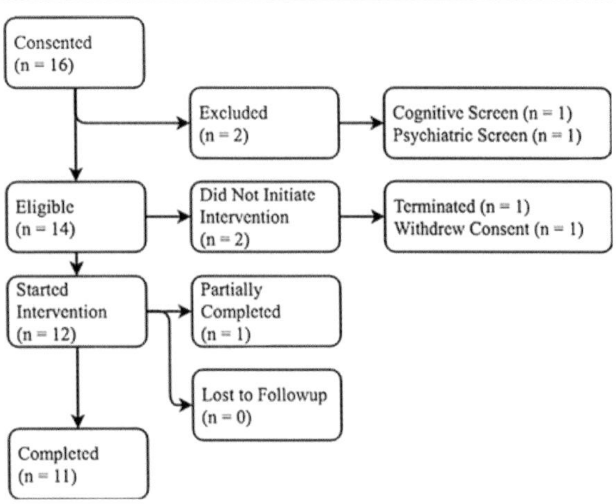

Fig. 3 Consort diagram

Table 1 Sample characteristics

	Total N=12	Male n=8	Female n=4
Demographics			
Age			
Mean (± SD)	31.33 (2.84)	31.13 (3.44)	31.75 (1.26)
[Range] years	[26–36]	[26–36]	[25–33]
Ethnicity, n (%)			
White	11 (91.7)	7 (87.5)	4 (100)
Other	1 (8.3)	1 (12.5)	0 (0)
Marital status, n (%)			
Single, never married	10 (83.3)	6 (75.0)	4 (100)
Married	2 (16.7)	2 (25.0)	0 (0)
Education, n (%)			
Some high school	3 (25.0)	3 (37.5)	0 (0)
High school graduate or GED	5 (41.7)	3 (37.5)	2 (50.0)
Some college or trade school	4 (33.3)	2 (25.0)	2 (50.0)
Employment, n (%)			
Employed	7 (58.3)	6 (75.0)	1 (25.0)
Unemployed	5 (41.7)	2 (25.0)	3 (75.0)
Comorbid mental health disorder			
Depression, n (%)			
Hx major depressive episode	5 (41.7)	3 (37.5)	2 (50.0)
Anxiety, n (%)			
Any anxiety disorder	7 (58.3)	4 (50.0)	3 (75.0)
PTSD, n (%)			
Subset of anxiety	3 (25.0)	2 (25.0)	1 (25.0)
Recent illicit substance use			
Cocaine, n (%)			
30 days prior to baseline	4 (33.3)	4 (50.0)	0 (0)
Benzodiazepines, n (%)			
30 days prior to baseline	7 (58.3)	3 (37.5)	4 (100)
Technology use			
Videoconference, n (%)			
Any use before study	4 (33.3)	4 (50.0)	0 (0)
Smartphone, n (%)			
Any use before study	12 (100)	8 (100)	4 (100)

Acceptability

Overall satisfaction during the last week of the study as reported on the weekly Monitoring Survey report was on average 6.5 ± 0.7 (maximum 7). Participants endorsed being comfortable with using the pill dispenser (6.8 ± 0.4), the videoconferencing programs (6.7 ± 0.6), as well as the texting application (6.6 ± 0.6). Participants endorsed "seeing the benefit of taking my medication using the *MySafeRx* process" (6.5 ± 0.7), feeling the platform is "helping me become more independent" (6.5 ± 0.7), and has had a "positive influence on my recovery" (6.4 ± 0.8). Also, on the *MySafeRx* Satisfaction Scale delivered at the end of the program, participants displayed adequate overall satisfaction with a mean score of 4.3 ± 0.7 (maximum 5). At the end of the 4-week program, 9 of the 12 participants expressed a desire to continue with the *MySafeRx* program.

Secondary analyses

Toxicology

All participants (100%) had at least one urine toxicology screen positive for an illicit opioid other than buprenorphine in the 30 days prior to starting the study. The average level of illicit opioid abstinence, which was measured by percent negative toxicology (representing physiologic confirmation of no illicit opioid usage) per week started at 41.7% during week 1, then peaked at 63.6% for weeks 3 and 4 of the study during the intervention, representing a 53% increase in the frequency of toxicology-confirmed illicit opioid abstinence after 2 weeks of *MySafeRx*. However, within 2 weeks of discontinuing the *MySafeRx* program, the average percent negative toxicology fell to 36.4% by weeks 7 and 8, representing a 43% reduction in the frequency of toxicology-confirmed illicit opioid abstinence just 3 weeks after discontinuation of *MySafeRx* (Fig. 4).

Adverse events

Two adverse events were reported during the study, and no serious adverse events were reported. The safety protocol indicated that emergency services should be contacted if suicidal or homicidal ideation is present, though this was not experienced in this pilot trial.

One participant's family petitioned for involuntary commitment for substance use disorder treatment under MA General Law §35 [62] after the second week in the program while in the middle of a parental custody conflict. The participant was forced to taper off of buprenorphine, but completed post-study acceptability and usability surveys about the program. Another participant reported a domestic abuse situation during a *MySafeRx* daily coaching session. The participant's study involvement was suspended while in crisis at a housing stabilization facility, which did not allow her to participate. She returned and completed participation in the study.

Technology events

We found evidence that 19 missed scheduled check-ins out of 336 scheduled check-ins (5.6%) were a result of technology failure or patient's loss of devices, and not related to ambivalence around medication taking. The *MySafeRx* manager was generally able to reach out to the patient outside of check-in hours by phone or meet the patient in the office. Two technology failures resulted in the participant only having a half dose of medication for the day: once because the lockbox was opened over the weekend; and once because after a phone crashed, the participant's dispenser jammed getting second half of the day's dose. The rescue box was used twice as a result of technology failure, both due to an error in the dose code generation for the MedicaSafe devices.

Notable evening and weekend events with MySafeRx manager

In addition to the *MySafeRx* manager's role with technology failure, device loss, and missed check-ins, the *MySafeRx* manager was accessible 24/7 by text and phone hotline, which played an important clinical role in several cases. There were three notable instances of remote *MySafeRx* manager contact with participants handling urgent issues that arose during evenings and weekends. The managers and MRCs were trained to respond to participant issues in accordance with severity: (1) One participant in emotional crisis sent a few erratic texts to the on-call manager on a weekend, who was able to alert the participant's prescriber. The prescriber was able to reach out to the participant by phone, provide therapeutic relational support, and stabilize the situation by encouraging the patient to go to sleep. (2) In another instance a participant was heading to a public restroom in a restaurant where he had overdosed the week before with a new bag of fentanyl after having missed a planned meeting that weekend morning, when the *MySafeRx* manager reached out to the participant and talked with him until he flushed the drugs down the toilet, preventing a likely opioid overdose. The *MySafeRx* manager encouraged the participant to seek help with emergency services and paged the prescriber. (3) In the domestic violence situation mentioned above, the *MySafeRx* manager helped the participant find her way to the emergency department in the middle of winter with no belongings except her phone, where she was then able to get sent to a crisis stabilization unit for people with housing needs.

Discussion

The *MySafeRx* platform provides remote medication adherence and motivational recovery support to individuals with OUD receiving OBOT with buprenorphine/naloxone. The results of the present study suggest that

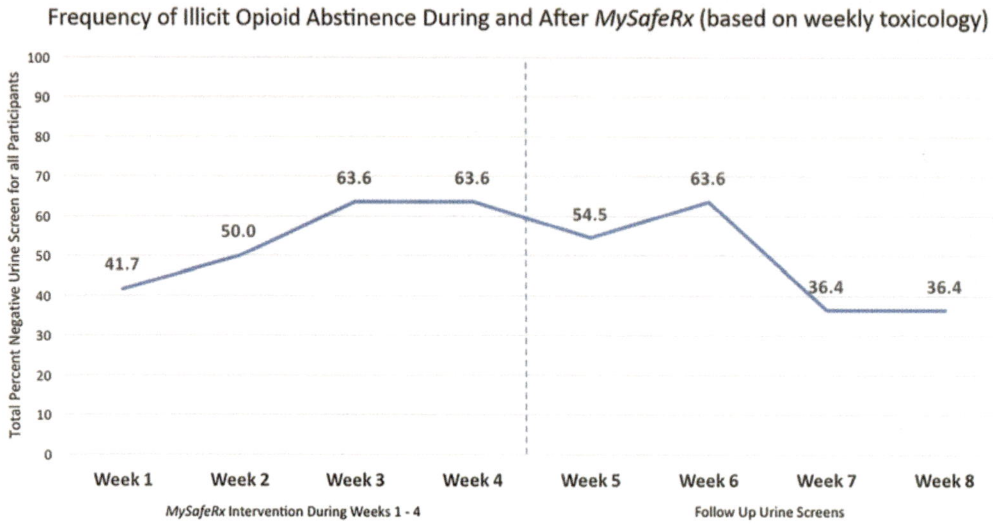

Fig. 4 Frequency of illicit opioid abstinence during and after *MySafeRx* (based on weekly toxicology)

the *MySafeRx* platform can be successfully integrated and utilized within a real-world outpatient buprenorphine treatment setting to bolster treatment during periods of instability. These pilot data demonstrate that the *MySafeRx* platform provides consistent and reliable visual confirmation of patients' buprenorphine self-administration. This study demonstrates that high-risk patients with OUD and co-morbid mental illness can learn to use the platform in a short amount of time, it is feasible to conduct training in a busy addiction clinic with overutilized space, and patients find the various components of the *MySafeRx* platform (e.g., app, pill dispenser) easy to use. Finally, the majority of participants were satisfied with this model of buprenorphine treatment delivery. In sum, *MySafeRx* is easy to use, amenable to patients prescribed buprenorphine in OBOT treatment and provides daily visual confirmation of B/N adherence without requiring substantial time or travel burden.

Should future studies confirm and extend these results to demonstrate robust clinical effectiveness, the *MySafeRx*-based buprenorphine treatment delivery model could potentially be utilized to address several opioid treatment-related shortcomings within the US healthcare system.

Taking the correct "blocking" dose of buprenorphine daily is important, because once buprenorphine binds to 90% of mu-opioid receptors (MOR) [63], it removes the possibility of euphoria or overdose from illicit opioids that day [19]—even most high-potency fentanyls [64]. For this reason, a daily patient-centered and motivation-focused intervention delivered during the critical moment of medication-taking each day could offer a new OBOT paradigm. Furthermore, taking the full dose of B/N as prescribed daily and reaching a steady-state can resolve dysregulation of the stress system that develops with chronic opioid use, and which contributes to ongoing depression, anxiety, and stress-related illness [65, 66] that can lead to relapse. By enhancing a person's focus on recovery and treatment goals during the period of time surrounding B/N dosing, which has both the highest treatment receptivity and largest clinical impact each day, and providing daily structure and external accountability, an intervention would offer an untapped therapeutic opportunity and could increase medication adherence and treatment retention while reducing illicit opioid use, overdose risk, dysregulation of the stress system, and diversion [67, 68].

Second, only a limited number of physicians have received a waiver to prescribe buprenorphine, and many who have received a waiver do not fill their treatment capacity [69]. This hesitancy is likely the consequence of several factors including lack of necessary clinical resources to manage complicated patients, insufficient support networks for counseling and mental health, and fears about medication misuse and diversion [36–38, 69, 70]. Clinicians regularly take multiple time-consuming steps to reduce diversion of medication with abuse potential like buprenorphine, using staff resources and possibly reducing access to treatment [71]. Because the *MySafeRx* platform provides daily medication adherence monitoring and rapidly alerts prescribers to events that suggest clinical destabilization (e.g. high-risk drug use events, suicidal ideation, persistent absence from daily sessions, etc.), clinicians anecdotally reported to the study team that they felt more confident in their ability to manage high-risk OUD patients in their under-resourced setting.

In an ongoing larger pilot trial among clinicians working in rural or underserved areas, where the availability of counseling support for primary care providers offering B/N has historically been more limited [72, 73], we are currently attempting to ascertain whether these anecdotal reports are supported with provider-level data. If providers feel this can help make treatment easier with their more difficult, high-risk patients, then *MySafeRx* might help contribute to a significant expansion of access to buprenorphine treatment by increasing the number of clinicians willing to prescribe buprenorphine and increasing access to buprenorphine in rural or underserved areas.

Third, non-adherence and partial adherence are associated with diversion behaviors, such as sharing and selling medication. One *MySafeRx* participant said, "I think the daily check-in and supervised taking of medication should be mandatory. Every person I've met on the Suboxone clinic sells their Suboxone and this will ensure they don't." Reducing opportunities for medication diversion can support medication adherence and improve treatment outcomes. Few existing office-based opioid treatment programs have the capacity for daily observed dosing needed to determine optimal stabilization doses for patients and prevent buprenorphine diversion. Other adherence technologies such as secure pill dispensers have recently been developed to address similar issues [74, 75]. However, without the ability to visually confirm medication adherence and dissolution with mouth checks, there remains a significant risk of diversion. Thus, stand-alone electronic pill dispensers may be an ineffective solution to address the rising rates of buprenorphine diversion. The daily medication monitoring provided by *MySafeRx* offers clinicians assurance that their patients are adherent to their medication and has the potential to support improvements in the patient-prescriber relationship and clinicians' capacity to effectively and confidently gauge the impacts of dose adjustments.

Finally, efforts to disseminate OBOT in the US are complicated by the prevalence of non-evidence-based buprenorphine dosing schedules and fears about medication diversion. A recent meta-analysis suggests that higher doses of buprenorphine may result in better clinical outcomes [76]. Allowing patients to take lower doses multiple times per day (i.e., "split-dosing"), can reduce the duration of MOR blockade and thus complicates treatment [77]. Patients using this dosing schedule may be unknowingly "reserving the option" to achieve euphoria through use of high-potency illicit opioids later in the day. Additionally, while sub-therapeutic dosing should be avoided, certain concerned prescribers in areas of high diversion, who are wary about providing large drug supplies to unstable patients, may unintentionally prescribe patients sub-therapeutic doses. Such doses do not provide full MOR blockade [29] and may not be sufficient to provide the full blocking effect needed for increasingly potent and prevalent fentanyls [78]. This can limit the potential of the medication, challenge the therapeutic alliance, and lead to distrust on both sides of the doctor-patient relationship. For this reason, an intervention which includes daily supervised medication administration may help prescribers feel comfortable providing patients with higher, once-daily doses of medication needed to prevent relapse and overdose.

Importantly, there was a large discrepancy between objective adherence data (where just 1 out of 12 participants achieved 100% visually-confirmed adherence) and the self-report surveys (where 10 out of 12 participants reports full adherence every day). This points to the difficulty inherent in relying on self-report of medication adherence behaviors and emphasizes the importance of more robust forms of adherence monitoring.

In this study, abstinence from illicit opioids fell by 43% within 3 weeks post-discontinuation of the 28-day *MySafeRx* intervention, which was often accompanied by relapse and treatment drop-out. This increase in illicit opioid use after abrupt completion of the program is concerning and could be interpreted in several ways. First, the rapid decrease in illicit opioid use during the intervention suggests that the program enhanced adherence and reduced substance use, but that a longstanding change in behavior was not created with just 1 month of the intervention. Second, it is possible that a longer version of *MySafeRx* with a less abrupt transition back to standard care (an intervention 'taper-down phase') may reduce the risk of return to opioid use. Alternatively, like long-term maintenance in methadone maintenance treatment programs, it is possible that the program will only work when some or all the components are integrated and provided in a continuous manner. Further studies with longer time periods and various tapering schedules will be necessary to ascertain whether an episodic model or continuous maintenance model of remote daily supervised self-administration of B/N will be most effective for patients.

Limitations

There were several limitations to this study. This pilot study had a small sample-size (n = 12) and was not designed to assess efficacy. Additionally, treatment drop-out led to substantial amount of missing urine toxicology data. Finally, the self-report survey on medication adherence had two-step logic with an initial dichotomous question, which may have enhanced the probability of a social desirability bias resulting in over-reporting of medication taking and under-reporting of diversion by participants. The study found substantially lower adherence rates measured by supervised self-administration than by self-report on weekly monitoring surveys, which was expected. A final limitation is that this study did not assess prescriber and delegate attitudes about the intervention.

Future research

Future studies with larger sample sizes are needed to evaluate efficacy outcomes, such as treatment retention, medication adherence, and illicit opioid use. In future studies, adding mobile technology to provide remote motivational engagement prior to medication treatment and to conduct observed induction are potential areas for future development. Additional data are needed to assess the impact of *MySafeRx* on both clinician attitudes toward increasing treatment capacity and medication doses as well as patient attitudes towards motivational mobile recovery coaching during daily dosing. In addition, cost analyses with larger samples will be important for evaluating actual real-world costs, which will be necessary in order to consider the potential for wide-scale dissemination. Patient, Mobile Recovery Coach, and clinician feedback should be incorporated into the design of future versions of the platform to further improve usability. Though roughly 63–76% of smartphone owners use an Android operating system [79] and Android had nearly an 82% market share worldwide in late 2016 [80], creating an iOS app version could provide even wider accessibility. Enhancing coordination with pharmacies and insurance providers as well as expanding platform accessibility are important challenges to address in the future to support dissemination.

Should future effectiveness trials yield positive results, the *MySafeRx* platform has the potential to provide the foundation for a nationwide adjunctive adherence support system for B/N treatment providers caring for vulnerable patients with OUD. In that case, it would be useful to evaluate whether the platform increases access to B/N treatment among high-risk groups. In conclusion, this study demonstrated the feasibility of integrating the MedicaSafe dispenser and *MySafeRx* and showed that the *MySafeRx* platform is acceptable to unstable young adults with OUD receiving buprenorphine treatment in a public-sector substance use disorder clinic.

Authors' contributions

Zev Schuman-Olivier, MD was principal investigator and directed all aspects of the Project. The Project was implemented by several authors (JB, QM, KB, JG) with close oversight from Zev Schuman-Olivier and Lisa A. Marsch. Data management and analysis was conducted by (MAG, HYX). The first draft of the manuscript was written by several authors (ZSO, JB, JG, JS), but all authors made a significant contribution to the final manuscript. All authors read and approved the final manuscript.

Author details

[1] Center for Technology and Behavioral Health, Geisel School of Medicine at Dartmouth, Hanover, USA. [2] Department of Psychiatry, Harvard Medical School, Boston, USA. [3] Cambridge Health Alliance, Outpatient Addiction Services, Department of Psychiatry, Harvard Medical School, 26 Central Street, Somerville, MA 02143, USA. [4] Boston University School of Medicine, Boston, USA. [5] Tufts University School of Medicine, Boston, USA.

Acknowledgements

We are grateful for the contribution by Theresa Moyer and Denise Ernst to the development of the *MySafeRx* Motivational Interviewing credentialing process. We are grateful to CHA Outpatient Addiction Services Team for assisting with study recruitment, especially the OBOT nurse care managers (Lolita Roland, Piter Jules). We appreciate the contribution and commitment of our first mobile recovery coaches Scott Graham, Kyle Butler, and Nancy Reilly. We appreciate Nellie Harvey, Diana Morrill, and Grace Janzow for their contributions to visual design and coach recruitment during the study. Finally, we deeply appreciate the commitment Kyle Butler had to caring for the participants in this study, for his tireless work helping to enhance the usability of the technology, and to his persistent effort refining this manuscript during the final days of his life. We dedicate this manuscript in honor of his memory with deep gratitude for how fully he applied his time and spirit to ensure the success of this project.

Competing interest

There are no competing interests. Several authors (ZSO, JB, LM, QM) hold either an officer or board position on MySafeRx Inc., which is a non-profit organization with a mission to support development, implementation, and dissemination of technological solutions for addiction treatment and medication adherence. MedicaSafe has not been involved in data collection, data analysis, or manuscript preparation. No data has been shared with MedicaSafe prior to manuscript completion. All conflicts of interest were reviewed by the Conflict of Interest Board at Geisel School of Medicine at Dartmouth, which declared that there was no financial conflict of interest in this study. All authors contributed in some way to the planning, execution, and manuscript development.

Funding

This study was funded by NIDA Grants P30DA029926 (PI: LM; Pilot Grant 014 from the Center for Technology and Behavioral Health) and R34DA040086 (PI: ZSO). We are also appreciative of an unrestricted investigator-initiated Grant from MedicaSafe and provision of dispenser devices for the study supported by SBIR Grant R43DA033702 (PI: Michael Davis).

References

1. Katz, J. Short answers to hard questions about the opioid crisis. The Upshot; 2017.
2. Center for Behavioral Health Statistics and Quality Key substance use and mental health indicators in the United States: Results from the 2015 National Survey on Drug Use and Health. HHS Publication No. SMA 16-4984, 2016. NSDUH Series H-51.
3. Fudala PJ, et al. Office-based treatment of opiate addiction with a sublingual-tablet formulation of buprenorphine and naloxone. N Engl J Med. 2003;349(10):949–58.
4. National Institute on Drug Abuse Effective Treatments for Opioid Addiction; 2016.
5. Fiellin DA, Rosenheck RA, Kosten TR. Office-based treatment for opioid dependence: reaching new patient populations. Am J Psychiatry. 2001;158(8):1200–4.
6. Comer SD, et al. Abuse liability of intravenous buprenorphine/naloxone and buprenorphine alone in buprenorphine-maintained intravenous heroin abusers. Addiction. 2010;105(4):709–18.

7. Sporer KA. Buprenorphine: a primer for emergency physicians. Ann Emerg Med. 2004;43(5):580–4.
8. Weiss RD, et al. Adjunctive counseling during brief and extended buprenorphine-naloxone treatment for prescription opioid dependence: a 2-phase randomized controlled trial. Arch Gen Psychiatry. 2011;68(12):1238–46.
9. Alford DP, et al. Collaborative care of opioid-addicted patients in primary care using buprenorphine: five-year experience. Arch Intern Med. 2011;171(5):425–31.
10. Fiellin DA, O'Connor PG. Office-based treatment of opioid-dependent patients. N Engl J Med. 2002;347(11):817–23.
11. LaBelle CT, et al. Office-based opioid treatment with buprenorphine (OBOT-B): statewide implementation of the massachusetts collaborative care model in community health centers. J Subst Abuse Treat. 2016;60:6–13.
12. Masand PS, et al. Partial adherence to antipsychotic medication impacts the course of illness in patients with schizophrenia: a review. Prim Care Companion J Clin Psychiatry. 2009;11(4):147–54.
13. Warden D, et al. Predictors of attrition with buprenorphine/naloxone treatment in opioid dependent youth. Addict Behav. 2012;37(9):1046–53.
14. Zhang Z, Friedmann PD, Gerstein DR. Does retention matter? treatment duration and improvement in drug use. Addiction. 2003;98(5):673–84.
15. Tkacz J, et al. Compliance with buprenorphine medication-assisted treatment and relapse to opioid use. Am J Addict. 2012;21(1):55–62.
16. Clausen T, Anchersen K, Waal H. Mortality prior to, during and after opioid maintenance treatment (OMT): a national prospective cross-registry study. Drug Alcohol Depend. 2008;94(1–3):151–7.
17. Roncero C, et al. Professionals' perception on the management of patients with dual disorders. Patient Prefer Adher. 2016;10:1855–68.
18. Bickel WK, et al. Buprenorphine: dose-related blockade of opioid challenge effects in opioid dependent humans. J Pharmacol Exp Ther. 1988;247(1):47–53.
19. Greenwald MK, Comer SD, Fiellin DA. Buprenorphine maintenance and mu-opioid receptor availability in the treatment of opioid use disorder: implications for clinical use and policy. Drug Alcohol Depend. 2014;144:1–11.
20. Tkacz J, et al. Relationship between buprenorphine adherence and health service utilization and costs among opioid dependent patients. J Subst Abuse Treat. 2014;46(4):456–62.
21. Hadland SE, Park TW, Bagley SM. Stigma associated with medication treatment for young adults with opioid use disorder: a case series. Addict Sci Clin Pract. 2018;13(1):15.
22. Fareed A, et al. Factors affecting noncompliance with buprenorphine maintenance treatment. J Addict Med. 2014;8(5):345–50.
23. Dayal P, Balhara YPS. A naturalistic study of predictors of retention in treatment among emerging adults entering first buprenorphine maintenance treatment for opioid use disorders. J Subst Abuse Treat. 2017;80:1–5.
24. Schuman-Olivier Z, et al. Emerging adult age status predicts poor buprenorphine treatment retention. J Subst Abuse Treat. 2014;47(3):202–12.
25. DiMatteo MR, Haskard KB, Williams SL. Health beliefs, disease severity, and patient adherence: a meta-analysis. Med Care. 2007;45(6):521–8.
26. Sussman S, Arnett JJ. Emerging adulthood: developmental period facilitative of the addictions. Eval Health Prof. 2014;37(2):147–55.
27. Arnett JJ. Emerging adulthood. A theory of development from the late teens through the twenties. Am Psychol. 2000;55(5):469–80.
28. Rosenblum A, et al. Distance traveled and cross-state commuting to opioid treatment programs in the United States. J Environ Public Health. 2011;2011:948789.
29. Lofwall MR, Walsh SL. A review of buprenorphine diversion and misuse: the current evidence base and experiences from around the world. J Addict Med. 2014;8(5):315–26.
30. Accurso AJ, Rastegar DA. The effect of a payer-mandated decrease in buprenorphine dose on aberrant drug tests and treatment retention among patients with opioid dependence. J Subst Abuse Treat. 2016;61:74–9.
31. Osterberg L, Blaschke T. Adherence to medication. N Engl J Med. 2005;353(5):487–97.
32. National Forensic Laboratory Information System Special Report: Methadone and Buprenorphine, 2003–2008; 2009.
33. Allen B, Harocopos A. Non-prescribed buprenorphine in New York City: motivations for use, practices of diversion, and experiences of stigma. J Subst Abuse Treat. 2016;70:81–6.
34. Lofwall MR, Havens JR. Inability to access buprenorphine treatment as a risk factor for using diverted buprenorphine. Drug Alcohol Depend. 2012;126(3):379–83.
35. Schuman-Olivier Z, et al. Self-treatment: illicit buprenorphine use by opioid-dependent treatment seekers. J Subst Abuse Treat. 2010;39(1):41–50.
36. Cicero TJ, Surratt HL, Inciardi J. Use and misuse of buprenorphine in the management of opioid addiction. J Opioid Manag. 2007;3(6):302–8.
37. Jones HE. Practical considerations for the clinical use of buprenorphine. Sci Pract Perspect. 2004;2(2):4–20.
38. Thomas CP, et al. Use of buprenorphine for addiction treatment: perspectives of addiction specialists and general psychiatrists. Psychiatr Serv. 2008;59(8):909–16.
39. Center for Substance Abuse Treatment, Clinical Guidelines for the Use of Buprenorphine in the Treatment of Opioid Addiction. Treatment Improvement Protocol (TIP) Series 40, 2004, Substance Abuse and Mental Health Services Administration: Rockville, MD.
40. Sigmon SC. Access to treatment for opioid dependence in rural America: challenges and future directions. JAMA Psychiatry. 2014;71(4):359–60.
41. Free C, et al. The effectiveness of mobile-health technology-based health behaviour change or disease management interventions for health care consumers: a systematic review. PLoS Med. 2013;10(1):e1001362.
42. Miller L, et al. Mobile technology interventions for asthma self-management: systematic review and meta-analysis. JMIR mHealth uHealth. 2017;5(5):e57.
43. Cooper V, et al. mHealth interventions to support self-management in HIV: a systematic review. Open AIDS J. 2017;11:119–32.
44. de Jongh T, et al. Mobile phone messaging for facilitating self-management of long-term illnesses. Cochrane Database Syst Rev. 2012;12:CD007459.
45. Amass L, Kamien JB, Mikulich SK. Thrice-weekly supervised dosing with the combination buprenorphine-naloxone tablet is preferred to daily supervised dosing by opioid-dependent humans. Drug Alcohol Depend. 2001;61(2):173–81.
46. Saulle R, Vecchi S, Gowing L. Supervised dosing with a long-acting opioid medication in the management of opioid dependence. Cochrane Database Syst Rev. 2017;4.CD011983.
47. Bangor A, Kortum PT, Miller JT. An empirical evaluation of the system usability scale. Int J Hum Comput Interact. 2008;24(6):574–94.
48. Bangor A, Kortum PT, Miller JT. Determining what individual SUS scores mean: adding an adjective rating scale. J Usability Stud. 2009;4(3):114–23.
49. Harris PA, et al. Research electronic data capture (REDCap)—a metadata-driven methodology and workflow process for providing translational research informatics support. J Biomed Inform. 2009;42(2):377–81.
50. Schuman-Olivier Z et al. MySafeRx: an integrated mobile platform for buprenorphine adherence. In: American academy of addiction psychiatry (AAAP) 27th annual meeting and symposium 2016. Bonita Springs: Wiley/Blackwell (10.1111).
51. Rollnick S, Miller WR. Motivational interviewing: helping people change. New York: The Guilford Press; 2013.
52. Moyers TB, et al. The motivational interviewing treatment integrity code (MITI 4): rationale, preliminary reliability and validity. J Subst Abuse Treat. 2016;65:36–42.
53. Zoom. Zoom Video Conferencing and Web Conferencing Service. 2017. Cited 2017 September 7, 2017. https://zoom.us/.
54. Palmer RS, et al. Substance user treatment dropout from client and clinician perspectives: a pilot study. Subst Use Misuse. 2009;44(7):1021–38.
55. Rosen LD, et al. The media and technology usage and attitudes scale: an empirical investigation. Comput Human Behav. 2013;29(6):2501–11.
56. First MB et al. Structured clinical interview for DSM-IV-TR axis I disorders, research version, patient edition. Vol. SCID-I/P. 2002, New York: Biometrics Research, New York State Psychiatric Institute.

57. Nasreddine ZS, et al. The montreal cognitive assessment, MoCA: a brief screening tool for mild cognitive impairment. J Am Geriatr Soc. 2005;53(4):695–9.
58. Brooke J. SUS—A quick and dirty usability scale. Usability Eval Ind. 1996;189(194):4–7.
59. Sauro, J. SUStisfied? little-known system usability scale facts; 2011. http://uxpamagazine.org/sustified/.
60. Schuman-Olivier Z et al. Feasibility for ActiWatch score (TM) for recording skills practice and conducting ecological momentary assessment in a RCT of mindfulness training vs. cognitive-behavioral therapy for tobacco smoking cessation. In: Poster presentation, international symposium on contemplative studies; 2012.
61. Hwang W, Salvendy G. Number of people required for usability evaluation. Commun ACM. 2010;53(5):130.
62. Commitment of Alcoholics or Substance Abusers. Massachusetts general law; 2016.
63. Dahan A, et al. Comparison of the respiratory effects of intravenous buprenorphine and fentanyl in humans and rats. Br J Anaesth. 2005;94(6):825–34.
64. Boas RA, Villiger JW. Clinical actions of fentanyl and buprenorphine. The significance of receptor binding. Br J Anaesth. 1985;57(2):192–6.
65. Bershad AK, et al. Opioid partial agonist buprenorphine dampens responses to psychosocial stress in humans. Psychoneuroendocrinology. 2015;52:281–8.
66. Vuong C, et al. The effects of opioids and opioid analogs on animal and human endocrine systems. Endocr Rev. 2010;31(1):98–132.
67. Koob GF. A role for brain stress systems in addiction. Neuron. 2008;59(1):11–34.
68. Sinha R. Chronic stress, drug use, and vulnerability to addiction. Ann N Y Acad Sci. 2008;1141:105–30.
69. Stein BD, et al. Physician capacity to treat opioid use disorder with buprenorphine-assisted treatment. JAMA. 2016;316(11):1211–2.
70. Substance Abuse and Mental Health Services Administration, National Survey of Stubstance Abuse Treatment Services (N-SSATS). 2017. BHSIS Series S-93 (HHS Publication No. (SMA) 17-5039), p. 1–213.
71. Yang A, Arfken CL, Johanson CE. Steps physicians report taking to reduce diversion of buprenorphine. Am J Addict. 2013;22(3):184–7.
72. New Freedom Commission on Mental Health Subcommittee on Rural Issues: Background Paper. DHHS Pub. No. SMA-04-3890; 2004.
73. Andrilla CHA, Coulthard C, Larson EH. Barriers rural physicians face prescribing buprenorphine for opioid use disorder. Ann Fam Med. 2017;15(4):359–62.
74. Sigmon SC, et al. Interim buprenorphine vs. waiting list for opioid dependence. N Engl J Med. 2016;375(25):2504–5.
75. Uosukainen H, Pentikainen H, Tacke U. The effect of an electronic medicine dispenser on diversion of buprenorphine-naloxone-experience from a medium-sized Finnish city. J Subst Abuse Treat. 2013;45(1):143–7.
76. Fareed A, et al. Effect of buprenorphine dose on treatment outcome. J Addict Dis. 2012;31(1):8–18.
77. Greenwald M, et al. Buprenorphine duration of action: mu-opioid receptor availability and pharmacokinetic and behavioral indices. Biol Psychiatry. 2007;61(1):101–10.
78. Daniulaityte R, et al. Overdose deaths related to fentanyl and its analogs—Ohio, January–February 2017. MMWR Morb Mortal Wkly Rep. 2017;66(34):904–8.
79. Fluent L. Devices and demographics; 2016. 2 Nov 2017. http://www.fluentco.com/wp-content/uploads/2016/01/Fluent2_DevicesandDemographics_2016.pdf.
80. Statista. Subscriber share held by smartphone operating systems in the United States from January 2012 to June 2017; 2017. 1 Dec 2017. https://www.statista.com/statistics/266572/market-share-held-by-smartphone-platforms-in-the-united-states/.

Delivery of screening and brief intervention for unhealthy alcohol use in an urban academic Federally Qualified Health Center

Marcus A. Bachhuber[1*], Megan A. O'Grady[2], Henry Chung[3], Charles J. Neighbors[2], Joseph DeLuca[1], Elenita M. D'Aloia[4], Arelis Diaz[4] and Chinazo O. Cunningham[1]

Abstract

Background: Screening and brief intervention (SBI) for unhealthy drinking has not been widely implemented in primary care partly due to reliance on physicians to perform it.

Methods: We implemented a model of nursing staff-delivered SBI for unhealthy drinking for adult patients receiving primary care at an academically-affiliated Federally Qualified Health Center in the Bronx, NY. Our model consisted of nursing staff screening all patients with the alcohol use disorders identification test consumption questions (AUDIT-C) and, if screening positive, providing BI or referral to specialty services. We developed a clinical decision support tool integrated into the electronic health record to guide nursing staff and record SBI provision. To evaluate this model, we determined overall SBI delivery to patients and factors associated with receiving SBI.

Results: Between October 2013 and September 2014, 9119 unique adult patients made 24,285 visits. Patients were majority women (67.5%) and Hispanic/Latino (54.5%). Overall, 46.2% were screened, with 19.0–35.8% of eligible patients screened in each month. Increasing age (OR: 0.82 [95% CI 0.80–0.85] for a 10-year increase), female sex (OR: 0.83 [95% CI 0.77–0.91]), and chronic conditions like hypertension (OR: 0.62 [95% CI 0.56–0.70]) and diabetes (OR: 0.66 [95% CI 0.58–0.75]), among others, were associated with a lower odds of being screened. Of all patients screened, 225 (5.3%) screened positive and of those patients, 122 (54.2%) received a BI. Patients with higher AUDIT-C scores were more likely to receive a BI (OR: 1.24 [95% CI 1.04–1.47] for a 1-point increase) and non-English speaking patients were less likely to receive a BI than those who spoke English (OR: 0.42 [95% CI 0.18–0.97]).

Conclusions: Our model of SBI resulted in screening of nearly half of all eligible patients and BI provision to over half of those screening positive. Future efforts to improve SBI delivery should focus on groups such as older adults, women, and those with chronic medical conditions.

Keywords: Alcohol use disorder, Unhealthy alcohol use, Screening and brief intervention, Primary care, Screening

Background

Unhealthy alcohol use, defined as drinking at a level that can lead to negative health consequences [1], is a leading cause of preventable morbidity and mortality in the US [2]. Screening and brief intervention for unhealthy drinking (SBI) can reduce self-reported drinking in primary care settings [3]. Despite the US Preventive Services Task Force recommendation that all adults receive SBI [4], it is uncommonly provided, resulting in missed opportunities to improve outcomes [5]. In a recent national study, while 71.1% of respondents reported that their doctor asked about alcohol use (not necessarily with standardized

*Correspondence: mbachhub@montefiore.org
[1] Division of General Internal Medicine, Department of Medicine, Montefiore Medical Center/Albert Einstein College of Medicine, 3300 Kossuth Ave, Bronx, NY 10467, USA
Full list of author information is available at the end of the article

validated screening tools), only 4.4% of those with heavy episodic (i.e., binge) drinking reported being advised to cut back [6]. This gap between evidence and practice is likely the result of several barriers, including competing clinical priorities, staff training and knowledge, and organizational factors [7].

In settings that deliver SBI, physicians have traditionally provided it during routine clinical care; however, physicians' competing priorities are a barrier to broader implementation of SBI [8–10]. In line with efforts to move toward team-based primary care, SBI delivery by non-physician providers—often nursing staff—is feasible and efficacious [11]. Two implementation trials in primary care settings found that non-physician-delivered SBI resulted in a higher percentage of patients screened than physician-delivered SBI (24 vs. 19% and 51 vs. 9%) [12, 13]. One trial found that non-physician-delivered SBI resulted in higher rates of BI provision among patients screening positive than physician-delivered SBI (73.1 vs. 57.1%) [12] and one found the opposite (3.4 vs. 44.0%) [13]. Despite intensive efforts, both studies also revealed that a significant percentage of patients did not receive SBI.

While many non-physician providers receive less training and feel less comfortable addressing unhealthy alcohol use than physicians [14], clinical decision support (CDS) tools—electronic health record (EHR)-based tools designed to aid clinicians in making diagnostic and treatment decisions—can mitigate these challenges and have been widely used to promote guideline-concordant care [15]. To increase provision of alcohol screening, the Veterans Health Administration (VA) successfully used a CDS tool (i.e., a clinical reminder) in combination with provider training and a national performance measure, resulting in very high rates of screening (93%) [16].

On an organizational level, incorporating new practices such as SBI into existing clinical systems can be challenging, but some strategies can improve this process. For example, piloting with teams including front-line clinicians, leadership, and administration can help ensure that everyone affected by a new practice has an opportunity to provide input and feedback [17]. Identifying and working with clinical champions can also promote implementation; specifically, physician and nursing champions can help to serve as opinion leaders promoting SBI [18].

With the goal of improving the delivery of evidence-based preventive care, we implemented routine SBI for unhealthy drinking at an adult medicine practice. To build on findings from previous research and utilize practices shown to enhance the success of implementation, our model consisted of nursing staff-delivered SBI with an SBI-focused CDS tool that was piloted and promoted by a physician and nurse champion. To target future improvements, we also conducted an evaluation of this model to determine overall SBI delivery and factors associated with receiving SBI.

Methods

Study setting and population

The study setting is a Federally Qualified Health Center affiliated with our academic institution in the Bronx, NY. It is a multispecialty practice with internal medicine, pediatrics, obstetrics/gynecology, dermatology, podiatry, and dentistry, with onsite behavioral health, laboratory, and radiology services. We implemented SBI in the internal medicine practice which includes 11 Licensed Practical Nurses, two Patient Care Technicians (similar to medical assistants), one Registered Nurse, 15 attending physicians, and 30 resident physicians. Over 9000 unique adult patients attend about 25,000 visits per year.

Model of care

Our model of SBI for unhealthy drinking consisted of annual screening by nursing staff followed by delivery of a BI for patients with unhealthy alcohol use. Patients eligible for screening included all adult patients seen for any type of visit. Nursing staff performed screening prior to patients' visits with physicians, at the same time they measured vital signs and weight. If a BI was warranted, nursing staff performed it immediately after screening, before physician encounters.

To improve delivery of SBI, we developed a CDS tool integrated into our EHR (Centricity Electronic Medical Record version 9.8) consisting of three components: (1) a clinical reminder for screening, (2) screening questions and fields to record answers, and (3) prompts for BI and a field to record delivery. For the clinical reminder, we integrated it into the note in the same location as reminders for other preventive services (e.g., colorectal cancer screening). The reminder was not a "hard stop" and could be ignored; if ignored, it would appear again at patients' next visit. If screening was performed, the reminder would not appear for 1 year. Clicking on the reminder activated the screening questions. While our model of SBI relied on nursing staff, the clinical reminder was visible to physicians and could be completed by them; however, anecdotally, this was rare due to competing clinical priorities.

To screen, nursing staff used the alcohol use disorders identification test consumption questions (AUDIT-C) [19, 20]: (1) "How often did you have a drink containing alcohol in the past year?"; (2) "How many drinks did you have on a typical day when you were drinking in the past year?"; and (3) "How often did you have six or more drinks on one occasion in the past year?" Each item is scored from 0 to 4 points (total possible score = 0–12 points). For women scoring ≥ 3 points, a question appeared asking, "Does the drinking level exceed 7 drinks per week?"; for men scoring ≥ 4 points, the question read "Does the drinking level exceed 14 drinks per week?" [21]. We included questions about exceeding weekly limits because the AUDIT-C does not map precisely on to recommended drinking limits. Based on the patient's score, nursing staff were prompted to provide a verbal BI, referral to behavioral health staff (e.g., social work), a verbal notification to the patient's physician, or combinations of the above. The SBI algorithm and the specific BI components delivered by nursing staff at each AUDIT-C score are shown in Fig. 1.

Prior to implementation, we piloted the CDS tool and screening procedure with a nurse champion. The purpose of this step was to test the CDS tool, determine if nursing staff would be able to screen patients while collecting vital signs and chief complaint, determine the time it took to screen, and gauge patients' responses. In addition to the nurse champion, an attending physician champion specializing in addiction medicine also took a lead role in testing and suggesting changes to the CDS tool. Furthermore, we involved the medical director and other administrative and clinical staff at the clinic throughout the piloting phase to ensure that all staff affected by this new practice could give feedback. After the pilot, we trained the 12 members of the nursing staff as well as attending and resident physicians in separate 1-h meetings. These meetings covered the rationale for screening for unhealthy alcohol use, best practices in administering the AUDIT-C, the evidence supporting the benefit of BI, the overall framework of BI and best practices in administering BI, and the practicalities of SBI at the clinic including the workflow.

Evaluation and data collection

To evaluate implementation, we extracted data on all adult medicine patients seen within 1 year after implementation of routine SBI (October 2013–September 2014). From the EHR, we extracted patient data (e.g., demographics), visit data (e.g., visit diagnoses), and results of the screener (e.g., the AUDIT-C score and whether a BI was performed).

Main outcome measures

Our main outcomes were documentation of screening, screening positive for unhealthy drinking, and documentation of BI provision. While nurses were instructed to provide BIs according to the algorithm (Fig. 1), we were unable to extract EHR data from the question about exceeding weekly limits; therefore, in the evaluation we considered an AUDIT-C score of ≥ 4 as a positive screen for both men and women. Of all women, 93 received an AUDIT-C score of 3 points and some of those would have ultimately been considered a positive screen at their visit (i.e., if they also exceeded weekly limits) and been eligible to receive a BI.

Visit and patient factors

From EHR data, we coded several visit and patient factor variables. For visits, we collected the type of visit (e.g., new patient, established patient, or urgent care/walk-in) and the month in which the visit occurred. New patient visits were defined as the patient's first ever visit to the

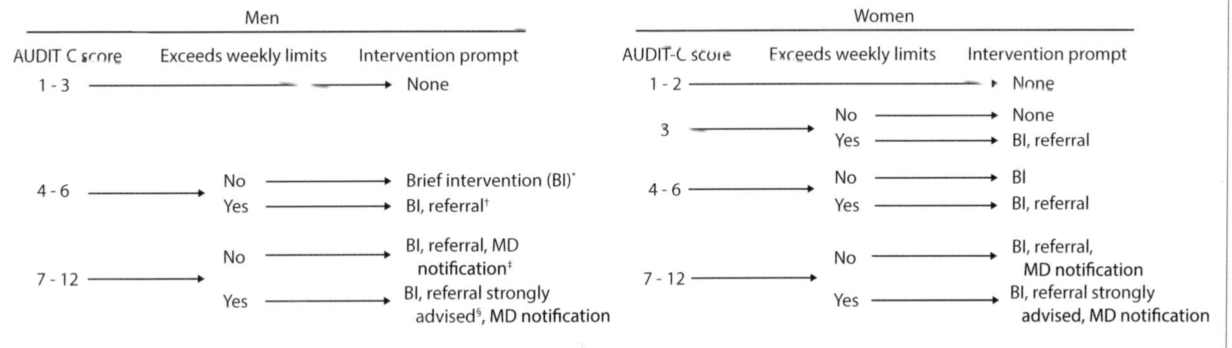

*Nursing staff provided with the following prompt: "Educate about the risks of drinking at this level; if patient is not ready, use motivational interviewing approach, i.e., 'If you were to cut down on your drinking, what might be some reasons you could think of?' or 'How might you try even though you might not be ready now?' Tell them you can assist and will work with them on cutting down and can discuss more in future visits."

†Nursing staff provided with the following prompt: "Offer a referral to a behavioral specialist or social worker/health educator at the site or off site if the patient is willing."

‡Nursing staff verbally notified the patient's physician.

§Nursing staff provided with the following prompt: "STRONGLY RECOMMEND a visit with a behavioral health specialist for a further assessment."

Fig. 1 Algorithm for screening and brief intervention for unhealthy drinking in an urban academic Federally Qualified Health Center

clinic or the patient's first visit with a new provider (i.e., transition of care). For patient sociodemographics, we collected age, sex, race/ethnicity, and preferred language. Finally, we identified patients' chronic medical conditions using visit diagnoses (i.e., diagnoses coded as actively addressed) grouped into clinically meaningful categories using established coding schemes [22].

Statistical analysis

First, we summarized patient characteristics using descriptive statistics. Next, we determined the number and percentage of patients screened overall and in each month, the number and percentage screening positive, and the number and percentage of patients screening positive who received a BI.

We then determined visit and patient factors associated with being screened, screening positive, and receiving a BI if screening positive. We created three separate multivariable logistic regression models. In the first model, to determine visit and patient factors associated with being screened, the dependent variable was whether the patient was screened. To account for the possibility of patients having multiple visits over the study period, we used person-visit as the unit of analysis, using a generalized estimating equations model accounting for clustering at the patient level and producing robust standard errors. We included visit type (new patient, established patient, or urgent care/walk-in), visit month, and all patient factors as independent variables. In the second model, to determine patient factors associated with screening positive for unhealthy drinking, the dependent variable was the presence of a positive screen among those who were screened. Because of a reduced sample size and collinearity, we removed race/ethnicity from the model and combined several categories for language, visit type, and chronic conditions. In the third model, to determine patient factors associated with receiving a BI among those screening positive, the dependent variable was the documentation of BI among those screening positive. The independent variables were similar to the previous model with the addition of AUDIT-C score. For the second and third model, we analyzed only the visit at which screening was performed (i.e., only one visit per patient); therefore, the unit of analysis in these models is the patient.

We evaluated the associations of patient factors with outcomes in terms of odds ratios and 95% confidence intervals (95% CIs). We also used predictive margins to describe each factor's association with outcomes in terms of the difference in probability of the outcome (in percentage points) compared to the referent group, after adjusting for all other factors. We conducted all analyses with SAS 9.4 (Cary, NC) and Stata 13.1 (College Station, TX).

Results

Between October 2013 and September 2014, 9119 adult patients attended one or more visit. The mean number of visits per patient was 2.7 (range 1–32). Patients were majority women (67.5%) and Hispanic/Latino (54.5%; Table 1). Most patients preferred English (71.5%), followed by Spanish (25.4%). The most common chronic conditions among patients were hypertension (26.5%), diabetes (14.8%), and depression (13.1%).

Overall, 4212 (46.2%) patients were screened with 19.0–35.8% of eligible patients screened in each month (Fig. 2). Of all patients screened, 2767 (65.6%) were screened on their first visit during the study period. Increasing age (10-year increment, OR: 0.82 [95% CI 0.80–0.85]), female sex (OR: 0.83 [95% CI 0.77–0.91]), and chronic conditions such as hypertension (OR: 0.62 [95% CI 0.56–0.70]) and diabetes (OR: 0.66 [95% CI 0.58–0.75]), among others, were associated with a lower odds of being screened (Table 2). Screening was also less likely at established patient visits (OR: 0.22 [95% CI 0.20–0.24]) and urgent care/walk-in visits (OR: 0.12 [95% CI 0.11–0.14]) compared to new patient visits. The odds of screening increased in each month during the study period (OR: 1.03 [95% CI 1.02–1.04]).

Table 1 Demographic and clinical characteristics of adult medicine patients of an urban academic Federally Qualified Health Center during implementation of a screening and brief intervention initiative (n = 9119)

Characteristic	n (%)
Age, median (IQR)	48.8 (33.7, 60.9)
Female sex	6153 (67.5)
Race/ethnicity	
Black, non-Hispanic	945 (10.4)
Hispanic, of any race	4965 (54.5)
Any other or undetermined race[a]	3209 (35.2)
Language	
English	6518 (71.5)
Spanish	2316 (25.4)
French	285 (3.1)
Chronic conditions	
Hypertension	2420 (26.5)
Diabetes	1345 (14.8)
Congestive heart failure	162 (1.8)
Chronic kidney disease	305 (3.3)
HIV	255 (2.8)
Hepatitis C virus	113 (1.2)
Depression	1194 (13.1)
Opioid or cocaine use disorder	460 (5.0)

[a] Includes White, Asian/Pacific Islander, Native American/Alaskan Native, or more than one race

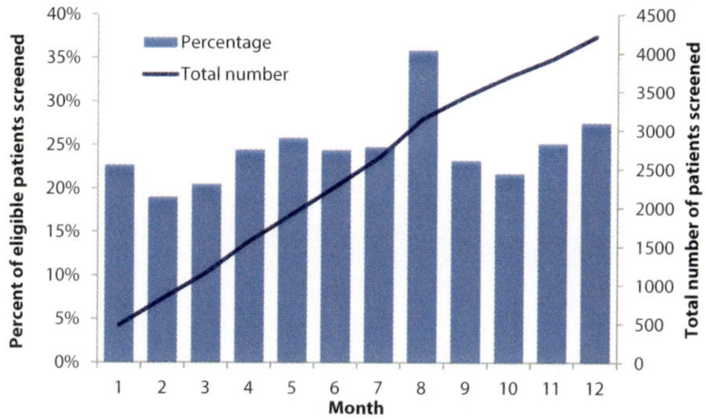

Fig. 2 Percent and cumulative number of eligible adult medicine patients screened for unhealthy alcohol use, by month, in an urban academic Federally Qualified Health Center. Light blue bars represent percentage of patients screened in each month of the study period (left axis). Dark blue line represents the cumulative number of patients screened (right axis)

Of all screened patients, 225 (5.3%) screened positive (≥ 4 points on the AUDIT-C; Table 3). Increasing age (OR: 0.79 [95% CI 0.71–0.87]), female sex (OR: 0.32 [95% CI 0.24–0.42]), and non-English language (OR: 0.50 [95% CI 0.33–0.75]) were associated with a lower odds of screening positive. Patients screened during established or urgent care visits were also less likely to screen positive than new patients (OR: 0.53 [95% CI 0.40–0.71]).

Of all patients screening positive, 122 (54.2%) received a BI (Table 4). Non-English speaking patients were less likely to receive a BI than those who spoke English (OR: 0.40 [95% CI 0.17–0.91]). Patients with higher AUDIT-C scores were more likely to receive a BI (OR: 1.24 [95% CI 1.04–1.47] for a 1-point increase in AUDIT-C).

Discussion

Using a model of nursing staff-delivered SBI with an integrated CDS tool, our adult medicine practice screened almost half of all patients and provided a BI to over half of patients who screened positive. Monthly rates of screening increased modestly over the 1-year study period. Our study is among the few published studies reporting SBI rates and factors associated with receipt of SBI, in which SBI is integrated into routine care and delivered by nursing staff that are not grant funded [16]. As most clinical settings would not have additional grant funding available for SBI implementation, our findings are significant by showing that SBI can be integrated into routine care in an urban safety net setting without additional funding by using team-based models along with other implementation facilitators such as clinical champions, EHR CDS tools, and getting feedback and buy-in among all team members of the clinic.

While significant room for improvement remains, the rates of screening and BI we achieved are in the range of previous studies [23]. However, our screening rates (46.2%) were lower than rates reported in the VA (93%) [16]. This may be due to several factors in the VA system such as high levels of clinician comfort with clinical reminders and use of a system-wide alcohol screening performance measure to provide feedback to clinicians. The rates of BI we achieved (54.2%) were higher than in the non-physician provider arm of one implementation trial (3.4%) [13]. In that trial, provision of BI was dependent on availability of additional staff and rooms, compared to our model where BI was performed within routine patient flow.

We identified specific visit and patient characteristics that were associated with lower odds of being screened, including older age, female sex, and chronic medical conditions. Lower rates of screening among older adults and women may be related to assumptions or inferences about patient responses without asking screening questions verbatim [24]. Lower rates of screening among those with chronic medical conditions may be due to competing clinical priorities. For example, nursing staff routinely measure blood capillary glucose for patients with diabetes. For patients with depression, nursing staff also routinely administer depression questionnaires and record them in the EHR. As unhealthy alcohol use affects all demographics and can exacerbate many chronic medical conditions [25–29], reinforcement of the importance of SBI for all patients is essential. Furthermore, adjusting clinical processes to allow for extra time (e.g., reducing the frequency of blood capillary glucose measurements) may be necessary to improve SBI delivery among those with chronic medical conditions. Beyond these factors, qualitative research with nursing staff could help identify other areas where SBI delivery can be improved.

In our evaluation, 5.3% of patients screened had a positive screen. While we had to modify our definition of a positive screen due to technical limitations (to ≥ 4 AUDIT-C points for men and women), this rate of positive screens is at the low end of what we would expect based on community surveys. In a 2014 survey, 4.6% of Bronx adults reported heavy drinking—defined in that survey as an average of > 2 drinks per day for men and > 1 drink per day for women; 14.6% reported binge drinking—defined as ≥ 5 drinks on one occasion for men and ≥ 4 drinks on one occasion for women in the past 30 days [30]. As our CDS tool only included screening questions in English, one potential explanation for a relatively low rate of positive screens may be language. While non-English speakers were screened at similar rates as English speakers, non-English language was associated

Table 2 Screening and factors associated with screening for unhealthy alcohol use among adult medicine patients at an urban academic Federally Qualified Health Center (n = 24,285 visits among 9119 patients)

Characteristic	Screened, n (%)[a]	Adjusted odds ratio, 95% CI	*p*	Adjusted difference in percent screened, % (95% CI)[b]
All	4212 (46.2)	–	–	–
Age[c]		0.82 (0.80–0.85)	< 0.001	– 2.5 (– 2.9 to – 2.1)
18–29 years	1022 (58.8)			
30–49	1493 (48.7)			
50–64	1079 (41.8)			
≥ 65	618 (35.6)			
Sex				
Male	1479 (49.9)	Ref.	< 0.001	Ref.
Female	2733 (44.4)	0.83 (0.77–0.91)		– 2.4 (– 3.5 to – 1.3)
Race				
Black, non-Hispanic	420 (44.4)	Ref.		Ref.
Hispanic, of any race	2298 (46.6)	0.95 (0.83–1.10)	0.53	– 6.0 (– 2.5 to 1.3)
Any other or undetermined race[d]	1494 (46.3)	1.00 (0.87–1.15)	0.99	0.02 (– 1.8–1.8)
Language				
English	3450 (47.1)	Ref.		Ref.
Spanish	1301 (43.8)	1.02 (0.92–1.14)	0.68	0.3 (– 1.1 to 1.7)
French	156 (45.3)	0.94 (0.75–1.18)	0.61	– 0.75 (– 3.6 to 2.1)
Visit type				
New patient	–	Ref.		Ref.
Established patient	–	0.22 (0.20–0.24)	< 0.001	– 28.3 (– 0.30.3 to – 26.4)
Urgent care or walk-in	–	0.12 (0.11–0.14)	< 0.001	– 34.3 (– 36.3 to – 32.3)
Visit month	–	1.03 (1.02–1.04)	< 0.001	0.4 (0.3–0.6)
Chronic conditions				
Hypertension				
No	3421 (51.1)	Ref.		Ref.
Yes	791 (32.7)	0.62 (0.56–0.70)	< 0.001	– 5.9 (– 7.3 to – 4.6)
Diabetes				
No	3790 (48.8)	Ref.		Ref.
Yes	422 (31.4)	0.66 (0.58–0.75)	< 0.001	– 5.1 (– 6.6 to – 3.7)
Congestive heart failure				
No	4152 (46.4)	Ref.		Ref.
Yes	60 (37.0)	1.08 (0.80–1.47)	0.60	1.1 (– 3.0 to 5.1)
Chronic kidney disease				
No	4114 (46.7)	Ref.		Ref.
Yes	98 (32.1)	0.96 (0.75–1.22)	0.74	– 0.5 (– 3.6 to 2.5)
HIV				
No	4135 (46.7)	Ref.		Ref.
Yes	77 (30.2)	0.36 (0.28–0.45)	< 0.001	– 10.5 (– 12.3 to – 8.6)
Hepatitis C virus				
No	4173 (46.3)	Ref.		Ref.
Yes	39 (34.5)	0.64 (0.44–0.93)	0.02	– 5.1 (– 8.9 to – 1.3)

Table 2 continued

Characteristic	Screened, n (%)[a]	Adjusted odds ratio, 95% CI	*p*	Adjusted difference in percent screened, % (95% CI)[b]
Depression				
No	3729 (47.1)	Ref.		Ref.
Yes	483 (40.5)	0.75 (0.66–0.84)	< 0.001	− 3.6 (− 5.0 to − 2.3)
Opioid or cocaine use disorder				
No	3983 (46.0)	Ref.		Ref.
Yes	229 (49.8)	0.76 (0.64–0.91)	0.002	− 3.3 (− 5.3 to − 1.3)

[a] Percentages calculated at the patient level (i.e., the percent of male patients). Regression models estimated using patient-visit as the unit of analysis

[b] Refers to the absolute difference in the probability of being screened, adjusting for all variables

[c] Age categories used for descriptive statistics, age used as a continuous variable in regression models with a 1-unit change representing 10 years

[d] Includes White, Asian/Pacific Islander, Native American/Alaskan Native, or more than one race

Table 3 Factors associated with screening positive for unhealthy drinking among adult medicine patients who were screened at an urban academic Federally Qualified Health Center (n = 4212 patients)

Characteristic	Screened positive, n (%)	Adjusted odds ratio, 95% CI	*p*	Adjusted difference in percent screened, % (95% CI)[a]
All	225 (5.3)	–	–	–
Age[b]		0.79 (0.71–0.87)	< 0.001	− 1.2 (− 1.7 to − 6.8)
18–29 years	78 (7.6)			
30–49	93 (6.2)			
50–64	46 (4.3)			
≥ 65	8 (1.3)			
Sex				
Male	139 (9.4)	Ref.		Ref.
Female	86 (3.2)	0.32 (0.24–0.42)	< 0.001	− 5.9 (− 7.5 to − 4.4)
Language				
English	195 (6.4)	Ref.		Ref.
Spanish or French	30 (2.6)	0.50 (0.33–0.75)	0.001	− 2.9 (− 4.2 to − 1.5)
Visit type				
New patient	148 (7.7)	Ref.		Ref.
Established patient or urgent care/ walk-in	77 (3.4)	0.53 (0.40–0.71)	< 0.001	− 3.0 (− 4.4 to − 1.6)
Chronic medical or mental health condition				
No	154 (5.7)	Ref.		Ref.
Yes	71 (4.7)	1.24 (0.91–1.70)	0.18	1.1 (− 0.05 to 2.7)

Defined as an AUDIT-C score of ≥ 4

[a] Refers to the absolute difference in the probability of screening positive, adjusting for all variables

[b] Age categories used for descriptive statistics, age used as a continuous variable in regression models with a 1-unit change representing 10 years

with a lower odds of screening positive, suggesting that nursing staff were able to translate screening questions ad hoc, but in doing so, they may have lost sensitivity. Further study is needed to compare the sensitivity of our routine screening to a reference standard. In VA facilities, for example, routine screening has had an unexpectedly low sensitivity [31, 32].

For BI, a higher AUDIT-C score was associated with a higher odds of receiving the intervention, suggesting that, while nursing staff were not providing a BI to all patients, they were prioritizing those with higher AUDIT-C scores. Non-English language was the only factor associated with a lower odds of receiving the intervention. This finding is similar to the VA, where Hispanic/Latino patients are less likely to receive services for unhealthy alcohol use than white and black patients after screening positive [33]. Specific to our clinic, while most nursing staff are bilingual English and Spanish or English and

Table 4 Delivery of brief intervention and factors associated with delivery among adult medicine patients who screened positive for unhealthy drinking at an urban academic Federally Qualified Health Center (n = 225 patients)

Characteristic	Received brief intervention, n (%)	Adjusted odds ratio, 95% CI	*p*	Adjusted difference in percent screened, % (95% CI)[a]
All	122 (54.2)	–	–	–
Age[b]		1.07 (0.87–1.32)	0.53	1.6 (− 3.4 to 6.6)
18–29 years	46 (59.0)			
30–49	43 (46.2)			
50–64	27 (58.7)			
≥ 65	6 (75.0)			
Sex				
Male	73 (52.5)	Ref.		Ref.
Female	49 (57.0)	1.24 (0.69–2.21)	0.47	5.0 (− 8.6 to 18.5)
Language				
English	111 (56.9)	Ref.		Ref.
Spanish or French	11 (36.7)	0.42 (0.18–0.97)	0.04	− 20.3 (− 38.9 to − 1.7)
Visit type				
New patient	84 (56.8)	Ref.		Ref.
Established patient or urgent care/walk-in	38 (49.4)	0.75 (0.42–1.32)	0.33	− 6.7 (− 19.9 to 6.6)
AUDIT-C score	–	1.24 (1.04–1.47)	0.01	5.1 (1.2–8.9)
Chronic medical or mental health condition				
No	82 (53.3)	Ref.		Ref.
Yes	40 (56.3)	1.01 (0.56–1.84)	0.96	0.3 (− 13.6 to 14.3)

Defined as an AUDIT-C score of ≥ 4

[a] Refers to the absolute difference in the probability of receiving a brief intervention, adjusting for all variables

[b] Age categories used for descriptive statistics, age used as a continuous variable in regression models with a 1-unit change representing 10 years

French speakers, they often care for patients who speak a different language. Although telephone interpreters are available on demand, this may create an unreasonable time delay; future work should examine alternatives such as interactive voice response or video-based BI for language-discordant encounters [34, 35]. More generally, future evaluations of this model of routine SBI should evaluate fidelity of nursing staff to the recommended BI framework and, most importantly, effects on clinical outcomes such as self-reported drinking and disease control.

This study has limitations. First, because of EHR limitations, we could not identify individual nursing staff or physicians providing SBI. As provider factors may be more important than visit and patient factors in determining which patients receive SBI, future research is needed to assess providers' impact. We also could not extract results for the question asking about weekly drinking limits which required us to use a nonstandard threshold for unhealthy drinking for women. This limitation of our data may have led to biased estimates of factors associated with screening positive and factors associated with receiving a BI; the bias could be in either direction. While BI provision was documented in the EHR, we did not assess fidelity to recommended BI framework. Our ability to examine the impact of race/ethnicity on screening and receipt of a BI was limited by the large number of patients with this variable recorded as "undetermined". Because our goal was to deliver SBI, we did not have a comparison group. Furthermore, SBI was not routinely provided prior to our study and the AUDIT-C questions were not available in the EHR, which also makes historical controls unavailable. Finally, during the study period, referrals to behavioral health providers were paper-based and therefore we cannot determine the number of patients referred after screening positive.

Conclusions

In a Bronx Federally Qualified Health Center without dedicated grant-funded personnel, we integrated a model of nursing staff-delivered routine SBI for unhealthy drinking into primary care. Almost half of the patients presenting for one or more visit were screened, and of those who screened positive, over half received a BI. Patient characteristics including older age, female sex, and chronic illnesses were associated with lower odds of screening; non-English language was associated with lower odds of receiving a BI. While integrating SBI into routine primary care by nursing staff can lead to moderate screening rates, it is important to ensure that SBI is delivered to patients who could clinically benefit most (e.g., those with chronic diseases impacted by unhealthy alcohol use). Health care facilities need to continue to integrate models of SBI that are comprehensively delivered to patients in routine primary care.

Abbreviations
SBI: screening and brief intervention; BI: brief intervention; EHR: electronic health record; CDS: clinical decision support; AUDIT-C: alcohol use disorders identification test consumption questions.

Authors' contributions
All authors contributed to the conception and design of this work; MB and CC acquired and analyzed the data; all authors contributed to the interpretation of the data as well as drafting and/or revising the work for important intellectual content. All authors read and approved the final manuscript.

Author details
[1] Division of General Internal Medicine, Department of Medicine, Montefiore Medical Center/Albert Einstein College of Medicine, 3300 Kossuth Ave, Bronx, NY 10467, USA. [2] Department of Health and Treatment Research and Analysis, The National Center on Addiction and Substance Abuse at Columbia University, 633 Third Avenue, 19th Floor, New York, NY 10017, USA. [3] Montefiore Care Management, Montefiore Medical Center, 200 Corporate Boulevard South, Yonkers, NY 10701, USA. [4] Montefiore Medical Group, Montefiore Medical Center, 305 E 161st St, Bronx, NY 10451, USA.

Competing interests
HC has served as a consultant to Merck Pharmaceuticals, Takeda Pharmaceuticals and Sunovion Pharmaceuticals. The authors declare that they have no competing interests.

Funding
This work was funded in part by research Grants from the National Institute on Drug Abuse of the National Institutes of Health (K24DA036955 and R01DA032110) and from The New York State Health Foundation (#3235651).

References
1. Saitz R. Clinical practice. Unhealthy alcohol use. N Engl J Med. 2005;352(6):596–607.
2. Stahre M, Roeber J, Kanny D, Brewer RD, Zhang X. Contribution of excessive alcohol consumption to deaths and years of potential life lost in the United States. Prev Chronic Dis. 2014;11:E109.
3. Kaner EF, Beyer F, Dickinson HO, et al. Effectiveness of brief alcohol interventions in primary care populations. Cochrane Database Syst Rev. 2007;(2):CD004148.
4. Jonas DE, Garbutt JC, Amick HR, et al. Behavioral counseling after screening for alcohol misuse in primary care: a systematic review and meta-analysis for the U.S. Preventive Services Task Force. Ann Intern Med. 2012;157(9):645–54.
5. Solberg LI, Maciosek MV, Edwards NM. Primary care intervention to reduce alcohol misuse ranking its health impact and cost effectiveness. Am J Prev Med. 2008;34(2):143–52.
6. Glass J, Bohnert K, Brown R. Alcohol screening and intervention among United States adults who attend ambulatory healthcare. J Gen Intern Med. 2016;31:739–45.
7. Nilsen P. Brief alcohol intervention—where to from here? challenges remain for research and practice. Addiction. 2010;105(6):954–9.
8. Aalto M, Pekuri P, Seppa K. Obstacles to carrying out brief intervention for heavy drinkers in primary health care: a focus group study. Drug Alcohol Rev. 2003;22(2):169–73.
9. Johnson M, Jackson R, Guillaume L, Meier P, Goyder E. Barriers and facilitators to implementing screening and brief intervention for alcohol misuse: a systematic review of qualitative evidence. J Public Health (Oxf). 2011;33(3):412–21.
10. Rahm AK, Boggs JM, Martin C, et al. Facilitators and barriers to implementing screening, brief intervention, and referral to treatment (SBIRT) in primary care in integrated health care settings. Subst Abus. 2015;36(3):281–8.
11. Sullivan LE, Tetrault JM, Braithwaite RS, Turner BJ, Fiellin DA. A meta-analysis of the efficacy of nonphysician brief interventions for unhealthy alcohol use: implications for the patient-centered medical home. Am J Addict. 2011;20(4):343–56.
12. Babor TE, Higgins-Biddle J, Dauser D, Higgins P, Burleson JA. Alcohol screening and brief intervention in primary care settings: implementation models and predictors. J Stud Alcohol. 2005;66(3):361–8.
13. Mertens JR, Chi FW, Weisner CM, et al. Physician versus non-physician delivery of alcohol screening, brief intervention and referral to treatment in adult primary care: the ADVISe cluster randomized controlled implementation trial. Addict Sci Clin Pract. 2015;10:26.
14. Harris BR, Yu J. Attitudes, perceptions and practice of alcohol and drug screening, brief intervention and referral to treatment: a case study of New York State primary care physicians and non-physician providers. Public Health. 2016;139:70–8.
15. Bright TJ, Wong A, Dhurjati R, et al. Effect of clinical decision-support systems: a systematic review. Ann Intern Med. 2012;157(1):29–43.
16. Bradley KA, Williams EC, Achtmeyer CE, Volpp B, Collins BJ, Kivlahan DR. Implementation of evidence-based alcohol screening in the Veterans Health Administration. Am J Manag Care. 2006;12(10):597–606.
17. Langley GJ, Moen R, Nolan KM, Nolan TW, Norman CL, Provost LP. The improvement guide: a practical approach to enhancing organizational performance. London: Wiley; 2009.
18. Salvalaggio G, Dong K, Vandenberghe C, et al. Enhancing screening, brief intervention, and referral to treatment among socioeconomically disadvantaged patients: study protocol for a knowledge exchange intervention involving patients and physicians. BMC Health Serv Res. 2013;13:108.
19. Bradley KA, DeBenedetti AF, Volk RJ, Williams EC, Frank D, Kivlahan DR. AUDIT-C as a brief screen for alcohol misuse in primary care. Alcohol Clin Exp Res. 2007;31(7):1208–17.
20. Bush K, Kivlahan DR, McDonell MB, Fihn SD, Bradley KA. The AUDIT alcohol consumption questions (AUDIT-C): an effective brief screening test for problem drinking. ambulatory care quality improvement project (ACQUIP). Alcohol use disorders identification test. Arch Intern Med. 1998;158(16):1789–95.
21. National Institute on Alcohol Abuse and Alcoholism. Helping patients who drink too much: a Clinician's guide (updated 2005 edition). Washington, DC: National Institutes of Health, U.S. Department of Health and Human Services; 2005.
22. Quan H, Sundararajan V, Halfon P, et al. Coding algorithms for defining comorbidities in ICD-9-CM and ICD-10 administrative data. Med Care. 2005;43(11):1130–9.
23. Williams EC, Johnson ML, Lapham GT, et al. Strategies to implement alcohol screening and brief intervention in primary care settings: a structured literature review. Psychol Addict Behav. 2011;25(2):206–14.
24. Williams EC, Achtmeyer CE, Thomas RM, et al. Factors underlying quality problems with alcohol screening prompted by a clinical reminder in primary care: a multi-site qualitative study. J Gen Intern Med. 2015;30(8):1125–32.
25. Ascherio A, Rimm EB, Giovannucci EL, et al. A prospective study of nutritional factors and hypertension among US men. Circulation. 1992;86(5):1475–84.
26. Forman JP, Stampfer MJ, Curhan GC. Diet and lifestyle risk factors associated with incident hypertension in women. JAMA. 2009;302(4):401–11.
27. McFadden CB, Brensinger CM, Berlin JA, Townsend RR. Systematic review of the effect of daily alcohol intake on blood pressure. Am J Hypertens. 2005;18(2 Pt 1):276–86.
28. Sullivan LE, Fiellin DA, O'Connor PG. The prevalence and impact of alcohol problems in major depression: a systematic review. Am J Med. 2005;118(4):330–41.
29. Howard AA, Arnsten JH, Gourevitch MN. Effect of alcohol consumption on diabetes mellitus: a systematic review. Ann Intern Med. 2004;140(3):211–9.

30. Epiquery: NYC interactive health data system—community health survey 2014. http://nyc.gov/health/epiquery. Accessed 14 Oct 2016.
31. Bradley KA, Lapham GT, Hawkins EJ, et al. Quality concerns with routine alcohol screening in VA clinical settings. J Gen Intern Med. 2011;26(3):299–306.
32. Hawkins EJ, Kivlahan DR, Williams EC, Wright SM, Craig T, Bradley KA. Examining quality issues in alcohol misuse screening. Subst Abus. 2007;28(3):53–65.
33. Williams EC, Lapham GT, Hawkins EJ, et al. Variation in documented care for unhealthy alcohol consumption across race/ethnicity in the Department of Veterans Affairs Healthcare System. Alcohol Clin Exp Res. 2012;36(9):1614–22.
34. Rose GL, Badger GJ, Skelly JM, Ferraro TA, MacLean CD, Helzer JE. A randomized controlled trial of IVR-based alcohol brief intervention to promote patient-provider communication in primary care. J Gen Intern Med. 2016;31(9):996–1003.
35. Rose GL, MacLean CD, Skelly J, Badger GJ, Ferraro TA, Helzer JE. Interactive voice response technology can deliver alcohol screening and brief intervention in primary care. J Gen Intern Med. 2010;25(4):340–4.

25

Convenience without disclosure: a formative research study of a proposed integrated methadone and antiretroviral therapy service delivery model in Dar es Salaam, Tanzania

Alexis Cooke[1*], Haneefa Saleem[2], Dorothy Mushi[3], Jessie Mbwambo[3], Saria Hassan[4] and Barrot H. Lambdin[4]

Abstract

Background: Though timely initiation of antiretroviral therapy (ART) is a vital component of effective HIV prevention, care and treatment, people who inject drugs are less likely to receive ART than their non-drug using counterparts. In an effort to increase access to ART for people who inject drugs, we examined perceived benefits, challenges, and recommendations for implementing an integrated methadone and ART service delivery model at an opioid treatment program (OTP) clinic in Dar es Salaam, Tanzania.

Methods: We conducted in-depth interviews with 12 providers and 20 HIV-positive patients at the Muhimbili National Hospital OTP clinic in early 2015. We used thematic content analysis to examine patient and provider perspectives of an integrated model.

Results: Respondents perceived that offering on-site CD4 testing and HIV clinical management at the OTP clinic would improve the timeliness and efficiency of the ART eligibility process, make HIV clinical care more convenient, mitigate stigma and discrimination in HIV care and treatment settings, and improve patient monitoring and ART adherence. However, perceived challenges included overburdened OTP clinic staff and limited space at the clinic to accommodate additional services. Limited privacy at the OTP clinic and its contribution to fear among HIV-positive patients of being stigmatized by their peers at the clinic was a common theme expressed particularly by patients, and often corroborated by providers. Co-dispensing ART and methadone at the clinic's pharmacy window was viewed as a potential deterrent for patients. Providers felt that an electronic health information system would help them better monitor patients' progress, but that this system would need to be integrated into existing health information systems. To address these potential barriers to implementing an integrated model, respondents recommended increasing OTP provider and clinic capacity, offering flexible ART dispensing options, ensuring privacy with ART dispensing, and harmonizing any new electronic health information systems with existing systems.

Conclusions: An integrated methadone and ART service delivery model at the MNH OTP clinic could improve access to HIV care and treatment for OTP patients. However, specific implementation strategies must ensure that OTP providers are not overburdened and confidentiality of patients is maintained.

*Correspondence: alexiscooke@ucla.edu
[1] Fielding School of Public Health Department of Community Health Sciences, University of California, Los Angeles, Los Angeles, CA, USA
Full list of author information is available at the end of the article

Background

An estimated 500,000 people in East Africa use opioids for non-medical reasons, and on the mainland of Tanzania, there are an estimated 30,000 people who inject drugs (PWID), primarily heroin [1, 2]. The rapid escalation of injection drug use, in the context of a generalized HIV epidemic, has resulted in a high burden of HIV among PWID. HIV prevalence among PWID in Tanzania is estimated at 35% compared to 5.1% among the general population in the country [2, 3].

Though timely initiation of antiretroviral therapy (ART) is a vital component of effective HIV prevention, care and treatment, PWID are less likely to receive ART than their non-drug using counterparts [4]. PWID consistently face barriers, such as laws and policies, which limit their access to HIV prevention and treatment interventions [5]. Where programs exist, many fail to reach those who could benefit due to requirements that make it difficult for people to enter and remain in services [6]. Individual and structural barriers, such as inadequate knowledge of ART, untreated mental illness, unstable housing, fear of criminalization, and stigmatization impact the use of HIV services among PWID [7–9]. In some settings, clinicians have delayed or withheld ART from people who use drugs for fear of non-adherence and development of drug resistance [10, 11]. As a result, only 4% of HIV-positive people who inject drugs receive ART globally [4].

To address the HIV epidemic among PWID, the government of Tanzania launched the first publicly-funded opioid treatment program (OTP) on the mainland of sub-Saharan Africa in February 2011, offering daily directly observed methadone services at Muhimbili National Hospital (MNH) in Dar es Salaam [12]. At the time of data collection, in order to be eligible for enrollment into OTP, individuals had to (1) present with opioid dependence, (2) have evidence of recent drug injection, and (3) test positive for opioids through urine screening. The estimated prevalence of HIV at 39% [13] and tuberculosis (TB) at 4% [14] among PWID enrolling into the MNH OTP clinic is over 7 and 20 times [15, 16], respectively, the prevalence in the general population. A strong body of evidence supports the integration of HIV treatment into OTPs in order to improve ART initiation and adherence, and HIV viral suppression [17–19].

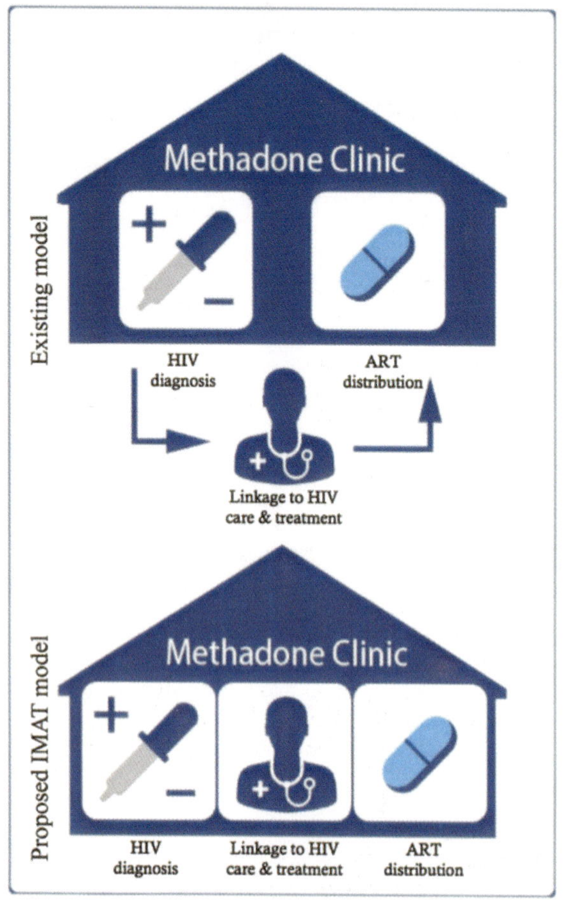

Fig. 1 Existing and proposed organization of HIV Care within the OTP clinic

Existing and proposed organization of HIV care within the MNH OTP clinic

The organization of HIV care within the MNH OTP clinic can be described in three major components: (1) HIV diagnosis, (2) linkage to HIV care and treatment, and (3) ART delivery (Fig. 1). At the time of this study, HIV care was partially integrated into the OTP clinic. For HIV diagnosis, the OTP clinic offered provider-initiated HIV testing and counseling for its patients at enrollment and after every 6 months. For linkage to HIV care and treatment, HIV-positive patients could have their blood drawn at the OTP clinic, which would be sent to the central pathology laboratory for CD4 assessment. Patients were then provided an escorted referral to the HIV care and treatment clinic at MNH, located about 500 meters from the OTP clinic on the same campus, for clinical visits to discuss CD4 results, co-morbidities, other aspects of clinical management, and to initiate people on ART once they became eligible. At the time of this study, Tanzania's national HIV management guidelines specified a CD4 count of less than 500 copies/mL to be eligible for ART [20]. Once initiated onto ART, patients could pick-up their monthly supply of ART medications from the methadone-dispensing window at the OTP clinic.

Despite daily encounters with the OTP clinic, less than half of all treatment-eligible patients at the MNH OTP clinic had initiated ART within 3 months of being deemed eligible for treatment [13]. To address delays in ART initiation and improve clinical outcomes, we proposed a more fully integrated HIV and methadone service delivery model at the MNH OTP clinic, which we called the integrated methadone and antiretroviral therapy (IMAT) model. At the time of data collection, the proposed IMAT model included four key components: (1) in-house point-of-care (POC) CD4 testing; (2) in-house HIV clinical management by OTP providers trained in comprehensive HIV management, with referrals to the HIV clinic for developing needs; (3) ART delivery through the OTP clinic; and (4) an electronic information system to help providers monitor OTP patients along the continuum of HIV care.

In this paper, we examine perceived benefits, challenges, and recommendations for the four key components of the proposed IMAT model from the perspective of patients and providers at the MNH OTP clinic as formative research, as part of a larger implementation study, to inform appropriate implementation strategies for this setting.

Methods

In February 2015, we conducted semi-structured interviews with 12 OTP clinic providers and 20 OTP patients living with HIV at the MNH OTP clinic in Dar es Salaam, Tanzania. Providers were eligible to participate if they had worked at the methadone clinic for at least 6 months. Patients were eligible to participate if they were currently enrolled in methadone treatment at the clinic, diagnosed and on record at the clinic as being HIV-positive, at least 18 years old, and willing and able to provide informed consent. We purposively sampled MNH OTP clinic providers based on job function in order to elicit insights from providers whose jobs would be directly affected by expanding HIV care and treatment services at the clinic, which included medical doctors (6), nurses (2), pharmacists (2), and social workers (2). We purposively sampled OTP patients based on sex and ART treatment status (10 women and 10 men; 10 on ART and 10 not on ART) in order to examine differences between women and men, and also between those patients who were, at the time of the interview, currently on ART and those who had not yet started ART. Among patients sampled, the median length of time enrolled at the OTP clinic was 3 years. Among those patients on ART, the median time on ART was 1 year and 4 months.

Interview guides included open-ended questions on the perceived benefits, challenges, and recommendations on strategies to further integrate HIV care, based on the four components of the proposed IMAT model, within the MNH OTP clinic. We obtained informed consent from participants before each interview. Interviews with providers were conducted in private offices in the OTP clinic, while interviews with OTP patients were conducted in a private room in a separate building at the hospital to ensure confidentiality.

Interviews were audio-recorded, transcribed word-for-word in Swahili by the research assistant who conducted the interview, and translated into English by independent, external translators. English translated transcripts were then reviewed by the original interviewer to assess for accuracy and completeness. Throughout data collection, the study team held weekly debriefing meetings to discuss emergent themes, which helped guide interview questions to further explore in subsequent interviews for an iterative data analysis process.

We adopted a thematic content analysis approach to data analysis, framed around identifying benefits, challenges and recommendations for the four proposed components of the IMAT model. The second author (HTS) developed a codebook using a priori descriptive codes based on the interview guides and other descriptive codes that emerged from an initial coding of six transcripts. A different member of the study team involved with data collection then used this codebook to code all transcripts, adding additional codes as they emerged after discussion with the second author. This study coder and the second author then conducted a second round of coding by using the first-order, descriptive codes to develop sub-codes that further categorized interview data for analysis [21]. All coding and data management were conducted using NVivo Version 11 (QSR International, Melbourne, Australia).

This study received ethical approval from the Tanzania National Institute for Medical Research, Muhimbili University of Health and Allied Sciences, and Ethical and Independent (E&I) Review Services in the United States.

Results

In-house POC CD4 testing

Both patients and providers commented that the previous process of sending blood samples to the central pathology laboratory for CD4 testing resulted in delays in ART initiation for methadone patients. An integrated model that includes POC CD4 testing and ART initiation at the MNH OTP clinic would eliminate delays resulting from off-site CD4 testing:

> *[Having CD4 testing capabilities at the methadone clinic]...would help us to control the timing of CD4 testing. You may find a client comes to you and you realize that he needs to undergo a CD4 test because he already has opportunistic diseases. But currently you have to draw blood and request to have him tested [at the central pathology laboratory]. You find you are wasting time waiting for the results. (Nurse)*

Though POC CD4 testing at the OTP clinic was widely reported among providers, in particular, as an opportunity to reduce delays in ART initiation, a few providers highlighted limited trained OTP personnel and space available at the clinic to house the machine as potential barriers to implementation and recommended increasing the number of OTP personnel trained in administering the CD4 tests and the clinic capacity to accommodate any new services. As one doctor at the OTP clinic explained:

[H]uman resources are very important to increase so that the services are maintained as they were before. Because you can't ask a person who was dressing [wounds] to dress [wounds] and at the same time to [administer a] CD4 [test], you see? But if there is another person allocated for that activity, it would be good. (Doctor)

In-house HIV clinical management

Integrating HIV clinical management at the OTP clinic, to create a "one-stop shop," was perceived by OTP patients as improving access to HIV care and treatment services, by making these services more convenient for patients. Mostly patients, though a few providers as well, reported having to seek HIV care and treatment at off-site HIV clinics as a deterrent for many OTP patients from initiating and adhering to ART medication, partly due to overcrowding. As one patient described:

Someone might go [to the HIV clinic] for treatment and find a long line with many people. He might think, "I'm late for my personal activities. I'll come back tomorrow." Tomorrow again he comes and finds the same long line: "Ah, let me come back tomorrow." And when you stay three days without taking ARTs, I heard there is a problem because every day you have to get your medicine. So [an integrated methadone and ART model] would help in some way. (Female patient on ART)

Another patient elaborated further:

At the HIV clinic, I don't know, most [methadone patients] when they are told to go and get medication, they say there is a long queue with a lot of disturbances. But I think that if [HIV treatment] services are brought here, most of [patients] would make the sacrifice themselves and decide to take [ARTs]. It would be faster. (Female patient on ART)

Stigma due to a history of opioid use and addiction was also reported by patients and providers as a deterrent to HIV care-seeking among OTP patients. Many patients and providers expressed that an integrated model of care would reduce OTP patients' exposure to stigma and discrimination when seeking HIV care and treatment at off-site HIV clinics, and ultimately increase their access to these services. Patients and providers hinted that the stigma encountered by OTP patients at outside HIV clinics was not just from other HIV-positive patients seeking care, but also HIV clinic providers. As one provider explained:

I am among those who fought for ART and methadone to be offered simultaneously [at the OTP clinic]. The first reason, I observed high rates of stigma when we started to offer methadone. We didn't have ART in our clinic; we did not have it in our pharmacy. What was happening was after we diagnosed [someone with] HIV and if that person was eligible to start ART, we referred that person to the [off-site] HIV clinic... For [patients] this was a big problem... They were being labeled and stigmatized. There was offensive and stigmatizing language that made many of them discontinue [HIV care and treatment]. And in the beginning, most did not use ART for that reason. (Senior doctor)

Many clinical personnel at the OTP clinic are trained mental health specialists, with primary appointments in the hospital's psychiatry and mental health ward. They have experience caring for patients with histories of opioid use and behavioral disorders. Many OTP patients expressed positive feelings toward the care they receive from providers at the OTP clinic, and viewed this as an advantage to receiving additional HIV clinical services as part of the proposed IMAT model at the OTP clinic:

I: [W]hat would be the advantages of getting HIV services from [the OTP clinic] rather than going somewhere else in the hospital or another hospital?
R: I mean, like here [at the OTP clinic] we are family. There is nothing like discrimination or humiliation. So it would be a relief for us because [the OTP providers] know us. (Female patient on ART)

Providers perceived that an integrated model at the OTP clinic could improve access and adherence to HIV treatment:

Many of our clients would agree to receive those HIV services because right now the majority refuses because HIV services are rendered from another clinic different from ours here. So I think many more would agree to start ARTs and they would agree to get those services because they are offered from one place. (Senior doctor)

According to providers, offering expanded HIV treatment services at the OTP clinic would not only make it easier for patients to initiate and remain on ARTs, but would also allow providers to better move patients along the HIV continuum of care by being more involved in and aware of their care.

The opportunities to increase access to HIV care and treatment among OTP patients that would be afforded by more fully integrating HIV clinical care at the OTP clinic were often expressed by providers alongside the need to adequately train OTP providers in the clinical management of HIV-positive patients and to take into consideration the current high volume of patients seen on a daily basis at the OTP clinic.

ART delivery through the OTP clinic

In the proposed IMAT model, ARTs would be co-dispensed at the pharmacy window where methadone is currently dispensed. Patients, especially, but providers as well, were concerned that the lack of privacy at the OTP clinic window (where patients take their methadone) could result in unintended HIV status disclosures to their fellow patients since the pharmacy windows at the OTP clinic are open to the waiting area:

> *I think this service needs to continue being confidential because most of them stigmatize. So there if you dispense from the window, it is when people [other OTP patients] will see that someone has what, has AIDS. And you should know that the patient's secret is between himself and the doctor. Now there you reveal it out for everyone to know. (Male patient not on ART)*

The disclosure of one's HIV status through a lack of privacy at the pharmacy window could result in stigma and discrimination by peers, as one patient explained:

> *It's not good because when someone finds out that you are infected, know that fingers will be pointed towards you. "Ah there he goes. He is taking medicine! There he goes!" Because now I am infected. Someone has only a chest problem and they talk about him. What about me who is infected [with HIV]? And again there is the issue of love. We fall in love among ourselves. So you see that if my lover sees me taking pills there at the window, that container, she would stare at me. She wouldn't love me anymore. She would run away from me. You see? For that small thing, stigma would persist. (Male patient on ARTs)*

As a way of addressing the privacy issues at the clinic's pharmacy window, patients echoed recommendations also made by providers to dispense ARTs in a separate, more private location at the OTP clinic to mitigate HIV-related stigma. When asked how to maintain confidentiality when offering ART at the clinic, one patient responded:

> *If someone knows your problem, it becomes a caning stick to you. Another window is required so that other people won't know what you are going to do or even to know that you are going there. You would just know yourself. (Female patient on ART)*

Patients also reported ART medication adherence as a potential challenge to co-dispensing ART medications and methadone in light of current clinic policies regarding late arrivals. Methadone is dispensed at the OTP clinic daily from 6 a.m. to 11 a.m. If a patient arrives after clinic dispensing hours, according to clinic policies, she or he is denied his or her methadone dose: "If you come late, they do not receive you. Which means if you miss a methadone dose, then you would have to miss an ART dose [as well]." (Male client not on ART) This was viewed as particularly problematic given the gravity of non-adherence to ART medication.

Patients, especially, expressed that if the proposed IMAT model is implemented at the OTP clinic, then there should be flexibility in clinic policies regarding ART dosing and dispensing. Methadone is administered once daily in the morning at the OTP clinic, however some patients reported a preference to take ART medications in the evening, in the privacy of their homes, or at a time they might be more likely to have food. An option for take-home dosing of ART medications—such as a monthly supply of medication as practiced at HIV clinics—rather than daily, observed therapy was described by patients as another option for ART dosing and dispensing to ensure privacy. One patient reported his preference for take-home dosing:

> *For me it is better because I take my [ART] pills [home]. I drink my [methadone], I take my pills and leave with them. Because I cannot take my pills [at the OTP clinic]. (Male patient on ART)*

Lack of privacy at the OTP clinic and its contribution to fear among HIV-positive patients of being stigmatized by their peers at the clinic because of their HIV status was a common theme expressed particularly by patients interviewed, and often corroborated by providers.

> *There is no privacy for patients, so it becomes a problem. So if people see him coming to the window for [ART] medicines, then it would be a problem. So there is the possibility that some may stop [coming to the OTP clinic] due to stigma. And so there is a need for privacy. (Pharmacist)*

Co-dispensing ART medications with methadone as part of the proposed IMAT model at the OTP clinic was also perceived by OTP providers as adding more work for already overburdened OTP clinic personnel, and might, consequently, lead to delays in ART, as well as methadone, delivery at the clinic.

To dispense methadone, I have to observe his behavior: has he taken alcohol; has he smoked weed; does he have a behavior that is not appropriate. It is very important that he is observed so that he can be assisted. Now when I am through observing him, I give him methadone. It takes like three minutes to do those observations, but later on I would need to give him ART medicine. He would need to go around to the window so that I could give him his medicine. So it may start to delay the rendering of services. (Pharmacist)

Electronic health information system to track OTP patients along the HIV care continuum

One of the proposed components of the IMAT model at the OTP clinic was an electronic health information system that would serve as a platform to: (1) store patients' HIV-related data, such as HIV testing, ART testing, and treatment results and status updates; (2) send out alerts to providers on any required testing needed; and (3) remind providers of the next steps to take to move patients along the continuum. Most providers reported that this type of electronic system would help them to better monitor patients' progress along the HIV continuum of care in real time and more effectively manage their HIV care, compared to the existing paper-based system, by improving their ability to quickly retrieve and access important patient HIV-related data to make clinical decisions. Yet providers stressed that OTP clinic's electronic health information system for managing HIV-positive patients would need to be harmonized with the existing methadone treatment data available at the clinic.

But if they could find a way to harmonize the information about HIV/AIDS [with the existing methadone data] it would be easy because the information would flow in the same manner. So when I open it, I would know now he is at a certain dosage of methadone, this one's CD4 information was taken on this date, okay, he has already started ART and is doing fine and he is due for another CD4 test... in general, to see progress and treatment failure. (Doctor)

Providers also recommended ensuring that any electronic HIV-related alert-and-reminder health information system adopted by the OTP clinic be interoperable with existing laboratory and national HIV electronic health information systems currently used at the hospital.

Providers perceived barriers to adopting an electronic health information system at the OTP clinic to manage the HIV care of patients that would need to be addressed when developing specific implementation strategies and protocols for the IMAT model. Electrical power outages were reported as sporadically occurring at the OTP clinic, which could affect the ability of OTP providers responsible for the management of HIV care of patients to access the information necessary to make clinical decisions. Problems with the computer server being down could also limit timely access to patient data. Providers revealed how the computer server that provided data sharing capabilities to the OTP clinic for managing patient's methadone treatment was non-functional for over a year. As a result, OTP providers had to revert back to using paper-based forms, which made retrieving and accessing patient data difficult and time-consuming. In light of this, some providers recommended developing plans and protocols for maintaining and repairing the electronic health information system and its associated equipment, when needed:

There should be a good system that when it is broken, maybe there should be a technician or someone who will be close to take care of it, so that when they are broken, they can be fixed and the service continues instantly, and not that the service should be halted for a long time. (Senior Doctor)

In concurrence with the cross-cutting theme around issues of privacy and confidentiality with fully integrating HIV services at the OTP clinic, to maintain patient-provider confidentiality a provider also recommended that security access certificates be provided to OTP providers based on the patient information required to carry out their assigned clinic duties.

Discussion

This study described the perceived benefits, challenges and recommendations for implementation regarding the integration of HIV care into the OTP clinic at Muhimbili National Hospital. Our findings highlight the importance of integrating HIV care into the OTP clinic setting in order to reduce stigma and discrimination and leverage the compassionate care offered by OTP clinic providers. However, specific attention will be needed to structure services so that providers are not overburdened and confidentiality regarding patients' HIV status is maintained.

At the time of data collection there were 17 clinicians, 6 postgraduate residents (that serve on a rotating basis) along with 3 nurses, 4 pharmacists and 3 social workers that served the OTP clinic. While the addition of HIV care and treatment would add to provider work responsibilities, the addition of these services alone would not increase the number of patients enrolled at the OTP clinic. The combination of OTP and HIV services would help to address patient concerns around the time required to receive both kinds of care. However, providers recognized the clinic level changes that would be needed to make these changes. Providers also felt that for integration to be successful, they would need a system to manage and monitor patient care, which would be fully functional and include technical assistance. Findings from this study have been used to inform the development of a model to integrate HIV care into OTP in Dar es Salaam, Tanzania.

The management of HIV among people who use drugs is key to addressing the intersecting epidemics of HIV and drug use [4]. This is especially important as existing research has demonstrated the spread of injection drug use in East Africa, along with a high burden of HIV [13, 22]. It is, therefore, critical to develop HIV care models that will facilitate utilization of HIV services for this key population. Engaging OTP patients who would access and providers who would implement HIV care and treatment is critical to build delivery approaches that factor in culture and context and respond to the needs of communities that interact with them [23]. The ability of OTP providers to care for patients is especially relevant as other (non-OTP) clinicians may be resistant to working with PWID. This creates an environment at the OTP clinic conducive to compassionate care based on respect for patients and that acknowledges their unique vulnerabilities and struggles.

Previous research conducted at the MNH OTP clinic has identified challenges around initiating HIV-positive OTP patients onto ART, including delays in CD4 testing, the inconvenience of off-site HIV clinics, and stigma [12]. The IMAT model was refined through this research to address many of the challenges identified with the intention of improving the provision of HIV care for OTP patients. OTP providers (clinicians and nurses) have medical expertise that can be enhanced with additional training to provide HIV care and treatment. HIV-positive OTP clients are familiar with, and comfortable in, the OTP clinic environment where they feel respected by OTP providers. For these reasons, the IMAT model is, potentially, a more feasible intervention than providing OTP in existing HIV clinics.

Patients and providers were broadly supportive of integrating HIV care into the OTP clinic. As a health service model, OTPs can facilitate the improvement of health-related outcomes for their patients and have proven to be a successful venue for treatment of infectious diseases such as HIV [24–27]. Additionally, research shows that combining OTPs, such as methadone maintenance, and ART is both cost effective and helps care providers to monitor and observe patient treatment [28]. OTP clinics in Tanzania provide a unique opportunity for comprehensive HIV care to this high-risk population for several reasons. First, the HIV burden among PWID is 7-fold greater than what is observed in the general population [13]. Second, methadone helps to stabilize PWID and can facilitate adherence and completion of treatment regimens [29, 30]. Third, methadone treatment decreases injecting behaviors and therefore decreases transmission and the potential for reinfection. Fourth, OTP providers are perfectly positioned to provide culturally competent services for PWID, compared to most other health care providers, and can assist in the cultivation of a welcoming environment for the provision of services. Fifth, as the majority of patients present daily for their methadone dose, OTP clinics are ideal venues to administer once-daily medication, monitor treatment, and provide proper follow-up care, including risk prevention counseling.

Researchers have engaged communities of interests in the interpretation of findings, to translate research findings into implementation strategies [31, 32]. Key stakeholders, including patients, community outreach workers, providers, and policymakers, played a key role in interpreting this study's findings and shaping the final design of the IMAT service delivery model through community and partner engagement meetings. For example, as part of the proposed IMAT strategy we originally planned to train two dedicated HIV care and treatment specialists within the OTP clinic. However, in light of feedback provided by key stakeholders during the engagement meetings, we realized that the original approach might be too limiting and that it would be more beneficial to build HIV care and treatment capabilities among more clinicians, including both physicians and nurses, within the OTP clinic to prevent increasing the workload and overburdening individual providers. Training several clinicians would also provide flexibility in scheduling patients for clinical visits and follow-up consultations, increasing the capacity of the MNH OTP clinic to provide HIV care to patients.

Perhaps the greatest concern of the patients and providers interviewed for the study was maintaining confidentiality regarding their HIV status. This concern was echoed during the community and partner engagement meetings. OTP patients concerns around HIV serostatus disclosure should be especially respected in terms of non-discrimination related to HIV care and treatment; however, this can be a problem in the context of non-disclosure to sex partners. Fear of inadvertent disclosure by accessing HIV care within an integrated setting has been previously reported in the literature [33]. To address this concern, the revised IMAT strategy allows patients to select one of three ART dispensing models: (1) directly administered ART by a clinician in a private setting, (2) directly administered ART at the methadone dispensing window, or (3) monthly supplies of ART, which is the standard of care in Tanzania.

This study has limitations. We only interviewed patients currently enrolled and providers working at the MNH OTP clinic. Patients who have defaulted or who were not currently enrolled in care for other reasons may have very different perspectives around these issues. The MNH OTP clinic is one of four OTP clinics in Tanzania. Findings from this study and the integrated HIV and methadone delivery model that was developed to address some of the challenges and recommendations identified by participants, may not be applicable to the other OTP clinics given the high-level of resources available at the MNH OTP clinic.

Conclusions

Building on our previous implementation science research [12, 13, 23, 33–38], this study sought examine how to best integrate HIV services into the MNH OTP clinic from the perspectives of OTP patients and providers. Our findings suggest broad support from patients and providers regarding integrating HIV care within OTP, but highlight that implementation strategies must ensure that the confidentiality of patients is maintained with an integrated model. As this study examined perceptions regarding a proposed integrated care model, future implementation research will focus on understanding the implementation of the integrated model and its impact on improved access to HIV services for OTP patients.

Abbreviations

PWID: people who inject drugs; ART: antiretroviral therapy; OPT: opioid treatment program; MNH: Muhimbili National Hospital; TB: tuberculosis; IMAT: integrated methadone and anti-retroviral therapy initiative; POC: point-of-care.

Authors' contributions

AC and HS analyzed interview data using thematic context analysis. Manuscript preparation was divided between AC and HS. Feedback and editing was provided by DM JM and BL, who contributed greatly to manuscript development. All authors read and approved the final manuscript.

Author details

[1] Fielding School of Public Health Department of Community Health Sciences, University of California, Los Angeles, Los Angeles, CA, USA. [2] Department of International Health, Johns Hopkins Bloomberg School of Public Health, 615 North Wolfe Street, E5033, Baltimore, MD 21205, USA. [3] Department of Psychiatry, Muhimbili University of Health and Allied Sciences, P.O. Box 65293, Dar es Salaam, Tanzania. [4] Behavioral Health and Criminal Justice Research Division, RTI International, 351 California Street, Suite 500, San Francisco, CA 94104, USA.

Acknowledgements

We would like to thank all research participants and our research assistants.

Competing interests

The authors declare that they have no competing interests.

Funding

This research was supported by the National Institutes of Health, National Institute on Drug Abuse.

References

1. Csete J, Kamarulzaman A, Kazatchkine M, Altice F, Balicki M, Buxton J, et al. Public health and international drug policy. Lancet. 2016;387:1427–80.
2. Dutta A, Barker C, Makyao N. Consensus estimates on key population size and HIV prevalence in Tanzania. National AIDS Control Programme (NACP), Ministry of Health and Social Welfare; 2014.
3. Tanzania Commission for AIDS (TACAIDS), Zanzibar AIDS Commission (ZAC), National Bureau of Statistics (NBS), Office of the Chief Government Statistician (OCGS), and ICF International 2013. Tanzania HIV/AIDS and Malaria Indicator Survey 2011–12. Dar es Salaam, Tanzania: TACAIDS, ZAC, NBS, OCGS, and ICF International.
4. Mathers BM, Degenhardt L, Ali H, Wiessing L, Hickman M, Mattick RP, et al. HIV prevention, treatment, and care services for people who inject drugs: a systematic review of global, regional, and national coverage. Lancet. 2010;375:1014–28.
5. Gruskin S, Ferguson L, Alfven T, Rugg D, Peersman G. Identifying structural barriers to an effective HIV response: using the National Composite Policy Index data to evaluate the human rights, legal and policy environment. J Int AIDS Soc 2013;16(1):18000. doi:10.7448/IAS.16.1.18000.
6. Keeney E, Saucier R. Lowering the threshold: models of accessible methadone and buprenorphine treatment. New York: Open Society Institute; 2010.
7. Mimiaga MJ, Safren SA, Dvoryak S, Reisner SL, Needle R, Woody G. "We fear the police, and the police fear us": structural and individual barriers and facilitators to HIV medication adherence among injection drug users in Kiev, Ukraine. AIDS Care. 2010;22:1305–13.
8. Wood E, Kerr T, Tyndall MW, Montaner JS. A review of barriers and facilitators of HIV treatment among injection drug users. AIDS. 2008;22:1247–56.
9. Krüsi A, Wood E, Montaner J, Kerr T. Social and structural determinants of HAART access and adherence among injection drug users. Int J Drug Policy. 2010;21:4–9.
10. Wolfe D, Carrieri MP, Shepard D. Treatment and care for injecting drug users with HIV infection: a review of barriers and ways forward. Lancet. 2010;376:355–66.
11. Rhodes T, Sarang A. Drug treatment and the conditionality of HIV treatment access: a qualitative study in a Russian city. Addiction. 2012;107:1827–36.
12. Lambdin BH, Masao F, Chang O, Kaduri P, Mbwambo J, Magimba A, et al. Methadone treatment for HIV prevention—feasibility, retention, and predictors of attrition in Dar es Salaam, Tanzania: a retrospective cohort study. Clin Infect Dis. 2014;59:735–42.
13. Tran OC, Bruce RD, Masao F, Ubuguyu O, Sabuni N, Mbwambo J, et al. Implementation and operational research: linkage to care among methadone clients living with HIV in Dar es Salaam, Tanzania. J Acquir Immune Defic Syndr. 2015;69:e43–8.
14. Gupta A, Mbwambo J, Mteza I, Shenoi S, Lambdin B, Nyandindi C, et al. Active case finding for tuberculosis among people who inject drugs on methadone treatment in Dar es Salaam, Tanzania. Int J Tuberc Lung Dis. 2014;18:793–8.
15. Global AIDS Response Country Progress Report. Tanzania Commission for AIDS; 2014. http://www.unaids.org/sites/default/files/country/documents/TZA_narrative_report_2014.pdf. Accessed 11 Oct 2016.
16. Global Tuberculosis Report. World Health Organization; 2012. http://apps.who.int/iris/bitstream/10665/75938/1/9789241564502_eng.pdf. Accessed 11 Oct 2016.
17. Milloy M, Kerr T, Buxton J, Rhodes T, Guillemi S, Hogg R, et al. Dose-response effect of incarceration events on nonadherence to HIV antiretroviral therapy among injection drug users. J Infect Dis. 2011;203:1215–21.
18. Palepu A, Tyndall MW, Joy R, Kerr T, Wood E, Press N, et al. Antiretroviral adherence and HIV treatment outcomes among HIV/HCV co-infected injection drug users: the role of methadone maintenance therapy. Drug Alcohol Depend. 2006;84:188–94.
19. Sullivan LE, Barry D, Moore BA, Chawarski MC, Tetrault JM, Pantalon MV, et al. A trial of integrated buprenorphine/naloxone and HIV clinical care. Clin Infect Dis. 2006;43(Supplement 4):S184–90.

20. National Guidelines for the Management of HIV and AIDS. The United Republic of Tanzania Ministry of Health and Social Welfare National Aids Control Programme; 2015. https://aidsfree.usaid.gov/sites/default/files/04_11_2016.tanzania_national_guideline_for_management_hiv_and_aids_may_2015._tagged.pdf. Accessed 11 Oct 2016.
21. Green LW, Kreuter MW. Health program planning: an educational and ecological approach. Boston: McGraw-Hill Companies; 2005.
22. Miles MB, Huberman A, Saldaña J. Qualitative data analysis: a methods sourcebook, Califorinia. Thousand Oaks: SAGE Publications, Inc.; 2014.
23. Kurth AE, Cleland CM, Des Jarlais DC, Musyoki H, Lizcano JA, Chhun N, et al. HIV prevalence, estimated incidence, and risk behaviors among people who inject drugs in Kenya. J Acquir Immune Defic Syndr. 2015;70:420–7.
24. Lambdin BH, Cheng B, Peter T, Mbwambo J, Apollo T, Dunbar M, et al. Implementing implementation science: an approach for HIV prevention, care and treatment programs. Curr HIV Res. 2015;13:244–6.
25. Kresina TF, Lubran R. Improving public health through access to and utilization of medication assisted treatment. Int J Environ Res Public Health. 2011;8:4102–17.
26. Lin C, Li L, Cao X. Client acceptability for integrating antiretroviral therapy in methadone maintenance therapy clinics in Sichuan, China. Subst Use Misuse. 2017;52(1):119–126.
27. Bachireddy C, Soule MC, Izenberg JM, Dvoryak S, Dumchev K, Altice FL. Integration of health services improves multiple healthcare outcomes among HIV-infected people who inject drugs in Ukraine. Drug Alcohol Depend. 2014;134:106–14.
28. Lucas GM, Mullen BA, Weidle PJ, Hader S, McCaul ME, Moore RD. Directly administered antiretroviral therapy in methadone clinics is associated with improved HIV treatment outcomes, compared with outcomes among concurrent comparison groups. Clin Infect Dis. 2006;42:1628–35.
29. Tran BX, Ohinmaa A, Duong AT, Nguyen LT, Vu PX, Mills S, et al. Cost-effectiveness of integrating methadone maintenance and antiretroviral treatment for HIV-positive drug users in Vietnam's injection-driven HIV epidemics. Drug Alcohol Depend. 2012;125:260–6.
30. Spire B, Lucas GM, Carrieri MP. Adherence to HIV treatment among IDUs and the role of opioid substitution treatment (OST). Int J Drug Policy. 2007;18:262–70.
31. Kapadia F, Vlahov D, Wu Y, Cohen MH, Greenblatt RM, Howard AA, et al. Impact of drug abuse treatment modalities on adherence to ART/HAART among a cohort of HIV seropositive women. Am J Drug Alcohol Abuse. 2008;34:161–70.
32. Cashman SB, Adeky S, Allen AJ III, Corburn J, Israel BA, Montaño J, et al. The power and the promise: working with communities to analyze data, interpret findings, and get to outcomes. Am J Public Health. 2008;98:1407–17.
33. Edelman EJ, Cole CA, Richardson W, Boshnack N, Jenkins H, Rosenthal MS. Stigma, substance use and sexual risk behaviors among HIV-infected men who have sex with men: a qualitative study. Prev Med Rep. 2016;3:296–302.
34. Saleem HT, Mushi D, Hassan S, Douglas Bruce R, Cooke A, Mbwambo J, et al. "Can't you initiate me here?" Challenges to timely initiation on antiretroviral therapy among methadone clients in Dar es Salaam, Tanzania. Int J Drug Policy. 2015. doi:10.1016/j.drugpo.2015.12.009.
35. Zamudio-Haas S, Mahenge B, Saleem H, Mbwambo J, Lambdin BH. Generating trust: programmatic strategies to reach women who inject drugs with harm reduction services in Dar es Salaam, Tanzania. Int J Drug Policy. 2016;30:43–51.
36. Lambdin BH, Nyandindi C, Bruce D, Sabuni N, Magimba A, Matiko E. Low threshold services for females who inject drugs: reducing gender inequities in methadone enrolment. J Int AIDS Soc. Int AIDS Society Avenue de France 23, Geneva, 1202, Switzerland; 2015.
37. Lambdin BH, Mbwamb JK, Josiah RM, Bruce RD. Service integration: opportunities to expand access to antiretroviral therapy for people who inject drugs in Tanzania. J Int AIDS Soc 2015;18(1):19936. doi:10.7448/IAS.18.1.19936.
38. Lambdin BH, Bruce RD, Chang O, Nyandindi C, Sabuni N, Zamudio-Haas S, et al. Identifying programmatic gaps: inequities in harm reduction service utilization among male and female drug users in Dar es Salaam, Tanzania. PLoS ONE. 2013;8:e67062.

Permissions

All chapters in this book were first published in AS&CP, by BioMed Central; hereby published with permission under the Creative Commons Attribution License or equivalent. Every chapter published in this book has been scrutinized by our experts. Their significance has been extensively debated. The topics covered herein carry significant findings which will fuel the growth of the discipline. They may even be implemented as practical applications or may be referred to as a beginning point for another development.

The contributors of this book come from diverse backgrounds, making this book a truly international effort. This book will bring forth new frontiers with its revolutionizing research information and detailed analysis of the nascent developments around the world.

We would like to thank all the contributing authors for lending their expertise to make the book truly unique. They have played a crucial role in the development of this book. Without their invaluable contributions this book wouldn't have been possible. They have made vital efforts to compile up to date information on the varied aspects of this subject to make this book a valuable addition to the collection of many professionals and students.

This book was conceptualized with the vision of imparting up-to-date information and advanced data in this field. To ensure the same, a matchless editorial board was set up. Every individual on the board went through rigorous rounds of assessment to prove their worth. After which they invested a large part of their time researching and compiling the most relevant data for our readers.

The editorial board has been involved in producing this book since its inception. They have spent rigorous hours researching and exploring the diverse topics which have resulted in the successful publishing of this book. They have passed on their knowledge of decades through this book. To expedite this challenging task, the publisher supported the team at every step. A small team of assistant editors was also appointed to further simplify the editing procedure and attain best results for the readers.

Apart from the editorial board, the designing team has also invested a significant amount of their time in understanding the subject and creating the most relevant covers. They scrutinized every image to scout for the most suitable representation of the subject and create an appropriate cover for the book.

The publishing team has been an ardent support to the editorial, designing and production team. Their endless efforts to recruit the best for this project, has resulted in the accomplishment of this book. They are a veteran in the field of academics and their pool of knowledge is as vast as their experience in printing. Their expertise and guidance has proved useful at every step. Their uncompromising quality standards have made this book an exceptional effort. Their encouragement from time to time has been an inspiration for everyone.

The publisher and the editorial board hope that this book will prove to be a valuable piece of knowledge for researchers, students, practitioners and scholars across the globe.

List of Contributors

Alex H. S. Harris, Thomas Bowe, Andrea Nevedal, Andrea K. Finlay, Risha Gidwani and Craig Rosen
Center for Innovation to Implementation, Health Services Research and Development, VA Palo Alto Health Care System, Menlo Park, CA, USA

Hildi Hagedorn
Center for Chronic Disease Outcomes Research, Health Services Research and Development, VA Minneapolis Health Care System, Minneapolis, MN, USA

Chad Kay and Melissa Christopher
Pharmacy Benefits M anagement, Academic Detailing Program, VA San Diego Health Care System, San Diego, CA, USA

Kelley Saia
Department of Obstetrics and Gynecology, Boston University School of Medicine, 85 East Concord Street, Boston, MA 02118, USA

Sarah M. Bagley
Section of General Internal Medicine, Boston University School of Medicine, Boston, MA, USA
Department of Pediatrics, Boston University School of Medicine, Boston, MA, USA

Elisha M. Wachman
Department of Pediatrics, Boston University School of Medicine, Boston, MA, USA

Payal P. Patel
Harvard Vanguard Medical Associates, Newton Wellesley Hospital, Newton, MA, USA

Marisa D. Nadas
Department of Obstetrics and Gynecology, Albert Einstein College of Medicine, Bronx, NY, USA

Susan B. Brogly
Department of Surgery, Queen's University, Kingston, Canada

Anna Lembke
Department of Psychiatry and Behavioral Sciences, Stanford University School of Medicine, 401 Quarry Road, Stanford, CA 94306, USA

Niushen Zhang
Department of Neurology, Stanford University School of Medicine, Stanford, CA 94306, USA

Christopher J. Cutter, Cheryl Danton and Patrick G. O'Connor
Yale University School of Medicine, 367 Cedar Street, ESH A, New Haven, CT 06510, USA

E. Jennifer Edelman, Lynn E. Fiellin and David A. Fiellin
Yale University School of Medicine, 367 Cedar Street, ESH A, New Haven, CT 06510, USA
Center for Interdisciplinary Research On AIDS, Yale University School of Public Health, 135 College Street, New Haven, CT 06510, USA

Nathan B. Hansen
Center for Interdisciplinary Research On AIDS, Yale University School of Public Health, 135 College Street, New Haven, CT 06510, USA
College of Public Health, University of Georgia, 131 Wright Hall, Health Sciences Campus, Athens, GA 30602, USA

Emily C. Williams
VA Puget Sound Health Care System, Center of Innovation for Veteran-Centered and Value-Driven Care, 1100 Olive Way, Suite 1400, Seattle, WA 98101, USA
Department of Health Services, University of Washington, 1959 NE Pacific S treet, Magnuson Health Sciences Center, Room H-664, Seattle, WA 98195, USA

Stephen A. Maisto
Syracuse University, 430 Huntington Hall, Syracuse, NY 13244, USA

Kendall J. Bryant
National Institute on Alcohol Abuse and Alcoholism HIV/AIDS Program, 5635 Fishers Lane, Bethesda, MD 20892-7003, USA

Blair Beadnell1 and Pamela A. Stafford
Prevention Research Institute, 841 Corporate Drive, Suite 300, Lexington, KY 40503, USA

Michele A. Crisafulli
University of Maryland, Baltimore County, 1000 Hilltop Circle, Baltimore, MD 21250, USA

Erin A. Casey
Social Work Program, University of Washington (Tacoma), 1900 Commerce Street, Box 358425, Tacoma, WA 98402, USA

Daniel M Blonigen
Center for Innovation to Implementation, Veterans Affairs Palo Alto Health Care System, 795 Willow Road (152-MPD), Menlo Park, CA 94025, USA
Family Research Center, VA Palo Alto Health Care System, 795 Willow Road (152-MPD), Menlo Park, CA 94025, USA

Christine Timko and Rudolf H Moos
Center for Innovation to Implementation, Veterans Affairs Palo Alto Health Care System, 795 Willow Road (152-MPD), Menlo Park, CA 94025, USA
Department of Psychiatry and Behavioral Sciences, Stanford University School of Medicine, 401 Quarry Road, Palo Alto, CA 94304, USA

Theodore Jacob
Family Research Center, VA Palo Alto Health Care System, 795 Willow Road (152-MPD), Menlo Park, CA 94025, USA
Palo Alto University, 1791 Arastradero Road, Palo Alto, CA 94304, USA

Leen Naji
Michael Degroote School of Medicine, McMaster University, Hamilton, Canada

Monica Bawor
St. George's University of London, London, UK.

Guillaume Pare
Department of Clinical Epidemiology and Biostatistics, McMaster University, Hamilton, Canada

Brittany Burns Dennis
St. George's University of London, London, UK.
Department of Clinical Epidemiology and Biostatistics, McMaster University, Hamilton, Canada

Michael Varenbut, Jeff Daiter, Carolyn Plater
Canadian Addiction Treatment Centres, Richmond Hill, Canada

David C. Marsh
Canadian Addiction Treatment Centres, Richmond Hill, Canada
Northern Ontario School of Medicine, Sudbury, ON, Canada

Andrew Worster
Canadian Addiction Treatment Centres, Richmond Hill, Canada
Department of Medicine, Hamilton General Hospital, Hamilton, Canada

Dipika Desai
Population Genomic Program, Chanchalani Research Centre, McMaster University, Hamilton, Canada

Zainab Samaan
Department of Clinical Epidemiology and Biostatistics, McMaster University, Hamilton, Canada
Population Genomic Program, Chanchalani Research Centre, McMaster University, Hamilton, Canada
Peter Boris Centre for Addictions Research, Hamilton, Canada
Department of Psychiatry and Behavioural Neuroscience, McMaster University, 100 West 5th Street, Hamilton, ON L8N 3K7, Canada

Lehana Thabane
Departments of Pediatrics and Anesthesia, McMaster University, Hamilton, Canada
Centre for Evaluation of Medicine, St Joseph's Healthcare, Hamilton, Canada
Biostatistics Unit, Father Sean O'Sullivan Research Centre, St Joseph's Healthcare, Hamilton, Canada

James MacKillop
Peter Boris Centre for Addictions Research, Hamilton, Canada
Department of Psychiatry and Behavioural Neuroscience, McMaster University, 100 West 5th Street, Hamilton, ON L8N 3K7, Canada

Karen Chan Osilla, David P. Kennedy, Sarah B. Hunter and Ervant Maksabedian
RAND Corporation, 1776 Main Street, Santa Monica, CA 90407-2138, USA

Wendee M. Wechsberg
Substance Use, Gender and Applied Research, RTI International, 3040 East
Cornwallis Road, Research Triangle Park, NC 27709-2194, USA

Health Policy and Management, UNC Gillings School of Global Public Health, Chapel Hill, NC, USA
Department of Psychology, North Carolina State University, Raleigh, NC, USA
Psychiatry and Behavioral Sciences, Duke University School of Medicine, Durham, NC, USA

Felicia A. Browne and William A. Zule
Substance Use, Gender and Applied Research, RTI International, 3040 East Cornwallis Road, Research Triangle Park, NC 27709-2194, USA

Charles van der Horst
School of Medicine, University of North Carolina, Chapel Hill, NC, USA

Jacqueline Ndirangu
Substance Use, Gender and Applied Research, RTI International, Pretoria, South Africa

Irene A. Doherty
UCB Biosciences, Raleigh, NC, USA

Tracy Kline
Statistics and Epidemiology, RTI International, 3040 East Cornwallis Road, Research Triangle Park, NC 27709-2194, USA

Jennifer M. Belus
Psychology Department, University of North Carolina, Chapel Hill, NC, USA

Robin Nance
Biostatistics, School of Public Health, University of Washington, 1410 NE Campus Parkway, Seattle, WA, USA

Edwin D. Boudreaux
Departments of Emergency Medicine, Psychiatry, and Quantitative Health Sciences, University of Massachusetts Medical School, LA-189, 55 Lake Avenue North, Worcester, MA 01655, USA

Beau Abar
Departments of Emergency Medicine, Psychiatry, and Public Health Sciences, University of Rochester Medical Center, Rochester, NY, USA

Brianna Haskins
Department of Emergency Medicine, University of Massachusetts Medical School, Worcester, MA, USA

Brigitte Bauman
Department of Emergency Medicine, Cooper Medical School of Rowan University, Camden, NJ, USA

Grant Grissom
Polaris Health Directions, Inc, Langhorne, PA, USA

Christina Nehlin and Caisa Öster
Department of Neuroscience, Psychiatry, Uppsala University, UAS ing 10, 75185 Uppsala, Sweden.
Division of Psychiatry, Uppsala University Hospital, UAS ing 10, 75185 Uppsala, Sweden

Margareta Wennberg
Division of Psychiatry, Uppsala University Hospital, UAS ing 10, 75185 Uppsala, Sweden

Traci Takahashi
Department of Veterans Affairs Puget Sound Health Care System, General Medicine Services, 1660 South Columbian Way (S-152), Seattle, WA 98108, USA
Department of Medicine, University of Washington, 1959 NE Pacific Street, Seattle, WA 98195, USA

Gwen Lapham
Health Services Research and Development (HSRandD), Seattle Center of Innovation for Veteran-Centered and Value-Driven Care, 1660 S. Columbian Way, Seattle, WA 98108, USA Kaiser Permanente Washington Health Research Institute, 1730 Minor Avenue, Ste. 1600, Seattle, WA 98101, USA

Laura J. Chavez
Health Services Research and Development (HSRandD), Seattle Center of Innovation for Veteran-Centered and Value-Driven Care, 1660 S. Columbian Way, Seattle, WA 98108, USA
Division of Health Services Management and Policy, College of Public Health, The Ohio State University, Columbus, OH, USA
Center for Innovation in Pediatric Practice, Nationwide Children's Hospital, Columbus, OH, USA

Amy K. Lee
Kaiser Permanente Washington Health Research Institute, 1730 Minor Avenue, Ste. 1600, Seattle, WA 98101, USA

Emily C. Williams
Health Services Research and Development (HSRandD), Seattle Center of Innovation for Veteran-Centered and Value-Driven Care, 1660 S. Columbian Way, Seattle, WA 98108, USA

Department of Health Services, University of Washington, 1959 Pacific Street, Seattle, WA 98195, USA

Julie E. Richards
Kaiser Permanente Washington Health Research Institute, 1730 Minor Avenue, Ste. 1600, Seattle, WA 98101, USA
Department of Health Services, University of Washington, 1959 Pacific Street, Seattle, WA 98195, USA

Diane Greenberg
Psychiatry and Behavioral Sciences, University of Washington, Seattle, WA, USA
Department of Veterans Affairs Puget Sound Health Care System, Mental Health Service, 1660 South Columbian Way (S-152), Seattle, WA 98108, USA

Anna Rubinsky
Health Services Research and Development (HSRandD), Seattle Center of Innovation for Veteran-Centered and Value-Driven Care, 1660 S. Columbian Way, Seattle, WA 98108, USA
Center of Excellence in Substance Abuse Treatment and Education (CESATE), Veterans Affairs (VA) Puget Sound Health Care System, S-123-PCC, 1660 S. Columbian Way, Seattle, WA 98108, USA
The Kidney Health Research Collaborative, San Francisco and San Francisco VA Medical Center, University of California, 4150 Clement Street (111A1), San Francisco, CA 94121, USA

Douglas Berger
Department of Veterans Affairs Puget Sound Health Care System, General Medicine Services, 1660 South Columbian Way (S-152), Seattle, WA 98108, USA
Department of Medicine, University of Washington, 1959 NE Pacific Street, Seattle, WA 98195, USA

Eric J. Hawkins
Health Services Research and Development (HSRandD), Seattle Center of Innovation for Veteran-Centered and Value-Driven Care, 1660 S. Columbian Way, Seattle, WA 98108, USA
Center of Excellence in Substance Abuse Treatment and Education (CESATE), Veterans Affairs (VA) Puget Sound Health Care System, S-123-PCC, 1660 S. Columbian Way, Seattle, WA 98108, USA
Psychiatry and Behavioral Sciences, University of Washington, Seattle, WA, USA

Joseph O. Merrill
Department of Medicine, University of Washington, 1959 NE Pacific Street, Seattle, WA 98195, USA

Katharine A. Bradley
Health Services Research and Development (HSRandD), Seattle Center of Innovation for Veteran-Centered and Value-Driven Care, 1660 S. Columbian Way, Seattle, WA 98108, USA
Center of Excellence in Substance Abuse Treatment and Education (CESATE), Veterans Affairs (VA) Puget Sound Health Care System, S-123-PCC, 1660 S. Columbian Way, Seattle, WA 98108, USA
Kaiser Permanente Washington Health Research Institute, 1730 Minor Avenue, Ste. 1600, Seattle, WA 98101, USA
Department of Health Services, University of Washington, 1959 Pacific Street, Seattle, WA 98195, USA
Department of Medicine, University of Washington, 1959 NE Pacific Street, Seattle, WA 98195, USA

Jennifer R. Mertens
Kaiser Permanente Northern California, 1800 Harrison, Oakland, CA 94612, USA

Felicia W. Chi, Thekla B. Ross, Steve Allen, Cynthia I. Campbell, Yun Wendy Lu and Stacy A. Sterling
Division of Research, Kaiser Permanente Northern California, 2000 Broadway, Oakland, CA 94612, USA

Constance M. Weisner and Derek D. Satre
Division of Research, Kaiser Permanente Northern California, 2000 Broadway, Oakland, CA 94612, USA
Department of Psychiatry, University of California, San Francisco, 401 Parnassus Ave, San Francisco, CA 94143, USA

David Pating
The Permanente Medical Group, Kaiser Northern California, 1201 Fillmore Street, San Francisco, CA 94115, USA

Pierre Poloméni
Hôpitaux Universitaires Paris Seine St Denis, Site René Muret, Avenue du Dr Schaeffner, Sevran 93270, France

Claude Bronner
rue de Haslach, 67200 Strasbourg, France

Fréderic Fry
CSAPA Dune, Parvis de la préfecture, Immeuble les Oreades, 95000 Cergy, France

Bruno Ravoninjatovo
151 Bis rue de Courcelles, 51100 Reims, France

Mélina Fatseas
Laboratoire de psychiatrie, Département d'addictologie, Centre hospitalier Charles Perrens, 146 bis, rue Léo Saignat, Bordeaux 33076, France

Alan R. Lifson and Rose Hilk
Division of Epidemiology and Community Health, University of Minnesota, 1300 S. Second Street, Suite 300, Minneapolis, MN 55454-1015, USA

Sale Workneh, Tibebe Shenie, Lemlem Bezabih, Hiwot Tekle Waktola and Behailu Dagne
Ethiopian Office, National Alliance of State and Territorial AIDS Directors, Addis Ababa, Ethiopia

Desalegn Admassu Ayana
College of Health and Medical Sciences, Haramaya University, Dire Dawa, Ethiopia

Zenebe Melaku
International Center for AIDS Care and Treatment Program, Addis Ababa, Ethiopia

Ken C. Winters
Oregon Research Institute, Eugene, OR, USA

Lucy Slater
Global Program, National Alliance of State and Territorial AIDS Directors, Washington, DC, USA

Shalini Gupta, Thomas Bowe, Laura S. Ellerbe, Tyler E. Phelps, Anna D. Rubinsky, John W. Finney, Steven M. Asch, Keith Humphreys and Jodie Trafton
Center for Innovation to Implementation, Health Services Research and Development Service, VA Palo Alto Health Care System, Menlo Park, CA, USA

Sokunny Muth, Aynar Len, Maly Phou and Song Ngak
FHI360, Phnom Penh, Cambodia

Jennifer L. Evans and Ellen S. Stein
Department of Epidemiology and Biostatistics, and Global Health, University of California, San Francisco, San Francisco, CA, USA

Sophal Chhit
Department of Mental Health and Substance Abuse, Ministry of Health, Phnom Penh, Cambodia

Yuthea Neak
National Authority for Combating Drugs, Phnom Penh, Cambodia

Adam W. Carrico
Public Health Sciences and Psychology, University of Miami, Coral Gables, FL, USA

Lisa Maher
The Kirby Institute for Infection and Immunity, UNSW Australia, Sydney, Australia

Kimberly Page
Division of Epidemiology, Biostatistics and Preventive Medicine, Department of Internal Medicine, University of New Mexico, Albuquerque, NM, USA

David C. Hodgins and Jonathan N. Stea
Department of Psychology, University of Calgary, 2500 University Drive NW, Calgary, AB T2N 1N4, Canada

Gitau Mburu
Division of Health Research, Lancaster University, Lancaster, UK

Chanrith Ngin, Sovannary Tuot, Pheak Chhoun and Khuondyla Pal
KHANA Center for Population Health Research, No. 33, Street 71, Phnom Penh, Cambodia

Siyan Yi
KHANA Center for Population Health Research, No. 33, Street 71, Phnom Penh, Cambodia.
Center for Global Health Research, Touro University California, Vallejo, CA, USA

Jennifer E. Hettema, Stephanie A. Cockrell and Valerie A. Carrejo
Department of Family and Community Medicine, University of New Mexico, Albuquerque, NM, USA

Abigail Reeves and Karen S. Ingersoll
Department of Psychiatry and Neurobehavioral Sciences, University of Virginia, Charlottesville, VA, USA

Paula J. Lum
Department of Medicine, University of California San Francisco, San Francisco, CA, USA

Richard Saitz
Department of Community Health Sciences, Boston University School of Public Health, Boston, MA, USA

Cristina M. Murray-Krezan
Department of Internal Medicine, University of New Mexico Health Sciences Center, Albuquerque, NM, USA

Pritika C. Kumar, Erica Sedlander and Christine Chollak
Department of Population Health, New York University School of Medicine, 550 First Avenue, VZ30 6th Floor, New York, NY 10016, USA

Jennifer McNeely
Department of Population Health, New York University School of Medicine, 550 First Avenue, VZ30 6th Floor, New York, NY 10016, USA
Division of General Internal Medicine, Department of Medicine, New York University School of Medicine, 550 First Avenue, New York, NY 10016, USA

Traci Rieckmann
Greenfield Health and Department of Psychiatry, Oregon Health and Science University, 9450 SW Barnes Suite 100, Portland, OR 97225, USA

Sarah Farkas and John Rotrosen
Department of Psychiatry, New York University School of Medicine, One Park Avenue, 8th Floor, New York, NY 10016, USA

Joseph L. Kannry, Aida Vega, Eva A. Waite and Lauren A. Peccoralo
Division of General Internal Medicine, Department of Medicine, Icahn School of Medicine at Mt. Sinai, One Gustave L. Levy Place, New York, NY 10029, USA

Richard N. Rosenthal
Department of Psychiatry, Icahn School of Medicine at Mt. Sinai, 1090 Amsterdam Avenue, New York, NY 10025, USA

Dennis McCarty
OHSU-PSU School of Public Health, Oregon Health and Science University, 3181 SW Sam Jackson Park Road, Portland, OR 97239, USA

R. L. Cook, Z. Zhou and N. E. Kelso-Chichetto
Department of Epidemiology, College of Public Health and Health Professions and College of Medicine, University of Florida, PO Box 100231, Gainesville, FL 32610, USA

J. Janelle
Department of Epidemiology, College of Public Health and Health Professions and College of Medicine, University of Florida, PO Box 100231, Gainesville, FL 32610, USA
Department of Medicine, University of Florida, Gainesville, FL, USA

N. Ennis and R. A. Cohen
Department of Clinical and Health Psychology, University of Florida, Gainesville, FL, USA

C. L. Cook
Department of Family, Community, and Health System Science, College of Nursing, University of Florida, Gainesville, FL, USA

B. Brumback
Department of Biostatistics, University of Florida, Gainesville, FL, USA

J. P. Morano
Division of Infectious Diseases and International Medicine, University
of South Florida Morsani College of Medicine, Tampa, FL, USA

C. Somboonwit
Department of Internal Medicine, University of South Florida Morsani College of Medicine, Tampa, FL, USA

W. Carter
Florida Department of Health, Orange County Office of Clinical Services, Disease Investigation and Research, Orlando, FL, USA

G. E. Ibanez
Department of Epidemiology, Florida International University, Miami, FL, USA

K. Bryant
National Institute on Alcohol Abuse and Alcoholism, Bethesda, MD, USA

Mandy D. Owens, Jessica A. Chen and Emily C. Williams
Health Services Research and Development, VA Puget Sound Health Care System, Department of Health Services, University of Washington, 1660 South Columbian Way, S-152, Seattle, WA 98108, USA

Tracy L. Simpson
Center for Substance Abuse Treatment and Education, VA Puget Sound Health Care System, Seattle, USA
Department of Psychiatry and Behavioral Sciences, University of Washington, Seattle, WA, USA

Christine Timko
Center for Innovation to Implementation, VA Palo Alto Health Care System, Palo Alto, USA
Department of Psychiatry and Behavioral Sciences, Stanford University, Palo Alto, CA, USA

Kara M. Bensley and Emily C. Williams
Department of Health Services, Magnuson Health Sciences Center, University of Washington School of Public Health, 1959 NE Pacific St, Box 357660, Seattle, WA 98195-7660, USA
VA Health Services Research and Development (HSRD) Denver Seattle Center of Innovation for Veteran-Centered and Value-Driven Care, VA Puget Sound Healthcare System, 1660 S. Columbian Way, Mailstop S-152, Seattle, WA 98108, USA

India J. Ornelas and K. C. Gary Chan
Department of Health Services, Magnuson Health Sciences Center, University of Washington School of Public Health, 1959 NE Pacific St, Box 357660, Seattle, WA 98195-7660, USA

Julie R. Gaither and Amy C. Justice
VA Connecticut Healthcare System, West Haven Campus, 950 Campbell Avenue, West Haven, CT 06516, USA
Yale School of Medicine, 333 Cedar St, New Haven, CT 06510, USA

Kathleen A. McGinnis
VA Connecticut Healthcare System, West Haven Campus, 950 Campbell Avenue, West Haven, CT 06516, USA

David A. Fiellin and E. Jennifer Edelman
Yale School of Medicine, 333 Cedar St, New Haven, CT 06510, USA

Adam J. Gordon
Salt Lake City VA, 500 Foothill Dr, Salt Lake City, UT 84148, USA
University of Utah, 201 Presidents Cir, Salt Lake City, UT 84112, USA

Kevin L. Kraemer
VA Pittsburgh Healthcare System, University Drive, Pittsburgh, PA 15240, USA
University of Pittsburgh School of Medicine, 3550 Terrace St, Pittsburgh, PA 15213, USA

Kendall J. Bryant
National Institute on Alcohol Abuse and Alcoholism, 5635 Fishers Ln, Rockville, MD 20852, USA

Stephen Crystal
Rutgers University, 7 College Ave, New Brunswick, NJ 08901, USA

P. Todd Korthuis
Oregon Health and Science University, 3181 SW Sam Jackson Park Rd, Portland, OR 97239, USA

Brandon D. L. Marshall and John C. Fortney
Brown University School of Public Health, 121 S Main St, Providence, RI 02903, USA

Julia C. Dombrowski
University of Washington School of Medicine, 1959 NE Pacific St, Seattle, WA 98195, USA

Zev Schuman-Olivier
Center for Technology and Behavioral Health, Geisel School of Medicine at Dartmouth, Hanover, USA
Department of Psychiatry, Harvard Medical School, Boston, USA.
Cambridge Health Alliance, Outpatient Addiction Services, Department of Psychiatry, Harvard Medical School, 26 Central Street, Somerville, MA 02143, USA

Jacob T. Borodovsky, Mary Ann Greene, Kyle Butler, Hai Yi Xie and Lisa A. Marsch
Center for Technology and Behavioral Health, Geisel School of Medicine at Dartmouth, Hanover, USA

Qays Munir
Center for Technology and Behavioral Health, Geisel School of Medicine at Dartmouth, Hanover, USA
Cambridge Health Alliance, Outpatient Addiction Services, Department of Psychiatry, Harvard Medical School, 26 Central Street, Somerville, MA 02143, USA

Jackson Steinkamp
Cambridge Health Alliance, Outpatient Addiction Services, Department of Psychiatry, Harvard Medical School, 26 Central Street, Somerville, MA 02143, USA
Boston University School of Medicine, Boston, USA

Jonah Goldblatt
Cambridge Health Alliance, Outpatient Addiction Services, Department of Psychiatry, Harvard Medical School, 26 Central Street, Somerville, MA 02143, USA
Tufts University School of Medicine, Boston, USA

Marcus A. Bachhuber, Joseph DeLuca and Chinazo O. Cunningham
Division of General Internal Medicine, Department of Medicine, Montefiore
Medical Center/Albert Einstein College of Medicine, 3300 Kossuth Ave, Bronx, NY 10467, USA

Megan A. O'Grady and Charles J. Neighbors
Department of Health and Treatment Research and Analysis, The National Center on Addiction and Substance Abuse at Columbia University, 633 Third Avenue, 19th Floor, New York, NY 10017, USA

Henry Chung
Montefiore Care Management, Montefiore Medical Center, 200 Corporate Boulevard South, Yonkers, NY 10701, USA

Elenita M. D'Aloia and Arelis Diaz
Montefiore Medical Group, Montefiore Medical Center, 305 E 161st St, Bronx, NY 10451, USA

Alexis Cooke
Fielding School of Public Health Department of Community Health Sciences, University of California, Los Angeles, Los Angeles, CA, USA

Haneefa Saleem
Department of International Health, Johns Hopkins Bloomberg School of Public Health, 615 North Wolfe Street, E5033, Baltimore, MD 21205, USA

Dorothy Mushi and Jessie Mbwambo
Department of Psychiatry, Muhimbili University of Health and Allied Sciences, Dar es Salaam, Tanzania

Saria Hassan and Barrot H. Lambdin
Behavioral Health and Criminal Justice Research Division, RTI International, 351 California Street, Suite 500, San Francisco, CA 94104, USA

Index

A

Acamprosate, 1-2, 4, 6, 25, 32

Addiction Treatment, 16-17, 20, 22-23, 26, 32, 50-51, 55, 103, 128-129, 133, 147, 154, 173-174, 180, 184, 197-198, 200, 202-204, 220, 230-231

Adherence Monitoring, 219, 221-223

Alcohol Abuse, 7, 25, 35-36, 55, 66, 82, 96, 102-103, 105, 116-120, 126, 171-172, 174, 187, 195, 205, 216, 241, 251

Alcohol Consumption, 25, 33, 35, 39, 49, 89, 115, 118, 120, 187-196, 216-218, 241-242

Alcohol Intervention, 48, 116, 118, 120, 165-166, 171, 186, 241

Alcohol Misuse, 103, 105-106, 118-119, 135, 171, 186-187, 195, 217-218, 241-242

Alcohol Screening, 37, 103-105, 108-109, 112-113, 115, 117-119, 167, 174, 186-187, 209, 217-218, 234, 237, 241-242

Alcohol Use Disorder, 1, 6-7, 28, 38, 94-95, 99, 103, 117, 139, 141, 167-168, 181, 187, 189, 199-200, 204, 209, 215, 217-218, 233

Amphetamine, 12, 16, 69, 121, 136, 144-145, 225

Antiretroviral Therapy, 24, 35-36, 68-70, 76-77, 127, 136, 144-145, 163-164, 188-189, 191, 195-196, 210, 216, 243-244, 250-251

Anxiety Disorder, 52-54, 97, 102, 190, 195, 226

B

Buprenorphine, 8-14, 34, 36-37, 55, 206, 219-221, 225, 227-232, 250

C

Cannabis Use Disorder, 146-147, 154

Catha Edulis, 121, 127

Clonidine, 8-9, 11, 13, 15

Cluster Randomized Trial, 105, 119

D

Detoxification, 17, 19, 21-22, 128, 130-131, 133

Disulfiram, 1-4, 25, 30

Drug Abuse Screening, 174

Drug Prevention, 136-137

Drug Use, 17-20, 22, 29, 34-35, 46, 48-49, 51, 54-55, 57, 62, 64, 66-72, 74, 79, 81, 83, 86, 119, 121, 124, 129, 144, 160, 163, 177, 179, 191-193, 195, 217, 228, 244, 249

E

Emergency Medicine, 78, 86

H

Healthcare, 1, 5, 26, 55, 79-80, 84, 86, 118, 120, 164, 166, 175, 179, 186, 195, 202, 204, 215-216, 218-220, 228, 241-242, 251

Heroin, 14, 16-23, 51, 55, 69-72, 147, 155, 159-160, 190, 230, 244

K

Khat, 121-127

M

Maintenance Therapy, 23, 50, 55, 250-251

Marijuana, 69-72, 74-75, 146, 148, 152, 154, 160, 190

Medication Assisted Treatment, 1, 207, 251

Mental Disorders, 36, 51, 55-56, 94, 102-103, 122, 154, 187

Mental Health, 2-3, 6-7, 32, 35, 54-56, 70, 72, 74-75, 77, 83, 94-103, 105, 118-122, 126-127, 135, 144-145, 148, 154, 171, 180, 189, 207, 223, 226, 230, 232, 246

Methadone, 8-23, 50-53, 55-56, 157, 159, 161-162, 199, 204, 220, 229, 243-251

Methamphetamines, 155, 160

Mortality Risk, 54, 133, 208-209, 212-216

N

Naloxone, 37, 219-220, 227, 230-232, 250

Naloxone Adherence, 219

Naltrexone, 1-4, 6, 25, 32, 37, 218

Natural Recovery, 146, 148-154

Neonatal Abstinence Syndrome, 8, 13-15

Neonatal Morphine, 8-9, 11, 14-15

O

Opiate, 23, 55, 71-72, 74-75, 230

Opioid Dependency, 8

Opioid Epidemic, 8

Opioid Use Disorder, 8-10, 14, 18, 50-51, 55, 206, 219-221, 231-232

Opioid-agonist Treatment, 14

P

Paranoia, 121, 178

Pharmacotherapy, 1-3, 6-7, 24-25, 29-30, 32-34, 56, 103, 184, 187, 203, 218

Phnom Penh, 139, 141, 143-145, 155-156, 158-159, 162-164

Prenatal Care, 8-14

Prenatal Treatment, 8, 11

Primary Care, 3, 25, 27, 31-32, 35-37, 55, 66-67, 77-78, 94, 97, 99, 101-110, 113-120, 153, 165-167, 169-171, 173-175, 177-178, 183-187, 190, 195, 215, 229, 240-242

Psychiatric Care, 88-89, 91-92

Psychological Dependence, 121-122

Psychological Distress, 136, 138-140, 143, 145

Q

Quality Improvement, 1-2, 5-7, 36, 105, 117, 119, 130, 241

R

Recovery Pathway, 148-152

Residential Treatment, 9, 128-129, 135, 198

S

Screening Tool, 106, 108, 232

Self-reflection, 88, 90, 92, 168

Sexual Behavior, 70, 160

Sexual Intercourse, 139-140, 142, 145, 155, 160, 164

Smoking Cessation, 78-81, 84-87, 167, 172, 179, 232

Substance Use Disorder, 6-7, 9, 37, 54, 89, 103, 119, 128, 134-135, 179, 197, 200, 218, 227

T

Tobacco Screening, 78, 177

Tobacco Treatment, 78, 80, 83-86

Topiramate, 1-4, 6, 25, 37, 103

Treatment Cascade, 68-71, 136-137, 144, 163

Treatment Fidelity, 165

V

Viral Suppression, 35, 76, 136, 138-141, 143, 156, 188-196, 244